Advances in Andrology

Eric Chung • Widi Atmoko
Edmund Ko • Ashok Agarwal
Editors

Advances in Andrology

New Developments and Innovations

Springer

Editors
Eric Chung
Department of Urology, Princess Alexandra Hospital
University of Queensland
Brisbane, QLD, Australia

AndroUrology Centre
Brisbane, QLD, Australia

Edmund Ko
Department of Urology
Kaiser Permanente Fontana
Fontana, CA, USA

Widi Atmoko
Department of Urology
Dr. Cipto Mangunkusumo Hospital, Faculty of Medicine, Universitas Indonesia
Jakarta, Jakarta, Indonesia

Ashok Agarwal
Global Andrology Forum
Moreland Hills, OH, USA

ISBN 978-3-032-29111-0 ISBN 978-3-032-29112-7 (eBook)
https://doi.org/10.1007/978-3-032-29112-7

This Springer imprint is published by the registered company Springer Nature Switzerland AG
The registered company address is: Gewerbestrasse 11, 6330 Cham, Switzerland

I like to dedicate this book to my family, specifically my loving wife, Jane, and my son, Etienne, who continue to inspire me with joy and love every day. I am indebted to my mentors, Professor Gerry Brock and Dr. Ross Cartmill, for their guidance and friendship. Last but not least, to Professor Ashok Agarwal and the entire Global Andrology Forum for their commitment to scientific knowledge and for breaking down barriers to form a truly international network of experts across various disciplines in andrology and beyond.

Eric Chung

I would like to dedicate this book to my parents for their unwavering support and guidance throughout my life. To my wife, Febrini, for her patience, understanding, and constant encouragement, and to our children, Aruna, Arkana, and Aliya, who continue to inspire me every day.
I am also deeply grateful to my mentors and colleagues, particularly Prof. Ashok Agarwal and the Global Andrology Forum, for their guidance, collaboration, and commitment to advancing the field of andrology. Finally, this

book is dedicated to our patients, whose trust and experiences continually remind us of the art and science of medicine.

Widi Atmoko

I would like to dedicate this book to my parents, who encouraged my journey into medicine; my wife, for weathering the storm of residency and fellowship; and our children, Ethan and Addy, for putting up with the late nights and early mornings in a surgical family.
I am forever indebted to my mentors, Drs. Donald Novicki and Scott Swanson (Mayo Clinic, Arizona), Edmund Sabanegh and Ashok Agarwal (Cleveland Clinic), Steve Stewart, Roger Hadley, and Herb Ruckle (Loma Linda University), who all provided the tools and opportunities for me to rise academically and inspired me to never stop seeking.

Edmund Ko

In cherished memory of my father, Professor R.C. Aggarwal, whose life of integrity, discipline, and unwavering commitment continues to illuminate my path. To my beloved wife, Meenu, and my sons, Rishi and Neil-Yogi, whose constant love, strength, and encouragement sustain me in every endeavor. With heartfelt gratitude to Professor Kevin Loughlin (Harvard Medical School) and the late Professor Anthony Thomas (Cleveland Clinic) for their enduring friendship, mentorship, and the profound influence they have had on my professional and personal journey. To the thousands of researchers, trainees, colleagues, and countless patients who have entrusted me over the past four decades, I extend my deepest gratitude. Your collaboration, confidence, and shared commitment to excellence have been both my greatest privilege and my enduring source of inspiration.

Ashok Agarwal

Foreword

Andrology is a rapidly evolving field with many advances in evaluation protocols, diagnostic tests, clinical interpretation, and therapeutic options. "Advances in Andrology: New Developments and Innovations" is a timely review of the latest advances in the field, covering both male infertility and male sexual dysfunction.

The book focuses on clinically relevant advances and emerging areas of interest, providing an in-depth coverage from fundamentals and pathophysiology to diagnostics and therapeutic decision-making. The book provides a strong interdisciplinary perspective and should be of interest to experts from all specialities that deal with male infertility or sexual dysfunction.

The book is divided into two parts. The first part focuses on male reproductive function. It starts with a detailed discussion of the latest edition of the WHO manual of semen examination and provides valuable clinical insights into the implications on the abandonment of a reference range that distinguishes between fertile and infertile semen samples. A detailed discussion provides clinical perspectives on various new tests including those for sperm DNA fragmentation and oxidative stress. With the increasing use of whole exome screening, numerous single gene defects are being identified as potential causes of azoospermia and other sperm defects; a chapter on genetics helps guide clinicians through the maze of these new findings.

The eternally controversial topics of varicocele and antioxidants also get due importance and are discussed in detail. Recently, onco-fertility and preservation of fertility in pre-adolescents have been gaining increasing importance and these topics find a niche focus in a special chapter dedicated to the subject. Advances and innovations in surgical techniques are also discussed. Finally, futuristic advances including male fertility regeneration, the role of artificial intelligence, and advances in sperm and embryo selection are presented. This wide range of clinically useful topics make the book mandatory reading for all those who deal with male infertility.

The second half of the book deals with male sexual dysfunction, and this is more focused on controversies and advances. While it includes chapters on pharmacological therapy and penile implantation, most of the topics are related to areas that clinicians are still uncertain about. It starts with a critical review of the role of hormone therapy for male hypogonadism, and this is followed by an in-depth discussion on the controversial topic of regenerative therapies for ED. Erection preservation in prostate cancer surgery and the surgical management of ED with incontinence are discussed in separate chapters.

Peyronie's disease presents in a variety of ways and its management can range from mere reassurance to patient-dependent treatments like penile traction to expensive options like collagenase injections or surgery. The chapter on advances in management of Peyronie's disease will help clinicians understand the indications for each of these treatments and their clinical utility.

Ejaculatory dysfunction encompasses a broad spectrum of clinical presentations ranging from early ejaculation to delayed ejaculation and even complete failure to reach orgasm. The chapter on ejaculatory dysfunctions explains the pathophysiology in detail so that the treatment options can be well understood. Chronic orchialgia and chronic prostatitis are a clinician's nightmare, and the two chapters on these topics provide valuable practical guidance. Finally, the oft-neglected topic of wearable devices to assist male sexual function and the controversial topic of penile enlargement surgery also receive detailed discussions.

I have no doubt that this very comprehensive textbook will provide timely guidance to the wide range of clinical specialists engaged in the management of either male infertility or male sexual dysfunction, and I congratulate the editors for an excellent reference textbook.

Global Andrology Forum
Moreland Hills, OH, USA

Division of Andrology, Department of
Urology, Lilavati Hospital and Research Centre
Mumbai, India
2026

Rupin Shah

Preface

Advances in Andrology: New Developments and Innovations is conceived as a comprehensive and contemporary resource for clinicians, scientists, and researchers engaged in the multidisciplinary field of andrology. This volume seeks to provide a reliable, evidence-based, and current reference that addresses the expanding spectrum of male reproductive, sexual, and urinary health. The 28 chapters are authored by internationally recognized experts who integrate clinical experience with scientific rigor and translational insight. Together, they reflect the growing need for a cohesive and interdisciplinary approach to personalized and evidence-based care for men seeking treatment for reproductive and sexual dysfunction. The contributors offer balanced perspectives that help bridge gaps in current knowledge while providing clarity on complex and evolving issues in male health.

The organization of this book follows a deliberate progression from fundamental principles and pathophysiological mechanisms to advanced diagnostics, contemporary therapeutic strategies, surgical innovations, and future directions. Although this volume is not intended to be exhaustive, it focuses on clinically relevant and emerging topics shaping modern andrology and likely to influence future clinical practice guidelines. A distinguishing strength of this text lies in its integration of clinical care, diagnostic evaluation, and translational research. By connecting foundational science with real-world application, the book aims to serve both as a practical guide for patient management and as a stimulus for continued scientific inquiry.

We extend our sincere gratitude to the 70 distinguished contributors from 28 countries whose scholarship and dedication have made this work possible. Their collective expertise and commitment to advancing male reproductive health have shaped this volume into an authoritative and meaningful resource. We also acknowledge with appreciation the invaluable guidance of Lillie Mae Gaurano, Springer Editor, Clinical Medicine Books, and the meticulous coordination of Janakiraman G, Production Editor, whose professionalism ensured the successful completion of this project.

This book is dedicated to our families, mentors, and patients whose encouragement, wisdom, and resilience continue to inspire our pursuit of excellence in andrology and male infertility. It is our hope that *Advances in Andrology* will serve not only as a valuable reference but also as a catalyst for continued dialogue, collaboration, and innovation, ultimately contributing to improved outcomes and quality of life for men worldwide.

Brisbane, QLD, Australia Eric Chung
Jakarta, Jakarta, Indonesia Widi Atmoko
Fontana, CA, USA Edmund Ko
Moreland Hills, OH, USA Ashok Agarwal

Contents

Editors and Contributors

About the Editors

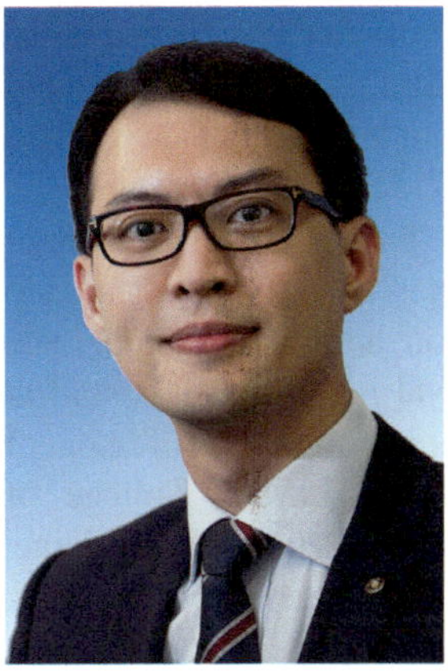

Eric Chung is a consultant urological surgeon at the AndroUrology Centre for Sexual, Urinary, and Reproductive Excellence and holds professorial academic appointments at the University of Queensland in Brisbane and Macquarie University Hospital in Sydney, Australia. He is an internationally recognized leader in the field of male sexual, urinary, and reproductive dysfunction. He holds several executive positions in scientific organizations and serves as a expert advisor to the Australian Government's Department of Health. He is the youngest recipient of the Urological Society of Australia and New Zealand (USANZ) Medal in recognition of exceptional service and leadership in the Society and served as the past chair of the Male LUTS and Andrology sections in USANZ.

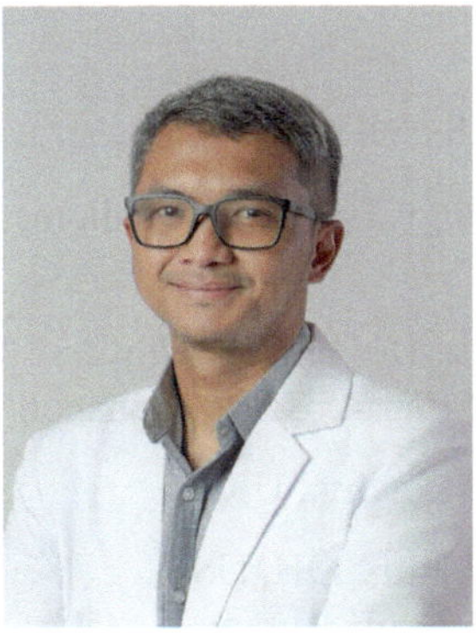

Widi Atmoko is an Indonesian urologist specializing in andro-urology at Universitas Indonesia and Cipto Mangunkusumo Hospital, Jakarta, Indonesia. He earned his medical and urology degrees with distinction and completed his PhD in medical science. A fellow of the European Committee of Sexual Medicine and the American College of Surgeons, he has authored over 90 scientific publications and is an active member of the Global Andrology Forum.

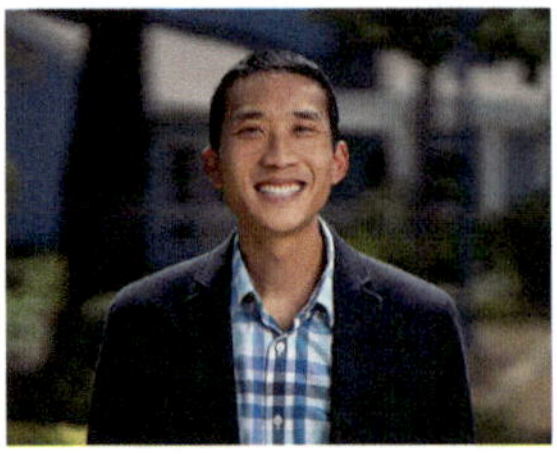

Edmund Ko, MD is a urologist at Kaiser Permanente in Fontana, CA, specializing in male infertility and men's health. He completed his residency in urology at Mayo Clinic, Arizona, and a fellowship in male infertility and andrology at the Arizona and the Cleveland Clinic under the mentorship of Drs. Ashok Agarwal, PhD, and Edmund Sabanegh, MD. Dr. Ko directed the male infertility program for the Department of Urology at Loma Linda University. During his time there, he was the residency program director. He was active in research with the residents and achieved the rank of a professor during his time in academia. Dr. Ko has since transitioned to a multispecialty system, where he continues to provide expertise in male infertility, andrology, and men's health.

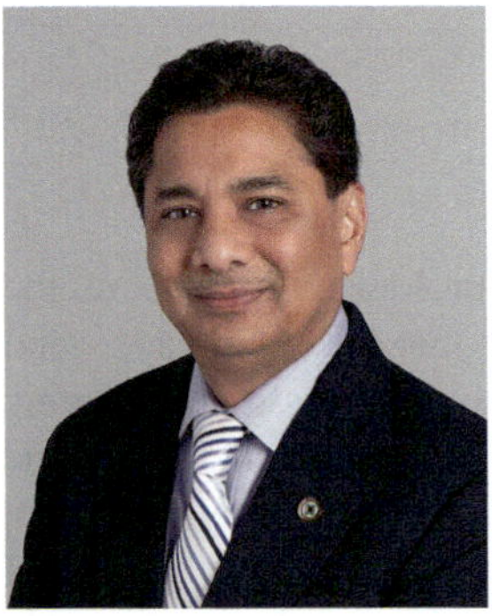

Ashok Agarwal, MSc, PhD, HCLD (Andrology), is an internationally recognized andrologist and reproductive scientist whose work has profoundly advanced the field of male infertility. He is the founder and president of the Global Andrology Forum (GAF), headquartered in Moreland Hills, Ohio, where he leads a global network of more than 850 members across 95 countries dedicated to collaborative research, education, and innovation in male reproductive health. Dr. Agarwal is an Emeritus staff at the Cleveland Clinic and the Emeritus professor of Urology at the Cleveland Clinic Lerner College of Medicine of Case Western Reserve School of Medicine. He continues to shape the global discourse on male infertility and reproductive health through scholarship, collaboration, and visionary leadership.

Contributors

Ashok Agarwal Global Andrology Forum, Moreland Hills, OH, USA

Hiva Alipour Department of Health Science and Technology, Faculty of Medicine, Aalborg University, Aalborg, Denmark

Marwan Alkassis Department of Urology, Hotel-Dieu De France University Hospital, Faculty of Medicine, Saint Joseph University of Beirut, Beirut, Lebanon

Hussain Alnajjar University College London Hospitals, London, UK

Ahmet Baris Altay Global Andrology Forum, Moreland Hills, OH, USA
Ege University School of Medicine, Urology Department, Izmir, Turkey

Christina Anagnostopoulou Future Life Akeso, Athens, Greece

Widi Atmoko Department of Urology, Dr. Cipto Mangunkusumo Hospital, Faculty of Medicine, Universitas Indonesia, Jakarta, Indonesia

Tomer Avidor-Reiss Global Andrology Forum, Moreland Hills, OH, USA
Department of Biological Sciences, University of Toledo, Toledo, OH, USA
Department of Urology, College of Medicine and Life Sciences, University of Toledo, Toledo, OH, USA

Kaan Aydos Department of Urology, Ankara University School of Medicine, Ankara, Turkey
Center for Research on Human Reproduction, Ankara University School of Medicine, Ankara, Turkey

Fahmi Bahar Faculty of Medicine, Muhammadiyah Palembang University, Palembang, Indonesia
Siloam Sriwijaya Palembang Hospital, Palembang, Indonesia

Balagobi Balasingam Department of Surgery, Faculty of Medicine, University of Jaffna, Jaffna, Sri Lanka

Ravi Banthia Global Andrology Forum, Moreland Hills, OH, USA
Department of Urology, Western General Hospital, Edinburgh, UK

Aykut Baser Department of Urology, Bandirma Onyedi Eylul University, Faculty of Medicine, Surgical Medical Sciences, Balikesir, Turkey

Ponco Birowo Department of Urology, Faculty of Medicine, Universitas Indonesia, Cipto Mangunkusumo Hospital, Jakarta, Indonesia

Kadir Bocu Department of Urology, Niğde Ömer Halisdemir University Faculty of Medicine, Niğde, Turkey

Luca Boeri IRCCS Fondazione Ca' Granda Ospedale Maggiore Policlinico, Milan, Italy

Kasonde Bowa University of Zambia, School of Medicine, Lusaka, Zambia

Selahittin Çayan Global Andrology Forum, Moreland Hills, OH, USA
Department of Urology, University of Mersin School of Medicine, Mersin, Türkiye

Matthew Chabot University of Massachusetts Chan Medical School, Worcester, MA, USA

Eric Chung Department of Urology, Princess Alexandra Hospital, University of Queensland, Brisbane, QLD, Australia
AndroUrology Centre, Brisbane, QLD, Australia

Fereshteh Dardmeh Department of Health Science and Technology, Faculty of Medicine, Aalborg, Denmark

Sulagna Dutta Basic Medical Sciences Department, College of Medicine, Ajman University, Ajman, UAE

Balantine Eze Global Andrology Forum, Moreland Hills, OH, USA
Urology Division, Department of Surgery, Enugu State University of Science and Technology Teaching Hospital, Enugu, Nigeria

Marco Falcone A.O.U. Città della Salute e della Scienza di Torino—Presidio Molinette—Clinica Urologica, Turin, Italy
Urology Department, Città della Salute e della Scienza, University of Torino, Torino, Italy
Urology Department, Biruni University, Istanbul, Turkey

Adriano Fregonesi Department of Surgery, Discipline/Area of Urology, Faculty of Medical Sciences, University of Campinas (UNICAMP), Campinas, São Paulo, Brazil

Chirag Gupta Matratva Fertility and Andrology Clinic, Jaipur, Rajasthan, India

Manaf Al Hashimi Department of Urology, Burjeel Hospital-Abu Dhabi, Abu Dhabi, UAE

Christopher C. K. Ho Department of Surgery, Taylor's University, Subang Jaya, Selangor, Malaysia

Zhongwei Huang NUS Bia Echo Asia Centre for Reproductive Longevity and Equality, National University of Singapore, Department of Obstetrics and Gynaecology, National University Health Systems, Singapore, Singapore

Muhammed Arif Ibis Department of Urology, Ankara University School of Medicine, Ankara, Turkey
Center for Research on Human Reproduction, Ankara University School of Medicine, Ankara, Turkey

Halil İbrahim İvelik Department of Urology, Faculty of Medicine, Kütahya Health Sciences University, Kütahya, Türkiye

Sunil Jindal Jindal Hospital, Meerut, Uttar Pradesh, India

Ates Kadıoglu Section of Andrology, Department of Urology, Istanbul School of Medicine, Istanbul, Turkey

Hussein Kandil Fakih IVF Fertility Center, Abu Dhabi, UAE

Global Andrology Forum (GAF), Moreland Hills, OH, USA

Dongsuk Kim Department of Urology, Ilsan Hospital, National Health Insurance Service, Goyang, South Korea

Christopher Chee Kong Ho Department of Surgery, School of Medicine, Taylor's University, Subang Jaya, Selangor, Malaysia

Raghavender Kosgi Department of Andrology and Men's Health, Apollo Hospitals, Jubilee Hills, Hyderabad, Telangana, India

Naveen Kumar Department of Urology, All India Institute of Medical Sciences, Patna, India

Tan V. Le Science Research and Training Department, Binh Dan Hospital, Ho Chi Minh City, Vietnam

Department of Surgery, Pham Ngoc Thach University of Medicine, Ho Chi Minh City, Vietnam

David K. W. Leung Division of Urology, Department of Surgery, Prince of Wales Hospital, The Chinese University of Hong Kong, Hong Kong, China

Charles A. Loeb Hoag Specialty Clinic, Hoag Memorial Hospital Presbyterian, Newport Beach, CA, USA

Asli Metin Mahmutoglu Department of Medical Biology, Faculty of Medicine, Yozgat Bozok University, Yozgat, Turkey

Israel Maldonado Citmer Reproductive Medicine, IVF LAB, Mexico City, Mexico

Vineet Malhotra VNA Hospital, New Delhi, India

Marlon Martinez Section of Urology, Department of Surgery, University of Santo Tomas Hospital, Manila, Philippines

Taymour Mostafa Department of Andrology, Sexology & STIs, Faculty of Medicine, Cairo University, Cairo, Egypt

Ayad Palani College of Medicine, University of Garmian, Kalar, Iraq

Dyandra Parikesit Urology Medical Staff Group, Universitas Indonesia Hospital, Universitas Indonesia, Depok, West Java, Indonesia

Hyun Jun Park Department of Urology, Pusan National University School of Medicine, Pusan National University Hospital, Busan, South Korea

Mirko Preto A.O.U. Città della Salute e della Scienza di Torino—Presidio Molinette—Clinica Urologica, Turin, Italy

Ana Puigvert Quiron Hospital, Barcelona, Spain

Nguyen Quang Center for Andrology and Sexual Medicine, VietDuc University Hospital, Hanoi, Vietnam
Department of Urology, Andrology and Sexual Medicine, University of Medicine and Pharmacy, Vietnam National University, Hanoi, Vietnam

Maged Ragab Department of Urology, Tanta University, Tanta, Egypt

Omer Raheem Cleveland Clinic Abu Dhabi, Abu Dhabi, UAE
Cleveland Clinic Lerner College of Medicine, Cleveland, OH, USA

Amarnath Rambhatla Vattikuti Urology Institute, Henry Ford Health, Detroit, MI, USA

Cesar Rojas-Cruz Global Andrology Forum, Moreland Hills, OH, USA
Urology Department University Hospital of Rostock, Rostock, Germany

Israel Maldonado Rosas Citmer Reproductive Medicine, IVF LAB, Mexico City, Mexico

Ramadan Saleh Ajyal IVF Center, Ajyal Hospital, Sohag, Egypt
Department of Dermatology, Venereology and Andrology, Faculty of Medicine, Sohag University, Sohag, Egypt

Selçuk Sarikaya University of Health Sciences, Gulhane Research and Training Hospital, Department of Urology, Ankara, Turkey

Missy Savira Department of Urology, Faculty of Medicine, Universitas Indonesia, Dr. Cipto Mangunkusumo Hospital, Jakarta Pusat, DKI Jakarta, Indonesia
Global Andrology Forum, Moreland Hills, OH, USA

Pallav Sengupta Department of Biomedical Sciences, College of Medicine, Gulf Medical University, Ajman, UAE

Rupin Shah Global Andrology Forum, Moreland Hills, OH, USA
Division of Andrology, Department of Urology, Lilavati Hospital and Research Centre, Mumbai, India

Akmal Taher Department of Urology, Faculty of Medicine, Universitas Indonesia, Jakarta, Indonesia Dr. Cipto Mangunkusumo Hospital, Jakarta, Indonesia

Charalampos Thomas Department of Urology, General Hospital of Corinth, Corinth, Greece

Manh Truong Nguyen Fertility Centre, Hanh Phuc International Hospital, Ho Chi Minh City, Vietnam
Department of Urology, School of Medicine, University of Medicine and Pharmacy, Ho Chi Minh City, Vietnam
Men's Health Centre, Ho Chi Minh City, Vietnam

Ranjit Vishwakarma Department of Urology, Lilavati Hospital and Research Centre, Mumbai, Spain

Paraskevi Vogiatzi Andromed Health and Reproduction, Fertility Diagnostics Laboratory, Maroussi, Greece

Faysal A. Yafi Department of Urology, University of California Irvine, Irvine, CA, USA

Mehmet Yilmaz Mediclin Kraichgau-Klinik, Urology, Bad Rappenau, Germany

Imad Ziouziou Department of Urology and Andrology, Mohammed VI University Hospital, College of Medicine and Pharmacy, Ibn Zohr University, Agadir, Morocco

Part I
Male Reproductive Function

Chapter 1
The WHO Sixth Edition: Understanding New Advances in Basic and Advanced Semen Preparation and Analysis

Missy Savira, Tomer Avidor-Reiss, Eric Chung, and Selahittin Çayan

Introduction

Infertility is defined as the inability to achieve clinical pregnancy despite regular, unprotected intercourse for at least 12 months [1]. The American Society for Reproductive Medicine further refines this definition, specifying that an evaluation should be conducted after 12 months for women under 35 and 6 months for those aged 35 or older [2]. This criterion facilitates earlier evaluation, recognizing that female reproductive potential declines significantly after age 35 due to various factors [3]. Globally, infertility affects approximately 15% of couples [4], with male-related factors contributing to 20–70% of cases [5]. A multicentric study

M. Savira
Department of Urology, Faculty of Medicine, Universitas Indonesia, Dr. Cipto Mangunkusumo Hospital, Jakarta Pusat, DKI Jakarta, Indonesia

Global Andrology Forum, Moreland Hills, OH, USA

T. Avidor-Reiss
Global Andrology Forum, Moreland Hills, OH, USA

Department of Biological Sciences, University of Toledo, Toledo, OH, USA

Department of Urology, College of Medicine and Life Sciences, University of Toledo, Toledo, OH, USA

E. Chung
Department of Urology, Princess Alexandra Hospital, University of Queensland, Brisbane, QLD, Australia

AndroUrology Centre, Brisbane, QLD, Australia

S. Çayan (✉)
Global Andrology Forum, Moreland Hills, OH, USA

Department of Urology, University of Mersin School of Medicine, Mersin, Türkiye

E. Chung et al. (eds.), *Advances in Andrology*,
https://doi.org/10.1007/978-3-032-29112-7_1

revealed that the percentage of infertility attributed to sole male factors was 23%, while the combination of male and female factors accounted for 45% [6]. Notably, the prevalence of male infertility has risen substantially, reaching 76.9% between 1990 and 2018 [7], although the evidence for this rise is still controversial [8]. Men aged 30–34 have the highest incidence of male infertility [7].

A comprehensive diagnosis approach in male infertility is crucial to minimize the incidence of idiopathic infertility to below 10%. Consequently, tailoring treatment based on the diagnosis enables over 40% of couples to achieve spontaneous pregnancy [6]. The initial evaluation of male infertility comprises a thorough history-taking, physical examination, and basic laboratory evaluation, including semen analysis [9]. Semen analysis assesses sperm quality through macroscopic and microscopic examination [10]. Advanced functional sperm tests may also be necessary for further evaluation in several clinical cases [11]. A study of over four thousand men who seek infertility treatment showed that 63% of them exhibit abnormal semen parameters [12]. The importance of semen analysis in male infertility evaluation is further highlighted by the temporal analysis by Levine et al., which revealed a concerning decline in sperm concentration by 51.6% from 1973 to 2018 [13].

Standardized testing and proper quality control of semen analysis are necessary to make sure that male infertility is correctly diagnosed and treated [14]. The WHO laboratory manual serves as a guide for semen analysis, which will benefit laboratory personnel, researchers, and clinicians [15]. The most recent manual, the sixth edition, was just released in 2021, providing several substantial updates on semen analysis [15]. This chapter aims to provide a comprehensive review of the latest development in basic and advanced semen analysis and preparation, as described in the 6th edition WHO Laboratory Manual for the Examination and Processing of Human Semen, offering deeper understanding into their clinical relevance and application.

Evolution of WHO Laboratory Manual for the Examination and Processing of Human Semen

The WHO laboratory manual for semen analysis was first published in 1980 [16], marking a pivotal step toward the standardization of semen analysis [17]. Since its inception, the manual has undergone continuous updates approximately every 8–10 years, resulting in five subsequent editions that were released in 1987, 1992, 1999, 2010, and, most recently, the 6th edition in July 2021 [15, 18–21]. Each edition incorporates new evidence, facilitating their validation and integration into both research and clinical practice [17].

The 6th edition of the manual introduces several updates and improvements over its previous edition, offering a more precise and detailed approach to semen analysis

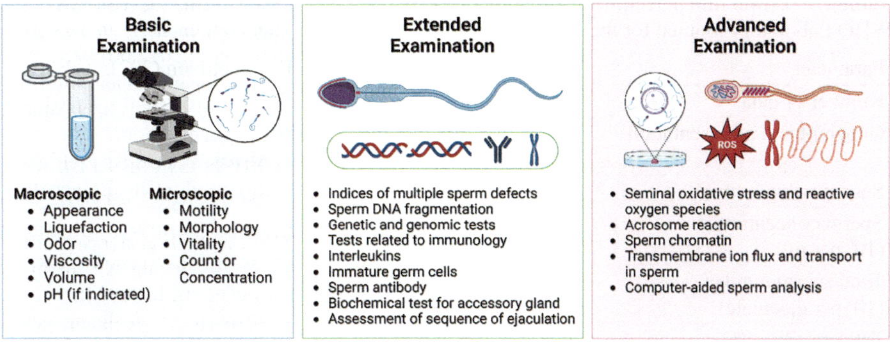

Fig. 1.1 Semen analysis based on the 6th edition of the WHO Laboratory Manual for the Examination and Processing of Human Semen

while refining terminology to enhance clarity and clinical relevance [22]. In the manual, sperm examination is categorized into three main classifications: basic, extended, and advanced examinations (Fig. 1.1) [15]. Compared to the prior edition, it integrates some novel tests, including semen odor assessment, while concurrently omitting obsolete procedures, such as human oocyte and zona pellucida binding and the oocyte penetration test [15]. Nevertheless, many other recently developed tests, such as sperm centriole evaluation, have not been included [23].

In response to the drawback of the 5th edition, which incorporated only a dataset of 1959 fertile men but no representation from Asia and Africa (Esteves 2014), the 6th edition has included new data from 5 studies that have representations from Asia and Africa while also use stricter inclusion criteria [15, 24]. Previously, criteria for cohort inclusion were voluntary, leading to regional imbalances and potential biases. In the new edition of the WHO manual, a total of 3589 men from couples who were able to achieve time-to-pregnancy (TTP) $\leq$ 12 months from 13 countries on five different continents were calculated for its distribution, resulting in several changes of lower five centiles of sperm parameters compared to the 5th edition (Table 1.1) [15, 21]. A particularly notable study found that when applying the new WHO manual's classification criteria, one in three infertile men experienced a downgraded semen classification compared to the 5th edition category [25].

Despite that, semen analysis could not be used to determine the fertility status of all men [26]. Fertility is instead an interplay of many factors, and normal semen analysis cannot be translated into fertile men [27]. In fact, real-world data showed that 12% of infertile men and only 41% of fertile men present with normal sperm parameters [27]. Therefore, one of the most notable changes in the latest edition is the abandonment of rigid reference thresholds of semen parameters but rather use it to complement the clinical assessment of male infertility [26]. A more extensive and global study of semen analysis parameters may provide more insight for the clinical evaluation of male infertility.

Table 1.1 Lower fifth percentile distribution of sperm parameters in the 5th and 6th editions of the WHO Laboratory Manual for the Examination and Processing of Human Semen

Parameter	WHO 5th edition (2010)	WHO 6th edition (2021)
Number of data	1953	3589
Geographical representation	Europe, Oceania, North America	Europe, Oceania, North America, Asia, Africa
Semen volume (ml)	1.5	1.4
Sperm concentration (10^6 per ml)	15	16
Total sperm number (10^6 per ejaculate)	39	39
Total motility (%)	42	42
Progressive motility (%)	30	30
Non-progressive motility (%)	1	1
Immotile spermatozoa (%)	22	20
Vitality (%)	58	54
Normal morphology (%)	4	4

Source
1. World Health Organization [15]
2. World Health Organization [21]
3. Campbell et al. [24]

Pre-examination Procedures

The recommendations for semen collection in the 6th edition of the WHO manual, in principle, remain the same as those in the previous edition [15]. Semen collection is generally performed through masturbation following an abstinence period of 2–7 days [15]. However, emerging evidence suggests that a shorter abstinence period may yield better sperm quality. A recent meta-analysis, which included 13 studies published between 2013 and 2022 and involved a total of 2315 patients, found that shorter ejaculatory abstinence is associated with a higher percentage of progressively motile sperm and lower levels of SDF [28]. In contrast, prolonged abstinence resulted in higher sperm concentrations but did not necessarily correlate with better overall sperm function [28]. Another meta-analysis also confirmed that very short abstinence, within 4 h, significantly reduced SDF levels [29]. These findings suggest that the WHO's recommended abstinence period may benefit from further refinement to consider the potential advantages of a shorter duration.

Once semen is collected, laboratory assessment should be performed within 30–60 min to ensure accurate evaluation. Studies have shown that sperm motility declines progressively, beginning 1 h after ejaculation, at a rate of approximately 5–10% per hour [30]. Notably, the proportion of sperm exhibiting rapid progressive motility is significantly higher when semen analysis is conducted within 30 min [31]. To maintain sample integrity, the transport temperature should be kept between 20 °C and 37 °C. Studies demonstrated that sperm motility significantly declines if semen is stored at 4 °C [32, 33]. Conversely, motility is highest, and reactive oxygen species (ROS) levels are lowest when the sample is maintained at 37 °C [33]. Therefore, in cases where semen is collected outside the laboratory, the WHO recommends that the specimen container be kept close to the body, such as in the armpit, during transport, most likely to help preserve optimal temperature conditions [15]. Proper patient education on semen collection protocols is essential to ensure the accuracy of semen analysis and the reliability of test results.

Semen analysis may need to be repeated, considering that the results are variable and uncertain. In recognition of this, the European Association of Urology (EAU) guidelines recommend repeating semen analysis if abnormal results are obtained [34]. In general, it is recommended to repeat semen analysis after 1 month. However, the optimal time frame for repeat testing should be individualized based on the findings of the initial analysis, as well as factors such as recent changes in medication, substance use (including alcohol and drug consumption), weight fluctuations, stress, and other lifestyle influences [35].

Basic Examination

The most fundamental evaluation in semen analysis is the basic examination, previously referred to as a standard test [22]. It primarily focuses on the macroscopic and microscopic characteristics of sperm, including the appearance of ejaculates, semen volume, pH, viscosity, sperm count or concentration, motility, morphology, and vitality assessment. While macroscopic evaluation may not always be emphasized in laboratory reports, it can reveal key clinical insights, such as whether the sample is a complete ejaculate or contains traces of blood or urine. Typically, the color of normal semen is cream/gray, opalescent, or off-white [36].

The 6th edition of the manual includes a new addition to the basic semen analysis, particularly for the macroscopic characteristics: the assessment of semen odor. The manual states that putrefactive odors may hold clinical significance, though standardizing this parameter remains challenging [15, 22]. A study reported a case of non-viscous, brown-hued semen with an unpleasant odor from men and revealed a significant quantity of Schistosoma haematobium eggs, considerable detritus, and numerous amorphous cells [37]. However, further reports are awaited to understand the benefit of odor assessment. For the measurement of ejaculate volume, the WHO manual recommends determining volume by weighing the empty sample container and then weighing it again with the semen sample rather than using pipettes or measuring cylinders, which may cause volume loss [15].

Concerning sperm motility, the 6th edition reintroduces the categorization used in the 4th edition, distinguishing progressive motility into two subcategories: rapid progressive and slow progressive motility [15]. Thus, sperm motility is now classified into rapid progressive (grade A), slow progressive (grade B), non-progressive (grade C), and immotile (grade D) [15]. The decision to reintroduce these motility grades has been criticized by some authors as justified by citing earlier studies that demonstrated the clinical value of rapid motility but does not include any recent studies [22]. Some studies mentioned the benefit of evaluating rapid progressive sperm motility to predict the successful outcome of IVF [38, 39]. Motility assessment requires pre-incubation of microscope slides at 37 °C to ensure accurate assessment. A rapid progressive motility is generally defined as one that moves more than five head-lengths per second [40] as sperm kinematics and velocity can only be assessed using computer-assisted sperm analysis (CASA) [41]. Training laboratory staff to recognize this distinction is essential for consistency.

The evaluation of sperm count has also been refined in the 6th edition. Semen dilutions have been simplified, and laboratories are now required to count at least 200 spermatozoa per replicate [15]. Previously, sperm concentration could be estimated by observing 0–4 spermatozoa per field at ×400 magnification (or 0–16 spermatozoa per field at ×200 magnification), allowing for a rough classification of samples with sperm concentrations below 2 × 10 [7]/mL [15]. This approach has been revised, and now, low sperm concentrations must be assessed with greater precision, acknowledging the significant errors associated with counting small numbers of spermatozoa [15, 22].

Despite appearing well-mixed macroscopically, liquefied semen samples can contain small compartments with variable sperm distributions. Proper dilution is essential for accurate counting, as it ensures that counting chambers fill correctly, preventing issues associated with viscous semen. Additionally, using a diluent that immobilizes spermatozoa allows for easier counting and reduces the likelihood of duplicate assessments of motile sperm. Compared to the 5th edition, the 6th edition of manual advocates for a more detailed approach to dilution to minimize variation and inaccurate results. It is recommended to use at least 50 μl of well-mixed ejaculate, and the total volume of sperm suspension should be at least 200 μl [15].

Sperm morphology assessment has also been enhanced with a more systematic approach based on a model presented initially by Rothmann et al. [42]. The manual also provided multiple high-quality micrographs of spermatozoa from unprocessed semen samples, categorized as normal, borderline, or abnormal [15]. These images are accompanied by detailed explanations to guide classification, making this edition a more useful reference for morphology assessment. Therefore, it will be easier to recognize specific defects in the head, neck/midpiece, tail, and cytoplasm of the sperm [15]. However, a recent review revealed that sperm morphology analysis may possess limited diagnostic and prognostic significance as recent studies do not demonstrate a correlation between sperm morphology and natural or aided reproductive outcomes, particularly with isolated abnormal sperm morphology [43, 44]. Nevertheless, certain abnormalities, such as midpiece or tail defects, may contribute to immotility, while acrosome defects may impair fertilization capacity.

For the overall interpretation, the reference thresholds for basic semen parameters used in the 5th edition have been omitted in the 6th edition of the WHO manual, as mentioned earlier. Specifically, the terms normozoospermia, asthenozoospermia, necrozoospermia, and teratozoospermia have been completely removed [15]. In clinical practice, the absence of clear reference values may confuse clinicians, who will need to rely on alternative sources in the literature to interpret semen analysis results. As highlighted in the EAU guidelines panel, this segregation of normal and abnormal semen analysis may still be clinically relevant in everyday clinical practice (EAU 2024).

Interestingly, an analysis of 3101 couples who underwent 4013 cycles of intracytoplasmic sperm injection revealed that, when sperm was categorized as <5th-percentile based or >5th-percentile according to WHO 2021 criteria, those with teratozoospermia, oligoteratozoospermia, oligoasthenoteratozoospermia, and azoospermia had lower fertilization rates compared to patients with all sperm parameters above the 5th-percentile [45]. Additionally, oligoasthenoteratozoospermia and obstructive azoospermia were also correlated with lower blastulation rates [45]. Nevertheless, there was no association found between semen parameters and day 5 blastocyst rates, Gardner's AA-grade blastocyst rates, euploidy rates per cohort of biopsied blastocysts, or live birth rates per first vitrified-warmed single euploid blastocyst transfer. Clinicians should always take a personalized approach to each infertility case while also attempting to improve semen parameters whenever possible.

Extended Examination

Tests deemed beneficial in clinical practices yet not classified in the basic examination for routine use are categorized as extended examinations. Tests that are included in examinations are assessment of sperm DNA fragmentation, genetic and genomic analyses, immunological assessments, interleukin levels, indices of multiple sperm defects, immature germ cells, sperm antibodies, biochemical evaluations of accessory glands, and the assessment of ejaculation sequence [15]. Among these tests, sperm DNA fragmentation (SDF) assessment is a test that was introduced in the new edition of the WHO manual for the first time [15].

SDF has been becoming a hot topic for the last few years and is regarded as one promising addition to male infertility evaluations [15]. A scientometric analysis showed that the number of publications on SDF tests for male infertility evaluations had consistently increased from 1999 to 2018 [46]. Evidence indicates that a high SDF rate is linked to lower spontaneous pregnancy rates, less successful ART outcomes, and higher miscarriage rates. However, these effects should be interpreted cautiously, particularly due to the weak evidence and methodological limitations in some studies [47–51]. The harmful impact of SDF is further exacerbated by poor oocyte quality, which may also increase the aneuploidy rate of embryos [52, 53]. In this regard, SDF served as a great addition to basic examination as it is not strongly correlated to conventional sperm parameters, and infertile men with normozoospermia can have high SDF rates [54, 55].

Four assays were mentioned in the WHO manual to evaluate the SDF rate. Those are Terminal deoxynucleotidyl transferase dUTP nick end labeling (TUNEL), Sperm Chromatin Structure Assay (SCSA), Sperm Chromatin Dispersion (SCD) or Halo, and Comet assay. Each test has its own principles and methods for interpreting results. While the WHO manual did not mention the superiority of one test over another test, a global survey by Global Andrology Forum (GAF) in 2023 found that

TUNEL assay is the most commonly ordered test among clinicians and researchers [56]. Regarding cut-off value, the WHO manual did not mention any range to define a high SDF rate. In a review of published articles, the commonly used cut-off was varied. It ranges from 20% to 35%, indicating that a single cut-off is not universally applicable [57].

The manual also lacks recommendations on the indication of SDF testing. Understandably, even other professional societies such as the American Urological Association (AUA) and EAU have not specified recommendations for SDF testing in many clinical scenarios [34, 58]. As an exception, SDF testing is strongly recommended by AUA and EAU in the cases of recurrent pregnancy loss. The lack of recommendations from professional guidelines resulted in the delayed implementation of SDF testing in clinical practice.

To address the controversies surrounding SDF testing, GAF has published its recommendations [59]. They recommend evaluating SDF in unexplained male infertility, idiopathic male infertility before ART, recurrent pregnancy loss, and clinical varicocele if ART is planned, failed medical therapy, or persistent infertility post-varicocelectomy. SDF testing is also possible for ART planning but should be used with caution because of its limitations. Finally, the decision to test SDF in sperm cryopreservation can be tailored to each case.

In general, clinicians should order SDF testing only if it affects the management plan. Modalities to reduce the SDF rate range from noninvasive methods like antioxidants and lifestyle modifications to more invasive techniques such as ICSI, varicocelectomy, and using testicular sperm for treatment [60, 61]. Nevertheless, the manual does not discuss therapeutic interventions to reduce SDF levels, which remains an area for further research.

Another component of the extended examination is the assessment of immature germ cells, which is conducted using a semen smear stained with the Papanicolaou method [15]. While there are other techniques, this stain is the most evaluated method. It allows for the identification of spermatogonia (nuclear size ~8 μm), spermatocytes (~10 μm), and spermatids (~5 μm) based on the nuclear size, although the size of the nucleus can be altered with degeneration and cell division. Previously considered a routine test in the 4th and 5th editions, this assessment has now been reclassified as an extended examination, and reference cut-off values have been removed. The identification of immature germ cells can sometimes be important, especially in men with non-obstructive azoospermia that failed to obtain spermatozoa even after microscopic testicular sperm extraction. Although controversial, some studies have reported successful live births from round spermatid injection into oocytes [62]. Another study also found the benefit of immature germ cell identification, as it was negatively correlated with total sperm count and motility [63].

Evaluation of antisperm antibodies and leukospermia was reclassified from a standard examination in the 5th edition to an extended examination in the 6th edition [15, 21]. In cases where more than 50% of motile spermatozoa exhibit adherent antibody particles, immune infertility is suspected [21]. However, the 6th edition now advises each laboratory to establish its own reference limits [15]. Based on the current evidence, the precise etiology of male infertility resulting from ASA remains unclear, and the management depends on the underlying cause [64]. For leukocytes, the peroxidase staining method for initial screening for granulocytes is useful in distinguishing polymorphonuclear leukocytes from multinucleated spermatids, which are peroxidase-free [15]. While this test is quick and inexpensive, it does not detect activated or other types of polymorphonuclear cells that do not contain peroxidase [15]. Alternatively, pan-leukocyte (CD45) immunocytochemical staining is an option, offering a clear distinction between leukocytes and germ cells, though it is more costly and time-consuming [15]. High quantities of seminal leukocytes are posited to impair sperm function, leading to lower progressive and total sperm motility percentages [65]. Nevertheless, the exact correlation of leukocytospermia and infertility is still a matter of debates with conflicting results on the effect treatment to sperm quality and pregnancy [66].

The inclusion of genetic and genomic testing is another major update in the 6th edition of the WHO manual. The sperm aneuploidy test detects chromosomal abnormalities that may arise due to meiotic segregation errors, which can occur even in men with a normal karyotype or Robertsonian translocations [67]. Infertile patients with abnormal sperm parameters exhibit a higher risk in sperm aneuploidy compared to fertile men [68]. Fluorescence in situ hybridization (FISH) is the primary technique for detecting aneuploidy [15]. Nevertheless, a lack of clear recommendations on when and how to apply these tests in clinical practice may lead to inconsistent usage. Moreover, this examination required specialized andrology laboratory facilities and therefore may limit its broad use.

Included in the extended examination are the assessments of accessory sex gland function. They are important for identifying potential dysfunctions caused by infection or other pathologies. The secretory capacity of the prostate, seminal vesicles, and epididymis can be evaluated using biochemical markers such as zinc ($\geq$2.4 μmol/ejaculate), fructose, and α-glucosidase ($\geq$13 μmol/ejaculate). The concentration of these seminal biomarkers has been found to be correlated with semen parameters [69, 70]. Additionally, the 6th edition of the WHO manual introduces indices for evaluating multiple sperm defects, including the Teratozoospermia Index (TZI), Multiple Anomalies Index (MAI), and Sperm Deformity Index (SDI) [15]. These indices help quantify sperm abnormalities; however, the literature that supported the clinical relevance of these indices was very scarce [71].

Advanced Examination

In the advanced examination, which was previously referred to as a research test, several tests have been removed due to its impracticality and low clinical value, which are the zona-free hamster oocyte penetration test, the human zona pellucida binding test, and the sperm-cervical interaction assessment [15]. On the other hand, the new edition introduces several updates of highly specialized tests in the advanced examination, including evaluation of seminal oxidative stress (OS), sperm acrosome reaction, transmembrane ion flux, sperm transport, and chromatin condensation [15].

Spermatozoa are particularly vulnerable to oxidative stress due to their limited DNA repair capacity [72]. At the same time, physiological levels of reactive oxygen species (ROS) are essential for processes like capacitation and acrosome reaction, an imbalance where ROS exceeds antioxidant defenses results in OS [73]. This leads to sperm damage through lipid peroxidation, DNA damage, and apoptosis, which has a detrimental impact on natural and assisted pregnancies (Agarwal et al. 2003; [74]). ROS can be from endogenous factors like varicocele and leukocytes or exogenous factors such as smoking, pollution, and alcohol [75].

Evaluation of OS can be done by assessing seminal ROS levels, antioxidant capacity, and the redox balance state. The WHO manual briefly outlines the descriptions of these procedures and their limitations. Seminal ROS can be evaluated using chemiluminescence, flow cytometry, thiobarbituric acid reactive substances, and nitroblue tetrazolium assays. Antioxidant capacity is assessed via the total antioxidant capacity assay, which is rapid but has limited sensitivity and specificity. Redox state evaluation utilizes oxidation–reduction potential (ORP), which can be tested using the MiOXSYS system. Data analysis from 2092 patients found that 1.36 mV/10^6 sperm/mL in MiOXSYS results could differentiate specimens with abnormal semen parameters [76]. On the other hand, another study found that the measurement of ORP with MiOXSYS was not correlated with semen parameters and inconsistently correlated with OS biomarkers and SDF rate [77]. Currently, no cut-off of OS is clearly endorsed in the WHO manual. It highlights the need for further evidence to determine the most reliable methodology for measuring seminal OS.

In congruence, the WHO manual also did not state the recommendation of any treatment for infertile men with high OS levels. While some studies found the benefit of antioxidants for improving sperm parameters, live birth rate, and ART outcomes [78], physicians must use them wisely as there is a lack of robust evidence of antioxidant use for male infertility due to the heterogeneity of the available studies. No single antioxidant can be used as a panacea for all male infertility cases; on the contrary, different antioxidant types may result in various improvements in sperm parameters [79]. Additionally, excessive use of antioxidants can lead to reductive stress, which poses risks such as cancer, cardiomyopathy, and potential negative impacts on male fertility [80]. This "antioxidant paradox" highlights the importance of balancing oxidative and reductive states to avoid harmful outcomes.

To assess sperm chromatin integrity, the new WHO manual describes assays such as aniline blue and chromomycin A3 to evaluate the degree of histone replacement by protamines in the sperm nucleus, which are critical from chromatin condensation. However, more advanced epigenetic assays that assess post-translational histone modifications, sperm DNA methylation, or small RNA expression are not included. Adopting these techniques in fertility laboratories will require further research and clinical validation to establish their diagnostic value. Similarly, sperm capacitation test and acrosome reaction examination also require extensive training, monitoring, and may not be cost-effective for routine use.

The next advanced examination is computer-aided sperm analysis (CASA) in clinical settings, which has been a topic of debate over years. While CASA systems are commonly used for automated semen analysis, their capabilities vary significantly depending on the specific task, such as basic sperm function assessment, live cell motility analysis, and fixed assays [15]. Recent studies have demonstrated high inter- and intra-rater reliability levels, indicating that certain automated semen analyzers, such as the new X1 PRO, can provide accurate and rapid test results in a clinical laboratory setting (Agarwal et al. 2021). The benefit of CASA lies in its ability to perform computational measurements such as sperm kinematics that may be difficult for the human eye to quantify, thereby enhancing but not replacing traditional sperm function assessments. Despite that, the CASA area is limited in differentiating sperm cells from debris or other cellular components within the semen sample, leading to misclassification errors [15]. The lack of standardization in CASA algorithms also results in inconsistency across laboratories. As such, CASA should be viewed as a supplementary tool rather than a replacement for manual semen analysis.

Sperm Preparations and Cryopreservation

While sperm cryopreservation and sperm preparation techniques were previously covered in a single chapter in the 5th edition of the WHO manual, the 6th edition presents them as two distinct topics, reflecting their growing significance in assisted reproductive technologies (ART). An ideal sperm preparation technique should recover a highly functional sperm population while minimizing DNA fragmentation and avoiding oxidative stress induced by reactive oxygen species (ROS) from sperm and leukocytes [15].

The WHO manual describes several well-established sperm selection techniques, including the direct swim-up and density gradient centrifugation (DGC), which differ in their ability to remove seminal plasma components, which can influence the final quality of the sperm preparation [15]. One of the important additions in this new manual is the introduction of magnetic-activated cell sorting (MACS). A meta-analysis of five studies found that sperm selection using MACS resulted in statistically significant higher pregnancy rates ((RR = 1.50, 95% CI 1.14–1.98) when compared to DGC and swim-up techniques with comparable implantation and miscarriage rates [81].

An emerging sperm selection option that is yet to be in the WHO manual is the microfluidics system. By applying the microscale fluid dynamic through diverse on-chips with mechanical and chemical stimuli [82], it can sort an unprocessed semen to find a highly motile sperm with a nearly undetectable SDF level for IVF/ICSI [83]. Compared to DGS and swim-up, it offers the benefit of a better selection of high-quality sperm with lower SDF and higher progressive motility rate from a raw semen sample without the need for an additional filtration step, hence reducing the hands-on time [83, 84]. Pooled analysis from 13 studies found that selected sperm from microfluid resulted in 52.7% clinical pregnancy out of 1646 embryo transfers with a 15.9% rate of miscarriage out of 598 confirmed clinical pregnancies [85]. More clinical studies are needed for this promising technique to be fully incorporated and recommended in clinical practices [86].

In the chapter on cryopreservation, the 6th edition of the WHO manual introduces the vitrification technique to cryopreserve ejaculated spermatozoa, detailing both open and closed systems. While vitrification has shown superiority to conventional freezing methods in the preservation of spermatozoa in terms of total and progressive motility, it comes from several small studies [87]. Moreover, the efficacy of vitrification is influenced by using different vitrification protocols and cryopreservation of different quality spermatozoa. In this regard, the WHO manual recommended considering vitrification as an experimental procedure.

Future Directions

The 6th edition of the WHO manual of human semen examination and processing has successfully addressed the issues from the previous edition. It improves the precision of semen analysis while simultaneously underscoring the necessity for additional scientific evidence. Many tests, particularly those in extended and advanced examinations, lack clinical indication and cut-off value. Therefore, the future area should focus on this aspect. Revisiting the established tests is also encouraged for a continuous confirmation of their relevance in clinical practice.

With more detailed and clear instructions on standardized semen analysis, future studies are expected to adhere more closely to the guidelines to avoid data misinterpretation. Emerging automated, cost-effective, and mobile-testing technologies for semen analysis will complement and not replace manual semen analysis. In addition, with increasing scientific knowledge and technological advancements, the future of sperm testing and processing will incorporate more molecular and cellular markers in spermatozoa function and the use of artificial intelligence to better identify and educate patients and clinicians while, at the same time, streamline the entire IVF process.

The WHO manual's 7th edition is anticipated to include a refined and updated manual of semen analysis. This manual should be released in several years and will likely incorporate more datasets from the remaining regions and continents that have not been involved.

References

1. Vander Borght M, Wyns C. Fertility and infertility: definition and epidemiology. Clin Biochem. 2018;62:2–10. https://doi.org/10.1016/j.clinbiochem.2018.03.012. Epub 2018 Mar 16. PMID: 29555319.
2. Practice Committee of the American Society for Reproductive Medicine. Definition of infertility: a committee opinion. Fertil Steril. 2023;120(6):1170.
3. Maheshwari A, Hamilton M, Bhattacharya S. Effect of female age on the diagnostic categories of infertility. Hum Reprod. 2008;23(3):538–42. https://doi.org/10.1093/humrep/dem431. PMID: 18308834.

4. Sharlip ID, Jarow JP, Belker AM, Lipshultz LI, Sigman M, Thomas AJ, Schlegel PN, Howards SS, Nehra A, Damewood MD, Overstreet JW, Sadovsky R. Best practice policies for male infertility. Fertil Steril. 2002;77(5):873–82. https://doi.org/10.1016/s0015-0282(02)03105-9. PMID: 12009338.
5. Agarwal A, Mulgund A, Hamada A, Chyatte MR. A unique view on male infertility around the globe. Reprod Biol Endocrinol. 2015;13:37. https://doi.org/10.1186/s12958-015-0032-1. PMID: 25928197; PMCID: PMC4424520.
6. Grande G, Garolla A, Graziani A, Astorri AL, Cammarota MV, Merola A, Polidori MP, Lulli E, Busato E, Pesce F, Pompa G, Pontecorvi A, Milardi D, Ferlin A. Comprehensive diagnostic and therapeutic approach to male factor infertility aimed at natural fertility: A multicentric retrospective cohort study. Andrology. 2025; https://doi.org/10.1111/andr.70006. Epub ahead of print. PMID: 39930939.
7. Huang B, Wang Z, Kong Y, Jin M, Ma L. Global, regional and national burden of male infertility in 204 countries and territories between 1990 and 2019: an analysis of global burden of disease study. BMC Public Health. 2023;23(1):2195. https://doi.org/10.1186/s12889-023-16793-3. PMID: 37940907; PMCID: PMC10631182.
8. Tong N, Witherspoon L, Dunne C, Flannigan R. Global decline of male fertility: fact or fiction? BC Med J. 2022;64(3):126–30.
9. Schlegel PN. Evaluation of male infertility. Minerva Ginecol. 2009;61(4):261–83. PMID: 19745794.
10. Baskaran S, Finelli R, Agarwal A, Henkel R. Diagnostic value of routine semen analysis in clinical andrology. Andrologia. 2021;53(2):e13614. https://doi.org/10.1111/and.13614. Epub 2020 May 12. PMID: 32400107.
11. Kızılay F, Altay B. Sperm function tests in clinical practice. Turk J Urol. 2017;43(4):393–400. https://doi.org/10.5152/tud.2017.96646. Epub 2017 Dec 1. PMID: 29201498; PMCID: PMC5687198.
12. Akhter A, Momen SHM, Fatema K, Nath SD. Prevalence of Abnormal Semen Parameters among the Infertile Couples Seeking Infertility Treatment. Mymensingh Med J. 2024;33(2):586–91. PMID: 38557544.
13. Levine H, Jørgensen N, Martino-Andrade A, Mendiola J, Weksler-Derri D, Jolles M, Pinotti R, Swan SH. Temporal trends in sperm count: a systematic review and meta-regression analysis of samples collected globally in the 20th and 21st centuries. Hum Reprod Update. 2023;29(2):157–76. https://doi.org/10.1093/humupd/dmac035. PMID: 36377604.
14. Agarwal A, Sharma R, Gupta S, Finelli R, Parekh N, Selvam MKP, Pompeu CP, Madani S, Belo A, Darbandi M, Singh N, Darbandi S, Covarrubias S, Sadeghi R, Arafa M, Majzoub A, Caraballo M, Giroski A, McNulty K, Durairajanayagam D, Henkel R. Standardized laboratory procedures, quality control and quality assurance are key requirements for accurate semen analysis in the evaluation of infertile male. World J Mens Health. 2022;40(1):52–65. https://doi.org/10.5534/wjmh.210022. Epub 2021 Apr 21. PMID: 33987999; PMCID: PMC8761242
15. World Health Organization. WHO laboratory manual for the examination and processing of human semen. 6th ed. Geneva: WHO Press; 2021.
16. World Health Organization. Laboratory manual for the examination of human semen and semen-cervical mucus interaction. Singapore: Press Concern; 1980.
17. Wang C, Mbizvo M, Festin MP, Björndahl L, Toskin I, other Editorial Board Members of the WHO Laboratory Manual for the Examination and Processing of Human Semen. Evolution of the WHO "Semen" processing manual from the first (1980) to the sixth edition (2021). Fertil Steril. 2022;117(2):237–45. https://doi.org/10.1016/j.fertnstert.2021.11.037. Epub 2022 Jan 5. PMID: 34996596; PMCID: PMC8842884.
18. World Health Organization. WHO Laboratory manual for the examination of human semen and semen-cervical mucus interaction. 2nd ed. Cambridge: Cambridge University Press; 1987.
19. World Health Organization. WHO Laboratory manual for the examination of human semen and sperm-cervical mucus interaction. 3rd ed. Cambridge: Cambridge University Press; 1992.

20. World Health Organization. WHO Laboratory manual for the examination of human semen and sperm-cervical mucus interaction. 4th ed. Cambridge: Cambridge University Press; 1999.
21. World Health Organization. WHO laboratory manual for the examination and processing of human semen. 5th ed. Geneva: WHO Press; 2010.
22. Boitrelle F, Shah R, Saleh R, Henkel R, Kandil H, Chung E, Vogiatzi P, Zini A, Arafa M, Agarwal A. The sixth edition of the WHO manual for human semen analysis: a critical review and SWOT analysis. Life (Basel). 2021;11(12):1368. https://doi.org/10.3390/life11121368. PMID: 34947899; PMCID: PMC8706130.
23. Turner KA, Fishman EL, Asadullah M, Ott B, Dusza P, Shah TA, Sindhwani P, Nadiminty N, Molinari E, Patrizio P, Saltzman BS, Avidor-Reiss T. Fluorescence-based ratiometric analysis of sperm centrioles (FRAC) finds patient age and sperm morphology are associated with centriole quality. Front Cell Dev Biol. 2021;9:658891. https://doi.org/10.3389/fcell.2021.658891. PMID: 33968935; PMCID: PMC8100587.
24. Campbell MJ, Lotti F, Baldi E, Schlatt S, Festin MPR, Björndahl L, Toskin I, Barratt CLR. Distribution of semen examination results 2020 – a follow up of data collated for the WHO semen analysis manual 2010. Andrology. 2021;9(3):817–22. https://doi.org/10.1111/andr.12983. Epub 2021 Mar 17. PMID: 33528873.
25. Boeri L, Fallara G, Pozzi E, Belladelli F, Corsini C, Raffo M, Schifano N, Capogrosso P, d'Arma A, Montorsi F, Salonia A. The impact of different WHO reference criteria for semen analysis in clinical practice: Who will benefit from the new 2021 thresholds for normal semen parameters? Andrology. 2022;10(6):1134–42. https://doi.org/10.1111/andr.13213. Epub 2022 Jun 30. PMID: 35726049; PMCID: PMC9541878
26. Wang C, Swerdloff RS. Limitations of semen analysis as a test of male fertility and anticipated needs from newer tests. Fertil Steril. 2014;102(6):1502–7. https://doi.org/10.1016/j.fertnstert.2014.10.021. Epub 2014 Nov 25. PMID: 25458617; PMCID: PMC4254491.
27. Boeri L, Belladelli F, Capogrosso P, Cazzaniga W, Candela L, Pozzi E, Valsecchi L, Papaleo E, Viganò P, Abbate C, Pederzoli F, Alfano M, Montorsi F, Salonia A. Normal sperm parameters per se do not reliably account for fertility: a case-control study in the real-life setting. Andrologia. 2021;53(1):e13861. https://doi.org/10.1111/and.13861. Epub 2020 Oct 30. PMID: 33125742.
28. Lo Giudice A, Asmundo MG, Cimino S, Cocci A, Falcone M, Capece M, Abdelhameed AS, Capogrosso P, Morgado A, Tsampoukas G, Manfredi C, Russo GI. Effects of long and short ejaculatory abstinence on sperm parameters: a meta-analysis of randomized-controlled trials. Front Endocrinol (Lausanne). 2024;15:1373426. https://doi.org/10.3389/fendo.2024.1373426. PMID: 38828413; PMCID: PMC11140051.
29. Barbagallo F, Cannarella R, Crafa A, Manna C, La Vignera S, Condorelli RA, Calogero AE. The impact of a very short abstinence period on conventional sperm parameters and sperm DNA fragmentation: a systematic review and meta-analysis. J Clin Med. 2022;11(24):7303. https://doi.org/10.3390/jcm11247303. PMID: 36555920; PMCID: PMC9782170.
30. Makler A, Zaidise I, Paldi E, Brandes JM. Factors affecting sperm motility. I. In vitro change in motility with time after ejaculation. Fertil Steril. 1979;31(2):147–54. https://doi.org/10.1016/s0015-0282(16)43815-x. PMID: 761677
31. Chua SC, Yovich SJ, Hinchliffe PM, Yovich JL. How well do semen analysis parameters correlate with sperm DNA fragmentation? A retrospective study from 2567 semen samples analyzed by the Halosperm test. J Pers Med. 2023;13(3):518. https://doi.org/10.3390/jpm13030518. PMID: 36983700; PMCID: PMC10056107.
32. Appell RA, Evans PR, Blandy JP. The effect of temperature on the motility and viability of sperm. Br J Urol. 1977;49(7):751–6. https://doi.org/10.1111/j.1464-410x.1977.tb04566.x. PMID: 23196
33. Esfandiari N, Saleh RA, Blaut AP, Sharma RK, Nelson DR, Thomas AJ Jr, Falcone T, Agarwal A. Effects of temperature on sperm motion characteristics and reactive oxygen species. Int J Fertil Womens Med. 2002;47(5):227–33. PMID: 12469709

34. Salonia A, Bettochhi P, Capogrosso P, Carvalho J, Corona G, Dinkelman-Smit M, et al. EAU Guidelines on Sexual and Reproductive Health. Arnhem: EAU Guidelines; 2024. Available at: https://uroweb.org/guidelines/sexual-and-reproductive-health. Last accessed 1 Feb 2025.
35. Punjani N, Wald G, Al-Hussein Alwamlh O, Feliciano M, Dudley V, Goldstein M. Optimal timing for repeat semen analysis during male infertility evaluation. F S Rep. 2021;2(2):172–5. https://doi.org/10.1016/j.xfre.2021.04.010. PMID: 34278350; PMCID: PMC8267395.
36. Mason MM, Schuppe K, Weber A, Gurayah A, Muthigi A, Ramasamy R. Ejaculation: the process and characteristics from start to finish. Curr Sex Health Rep. 2023;15(1):1–9. https://doi.org/10.1007/s11930-022-00340-z. Epub 2022 Sep 14. PMID: 36908762; PMCID: PMC9997041.
37. Chohan KR, Kling CA, Byler TK. *Schistosoma haematobium* ova in human semen: a case report. F S Rep. 2020;2(1):126–8. https://doi.org/10.1016/j.xfre.2020.10.004. PMID: 34223283; PMCID: PMC8244270.
38. Verheyen G, Tournaye H, Staessen C, De Vos A, Vandervorst M, Van Steirteghem A. Controlled comparison of conventional in-vitro fertilization and intracytoplasmic sperm injection in patients with asthenozoospermia. Hum Reprod. 1999;14(9):2313–9. https://doi.org/10.1093/humrep/14.9.2313. PMID: 10469701
39. Sifer C, Sasportes T, Barraud V, Poncelet C, Rudant J, Porcher R, Cedrin-Durnerin I, Martin-Pont B, Hugues JN, Wolf JP. World Health Organization grade 'a' motility and zona-binding test accurately predict IVF outcome for mild male factor and unexplained infertilities. Hum Reprod. 2005;20(10):2769–75. https://doi.org/10.1093/humrep/dei118. Epub 2005 Jun 15. PMID: 15958402.
40. Vasan SS. Semen analysis and sperm function tests: How much to test? Indian J Urol. 2011;27(1):41–8. https://doi.org/10.4103/0970-1591.78424. PMID: 21716889; PMCID: PMC3114587.
41. Aghazarian A, Huf W, Pflüger H, Klatte T. Standard semen parameters *vs.* sperm kinematics to predict sperm DNA damage. World J Mens Health. 2021;39(1):116–22. https://doi.org/10.5534/wjmh.190095. Epub 2019 Oct 17. PMID: 31749338; PMCID: PMC7752507.
42. Rothmann SA, Bort AM, Quigley J, Pillow R. Sperm morphology classification: a rational method for schemes adopted by the world health organization. Methods Mol Biol. 2013;927:27–37. https://doi.org/10.1007/978-1-62703-038-0_4. PMID: 22992901
43. Pelzman DL, Sandlow JI. Sperm morphology: evaluating its clinical relevance in contemporary fertility practice. Reprod Med Biol. 2024;23(1):e12594. https://doi.org/10.1002/rmb2.12594. PMID: 38915912; PMCID: PMC11194684.
44. Atmoko W, Savira M, Shah R, Chung E, Agarwal A. Isolated teratozoospermia: revisiting its relevance in male infertility: a narrative review. Transl Androl Urol. 2024;13(2):260–73. https://doi.org/10.21037/tau-23-397. Epub 2024 Feb 26. PMID: 38481866; PMCID: PMC10932644
45. Mazzilli R, Cimadomo D, Innocenti F, Taggi M, Cermisoni GC, Ginesi S, Dovere L, Albricci L, Guido M, Campitiello MR, Ferrero S, Capalbo A, Vaiarelli A, Ubaldi FM, Ferlin A, Rienzi L, Gennarelli G. A WHO 2021-based comprehensive scheme outlining sperm parameters' associations with IVF outcomes in PGT-A cycles. Andrology. 2024; https://doi.org/10.1111/andr.13811. Epub ahead of print. PMID: 39609097.
46. Baskaran S, Agarwal A, Panner Selvam MK, Finelli R, Robert KA, Iovine C, Pushparaj PN, Samanta L, Harlev A, Henkel R. Tracking research trends and hotspots in sperm DNA fragmentation testing for the evaluation of male infertility: a scientometric analysis. Reprod Biol Endocrinol. 2019;17(1):110. https://doi.org/10.1186/s12958-019-0550-3. PMID: 31878936; PMCID: PMC6931248.
47. Tan J, Taskin O, Albert A, Bedaiwy MA. Association between sperm DNA fragmentation and idiopathic recurrent pregnancy loss: a systematic review and meta-analysis. Reprod Biomed Online. 2019;38(6):951–60. https://doi.org/10.1016/j.rbmo.2018.12.029. Epub 2018 Dec 22. PMID: 30979611.
48. Simon L, Zini A, Dyachenko A, Ciampi A, Carrell DT. A systematic review and meta-analysis to determine the effect of sperm DNA damage on in vitro fertilization and intracytoplasmic

sperm injection outcome. Asian J Androl. 2017;19(1):80–90. https://doi.org/10.4103/1008-682X.182822. PMID: 27345006; PMCID: PMC5227680
49. Maghraby H, Elsuity MA, Adel N, Magdi Y, Abdelbadie AS, Rashwan MM, Ahmed OY, Elmahdy M, Khan KS, Fawzy M. Quantifying the association of sperm DNA fragmentation with assisted reproductive technology outcomes: an umbrella review. BJOG. 2024;131(9):1181–96. https://doi.org/10.1111/1471-0528.17796. Epub 2024 Mar 7. PMID: 38450853.
50. Cissen M, Wely MV, Scholten I, Mansell S, Bruin JP, Mol BW, Braat D, Repping S, Hamer G. Measuring sperm DNA fragmentation and clinical outcomes of medically assisted reproduction: a systematic review and meta-analysis. PLoS One. 2016;11(11):e0165125. https://doi.org/10.1371/journal.pone.0165125. PMID: 27832085; PMCID: PMC5104467.
51. Malić Vončina S, Golob B, Ihan A, Kopitar AN, Kolbezen M, Zorn B. Sperm DNA fragmentation and mitochondrial membrane potential combined are better for predicting natural conception than standard sperm parameters. Fertil Steril. 2016;105(3):637–644.e1. https://doi.org/10.1016/j.fertnstert.2015.11.037. Epub 2015 Dec 13. PMID: 26696300.
52. Meseguer M, Santiso R, Garrido N, García-Herrero S, Remohí J, Fernandez JL. Effect of sperm DNA fragmentation on pregnancy outcome depends on oocyte quality. Fertil Steril. 2011;95(1):124–8. https://doi.org/10.1016/j.fertnstert.2010.05.055. Epub 2010 Jul 18. PMID: 20643402.
53. Fu W, Cui Q, Bu Z, Shi H, Yang Q, Hu L. Elevated sperm DNA fragmentation is correlated with an increased chromosomal aneuploidy rate of miscarried conceptus in women of advanced age undergoing fresh embryo transfer cycle. Front Endocrinol (Lausanne). 2024;15:1289763. https://doi.org/10.3389/fendo.2024.1289763. PMID: 38650716; PMCID: PMC11033384.
54. Le MT, Nguyen TAT, Nguyen HTT, Nguyen TTT, Nguyen VT, Le DD, Nguyen VQH, Cao NT. Does sperm DNA fragmentation correlate with semen parameters? Reprod Med Biol. 2019;18(4):390–6. https://doi.org/10.1002/rmb2.12297. PMID: 31607800; PMCID: PMC6780033.
55. Belloc S, Benkhalifa M, Cohen-Bacrie M, Dalleac A, Amar E, Zini A. Sperm deoxyribonucleic acid damage in normozoospermic men is related to age and sperm progressive motility. Fertil Steril. 2014;101(6):1588–93. https://doi.org/10.1016/j.fertnstert.2014.02.006. Epub 2014 Mar 29. PMID: 24690240.
56. Farkouh A, et al. Controversy and consensus on the management of elevated sperm DNA fragmentation in male infertility: a global survey, current guidelines, and expert recommendations. World J Mens Health. 2023;41(4):809–47.
57. Cho CL, Agarwal A, Majzoub A, Esteves SC. A single cut-off value of sperm DNA fragmentation testing does not fit all. Transl Androl Urol. 2017;6(Suppl 4):S501–3. https://doi.org/10.21037/tau.2017.08.12.
58. Brannigan RE, Hermanson L, Kaczmarek J, Kim SK, Kirkby E, Tanrikut C. Updates to male infertility: AUA/ASRM Guideline (2024). J Urol. 2024;212(6):789–99. https://doi.org/10.1097/JU.0000000000004180.
59. Agarwal A, Farkouh A, Saleh R, Hamoda TAA, Salvio G, Boitrelle F, Harraz AM, Ghayda RA, Kavoussi P, Gül M, Toprak T, Russo GI, Durairajanayagam D, Rambhatla A, Birowo P, Cannarella R, Phuoc NHV, Zini A, Arafa M, Wyns C, Tremellen K, Sarıkaya S, Lewis S, Evenson DP, Ko E, Calogero AE, Bahar F, Martínez M, Ambar RF, Colpi GM, Bakircioglu ME, Henkel R, Kandil H, Serefoglu EC, Alfakhri A, Tsujimura A, Kheradmand A, Marino A, Adamyan A, Zilaitiene B, Ozer C, Pescatori E, Vogiatzi P, Busetto GM, Balercia G, Elbardisi H, Akhavizadegan H, Sajadi H, Taniguchi H, Park HJ, Maldonado Rosas I, Al-Marhoon M, Sadighi Gilani MA, Alhathal N, Quang N, Pinggera GM, Kothari P, Micic S, Homa S, Long TQT, Zohdy W, Atmoko W, Ibrahim W, Sabbaghian M, Abumelha SM, Chung E, Ugur MR, Ozkent MS, Selim O, Darbandi M, Fukuhara S, Jamali M, de la Rosette J, Kuroda S, Smith RP, Baser A, Kalkanli A, Tadros NN, Aydos K, Mierzwa TC, Khalafalla K, Malhotra V, Moussa M, Finocchi F, Rachman RI, Giulioni C, Avidor-Reiss T, Kahraman O, Çeker G, Zenoaga-Barbăroşie C, Barrett TL, Yilmaz M, Kadioglu A, Jindal S, Omran H, Bocu K, Karthikeyan VS, Franco G, Solorzano JF, Vishwakarma RB, Arianto E, Garrido N, Jain D, Gherabi N, Sokolakis

I, Palani A, Calik G, Kulaksiz D, Simanaviciene V, Simopoulou M, Güngör ND, Blecher G, Falcone M, Jezek D, Preto M, Amar E, Le TV, Ahn ST, Rezano A, Singh K, Rocco L, Savira M, Rajmil O, Darbandi S, Sogutdelen E, Boeri L, Hernández G, Hakim L, Morimoto Y, Japari A, Sofikitis N, Altay B, Metin Mahmutoglu A, Al Hashimi M, Ziouziou I, Anagnostopoulou C, Lin H, Shah R. Technical aspects and clinical limitations of sperm DNA fragmentation testing in male infertility: a global survey, current guidelines, and expert recommendations. World J Mens Health. 2024;42:202.

60. Agarwal A, Barbăroşie C, Ambar R, Finelli R. The Impact of Single- and Double-Strand DNA Breaks in Human Spermatozoa on Assisted Reproduction. Int J Mol Sci. 2020a;21(11):3882. https://doi.org/10.3390/ijms21113882. PMID: 32485940; PMCID: PMC7312948.
61. Agarwal A, Majzoub A, Baskaran S, Panner Selvam MK, Cho CL, Henkel R, Finelli R, Leisegang K, Sengupta P, Barbarosie C, Parekh N, Alves MG, Ko E, Arafa M, Tadros N, Ramasamy R, Kavoussi P, Ambar R, Kuchakulla M, Robert KA, Iovine C, Durairajanayagam D, Jindal S, Shah R. Sperm DNA Fragmentation: A New Guideline for Clinicians. World J Mens Health. 2020b;38(4):412–71. https://doi.org/10.5534/wjmh.200128. Epub 2020 Aug 6. PMID: 32777871; PMCID: PMC7502318
62. Tanaka A, Suzuki K, Nagayoshi M, Tanaka A, Takemoto Y, Watanabe S, Takeda S, Irahara M, Kuji N, Yamagata Z, Yanagimachi R. Ninety babies born after round spermatid injection into oocytes: survey of their development from fertilization to 2 years of age. Fertil Steril. 2018;110(3):443–51. https://doi.org/10.1016/j.fertnstert.2018.04.033. PMID: 30098696
63. Patil PS, Humbarwadi RS, Patil AD, Gune AR. Immature germ cells in semen – correlation with total sperm count and sperm motility. J Cytol. 2013;30(3):185–9. https://doi.org/10.4103/0970-9371.117682. PMID: 24130411; PMCID: PMC3793356.
64. Mukherjee AG, Gopalakrishnan AV. Anti-sperm antibodies as an increasing threat to male fertility: immunological insights, diagnostic and therapeutic strategies. Reprod Sci. 2024;31(11):3303–22. https://doi.org/10.1007/s43032-024-01610-y. Epub 2024 Jun 3. Erratum in: Reprod Sci. 2024;31(8):2537. 10.1007/s43032-024-01622-8. PMID: 38831152.
65. Moubasher A, Sayed H, Mosaad E, Mahmoud A, Farag F, Taha EA. Impact of leukocytospermia on sperm dynamic motility parameters, DNA and chromosomal integrity. Cent European J Urol. 2018;71(4):470–5. https://doi.org/10.5173/ceju.2018.1724x. Epub 2024 Jun 3. Erratum in: Reprod Sci. 2024;31(8):2537. 10.1007/s43032-024-01622-8. PMID: 38831152.
66. Brunner RJ, Demeter JH, Sindhwani P. Review of Guidelines for the Evaluation and Treatment of Leukocytospermia in Male Infertility. World J Mens Health. 2019;37(2):128–37. https://doi.org/10.5534/wjmh.180078. Epub 2018 Dec 31. PMID: 30644236; PMCID: PMC6479086
67. Piomboni P, Stendardi A, Gambera L. Chromosomal aberrations and aneuploidies of spermatozoa. Adv Exp Med Biol. 2014;791:27–52. https://doi.org/10.1007/978-1-4614-7783-9_3. PMID: 23955671
68. Gianaroli L, Magli MC, Cavallini G, Crippa A, Nadalini M, Bernardini L, Menchini Fabris GF, Voliani S, Ferraretti AP. Frequency of aneuploidy in sperm from patients with extremely severe male factor infertility. Hum Reprod. 2005;20(8):2140–52. https://doi.org/10.1093/humrep/dei033. Epub 2005 Apr 21. PMID: 15845594.
69. Mankad M, Sathawara NG, Doshi H, Saiyed HN, Kumar S. Seminal plasma zinc concentration and alpha-glucosidase activity with respect to semen quality. Biol Trace Elem Res. 2006;110(2):97–106. https://doi.org/10.1385/BTER:110:2:97. PMID: 16757839
70. Gruhl SL, Ho LM, Sim MYX, Lee SN, Yu SL, Yong TT, Lim LS, Rajesh H. Seminal biomarkers and their correlations to semen parameters in subfertile men. Eur J Obstet Gynecol Reprod Biol X. 2023;19:100229. https://doi.org/10.1016/j.eurox.2023.100229. PMID: 37700886; PMCID: PMC10493244.
71. Gatimel N, Moreau J, Parinaud J, Léandri RD. Sperm morphology: assessment, pathophysiology, clinical relevance, and state of the art in 2017. Andrology. 2017;5(5):845–62. https://doi.org/10.1111/andr.12389. Epub 2017 Jul 10. PMID: 28692759.
72. Li N, Wang H, Zou S, Yu X, Li J. Perspective in the mechanisms for repairing sperm DNA damage. Reprod Sci. 2025;32(1):41–51. https://doi.org/10.1007/s43032-024-01714-5. Epub 2024 Sep 27. PMID: 39333437; PMCID: PMC11729216.

73. de Lamirande E, Jiang H, Zini A, Kodama H, Gagnon C. Reactive oxygen species and sperm physiology. Rev Reprod. 1997;2(1):48–54. https://doi.org/10.1530/ror.0.0020048. PMID: 9414465
74. Takeshima T, Usui K, Mori K, Asai T, Yasuda K, Kuroda S, Yumura Y. Oxidative stress and male infertility. Reprod Med Biol. 2020;20(1):41–52. https://doi.org/10.1002/rmb2.12353. PMID: 33488282; PMCID: PMC7812476.
75. Sengupta P, Pinggera GM, Calogero AE, Agarwal A. Oxidative stress affects sperm health and fertility-Time to apply facts learned at the bench to help the patient: Lessons for busy clinicians. Reprod Med Biol. 2024;23(1):e12598. https://doi.org/10.1002/rmb2.12598. PMID: 39224210; PMCID: PMC11366688.
76. Agarwal A, Panner Selvam MK, Arafa M, Okada H, Homa S, Killeen A, Balaban B, Saleh R, Armagan A, Roychoudhury S, Sikka S. Multi-center evaluation of oxidation-reduction potential by the MiOXSYS in males with abnormal semen. Asian J Androl. 2019;21(6):565–9.
77. Furtado TP, Osadchiy V, Furtado MH. Semen static oxidation-reduction potential is not helpful in evaluating male fertility. Andrology. 2024; https://doi.org/10.1111/andr.13759. Epub ahead of print. PMID: 39388524.
78. Majzoub A, Agarwal A. Systematic review of antioxidant types and doses in male infertility: Benefits on semen parameters, advanced sperm function, assisted reproduction and live-birth rate. Arab J Urol. 2018;16(1):113–24. https://doi.org/10.1016/j.aju.2017.11.013. PMID: 29713542; PMCID: PMC5922223.
79. Barbonetti A, Tienforti D, Castellini C, Giulio FD, Muselli M, Pizzocaro A, Vena W, Baroni MG, Pivonello R, Isidori AM, Maggi M, Corona G. Effect of antioxidants on semen parameters in men with oligo-astheno-teratozoospermia: a network meta-analysis. Andrology. 2024;12(3):538–52. https://doi.org/10.1111/andr.13498. Epub 2023 Jul 26. PMID: 37495550.
80. Henkel R, Sandhu IS, Agarwal A. The excessive use of antioxidant therapy: a possible cause of male infertility? Andrologia. 2019;51(1):e13162.
81. Gil M, Sar-Shalom V, Melendez Sivira Y, Carreras R, Checa MA. Sperm selection using magnetic activated cell sorting (MACS) in assisted reproduction: a systematic review and meta-analysis. J Assist Reprod Genet. 2013;30(4):479–85. https://doi.org/10.1007/s10815-013-9962-8. Epub 2013 Mar 7. PMID: 23468098; PMCID: PMC3644127
82. Olatunji O, More A. A review of the impact of microfluidics technology on sperm selection technique. Cureus. 2022;14(7):e27369. https://doi.org/10.7759/cureus.27369. PMID: 36046322; PMCID: PMC9419845.
83. Quinn MM, Jalalian L, Ribeiro S, Ona K, Demirci U, Cedars MI, Rosen MP. Microfluidic sorting selects sperm for clinical use with reduced DNA damage compared to density gradient centrifugation with swim-up in split semen samples. Hum Reprod. 2018;33(8):1388–93. https://doi.org/10.1093/humrep/dey239. PMID: 30007319
84. Sheibak N, Amjadi F, Shamloo A, Zarei F, Zandieh Z. Microfluidic sperm sorting selects a subpopulation of high-quality sperm with a higher potential for fertilization. Hum Reprod. 2024;39(5):902–11. https://doi.org/10.1093/humrep/deae045. PMID: 38461455
85. Ferreira Aderaldo J, da Silva Maranhão K, Ferreira Lanza DC. Does microfluidic sperm selection improve clinical pregnancy and miscarriage outcomes in assisted reproductive treatments? A systematic review and meta-analysis. PLoS One. 2023;18(11):e0292891. https://doi.org/10.1371/journal.pone.0292891. PMID: 37983267; PMCID: PMC10659219.
86. Jahangiri AR, Ziarati N, Dadkhah E, Bucak MN, Rahimizadeh P, Shahverdi A, Sadighi Gilani MA, Topraggaleh TR. Microfluidics: The future of sperm selection in assisted reproduction. Andrology. 2024;12(6):1236–52. https://doi.org/10.1111/andr.13578. Epub 2023 Dec 26. PMID: 38148634.
87. Li YX, Zhou L, Lv MQ, Ge P, Liu YC, Zhou DX. Vitrification and conventional freezing methods in sperm cryopreservation: a systematic review and meta-analysis. Eur J Obstet Gynecol Reprod Biol. 2019;233:84–92. https://doi.org/10.1016/j.ejogrb.2018.11.028. Epub 2018 Dec 14. PMID: 30580229.

Chapter 2
Future Diagnostic Tools and Tests for Male Infertility

Hiva Alipour, Fereshteh Dardmeh, and Paraskevi Vogiatzi

Advanced Semen Analysis Techniques

Semen analysis is the principal and often the first diagnostic approach to assess male fertility. The World Health Organization (WHO) laboratory manual for the examination of semen [1] is a globally recognized source of reliable techniques for semen examination [2]. Semen analysis has traditionally been carried out in an andrology lab, with trained technicians manually assessing sperm parameters. This procedure can be very demanding and time-consuming and has been shown to have intra- and inter-operator variability [3]. Furthermore, not adhering to the established guidelines and protocols could also lead to unreliable results [4]. Semen analysis plays a crucial role in diagnosing pathologies, emphasizing the critical need for accurate and precise results due to their impact on clinical decisions [3]. The previous versions of the WHO laboratory examinations for sperm analysis have mainly focused on manual assessment of various sperm quality parameters, such as motility categorization and the determination of the percentage of morphologically normal sperm, as examples.

The field of male infertility has advanced significantly in the last few decades, especially in the area of novel diagnostic tools and techniques. Thus, the most recently published WHO manual of semen analysis [1] has also undergone some modifications to further clarify and standardize basic analysis methods, while introducing more advanced technology, such as sperm functional tests and a more

H. Alipour (✉) · F. Dardmeh
Department of Health Science and Technology, Faculty of Medicine, Aalborg University, Aalborg, Denmark
e-mail: hiva@hst.aau.dk; feda@hst.aau.dk

P. Vogiatzi
Andromed Health and Reproduction, Fertility Diagnostics Laboratory, Maroussi, Greece

E. Chung et al. (eds.), *Advances in Andrology*,
https://doi.org/10.1007/978-3-032-29112-7_2

sophisticated generation of Computer-Aided Sperm Analysis (CASA) systems [5]. The recent introduction of at-home tests and the application of artificial intelligence is further revolutionizing semen analysis. Furthermore, novel genomic and epigenomic analysis, functional tests, non-invasive biomarker tests, multi-omics approaches, single-cell analysis, specialized imaging techniques, microbiome analysis, sperm sorting techniques, and personalized medicine are also being evaluated for their potential in male infertility diagnosis.

Advanced Computer-Aided Sperm Analysis (CASA) Systems

CASA systems have exhibited numerous advantages, particularly in the last decade, including repeatability, reliability, and the capacity to evaluate detailed parameters [5, 6], making them an essential tool in assessing sperm quality. These systems employ state-of-the-art technology and enable scientists and medical professionals to assess sperm characteristics with great precision and accuracy.

Modern semi-automated CASA systems typically feature digital optical microscopes that capture sequential static images subsequently transferred to a computer or processing unit and analyzed using automated algorithms to conduct objective and quantitative analyses of several sperm structures and functional quality parameters [3]. CASA systems enhance throughput capacity by utilizing digital image processing tools such as noise filtering, image segmentation, localization, multi-object tracking, and machine learning [7] while ensuring consistent, accurate, and reproducible results. By minimizing inter- and intra-laboratory variations associated with manual assessment, CASA systems contribute significantly to standardizing sperm analysis procedures [8]. Accurate assessment of sperm motility is fundamental in understanding and determining factors that impact fertility. CASA and manual assessment of sperm concentration and motility have presented a good correlation [9], while CASA shows higher predictive power for the presence of sperm in affected samples such as in oligospermia patients, and provided more reliable semen analysis results than manual counting [10].

The progressive motility, as categorized by CASA, was significantly linked to both in vivo and in vitro fertilization rates [11–14]. The full diagnostic and prognostic potential of the detailed kinematic parameters provided by these systems is still under debate as there is no clear consensus on the robustness and reliability of these parameters for use in clinical diagnosis and outcome prediction, necessitating further investigation and validation. Moreover, significant advancements in the technology of CASA systems over the past decades have markedly improved the reliability and validity of the assessments, warranting investigations to identify the potential correlations between the detailed parameters provided by CASA and fertility potential and outcomes.

In contrast to motility and concentration, most CASA systems require the sperm to be manually stained before morphological evaluation. The variability in staining, the potential diversity within a specific semen sample, and the subjective aspect of interpretation have led to a lack of strong correlation between morphological evaluations conducted by CASA and manual assessments [15].

In addition to the well-established sperm concentration/motility and morphology CASA modules, certain CASA systems, such as the Sperm Class Analyzer® (Microptic S.L., Barcelona), have started introducing automated modules for vitality, fragmentation, acrosome reaction, and leukocyte count. All these modules (except motility and concentration) require the samples to be manually prepared and stained before detection and assessment, which can lead to variability and subjectivity, potentially affecting the reliability of results. Therefore, although these advanced modules hold promise for research applications, their integration into clinical settings demands further optimization to guarantee standardization, efficiency, and accuracy.

With the advancement of technology and increasing integration of AI into the medical field, we are observing a paradigm shift toward the full automation of sperm analysis, with far-reaching implications for clinical practice and research. In line with this goal, the "SCAScope®" (Microptic S.L., Barcelona) stands out with the capability to simultaneously evaluate motility and concentration, Vitality, Morphology, DNA Fragmentation, and leukocyte assessments, all at the same time with no need for user interaction with the system during the analysis; however, the sample still has to be prepared on separate slides and stained using the relevant staining process for each of the modules (except for motility and concentration) prior to running the analysis.

Further advancement and the emergence of fully automated CASA systems providing automated preparation of the samples would begin a new era of streamlined and optimized workflow, enhanced reproducibility and standardization, minimized variability, and eliminated subjectivity, which is a significant advancement in the field of male fertility assessment.

In summary, semi-automated CASA systems offer several advantages due to their capacity to compute more precise parameters in a more repeatable and reliable manner; however, they are also limited by the need for manual input and oversight for accurate results (especially in severe oligospermia) due to biological factors (like excess debris in ejaculate) or technical issues such as the inability to classify micro-aggregates or fragmented sperm [16] or inconsistency of results when using different slides [17]. These limitations leave room for human error and the possibility of misinterpretation. Technological advancements and the adoption of artificial intelligence are moving CASA systems toward improved accuracy, portability, and fully automated analysis, which could decrease inter- and intra-operator variability and error [18] and allow for broader adoption of CASA machines in clinical and research settings. Ultimately, the full automation of the entire process, from sample preparation to data interpretation, would revolutionize male fertility assessment and improve patient care outcomes.

Utilization of Artificial Intelligence (AI) Algorithms to Provide more Accurate and Detailed Assessments of Sperm Motility, Morphology, and Concentration

Artificial intelligence (AI) algorithms have demonstrated promising potential in reproductive medicine diagnostic tools, particularly in assessing sperm motility, morphology, and concentration. By leveraging advanced computational techniques, AI offers the potential to provide more accurate and detailed evaluations, thereby enhancing the understanding and management of male infertility.

AI tools already demonstrated a high accuracy of 90% in predicting sperm concentration or count, along with other seminal parameters in a study in 2013 [19]. With the advancement of AI and its increased integration in CASA systems, we can look forward to even more accurate and consistent results. Table 2.1 presents a selection of the AI and machine learning (ML) algorithms tested to evaluate sperm concentration and counts, motility, and morphology in semen samples or different datasets [20]. Additionally, a recent study using a full-spectrum neural network (FSNN) model trained by examining the absorption response of spermatozoa in 41 human samples to different light spectra (wavelength from 390 to 1100 nm)

Table 2.1 Artificial intelligence (AI) and machine learning (ML) algorithms used to evaluate sperm concentration/count, motility, and morphology in semen samples or different datasets

Algorithm or model	Dataset/sample	Performance or outcomes	Refs.
Concentration/counts			
Logistic regression, SVM, and RF	Semen	Good predictive accuracy with AUC = 0.72	[22]
FSNN, SPNN	Semen	Prediction accuracy: SPNN = 86%, FSNN = 93%	[21]
Image recognition algorithm	Semen	AI algorithm vs. manual analysis: sperm concentration ($r = 0.65$, $p < 0.001$), motile sperm concentration ($r = 0.84$, $p < 0.001$)	[23]
ANN	Semen	Accuracy = 90%, sensitivity = 95.45%, specificity = 50%, PPV = 93.33%, NPV = 60%	[19]
Motility			
SVR, MLP, CNN, RNN	VISEM	Mean absolute error (MAE): SVR = 9.29, MLP = 9.50, CNN = 9.22, RNN = 9.86	[24]
THMA	Semen	Accuracy = 97.37%, with a minimum execution time of 1.12 s.	[25]
Bemaner AI algorithm	Semen	AI algorithm vs. manual analysis: $r = 0.90$, $p < 0.001$	[23]
CNN	VISEM	MAE for predicted sperm motility = 2.92	[26]
SVM	Semen	Accuracy = 89.9%	[27]
ANN	Semen	Accuracy = 82%, sensitivity = 89.29%, specificity = 43.75%, PPV = 89.29%, NPV = 43.75%	[19]

(continued)

Table 2.1 (continued)

Algorithm or model	Dataset/sample	Performance or outcomes	Refs.
Morphology			
DL	JSD	Abnormal sperm: Sensitivity = 0.881 and PPV = 0.853; Normal sperm: Sensitivity = 0.794 and PPV = 0.689	[28]
DTL DMTL	MHSMA	Detection accuracy: Head = 84.0%, acrosome = 80.66%, and vacuole = 94.0%	[29]
DL, U-Net, and Mask-R-CNN	SCIAN-SpermSegGS	Dice coefficient using U-net with transfer learning: Head = 0.96, acrosome = 0.94, and nucleus = 0.95	[30]
DL, HoloStain	Semen	Virtual (holostain) vs. chemical staining: Structural similarity (SSIM) = 0.85 ± 0.03	[31]
CNN	VISEM	Accuracy of sperm head detection = 91.77%	[26]
SVM	Semen	Accuracy = 89.93%, sensitivity = 91.18%, and specificity = 88.61%	[32]
DL	MHSMA	Detection accuracy: Acrosome = 76.67%, head = 77.00%, vacuole = 91.33%	[33]
CNN and SVM	SCIAN	Dice coefficient: Head = 0.90, axial filament = 0.77, acrosome = 0.77, nucleus = 0.78, tail = 0.75, and mid-piece = 0.64	[34]
Deep CNN, VGG16	HuSHeM and SCIAN	Increased true positive rate: HuSHeM dataset = 94.1%, SCIAN dataset = 62%	[35]
SVM	Semen	Good accuracy with AUC = 89.59%	[36]
Dictionary learning	SCIAN and HuSHeM	Detection accuracy: HuSeM dataset = 92%, SCIAN dataset = 62%	[37]
Tail point algorithm	Semen	Dice coefficient accuracy: Heads = 92%, acrosome = 84%, nucleus = 87%, and tail = 96%	[38]

Adapted from Panner Selbam et al. [20]. (Under a Creative Commons Attribution 4.0 International License)

ANN artificial neural network, *FSNN* full-spectrum neural network, *NPV* negative predictive value, *PPV* positive predictive value, *RF* random forest, *SPNN* selected peak neural network, *SVM* support vector machine, *CNN* convolutional neural network, R-*CNN* region-based convolutional neural network, *MLP* multilayer perceptron, *RNN* recurrent neural network, *SVR* linear support vector regressor, *THMA* tail-to-head movement algorithm, *AUC* area under the curve, *DL* deep learning, *DTL* deep transfer learning, *DMTL* deep multi-task transfer learning, *HuSHeM* Human Sperm Head Morphology, *JSD* Jikei sperm data set, *MHSMA* Modified Human Sperm Head Morphology analysis, *VISEM* video dataset of human spermatozoa, *SCIAN-MorphoSpermGS* Gold-standard for Morphological Sperm Analysis

demonstrated over 93% prediction accuracy and 100% agreement with clinical assessments in the differentiation of healthy donor and patient samples [21]. Development, advanced machine learning (ML) algorithms have shown a strong correlation among semen parameters like total sperm count and total motile sperm when automatically evaluated using AI compared to manual assessment. AI-based models have also successfully forecasted the potential increase in sperm concentration post-varicocele repair, indicating the potential for AI to enhance diagnostic and prognostic capabilities in reproductive medicine [22].

AI and ML have always played a crucial role in sperm motility and morphology assessment by CASA [9, 24, 39]. However, recent studies [24, 39] have demonstrated the higher effectiveness and reproducibility of more developed AI algorithms, particularly deep learning convolutional neural networks (CNNs), in analyzing sperm video sequences to predict motility parameters and distinguish between progressive, non-progressive, and immotile spermatozoa. Moreover, the incorporation of temporal analysis has been shown to outperform traditional machine learning approaches, highlighting the potential of AI to capture nuanced motility patterns [15]. Table 2.2 presents selected studies using artificial intelligence to assess sperm motility and morphology, including their outcomes of interest, used datasets, AI methods, and results [15].

AI software may soon be able to correlate kinetic motility patterns with other critical factors, such as morphology, fertilization potential, or blastocyst formation, with the potential as a tool for real-time selection of sperm for intracytoplasmic sperm injection [40].

In addition to motility, AI plays a crucial role in sperm morphology assessment. Poor evaluation of sperm morphology by CASA remains a major drawback that can be improved by artificial intelligence and machine learning [15, 33]. A recent study demonstrated that the sequential deep learning algorithm could detect the acrosome and head of the sperm more accurately than current state-of-the-art approaches while requiring less execution time, even on a low-specification computer/laptop. Additionally, it can classify photos in real-time. Based on the results of our study, this tool could be an aid to the embryologist in deciding whether a spermatozoon in functional or not [41].

Current methods of determining sperm morphological abnormalities require staining of the spermatozoa structural components, which leaves them unusable for fertility treatments [42]. The pursuit of non-damaging methods to evaluate individual sperm morphology would highly benefit cases with extremely low sperm counts or in treatments that require isolating a single sperm [43]. Advanced CNNs have shown promise in identifying deformities in sperm head, acrosome, and vacuole in real-time, using low-magnification microscopes, without staining, and with improved objectivity [29, 33].

Non-invasive AI methods can also evaluate viability characteristics of frozen-thawed or immotile spermatozoa that may not be possible to identify manually. A recently introduced AI system could detect viable sperm using a sole bright-field image without any sample processing or reagents [44]. The model achieved impressive metrics, with 94.9% accuracy, 97.0% sensitivity, and 93.3% specificity, focusing on subtle changes in the cell nucleus morphology. Integrating such AI models into current CASA setups could notably diminish reliance on sperm staining, particularly for necrozoospermic samples, surgically retrieved or cryopreserved sperm of uncertain viability.

Furthermore, AI has contributed to sperm viability assessment by leveraging deep learning techniques to predict viability from morphological features. The non-invasive model developed by Jiang et al. [44] proved to be capable of accurately predicting sperm viability using a single bright-field image [44] by detecting subtle

Table 2.2 Selected studies using artificial intelligence for the assessment of sperm motility and morphology

ART process	Outcomes of interest	Dataset	AI methods	Results	Refs.
Motility assessment	Use sperm video sequences to predict motility, categorized as progressive, non-progressive, and immotile spermatozoa Combined with participant data in multimodal analysis for automated prediction of motility parameters	VISEM—live spermatozoa videos from 85 different participants	Deep learning-CNN	Deep learning algorithms are capable of predicting sperm motility efficiently and reproducibly Combining participant clinical information did not improve prediction Incorporation of temporal analysis outperformed the traditional machine learning approach The best MAE achieved with CNN was 8.74	[39]
Motility assessment	Extraction of temporal features from sequential video frames can predict motility and train traditional CNN models	VISEM	Deep learning-CNN	Increased number of stacked video frames from 9 to 18 improved motility prediction, implying this model could learn temporal features from different video frames The best MAE achieved with CNN was 8.74	[47]
Motility assessment	Automatic sperm motility assessment using a framework of unsupervised spermatozoa tracking, feature extraction, and ML	VISEM	Linear support vector regression	Able to predict the percentage of progressive, non-progressive, and immotile spermatozoa in a given sample MAE reduced to 7.31; an improvement compared to previous papers	[24]
Motility assessment	Individual operator-assessed single sperm morphology linked to motility patterns assessed by vision-based AI software in ICSI-ready sperm	2154 individual sperm video recordings	Vision-based AI Software SiD1 (IVF2.0 Ltd.)	Spermatozoa classified as morphologically normal showed better motility variables (higher linear movement, straight-line velocity) Sperm tail morphology defects had the most significant impact on motility variables AI-driven sperm motility assessment may be sufficient to assess morphological features for sperm selection	[40]*

(continued)

Table 2.2 (continued)

ART process	Outcomes of interest	Dataset	AI methods	Results	Refs.
Motility assessment	Vision-based AI software assessing progressive motility parameters (straight-line velocity, linearity of curvilinear path, head movement patterns) to predict successful fertilization and blastocyst formation	383 individual spermatozoa videos from 78 ICSI cycles	Vision-based AI Software SiD1 (IVF2.0 Ltd.)	Significant differences in progressive motility patterns measured by SiD1 between successful and unsuccessful fertilization and blastocyst formation Possible avenue for real-time analysis of individual spermatozoa during selection for ICSI	[46]
Morphology assessment	Sperm images labeled with a class were divided into patches to identify important features in the sperm Dictionary learning is more effective for sperm head classification than previously published shape-based feature recognition Developed HuSHeM dataset with consensus classification and freely available for research purposes	HuSHeM—includes 216 sperm head images (54 normal, 53 tapered, 57 pyriform, and 52 amorphous). SCIAN-MorphoSpermGS—Includes 1862 images of sperm shapes (100 normal, 228 tapered, 76 pyriform, 73 small, and 656 amorphous), with partial consensus among three experts	Traditional ML with adaptive patch dictionary learning	62% accuracy with SCIAN-MorphoSpermGS dataset 92.3% accuracy, 93.5% precision, and 92.3% recall with the new HuSHeM dataset	[37]
Morphology assessment	Deep CNN trained to detect head, acrosome, and vacuole morphological deformities Developed MHSMA dataset labeled with normal sperm (acrosome, head, vacuole, tail, and neck)	MHSMA—includes 1540 sperm images from 235 subjects with male factor infertility	Deep learning-CNN	High accuracy for detecting morphological deformities in sperm acrosome, head, and vacuole Accuracy scores of 76.7%, 77%, and 91.3% in acrosome, head and vacuole abnormality, respectively, require improvement Able to classify images in real time, aiding in the sperm selection for ICSI	[33]

Morphology assessment	Deep CNN algorithms trained to detect head, acrosome, and vacuole morphological deformities	MHSMA	Deep learning-CNN	AI models can predict sperm head features more accurately than previous studies (84%, 80.7%, and 94% for sperm head, acrosome, and vacuole, respectively)	[29]
Morphology and viability assessment	Deep learning AI technique to predict the viability of immotile sperm through morphology assessment with a single bright-field image	1471 images of immotile sperm from 15 semen samples for training 10 new semen samples for validation	Deep learning-CNN	The AI model can accurately predict sperm viability non-invasively without sample processing or staining AI detects subtle morphological changes to the sperm nucleus; otherwise, it is challenging to identify with the naked eye Yet to be externally validated	[44]*

Adapted from Hanassab [15]. (Under a Creative Commons Attribution 4.0 International License).

Summary of studies using artificial intelligence (AI) and machine learning (ML) methods for sperm assessment and selection. The asterisk (*) indicates studies from conference proceedings. *MAE* mean absolute error, *CNN* convolutional neural network, *ICSI* intracytoplasmic sperm injection morphological changes indicative of viability. This approach offers a convenient and efficient alternative to conventional viability assays, often requiring sample processing and staining. Additionally, the real-time classification capability of AI facilitates rapid decision-making in selecting viable sperm for fertilization procedures.

Overall, using AI algorithms in sperm assessment represents a significant advancement in reproductive medicine. By providing more accurate and detailed evaluations of motility, morphology, concentration, and viability, AI enhances our understanding of male infertility and improves the success rates of assisted reproductive technologies. However, further research and validation are needed to optimize AI algorithms and integrate them into clinical practice seamlessly, a process that involves developing and comparing methods, necessitating external validation and improvement in accuracy [15, 33]. An increasing number of accessible open datasets can be used to develop, test, and benchmark the different AI models against one another [33]. Furthermore, simulation-based approaches have provided a powerful tool for developing and evaluating CASA systems, offering an alternative to manual semen collection and assessment. A recent article by Chio et al. in 2022 presented a simulation-based approach for developing and enhancing such systems. The authors provided models for the image of a sperm cell and four different swimming modes of sperm cells. These models were used to generate simulated semen images that could be used to assess and validate CASA algorithms. The simulation models were also used to study algorithms for segmenting, localization, and tracking sperm cells. The performance of different algorithms is evaluated using metrics such as precision, recall, and the optimal sub-pattern assignment (OSPA) metric [7].

In summary, AI has been instrumental in andrology, extending from semen analysis to image diagnostics [45]. Further integration of AI in CASA software could allow and reveal the correlation of kinetic motility patterns with other crucial factors such as sperm morphology, likelihood of fertilization, or blastocyst formation to aid in the selection of sperm for intracytoplasmic sperm injection (ICSI) in real time [40, 46].

AI-Driven Algorithms to Analyze Semen Samples and Medical Records to Identify Patterns and Predict Male Infertility More Accurately

The use of AI-driven algorithms in analyzing semen samples along with medical records to identify patterns and predict male infertility more accurately has gained significant attention in recent research [48]. AI tools such as support vector machines, adaptive boosting, conventional extreme gradient boost, random forest, and extra tree algorithms have been successfully deployed to predict male fertility using explainable AI models [49]. These models offer a deeper understanding of the prediction process, enabling more informed decisions based on a balanced and imbalanced dataset. The examination and selection of sperm by andrologists and embryologists have greatly benefited from AI algorithms, paving the way for more accurate and objective selection processes [20]. As larger and more reliable datasets become available for training, these algorithms are expected to improve continuously over time, enhancing their predictive capabilities in identifying male infertility factors more effectively [20].

Furthermore, a multi-center analysis demonstrated the utility of AI-based machine learning models in predicting sperm parameter upgrading post-varicocele repair, marking an innovative approach to assessing male fertility [22]. This study highlighted the significance of hormonal data in predicting clinically meaningful upgrading and underlined the potential of machine learning models in enhancing predictive outcomes for men with varicocele [22].

The advanced predictive capabilities of AI models hold promise for improving diagnostic and treatment strategies, contributing to more effective interventions in cases of male infertility.

AI-driven algorithms have also been employed to analyze semen samples and medical data, aiming to identify patterns that can predict male infertility more accurately. GhoshRoy et al. [49] introduced an explainable AI model utilizing the Extreme Gradient Boosting Algorithm to predict male fertility, highlighting the potential of AI tools in this field [49]. Furthermore, a study by Yuan et al. [50] emphasized the importance of using innovative biomarkers such as sperm telomere length to diagnose male infertility and predict embryonic development outcomes [50]. Another study demonstrated a significantly increased risk of infertility associated with human papillomavirus (HPV) infection in semen, shedding light on the multifactorial nature of male infertility [51]. Omolaoye et al. [52] discussed the application of omics data to identify biomarkers for male infertility diagnosis, underlining the potential of leveraging comprehensive datasets for personalized treatment strategies [52]. Recently, the utilization of AI and machine learning in semen analysis was explored by Selvam et al. [20], suggesting that these algorithms could enhance sperm selection processes in clinical settings [52].

The integration of electronic medical records (EMRs) has also played a crucial role in understanding male infertility etiology. Woldemariam et al. [53] leveraged EMRs to reveal comorbidities significantly associated with male infertility, emphasizing the importance of comprehensive data analysis in this field [53].

In conclusion, the integration of AI-driven algorithms in semen analysis and medical records has revolutionized the field of male infertility prediction, offering more accurate and reliable diagnosis, prediction, and treatment of male infertility, paving the way for more personalized and effective interventions.

Three-Dimensional Sperm Surface Reconstruction

Assessing sperm morphology is a crucial aspect of understanding reproductive health. Traditional approaches often involve two-dimensional assessments, but recent technological advancements have paved the way for more sophisticated techniques. One such innovation is the three-dimensional sperm surface reconstruction, which offers a novel approach to evaluating sperm morphology [54]. This proof-of-principle study maintained spermatozoa in a fluid environment, allowing for the creation of automated reconstructions with minimal computing power [54]. A review paper by De Angelis [55] proposed a promising optical approach based on the combination of digital holography and Raman spectroscopy technologies, which would allow for the retrieval of 3D quantitative imaging of the sample with a single-shot acquisition directly in its native environment, providing detailed information about the morphology and physiology of the sperm cells [55].

Another cutting-edge technology in the field is Digital holographic microscopy (DHM), enabling the morphological assessment of live intact spermatozoa [56] by expanding the number of morphological parameters and incorporating simultaneous assessment of sperm motility. The integration of three-dimensional sperm surface reconstruction and DHM represents a substantial leap forward in sperm morphology assessment. In the future, these innovative approaches could provide researchers and clinicians with powerful tools to gain deeper insights into sperm structure and function, ultimately contributing to advancements in reproductive health research.

Three Dimensional (3D) Analyzes of Sperm Motility Tracks (in X, Y, and Z Axes)

The intricate chiral memory within sperm flagella has been suggested as a crucial property for understanding spermatozoa motility patterns. Muschol et al. [57] proposed a chiral memory in sperm flagella that stores torque for subsequent rolls, shedding light on the dynamic nature of sperm movement [57]. Another study by Powar et al. [58] focused on the kinematics of sperm motion by reconstructing flagellar wave motion in 3D, revealing the rolling beating behavior of mouse sperm in three dimensions [58]. This work highlighted the complexity of sperm motion and the significance of analyzing their movement in a three-dimensional space. Hernández et al. [59] introduced a 3D + t feature-based descriptor for the unsupervised classification of human sperm flagellar motion, offering a promising tool for determining sperm viability for fertilization [59]. Additionally, Soler et al. [60] explored the effect of counting chamber depth on the accuracy of lensless microscopy for evaluating boar sperm, highlighting the importance of analyzing the natural three-dimensional pattern of sperm movement for predicting male fertility motility [60]. In another study, Hernández-Herrera et al. [61] developed an algorithm for tracing sperm flagellum center lines in fluorescence 3D + t stacks with low signal-to-noise ratios, surpassing existing methods and achieving high precision and recall rates [61]. This advancement provides essential insights into the 3D motility analysis of sperm cells. In conclusion, the literature reflects a growing interest in leveraging three-dimensional analyses to unravel the complexities of sperm motility, offering valuable insights into the dynamic behavior of sperm cells.

Home Testing Kits

Home testing kits for sperm/semen quality assessment have recently gained popularity due to their convenience and potential cost-effectiveness, and a solution for patients who are too embarrassed to ejaculate in the clinics or where clinics do not have a dedicated semen collection room [62].

These kits offer a simple way for men to assess their fertility status in the comfort of their homes, thereby eliminating the need for repeated visits to a clinic for semen analysis [63]. One such at-home sperm testing device, the Trak System, has been evaluated for its utility in population-based epidemiological fertility studies [63]. An observational study on the variability in semen parameters, as measured from at-home semen collection kit samples, showed that semen quality can vary significantly among users of at-home sperm testing kits, emphasizing the need for multiple samples to provide a robust evaluation of male fertility [64]. Semen collection at home has been found to positively affect sperm quality compared to the collection at a clinic, with superior sample volume, sperm concentration, and total sperm count observed [65]. This finding underscores the potential benefits of at-home sample collection for fertility assessment [65]. Overall, the use of home testing kits for sperm/semen quality assessment presents a promising approach to fertility evaluation, offering convenience and potential benefits for population-based studies and individual fertility assessments. However, the variability in user semen parameters underscores the importance of thorough and accurate assessment methods to ensure reliable results and informed decision-making regarding male fertility [64, 65]. Home semen analysis can be instrumental in making semen analysis well known, screening men, and helping society in identifying and accepting male infertility as a significant cause of couple infertility [66] Further research and standardization in at-home sperm testing are necessary to enhance the effectiveness and reliability of these kits for fertility assessment [65].

Smartphone Apps for Screening of Male Infertility (Sperm Quality)

With the advancement of cell phone technology and the general availability of smartphones, numerous applications and features have been developed to facilitate health monitoring and management. Smartphone technology is already utilized to increase productivity, patient empowerment, and satisfaction in several medical specialties, including ophthalmology, hematology, pediatrics, and obstetrics [67]. Recently, apps that leverage smartphones' portability and high-quality cameras have been developed to offer cost-effective and convenient solutions for analyzing semen samples [68]. The smartphone-based CASA system has been validated for clinical semen diagnosis, possibly motivating infertile males to seek early medical intervention [69]. In low-resource settings, the Foldscope microscope has been proposed as a preliminary screening tool for male infertility, providing a quick and economical referral option for men with reproductive issues [70]. Additionally, smartphone-based home screening tests offer a niche solution for men without access to traditional andrology lab testing or those who prefer testing at home [71].

Another study evaluating the usefulness of the smartphone-based sperm quality test in 200 men showed significant correlations between sperm count and motility when measured by OVIEW-M tests ($r = 0.893$, $p < 0.01$) and standard microscope examination ($r = 0.883$, $p < 0.01$), suggesting it as a useful tool for sperm testing [72].

While existing smartphone tools and applications are promising and may potentially revolutionize the screening of male infertility by offering accessible, user-friendly, and cost-effective solutions, the authors do not recommend this course of examination as a replacement for visiting a specialist since the results are subjective and may not be accurate. Further research and development in this area are crucial to enhance the diagnostic capabilities of this method and its applications and validate the adoption of smartphone-based sperm quality assessment in clinical and home settings.

Molecular Methods in Semen Microbiological Testing, qPCR, and NGS

Real-time polymerase chain reaction (qPCR) has become a prominent technique due to its rapidity and increased accuracy in identifying trace amounts of pathogens [73]. In a retrospective study examining North African men, the investigation of bacterial semen infections highlighted the stable annual variation rate from 2013 to 2022, shedding light on the prevalence of different types of bacteria analyzed [74], which demonstrated the importance of comprehensive testing over an extended period.

Additionally, a study on cryptozoospermia associated with a recessive mutation emphasized the significance of genetic factors in male infertility, indicating the complexity of reproductive issues [75]. Understanding genetic mutations like the TEX15 nonsense mutation can provide valuable insights into the underlying causes of certain conditions.

Furthermore, the detection of specific microRNAs like miRNA-181a and miRNA-429 in non-obstructive azoospermia (NOA) patients suggests the potential of using these miRNAs as non-invasive biomarkers for diagnosing NOA, showcasing the potential for molecular biomarkers in male infertility diagnostics [76]. Moreover, investigations into the impact of bacterial colonization in asymptomatic infertile men elucidated the effects on semen quality, highlighting the importance of considering asymptomatic infections as contributing factors to male infertility [77]. Such studies underscore the need for comprehensive screening methods beyond traditional assessments. Lastly, the use of multiplex PCR assays for detecting genital mycoplasmas and ureaplasmas in infertile males demonstrated the efficiency of this molecular technique in diagnosing these pathogens, reflecting the increasing preference for molecular-based testing for microbial agents in semen samples [78].

In conclusion, integrating qPCR and other molecular techniques in andrology research presents a promising pathway for identifying microorganisms and genetic factors contributing to male infertility, ultimately improving diagnostic precision and potentially guiding personalized treatment strategies.

Sperm Functional Tests

DNA Fragmentation

AI in the Evaluation of Sperm DNA Integrity or Damage

While conventional semen analysis provides valuable information, it often falls short in evaluating specific aspects of sperm function that are crucial for successful fertilization. Recent advancements in male fertility research have led to the development of new tests that go beyond traditional semen analysis, aiming to evaluate sperm function more comprehensively. These novel tests assess various aspects of sperm function, including nuclear DNA fragmentation, mitochondrial function, capacitation, acrosome reaction, oocyte receptor binding and penetration, oxidative stress (OS), sperm oxidation-reduction potential (SORP), and the effects of reductive stress.

Previous studies have emphasized the significance of assessing sperm DNA fragmentation (SDF) as a key indicator of male fertility potential [79]. A variety of laboratory tests such as single-cell gel electrophoresis or Comet assay, terminal deoxynucleotidyl transferase dUTP nick end labeling (TUNEL) assay, sperm chromatin dispersion (SCD) assay, sperm chromatin structure assay (SCSA), and acridine orange (AO) assay are available to measure the DNA integrity of spermatozoa [80].

Recently, SDF has been increasingly recognized as a critical factor in male reproductive capability, and emerging evidence suggests a link between SDF and male infertility [81].

A large-scale study evaluating sperm DNA fragmentation using two frequently used assays, the TUNEL assay and the SCSA, across a wide age range demonstrated that SDF is negatively associated with sperm survival rate, sperm concentration, and percentage of progressively motile sperm, while its significance as a predictor of pregnancy outcomes following assisted reproduction technologies (ART) requires further investigation [82].

Table 2.3 summarizes artificial intelligence (AI) algorithms developed to measure or predict sperm DNA integrity or damage.. AI-assisted CASA was used to evaluate the degree of chromatin dispersion in a large number of sperm samples with less inter-observer variability, also showing a substantially stronger association

Table 2.3 Artificial intelligence (AI) algorithms developed to measure or predict sperm DNA integrity or damage

Algorithm or model	Dataset/ sample	Performance or outcomes	Refs.
CNN	Semen	AI algorithm vs. manual scoring ($r = 0.97$, $p < 0.001$)	[83]
MobileNet CNN	Semen	Prediction accuracy = 90%, sensitivity = 0.93, specificity = 0.9	[85]
Deep CNN	Semen	Sperm cell image vs. DNA quality (bivariate correlation ~0.43)	[84]
Logistic regression	Semen	Test accuracy = 82.7%	[89]

Adapted from Panner Selbam et al. [20]. (Under a Creative Commons Attribution 4.0 International License).
CNN Convolutional Neural Network

between the manual and AI-assisted results of DNA fragmentation index (DFI) ($r = 0.97$, $p < 0.001$) [83].

Despite the good diagnostic value, the spermatozoa analyzed using these advanced techniques cannot be selected or used in ART procedures, mainly because of the fixation and staining processes that limit cell viability or the complete lysation of the cells [84]. Hence, it is important to construct novel AI-based algorithms to measure or predict DNA fragmentation levels in live spermatozoa without compromising their biological activity in order to increase the success rate of IVF and ICSI procedures [85].

Despite the available guidelines for SDF testing [86, 87], these tests are still not included in the routine clinical diagnostic work-up mainly due to the methodological variations that require further optimization and standardization but are proposed for certain infertility cases [1, 88]. Once this standardization has been achieved, machine learning (ML) algorithms integrating morphological, motility, and DNA fragmentation data with fertilization, miscarriage, and live birth rates could significantly improve single sperm assessment and selection. These ML algorithms could streamline and improve the ART process by reducing subjective and inter-variable outcomes between embryologists.

While AI models trained on sperm images have shown promise in predicting DNA integrity [84], technical restrictions, in particular the use of various staining techniques, microscopes, and DNA fragmentation assays, can make it difficult to train an accurate AI model for SDF assessment; therefore, further validation is needed [84].

Development of Sperm Function Tests Beyond Traditional Semen Analysis

Another crucial aspect that has gained attention in recent research is the role of oxidative stress (OS) in sperm function. OS has been identified as a significant contributor to male factor infertility [90], and various studies have studied the impact of

OS on sperm function, exploring the effects of in vitro manipulation on sperm functional ability and embryo development [91, 92], as well as the detrimental effects of oxidative stress Variably-induced, or through extrinsic or environmental/lifestyle factors and mitochondrial dysfunction on sperm quality [93]. Moreover, the field has expanded to investigate the mechanisms underlying the inflammatory-associated impairment of sperm function, spermatogenesis, and steroidogenesis [94]. Understanding these intricate pathways is essential for developing targeted interventions to address male infertility issues associated with inflammation. In parallel, advancements have been made in assessing key mitochondrial parameters to reflect sperm quality and exploring therapeutic strategies, such as mitochondrial-targeted antioxidants, to enhance sperm function in various scenarios, including after sperm cryopreservation [95]. Mitochondrial function in sperm is crucial for oxidative homeostasis and overall functionality, underscoring the importance of evaluating this aspect in male fertility assessments [96]. Furthermore, studies focusing on specific sperm functions like capacitation and acrosome reaction have proposed innovative approaches for evaluation, such as utilizing combined Raman and polarization-sensitive holographic imaging for a multimodal, label-free assessment of human sperm function [97]. Additionally, dynamic elementomics of single-cell signals has shown promise in revealing ionic dysregulation in sperm and can be instrumental in the functional analysis of viable sperm during capacitation [98].

In conclusion, the contemporary landscape of sperm function evaluation encompasses many parameters beyond conventional semen analysis, emphasizing the diagnostic value and impact of OS, mitochondrial function, inflammation, and specific functional processes like capacitation and acrosome reaction. Integrating these advancements into clinical practice can offer more precise diagnostics and targeted interventions to address male factor infertility effectively.

Flow Cytometry Assessment for Sperm Function and DNA Integrity Assessment

Flow cytometry methods, such as the SCSA, have been utilized to assess sperm DNA fragmentation in large cohorts, demonstrating its effectiveness in evaluating age-related changes in sperm quality [82]. While flow cytometry offers many advantages in sperm analysis, it is essential to note that certain factors can impact its accuracy. For instance, the presence of apoptotic M540 bodies in human semen samples has been shown to interfere with flow cytometry-based assessments of sperm DNA fragmentation and oxidation [99]. On the other hand, a novel method utilizing quantitative image-based analysis to measure apoptosis has been proposed as a reliable alternative to traditional photometric methods, showcasing the potential of flow cytometry in assessing sperm apoptosis [99]. In conclusion, while flow cytometry-based assessments can be used for evaluating sperm function and DNA integrity, it is essential to consider the potential limitations and factors that may affect the accuracy of such tests.

Applications of NGS in Male Infertility

The current state of the art in genomic and epigenomic analysis in male infertility has shown promising findings and has the potential to revolutionize our understanding of the underlying causes of infertility in men. Several studies have utilized next-generation sequencing (NGS) technologies to identify genetic variants associated with male infertility. For example, a study by Patel et al. [100] used comprehensive genetic testing with NGS to identify novel genetic variants in both male and female infertility, revealing that NGS can provide valuable insights into the genetic causes of infertility and help guide personalized treatment options [100]. In addition to NGS, other genomic approaches have been employed to study male infertility. Copy number variants (CNVs) have been identified in patients with severe oligozoospermia and Sertoli-cell-only (SCO) syndrome [101]. These CNVs may play a role in spermatogenic failure and provide important diagnostic information for male infertility.

Furthermore, epigenomic analysis has also been explored in the context of male infertility. DNA fragmentation analysis, such as DNA breakage detection fluorescence in situ hybridization (DBD-FISH) and in situ nick translation (ISNT), has been used to assess sperm DNA integrity and predict male infertility diagnosis [102]. These techniques can provide valuable information about the quality of sperm DNA and its impact on fertility.

Large-scale sequencing approaches, such as NGS, have allowed for identifying monogenic forms of male infertility [103]. The Genetics of Male Infertility Initiative (GEMINI) and the International Male Infertility Genomics Consortium (IMIGC) have made significant progress in identifying genetic variants associated with male infertility [104]. Despite these advancements, there are still many cases of male infertility that lack a specific causal diagnosis. This highlights the need for further research and the exploration of additional genomic and epigenomic approaches. For example, whole-exome sequencing has been used to identify potential monogenic or oligogenic mutations in patients with non-obstructive azoospermia [105]. This approach has the potential to uncover novel genetic causes of male infertility.

In summary, genomic and epigenomic analysis has provided valuable insights into the genetic causes of male infertility. NGS technologies, CNV analysis, and DNA fragmentation analysis contributed to our understanding of male infertility. However, further research is needed to fully uncover the genetic and epigenetic factors contributing to male infertility and to develop personalized treatment options.

Microbiome Analysis

The Role of the Microbiome in Male Reproductive Health

Advancements in NGS have opened up exciting possibilities for exploring the sperm microbiome in various applications, such as microbiome studies and microbiological tests. NGS technology has enabled researchers to focus on the intricate microbial communities in sperm samples, providing valuable insights into male reproductive health and fertility potential. Corral-Vazquez et al. conducted a pioneering study [106] on the human sperm microbiome using transcriptomic analysis through NGS. The research identified distinct viruses and bacteria present in the sperm microbiome, shedding light on the diversity and commonalities among individuals. Similarly, Davies et al. [107] explored the semen microbiome in male reproductive disorders utilizing NGS, emphasizing the need for larger studies to inform clinical practices. Furthermore, Farahani et al. [108] investigated the seminal microbiome in male partners of women with recurrent pregnancy loss, elucidating the impact of microbiota on sperm DNA damage and fertility outcomes. In a study by Vajpeyee et al. [109], the characterization of the seminal microbiota in patients with different sperm conditions demonstrated the potential of NGS to enhance assisted reproductive technologies. Additionally, Yatsentyuk [110] delved into the sperm microbiome of bulls using metagenomic analysis, highlighting the associations between specific bacterial taxa and sperm quality indicators. Overall, these studies underscore the significant role of NGS in unraveling the complexities of the sperm microbiome and its implications for male reproductive health. By harnessing the power of NGS technology, researchers are poised to unlock new frontiers in understanding the impact of microbial communities on sperm quality and fertility outcomes.

Recent studies have shed light on the crucial role of the microbiome in male reproductive health, particularly in cases of infertility [111]. The interplay between microbial dysbiosis and male infertility has been explored, emphasizing the potential of precision medicine and personalized treatment strategies in addressing infertility linked to microbial factors [112]. Furthermore, investigations into the semen microbiome have revealed common bacterial clusters, indicating the need for larger studies to inform clinical practice [107]. Probiotics have emerged as a promising approach to potentially improve male infertility by enhancing sperm quality and addressing microbial factors [113]. The potential benefits of probiotics for male infertility have been highlighted, emphasizing the need for more extensive research in this area [114]. These studies emphasize the intricate relationship between the microbiome and male reproductive health, offering valuable insights for future research directions.

Genomic and Epigenomic Analysis

Recent research has emphasized the significance of genomic and epigenomic analyses in developing diagnostic tests for male infertility [115]. A comprehensive review by Wagner et al. [115] highlighted the importance of integrating multiple omics levels, including genomics and epigenomics, in understanding the factors associated with male infertility [115]. Furthermore, the study by Govindkumar et al. [116] focused on exploring the molecular basis of human spermatogenesis and non-obstructive azoospermia (NOA) through transcriptomics using next-generation sequencing methods [116]. This research identified a strong association of genes with human spermatogenesis and NOA, providing insights into potential diagnostic markers for male infertility [116]. In addition, Rajiwate [117] investigated the determination of diagnostic molecular markers in NOA through next-generation sequencing methods, emphasizing the differences in gene expression profiles between NOA patients and those with normal spermatogenesis [117]. This approach contributes to developing more targeted and effective diagnostic tests for male infertility. Overall, these studies underscore the importance of genomic and epigenomic analyses in unraveling the complexities of male infertility and paving the way for advancing diagnostic tools in this field. By integrating multi-omics approaches and exploring candidate diagnostic markers, researchers are moving closer to improving the understanding and diagnosis of male infertility.

The exploration of genetic mutations, chromosomal abnormalities, and epigenetic modifications in male infertility has also opened up new avenues for personalized treatment strategies. Rotondo et al. [118] reported that epigenetic modifications associated with male infertility, particularly DNA methylation, can be influenced by microbial dysbiosis, and sperm DNA epigenetic biomarkers can be measured to evaluate changes associated with dysbiosis [118]. This underlines the importance of tailored approaches for treatment based on individual characteristics and etiology. Epigenetic alterations have been identified as crucial factors in male infertility etiology, especially in couples requiring ART [119]. Marzouni et al. [119] noted the need for further research to understand abnormal epigenetic patterns and their transmission risks [119]. This sheds light on the necessity of personalized treatment strategies that consider the epigenetic profiles of infertile couples undergoing ART procedures.

Furthermore, genetic causes of male infertility, particularly in the Middle East and North Africa regions, have been extensively studied [120]. Duvuru et al. [120] identified common genetic aberrations leading to male infertility in these populations, emphasizing the importance of genetic testing in evaluating male infertility [120]. This emphasizes the relevance of genomic profiling in identifying genetic mutations associated with male infertility, paving the way for personalized treatment approaches.

A recent field of interest in male infertility research is single-cell analysis. This approach has provided crucial insights into factors affecting male fertility and opened up new insights for the development of future diagnostic tools and tests for male infertility. In particular, a study by Luo et al. [121] focused on the essential roles of CATSPER in mediating progesterone response and its association with idiopathic male infertility [121], highlighting the importance of understanding the genetic variations contributing to male infertility, with particular emphasis on the significance of single-cell sequencing techniques in uncovering subtle issues that traditional methods may overlook [121]. Combining genetic insights from studies like those by Luo et al. [121] with established genetic testing methods advocated by Hotaling and Carrell [122], researchers can pave the way for more precise diagnostic tools tailored to individual variability in male infertility [121, 122].

In conclusion, utilizing genomic and epigenomic profiling is instrumental in identifying underlying factors contributing to male infertility. By understanding genetic mutations, chromosomal abnormalities, and epigenetic modifications, personalized treatment strategies can be tailored to address the specific needs of individuals struggling with infertility. This holistic approach, considering both genetic and epigenetic factors, opens up possibilities for more effective interventions and improved outcomes for male infertility.

Non-invasive Biomarker Testing

Another promising intervention for diagnostic testing in male infertility is the identification of non-invasive biomarkers that can assess male reproductive health and predict fertility potential. Recent studies have explored different biomarkers and techniques to understand male infertility better. Gvozdjáková et al. [123] investigated the potential of Coenzyme Q10, α-Tocopherol, and oxidative stress as metabolic biomarkers for male infertility [123]. Chen et al. [124] delved into using human sperm tsRNA as a potential clinical target for male infertility, highlighting the importance of molecular markers [124].

Furthermore, Pandruvada et al. [125] emphasized the need for reliable diagnostic tools for male infertility, addressing the lack of standardized testing beyond conventional semen analysis [125]. Additionally, ongoing research focuses on seminal plasma metabolomic analysis to unearth emerging markers associated with male reproductive disorders [126]. Vashisht and Gahlay [127] provided a comprehensive overview of seminal plasma's diagnostic potential and highlighted the role of DNA Methylation of some imprinted non-imprinted genes in male infertility diagnosis [127]. Hao et al. [128] conducted a systematic review of microRNAs' roles in different types of male infertility, suggesting their potential as new biomarkers for enhanced diagnostic accuracy [128]. By exploring these biomarkers and methodologies across different bodily fluids and tissues, researchers are paving the way for future diagnostic tools that can revolutionize the field of male infertility assessment.

Multi-omics Approaches

The investigation of male infertility has seen significant progress through multi-omics approaches, encompassing genomics, proteomics, metabolomics, and epigenomics data. These integrated omics analyses provide a comprehensive understanding of the underlying factors contributing to male infertility [126], with some moving toward personalized treatment strategies [52]. By incorporating transcriptomic data, it becomes feasible to pinpoint biomarkers crucial for diagnosing male infertility and potentially shedding light on previously unexplained cases [52]. Furthermore, the role of artificial intelligence (AI) algorithms in processing vast amounts of data from diagnostic tests such as semen analysis, genetic data, hormonal profiles, and multi-omics approaches is crucial for detecting patterns and correlations that aid in diagnosing male infertility, as well as predicting treatment outcomes [20]. In line with these advancements, a study emphasizes the importance of the clinician's role in the multi-omics era, acting as a vital link between physicians, laboratory experts, and researchers to validate omics discoveries and improve clinical outcomes [20]. Moreover, exploring patient-specific multi-omics models and their application in personalized therapy highlights the potential of integrating different omics platforms and data integration techniques for tailored treatment regimens [129]. The continuous advancements in the field of male infertility research underscore the significance of embracing a multi-omics approach to unravel the complexity of the condition and improve patient outcomes. By merging various omics levels and harnessing the power of AI algorithms, researchers and clinicians are moving closer to personalized and more effective strategies in addressing male infertility.

Imaging

Non-invasive imaging techniques, such as multiphoton microscopy and magnetic resonance imaging (MRI) enable a detailed assessment of testicular function and structure and the identification of structural abnormalities or blockages within the male reproductive tract [130]. One study by Zupin et al. in 2020 [131] utilized synchrotron radiation soft X-ray microscopy and low-energy X-ray fluorescence to investigate elemental changes in spermatozoa following photobiomodulation therapy. This research sheds light on the potential of advanced imaging modalities to assess and track alterations in sperm characteristics, which could be invaluable for diagnosing male infertility. In a similar attempt, Gordon et al. [132] demonstrated the application of four-dimensional flow magnetic resonance imaging for quantifying blood flow in the thoracic aorta, showcasing the capability of MRI in assessing vascular health. This study highlights the utility of MRI beyond traditional structural imaging, opening new avenues for evaluating reproductive system functionality in male infertility.

Furthermore, the work by Pownder et al. in 2020 [133] presented the use of magnetic resonance imaging to monitor the healing process of canine patellar tendons, indicating the potential of MRI in tracking tissue recovery and health. This approach could be adapted for studying the structural integrity of male reproductive organs and their role in infertility. In conclusion, integrating cutting-edge imaging technologies such as multiphoton microscopy and MRI into the field of male infertility diagnostics holds great promise for enhancing our understanding of the condition and improving clinical outcomes. By harnessing the power of advanced imaging modalities, researchers are paving the way for more effective and tailored diagnostic approaches in addressing male infertility concerns.

Sperm Sorting Techniques

An area of significant advancement is sperm sorting techniques, where innovative methods such as microfluidics and magnetic-activated cell sorting (MACS) are promising. Mantravadi et al. [134] conducted a randomized control trial that demonstrated that microfluidics significantly reduced the DNA fragmentation index (DFI) and led to improved reproductive outcomes [134]. Similarly, novel sperm sorting techniques such as MACS have shown promise in improving sperm retrieval rates after microdissection TESE [135]. MACS has effectively reduced DNA fragmentation in infertile varicocele patients, making it a valuable method prior to ART procedures [135]. In the realm of ART, microfluidics has opened up new possibilities. Kashaninejad et al. [136] categorized various ART methods based on microfluidic technologies and highlighted their potential in infertility diagnosis, sperm selection, oocyte selection, and embryo culture, among other applications [137].

Similarly, Faraghat et al. [138] introduced a high-throughput cell separation method based on electrophysiology that significantly improved the efficiency and cost-effectiveness of cell separation [138]. Furthermore, a study by Berteli et al. [139] explored the combined use of MACS and density gradient centrifugation (DGC) to enhance the recovery of high-quality spermatozoa, indicating the clinical value of such combined protocols in ART settings [139]. Additionally, Ahmadi et al. [140] conducted a comparison between MACS and physiological intracytoplasmic sperm injection (PICSI) for sperm selection in cases of unexplained infertility, highlighting the efficiency of MACS in reducing sperm DNA fragmentation rates [140]. Overall, integrating advanced sperm sorting techniques such as microfluidics and MACS holds great promise for improving ART outcomes. These techniques offer more precise and effective methods for sperm selection, ultimately contributing to enhanced reproductive success in ART procedures.

Personalized Medicine

Personalized medicine in male infertility involves the integration of genetic and biomarker data, coupled with AI-driven analysis, to pave the way for tailored treatment plans addressing the specific underlying causes in each case. Kaltsas et al. [112] focused on microbial dysbiosis and male infertility, advocating for personalized treatment strategies rooted in precision medicine principles to address infertility related to microbial factors [112]. Omolaoye et al. [52] shed light on the application of omics in male fertility, suggesting that available data in this domain can aid in identifying biomarkers for diagnosing male infertility and potentially unraveling idiopathic cases [52]. Additionally, Xi et al. [141] provided evidence of a causal relationship between gut microbiota and male infertility, advocating[141] for preventive and personalized strategies based on microbiota abundance in feces to benefit infertility patients . Furthermore, the study by Bruno et al. [142] underscores the importance of inflammation and oxidative stress biomarkers in seminal plasma as potential clinical markers for male infertility, emphasizing their application in personalized medicine [142]. Santacroce et al. [143] discuss testicular immunity and its connection with the microbiota, highlighting the physiological and clinical implications for male infertility within personalized medicine [143]. In the context of genetic factors, Zamani-Badi et al. [144] suggest that the C3953T polymorphism in the interleukin 1β gene could serve as a potential biomarker for a genetic diagnosis of male infertility [144]. Aras-Tosun [145] also explored genetic alterations in azoospermia patients to unveil potential biomarkers for male infertility, pointing out the need to further validate the data presented [145]. Overall, personalized medicine in male infertility is a burgeoning field that holds promise for tailoring treatment approaches to the specific genetic and biomarker profiles of individuals, thereby revolutionizing the management of male infertility.

SWOT Analysis

Figure 2.1 illustrates the strengths, weaknesses, opportunities, and threats (SWOT) analysis for the use of AI and ML in andrology [20].

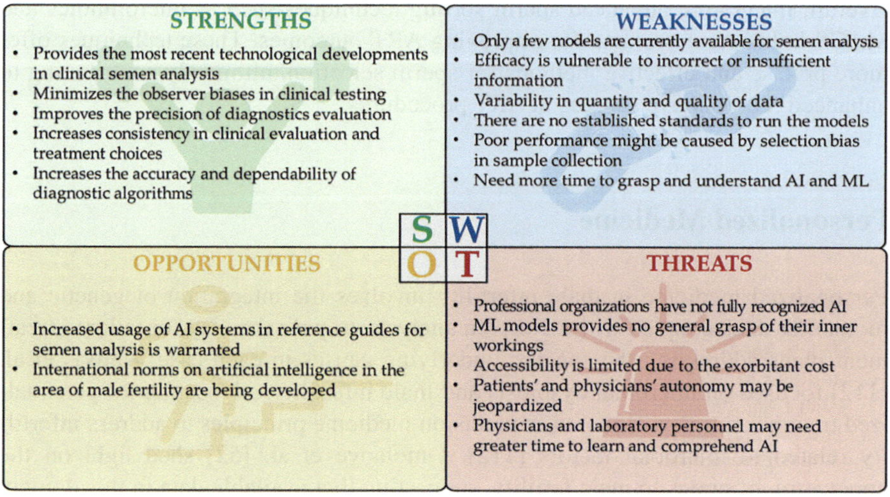

Fig. 2.1 Strengths, weaknesses, opportunities, and threats (SWOT) analysis of artificial intelligence (AI) and machine learning (ML) in andrology. (Figure reproduced from Panner Selbam et al. [20]. CC BY 4.0 DEED)

References

1. World Health Organization. WHO laboratory manual for the examination and processing of human semen. World Health Organization; 2021.
2. Björndahl L. A paradigmatic shift in the care of male factor infertility: how can the recommendations for basic semen examination in the sixth edition of the WHO manual and the ISO 23162: 2021 standard help? Reprod Biomed Online. 2022;45:731–6.
3. Diaz P, Dullea A, Chu KY, Zizzo J, Loloi J, Reddy R, et al. Future of male infertility evaluation and treatment: brief review of emerging technology. Urology. 2022;169:9–16.
4. Tomlinson MJ. Uncertainty of measurement and clinical value of semen analysis: has standardisation through professional guidelines helped or hindered progress? Andrology. 2016;4:763–70.
5. Schubert B, Badiou M, Force A. Computer-aided sperm analysis, the new key player in routine sperm assessment. Andrologia. 2019;51:e13417.
6. Pakpahan C. Computer assisted sperm analysis: a review. Indonesian Androl Biomed J. 2020;1:60–6.
7. Choi J, Alkhoury L, Urbano LF, Masson P, VerMilyea M, Kam M. An assessment tool for computer-assisted semen analysis (CASA) algorithms. Sci Rep. 2022;12:16830.
8. Agarwal A, Henkel R, Majzoub A. Standard semen analysis: computer-assisted semen analysis. Arch Androl. 2021;30:11–22.
9. Finelli R, Leisegang K, Tumallapalli S, Henkel R, Agarwal A. The validity and reliability of computer-aided semen analyzers in performing semen analysis: a systematic review. Transl Androl Urol. 2021;10:3069.
10. Agarwal A, Selvam MKP, Ambar RF. Validation of LensHooke® X1 PRO and computer-assisted semen analyzer compared with laboratory-based manual semen analysis. World J Mens Health. 2021;39:496.
11. Dearing C, Jayasena C, Lindsay K. Can the sperm class analyser (SCA) CASA-mot system for human sperm motility analysis reduce imprecision and operator subjectivity and improve semen analysis? Hum Fertil (Camb). 2019;24(3):208–18.
12. Larsen L, Scheike T, Jensen TK, Bonde JP, Ernst E, Hjollund NH, et al. Computer-assisted semen analysis parameters as predictors for fertility of men from the general population. Hum Reprod. 2000;15:1562–7.
13. Garrett C, Liu DY, Clarke GN, Rushford DD, Baker H. Automated semen analysis:'zona pellucida preferred'sperm morphometry and straight-line velocity are related to pregnancy rate in subfertile couples. Hum Reprod. 2003;18:1643–9.
14. Shibahara H, Obara H, Ayustawati, Hirano Y, Suzuki T, Ohno A, et al. Prediction of pregnancy by intrauterine insemination using CASA estimates and strict criteria in patients with male factor infertility. Int J Androl. 2004;27:63–8.
15. Hanassab S, Abbara A, Yeung AC, Voliotis M, Tsaneva-Atanasova K, Kelsey TW, et al. The prospect of artificial intelligence to personalize assisted reproductive technology. NPJ Digit Med. 2024;7:55.
16. Mortimer ST, Van der Horst G, Mortimer D. The future of computer-aided sperm analysis. Asian J Androl. 2015;17:545–53.
17. Dardmeh F, Heidari M, Alipour H. Comparison of commercially available chamber slides for computer-aided analysis of human sperm. Syst Biol Reprod Med. 2021;67:168–75.
18. Agarwal A, Sharma R, Gupta S, Finelli R, Parekh N, Selvam MKP, et al. Standardized laboratory procedures, quality control and quality assurance are key requirements for accurate semen analysis in the evaluation of infertile male. World J Mens Health. 2022;40:52.
19. Girela JL, Gil D, Johnsson M, Gomez-Torres MJ, De Juan J. Semen parameters can be predicted from environmental factors and lifestyle using artificial intelligence methods. Biol Reprod. 2013;88(99):1–8.
20. Selvam MKP, Moharana AK, Baskaran S, Finelli R, Hudnall MC, Sikka SC. Current updates on involvement of artificial intelligence and machine learning in semen analysis. Medicina. 2024;60:279.

21. Lesani A, Kazemnejad S, Zand MM, Azadi M, Jafari H, Mofrad MR, et al. Quantification of human sperm concentration using machine learning-based spectrophotometry. Comput Biol Med. 2020;127:104061.
22. Ory J, Tradewell MB, Blankstein U, Lima TF, Nackeeran S, Gonzalez DC, et al. Artificial intelligence based machine learning models predict sperm parameter upgrading after varicocele repair: a multi-institutional analysis. World J Mens Health. 2022;40:618.
23. Tsai VF, Zhuang B, Pong Y, Hsieh J, Chang H. Web-and artificial intelligence–based image recognition for sperm motility analysis: verification study. JMIR Med Inform. 2020;8:e20031.
24. Ottl S, Amiriparian S, Gerczuk M, Schuller BW. motilitAI: a machine learning framework for automatic prediction of human sperm motility. iScience. 2022;25:104644.
25. Somasundaram D, Nirmala M. Faster region convolutional neural network and semen tracking algorithm for sperm analysis. Comput Methods Prog Biomed. 2021;200:105918.
26. Valiuškaitė V, Raudonis V, Maskeliūnas R, Damaševičius R, Krilavičius T. Deep learning based evaluation of spermatozoid motility for artificial insemination. Sensors (Basel). 2020;21:72.
27. Goodson SG, White S, Stevans AM, Bhat S, Kao C, Jaworski S, et al. CASAnova: a multiclass support vector machine model for the classification of human sperm motility patterns. Biol Reprod. 2017;97:698–708.
28. Sato T, Kishi H, Murakata S, Hayashi Y, Hattori T, Nakazawa S, et al. A new deep-learning model using YOLOv3 to support sperm selection during intracytoplasmic sperm injection procedure. Reprod Med Biol. 2022;21:e12454.
29. Abbasi A, Miahi E, Mirroshandel SA. Effect of deep transfer and multi-task learning on sperm abnormality detection. Comput Biol Med. 2021;128:104121.
30. Marín R, Chang V. Impact of transfer learning for human sperm segmentation using deep learning. Comput Biol Med. 2021;136:104687.
31. Nygate YN, Levi M, Mirsky SK, Turko NA, Rubin M, Barnea I, et al. Holographic virtual staining of individual biological cells. Proc Natl Acad Sci USA. 2020;117:9223–31.
32. Dubey V, Popova D, Ahmad A, Acharya G, Basnet P, Mehta DS, et al. Partially spatially coherent digital holographic microscopy and machine learning for quantitative analysis of human spermatozoa under oxidative stress condition. Sci Rep. 2019;9:3564.
33. Javadi S, Mirroshandel SA. A novel deep learning method for automatic assessment of human sperm images. Comput Biol Med. 2019;109:182–94.
34. Movahed RA, Mohammadi E, Orooji M. Automatic segmentation of Sperm's parts in microscopic images of human semen smears using concatenated learning approaches. Comput Biol Med. 2019;109:242–53.
35. Riordon J, McCallum C, Sinton D. Deep learning for the classification of human sperm. Comput Biol Med. 2019;111:103342.
36. Mirsky SK, Barnea I, Levi M, Greenspan H, Shaked NT. Automated analysis of individual sperm cells using stain-free interferometric phase microscopy and machine learning. Cytometry A. 2017;91:893–900.
37. Shaker F, Monadjemi SA, Alirezaie J, Naghsh-Nilchi AR. A dictionary learning approach for human sperm heads classification. Comput Biol Med. 2017;91:181–90.
38. Shaker F, Monadjemi SA, Naghsh-Nilchi AR. Automatic detection and segmentation of sperm head, acrosome and nucleus in microscopic images of human semen smears. Comput Methods Prog Biomed. 2016;132:11–20.
39. Hicks SA, Andersen JM, Witczak O, Thambawita V, Halvorsen P, Hammer HL, et al. Machine learning-based analysis of sperm videos and participant data for male fertility prediction. Sci Rep. 2019;9:16770.
40. Farías AFS, Sakkas D, Chavez-Badiola A, Ocali O, Mendizabal G, Valencia R, et al. Single-sperm motility analysis during ICSI using an artificial intelligence sperm identification software (SID) and correlation with morphology. Fertil Steril. 2022;118:e56–7.
41. Shahzad S, Ilyas M, Lali MIU, Rauf HT, Kadry S, Nasr EA. sperm abnormality detection using sequential deep neural. Network. 2023;11:515.

42. You JB, McCallum C, Wang Y, Riordon J, Nosrati R, Sinton D. Machine learning for sperm selection. Nat Rev Urol. 2021;18:387–403.
43. Riegler MA, Stensen MH, Witczak O, Andersen JM, Hicks SA, Hammer HL, et al. Artificial intelligence in the fertility clinic: status, pitfalls and possibilities. Hum Reprod. 2021;36:2429–42.
44. Jiang A, Jiaqi W, Zhao H, Zhang Z, Sun Y. Identifying viability of immotile sperm at one glance: Sperm viability classifier powered by deep learning. Fertil Steril. 2022;118:e297–8.
45. Abou Ghayda R, Cannarella R, Calogero AE, Shah R, Rambhatla A, Zohdy W, et al. Artificial intelligence in andrology: from semen analysis to image diagnostics. World J Mens Health. 2024;42:39.
46. Mendizabal-Ruiz G, Chavez-Badiola A, Figueroa IA, Nuño VM, Farias AF, Valencia-Murilloa R, et al. Computer software (SiD) assisted real-time single sperm selection associated with fertilization and blastocyst formation. Reprod Biomed Online. 2022;45:703–11.
47. Thambawita V, Halvorsen P, Hammer H, Riegler M, Haugen TB. Extracting temporal features into a spatial domain using autoencoders for sperm video analysis. Comput Vis Patt Recog. 2019;19:27–9.
48. Goyal A, Kuchana M, Ayyagari KPR. Machine learning predicts live-birth occurrence before in-vitro fertilization treatment. Sci Rep. 2020;10:20925.
49. GhoshRoy D, Alvi PA, Santosh KC. Explainable AI to predict male fertility using extreme gradient boosting algorithm with SMOTE. Electronics. 2022;12:15.
50. Yuan Y, Tan Y, Qiu X, Luo H, Li Y, Li R, et al. Sperm telomere length as a novel biomarker of male infertility and embryonic development: a systematic review and meta-analysis. Front Endocrinol (Lausanne). 2023;13:1079966.
51. Lyu Z, Feng X, Li N, Zhao W, Wei L, Chen Y, et al. Human papillomavirus in semen and the risk for male infertility: a systematic review and meta-analysis. BMC Infect Dis. 2017;17:1–9.
52. Omolaoye TS, Omolaoye VA, Kandasamy RK, Hachim MY, Du Plessis SS. Omics and male infertility: highlighting the application of transcriptomic data. Life (Basel). 2022;12:280.
53. Woldemariam S, Xie F, Roldan A, Roger J, Tang A, Oskotsky T, et al. Leveraging electronic medical records reveals comorbidities significantly associated with male infertility. Fertil Steril. 2023;120:e53–4.
54. Levine BA, Feinstein J, Neri QV, Goldschlag D, Rosenwaks Z, Belongie S, et al. Three-dimensional sperm surface reconstruction: a novel approach to assessing sperm morphology. Fertil Steril. 2015;104:e14–5.
55. De Angelis A, Managò S, Ferrara MA, Napolitano M, Coppola G, De Luca AC. Combined Raman spectroscopy and digital holographic microscopy for sperm cell quality analysis. J Spectroscopy. 2017;2017:1–14.
56. Kamieniczna M, Stachowska E, Augustynowicz A, Woźniak T, Kurpisz MK. Human live spermatozoa morphology assessment using digital holographic microscopy. Sci Rep. 2022;12:4846.
57. Muschol M, Wenders C, Wennemuth G. Four-dimensional analysis by high-speed holographic imaging reveals a chiral memory of sperm flagella. PLoS One. 2018;13:e0199678.
58. Powar S, Parast FY, Nandagiri A, Gaikwad AS, Potter DL, O'Bryan MK, et al. Unraveling the kinematics of sperm motion by reconstructing the flagellar wave motion in 3d. Small Meth. 2022;6:2101089.
59. Hernández HO, Hernández-Herrera P, Montoya F, Olveres J, Bloomfield-Gadêlha H, Darszon A, et al. 3D t feature-based descriptor for unsupervised flagellar human sperm beat classification. In: Annu Int Conf IEEE Eng Med Biol Soc; 2022. p. 488–92.
60. Soler C, Picazo-Bueno JÁ, Micó V, Valverde A, Bompart D, Blasco FJ, et al. Effect of counting chamber depth on the accuracy of lensless microscopy for the assessment of boar sperm motility. Reprod Fertil Dev. 2018;30:924–34.
61. Hernandez-Herrera P, Montoya F, Rendón JM, Darszon A, Corkidi G. Sperm flagellum center-line tracing in fluorescence 3D t low SNR stacks using an iterative minimal path method. Image Anal Recog. 2017;2017:437–45.

62. Gonzalez D, Narasimman M, Best JC, Ory J, Ramasamy R. Clinical update on home testing for male fertility. World J Mens Health. 2021;39:615.
63. Sommer GJ, Wang TR, Epperson JG, Hatch EE, Wesselink AK, Rothman KJ, et al. At-home sperm testing for epidemiologic studies: Evaluation of the Trak male fertility testing system in an internet-based preconception cohort. Paediatr Perinat Epidemiol. 2020;34:504–12.
64. Aznavour Y, Navarrete F, Badreddine J, Simon PH, Gowda V, Rhodes S, et al. Semen parameter variability among users of at-home sperm testing kits. BMC Urol. 2022;22:184.
65. Scaruffi P, Bovis F, Massarotti C, Maccarini E, Stigliani S, DE Leo C, Gazzo I, Sozzi F, Anserini P. Collecting semen samples at home for fertility assessment: time for a new standard? Minerva Obstet Gynecol. 2023 Dec;75(6):535-543. doi: 10.23736/S2724-606X.23.05165-5. Epub 2023 May 4. PMID: 37140587.
66. Kobori Y. Home testing for male factor infertility: a review of current options. Fertil Steril. 2019;111:864–70.
67. Van Den Heuvel JF, Groenhof TK, Veerbeek JH, Van Solinge WW, Lely AT, Franx A, et al. eHealth as the next-generation perinatal care: an overview of the literature. J Med Internet Res. 2018;20:e202.
68. Kobori Y, Pfanner P, Prins GS, Niederberger C. Novel device for male infertility screening with single-ball lens microscope and smartphone. Fertil Steril. 2016;106:574–8.
69. Cheon WH, Park HJ, Park MJ, Lim MY, Park JH, Kang BJ, et al. Validation of a smartphone-based, computer-assisted sperm analysis system compared with laboratory-based manual microscopic semen analysis and computer-assisted semen analysis. Investig Clin Urol. 2019;60:380.
70. Errázuriz, J., Castillo, C., Sepúlveda-Martínez, A., Filselcker, I., & Alwane, E. (2023). Validation of the origami "foldscope" microscope as a preliminary screening tool for male infertility. Journal of Reproductive Medicine, Gynecology & Obstetrics, 8(3), Article 144. doi.org
71. Vij SC, Kumar PSM, Agarwal A. Smartphone-based home screening tests for male infertility. Panminerva Med. 2019;61:104–7.
72. Kim KS, Kim JH, Roh JH, Kim D, Kim HM, Jo JK. Ability and accuracy of the smartphone-based OVIEW-M® sperm test: Useful tool in the era of Covid-19. PLoS One. 2022;17:e0269894.
73. Pochernikov DG, Postovoytenko NT, Strelnikov AI. Comparative analysis of cell culture and molecular genetic testing of semen microbiota in male infertility. Int J Mol Sci. 2019;20:40–7.
74. Benkhalifa M, Zidi W, Fourati K, Bahri H. P-453 Bacterial semen infections of North-African men: a 10-year retrospective study of 10.386 semen samples between January, 2013 and December, 2022. Hum Reprod. 2023;38:dead093. 801.
75. Wang X, Jin H, Cui Y, Chen J, Sha Y, Gao Z. Case study of a patient with cryptozoospermia associated with a recessive TEX15 nonsense mutation. Asian J Androl. 2018;20:101–2.
76. Mostafa RM, Abdallah HY, Eissa HM, Ibrahim DR, Ibrahim SM. Assessment of expression profiles of three microRNAs and their clinical, laboratory, and histopathological correlations in non-obstructive azoospermia: a controlled study. Fam J. 2022;12:1–8.
77. Veiga E, Treviño M, Romay AB, Navarro D, Trastoy R, Macía M. Colonisation of the male reproductive tract in asymptomatic infertile men: Effects on semen quality. Andrologia. 2020;52:e13637.
78. Al-Musawi HS, Al-Talqani IA. Using multiplex PCR assay for detection of genital mycoplasmasand ureaplasmaspp in an infertility males. J Clin Microbiol. 2015;5:1528–33.
79. Majzoub A, Esteves SC, Gosálvez J, Agarwal A. Specialized sperm function tests in varicocele and the future of andrology laboratory. Asian J Androl. 2016;18:205–12.
80. Evenson DP. The sperm chromatin structure assay (SCSA®) and other sperm DNA fragmentation tests for evaluation of sperm nuclear DNA integrity as related to fertility. Anim Reprod Sci. 2016;169:56–75.
81. Peng T, Liao C, Ye X, Chen Z, Li X, Lan Y, et al. Machine learning-based clustering to identify the combined effect of the DNA fragmentation index and conventional semen parameters on in vitro fertilization outcomes. Reprod Biol Endocrinol. 2023;21:26.

82. Behdarvandian P, Nasr-Esfahani A, Tavalaee M, Pashaei K, Naderi N, Darmishonnejad Z, et al. Sperm chromatin structure assay (SCSA®) and flow cytometry-assisted TUNEL assay provide a concordant assessment of sperm DNA fragmentation as a function of age in a large cohort of approximately 10,000 patients. Basic Clin Androl. 2023;33:33.
83. Kuroda S, Karna KK, Kaiyal RS, Cannarella R, Lundy SD, Vij SC, et al. Novel sperm chromatin dispersion test with artificial intelligence-aided halo evaluation: a comparison study with existing modalities. Andrology. 2023;11:1581–92.
84. McCallum C, Riordon J, Wang Y, Kong T, You JB, Sanner S, et al. Deep learning-based selection of human sperm with high DNA integrity. Commun Biol. 2019;2:250.
85. Noy L, Barnea I, Mirsky SK, Kamber D, Levi M, Shaked NT. Sperm-cell DNA fragmentation prediction using label-free quantitative phase imaging and deep learning. Cytometry A. 2023;103:470–8.
86. Agarwal A, Majzoub A, Baskaran S, Selvam MKP, Cho CL, Henkel R, et al. Sperm DNA fragmentation: a new guideline for clinicians. World J Mens Health. 2020;38:412.
87. Esteves SC, Zini A, Coward RM, Evenson DP, Gosálvez J, Lewis SE, et al. Sperm DNA fragmentation testing: summary evidence and clinical practice recommendations. Andrologia. 2021;53:e13874.
88. Tharakan T, Bettocchi C, Carvalho J, Corona G, Jones TH, Kadioglu A, et al. European Association of Urology guidelines panel on male sexual and reproductive health: a clinical consultation guide on the indications for performing sperm DNA fragmentation testing in men with infertility and testicular sperm extraction in nonazoospermic men. Eur Urol Focus. 2022;8:339–50.
89. Wang Y, Riordon J, Kong T, Xu Y, Nguyen B, Zhong J, et al. Prediction of DNA integrity from morphological parameters using a single-sperm DNA fragmentation index assay. Adv Sci (Weinh). 2019;6:1900712.
90. Dutta S, Majzoub A, Agarwal A. Oxidative stress and sperm function: a systematic review on evaluation and management. Arab J Urol. 2019;17:87–97.
91. Gualtieri R, Kalthur G, Barbato V, Longobardi S, Di Rella F, Adiga SK, et al. Sperm oxidative stress during in vitro manipulation and its effects on sperm function and embryo development. Antioxidants (Basel). 2021;10:1025.
92. Rasmussen JMK, Dalgaard MIR, Alipour H, Dardmeh F, Christiansen OB. Seminal oxidative stress and sperm DNA fragmentation in men from couples with infertility or unexplained recurrent pregnancy loss. J Clin Med. 2024;13:833.
93. Jing J, Peng Y, Fan W, Han S, Peng Q, Xue C, et al. Obesity-induced oxidative stress and mitochondrial dysfunction negatively affect sperm quality. FEBS Open Bio. 2023;13:763–78.
94. Hasan H, Bhushan S, Fijak M, Meinhardt A. Mechanism of inflammatory associated impairment of sperm function, spermatogenesis and steroidogenesis. Front Endocrinol (Lausanne). 2022;13:897029.
95. Escada-Rebelo S, Cristo MI, Ramalho-Santos J, Amaral S. Mitochondria-targeted compounds to assess and improve human sperm function. Antioxid Redox Signal. 2022;37:451–80.
96. de Agostini Losano JD, Angrimani DSR, Leite RF, da Silva BCS, Barnabe VH, Nichi M. Spermatic mitochondria: role in oxidative homeostasis, sperm function and possible tools for their assessment. Zygote. 2018;26:251–60.
97. De Angelis A, Ferrara MA, Coppola G, Di Matteo L, Siani L, Dale B, et al. Combined Raman and polarization sensitive holographic imaging for a multimodal label-free assessment of human sperm function. Sci Rep. 2019;9:4823.
98. Zhang BL, Zhang ZP, Shi SM, Shi HJ, DeLeon PA, Shum W. Dynamic elementomics of single-cell ICP–MS-derived signals in normal and calcium pump PMCA4-deficient mouse epididymal sperm during capacitation. Metallomics. 2023;15:mfad059.
99. Henery S, George T, Hall B, Basiji D, Ortyn W, Morrissey P. Quantitative image based apoptotic index measurement using multispectral imaging flow cytometry: a comparison with standard photometric methods. Apoptosis. 2008;13:1054–63.

100. Patel B, Parets S, Akana M, Kellogg G, Jansen M, Chang C, et al. Comprehensive genetic testing for female and male infertility using next-generation sequencing. J Assist Reprod Genet. 2018;35:1489–96.
101. Tüttelmann F, Simoni M, Kliesch S, Ledig S, Dworniczak B, Wieacker P, et al. Copy number variants in patients with severe oligozoospermia and Sertoli-cell-only syndrome. PLoS One. 2011;6:e19426.
102. Oud MS, Volozonoka L, Smits RM, Vissers LE, Ramos L, Veltman JA. A systematic review and standardized clinical validity assessment of male infertility genes. Hum Reprod. 2019;34:932–41.
103. Mitchell MJ, Metzler-Guillemain C, Toure A, Coutton C, Arnoult C, Ray PF. Single gene defects leading to sperm quantitative anomalies. Clin Genet. 2017;91:208–16.
104. Schilit SLP. Recent advances and future opportunities to diagnose male infertility. Curr Sex Health Rep. 2019;11(4):331–341. https://doi.org/10.1007/s11930-019-00225-8.
105. Nakamura S, Miyado M, Saito K, Katsumi M, Nakamura A, Kobori Y, et al. Next-generation sequencing for patients with non-obstructive azoospermia: implications for significant roles of monogenic/oligogenic mutations. Andrology. 2017;5:824–31.
106. Corral-Vazquez C, Blanco J, Cigliano RA, Zaida S, Vidal F, Anton E. A transcriptomic insight into the human sperm microbiome through next-generation sequencing. Syst Biol Reprod Med. 2023;69:188–95.
107. Davies R, Minhas S, Jayasena CN. Next-generation sequencing to elucidate the semen microbiome in male reproductive disorders. Medicina (Kaunas). 2023;60:25.
108. Farahani L, Mowla S, Tharakan T, Lee Y, Kundu S, Khanjani S, et al. O-252 Next generation sequencing analysis of the seminal microbiome in male partners of women with idiopathic recurrent pregnancy loss: results of a prospective cohort study. Hum Reprod. 2022;37:deac106. 034.
109. Vajpeyee M, Tiwari S, Yadav LB, Chimote N. P-067 Characterization of seminal microbiota in patients with asthenozoospermic and normozoospermic using next-generation sequencing. Hum Reprod. 2023;38:dead093.432.
110. Yatsentyuk SP. Study of the sperm microbiome of bulls using metagenomic analysis. Innov Food Safety. 2023, 31 https://doi.org/10.31677/2311-0651-2023-41-3-31-38.
111. Magill RG, MacDonald SM. Male infertility and the human microbiome. Front Reprod Health. 2023;5:1166201.
112. Kaltsas A, Zachariou A, Markou E, Dimitriadis F, Sofikitis N, Pournaras S. Microbial dysbiosis and male infertility: understanding the impact and exploring therapeutic interventions. J Pers Med. 2023;13:1491.
113. Younis N, Mahasneh A. Probiotics and the envisaged role in treating human infertility. Middle East Fertility Soc J. 2020;25:1–9.
114. Wang H, Li X. The microbiome, an important factor that is easily overlooked in male infertility. Front Microbiol. 2022;13:831272.
115. Wagner AO, Turk A, Kunej T. Towards a multi-omics of male infertility. World J Mens Health. 2023;41:272.
116. Govindkumar B, Kavyashree B, Bajpai AK, Davuluri S, Shruthi K, Vasan SS, et al. Listing candidate diagnostic markers and transcriptomic exploration of the molecular basis of a type of male infertility (Non-Obstructive Azoospermia), via next generation sequencing methods. 2019; https://doi.org/10.1101/778670.
117. Rajiwate F. (086) Determination of diagnostic molecular markers in non-obstructive azoospermia-male infertility via next generation sequencing methods. J Sex Med. 2023;20:qdad060. 082.
118. Rotondo JC, Lanzillotti C, Mazziotta C, Tognon M, Martini F. Epigenetics of male infertility: the role of DNA methylation. Front Cell Dev Biol. 2021;9:689624.
119. Marzouni ET, Ilkhani H, Harchegani AB, Shafaghatian H, Layali I, Shahriary A. Epigenetic modifications, a new approach to male infertility etiology: a review. Int J Fertil Steril. 2022;16:1–9.
120. Duvuru R, Halabi M, Omolaoye TS, Du Plessis SS. The genetic causes of male infertility: a Middle East and North Africa perspective. F1000Res. 2022;11:125.

121. Luo T, Chen H, Zou Q, Wang T, Cheng Y, Wang H, et al. A novel copy number variation in CATSPER2 causes idiopathic male infertility with normal semen parameters. Hum Reprod. 2019;34:414–23.
122. Hotaling J, Carrell DT. Clinical genetic testing for male factor infertility: current applications and future directions. Andrology. 2014;2:339–50.
123. Gvozdjáková A, Kucharská J, Dubravicky J, Mojto V, Singh RB. Coenzyme Q 10, α-tocopherol, and oxidative stress could be important metabolic biomarkers of male infertility. Dis Markers. 2015;2015:827941.
124. Chen X, Sun Q, Zheng Y, Liu Z, Meng X, Zeng W, et al. Human sperm tsRNA as potential biomarker and therapy target for male fertility. Reproduction. 2021;161:111–22.
125. Pandruvada S, Royfman R, Shah TA, Sindhwani P, Dupree JM, Schon S, et al. Lack of trusted diagnostic tools for undetermined male infertility. J Assist Reprod Genet. 2021;38:265–76.
126. Alipour H, Duus RK, Wimmer R, Dardmeh F, Du Plessis SS, Jørgensen N, et al. Seminal plasma metabolomics profiles following long (4–7 days) and short (2 h) sexual abstinence periods. Eur J Obstet Gynecol Reprod Biol. 2021;264:178–83.
127. Vashisht A, Gahlay GK. Understanding seminal plasma in male infertility: emerging markers and their implications. Andrology. 2023;12(5):1058–77.
128. Hao H, Chen S, Wu Y, Jiang X, Jiang X, Xiao M, et al. Research progress of micro-RNA in pathogenesis and diagnosis of male infertility. Cells. 2023;6:306.
129. John A, Qin B, Kalari KR, Wang L, Yu J. Patient-specific multi-omics models and the application in personalized combination therapy. Future Oncol. 2020;16:1737–50.
130. Li M, Chen L, Yan J, Jayasena CN, Liu Z, Li J, et al. Super-resolution ultrasound localization microscopy for the non-invasive imaging of human testicular microcirculation and its differential diagnosis role in male infertility. 2024;5(2) https://doi.org/10.1002/VIW.20230093.
131. Zupin L, Pascolo L, Gianoncelli A, Gariani G, Luppi S, Giolo E, et al. Synchrotron radiation soft X-ray microscopy and low energy X-ray fluorescence to reveal elemental changes in spermatozoa treated with photobiomodulation therapy. Anal Meth. 2020;12:3691–6.
132. Gordon DZ, Abbasi MA, Lee J, Sarnari R, Sojoudi A, Wei Q, et al. Four-dimensional flow magnetic resonance imaging quantification of blood flow in bicuspid aortic valve. J Thorac Imaging. 2020;35:383–8.
133. Pownder SL, Hayashi K, Lin BQ, Meyers KN, Caserto BG, Breighner RE, et al. Differences in the magnetic resonance imaging parameter T2* may be identified during the course of canine patellar tendon healing: a pilot study. Quant Imaging Med Surg. 2021;11:1234.
134. Mantravadi KC, Gedela DR, Sambangi M, Manepalli V. P-007 A four arm prospective randomized control trial to investigate the role of advance sperm selection techniques for raised sperm DNA fragmentation index. Hum Reprod. 2023;38:dead093. 377.
135. Mangum CL, Patel DP, Jafek AR, Samuel R, Jenkins TG, Aston KI, et al. Towards a better testicular sperm extraction: novel sperm sorting technologies for non-motile sperm extracted by microdissection TESE. Transl Androl Urol. 2020;9:S206.
136. Kashaninejad N, Shiddiky MJA, Nguyen NT, Adv. Biosys. 2018;2:1700197. https://doi.org/10.1002/adbi.201700197.
137. Degheidy T, Abdelfattah H, Seif A, Albuz FK, Gazi S, Abbas S. Magnetic activated cell sorting: an effective method for reduction of sperm DNA fragmentation in varicocele men prior to assisted reproductive techniques. Andrologia. 2015;47:892–6.
138. Faraghat SA, Hoettges KF, Steinbach MK, Van Der Veen DR, Brackenbury WJ, Henslee EA, et al. High-throughput, low-loss, low-cost, and label-free cell separation using electrophysiology-activated cell enrichment. Proc Natl Acad Sci U S A. 2017;114:4591–6.
139. Berteli TS, Da Broi MG, Martins WP, Ferriani RA, Navarro PA. Magnetic-activated cell sorting before density gradient centrifugation improves recovery of high-quality spermatozoa. Andrology. 2017;5:776–82.
140. Ahmadi A, Sobhani A, Khalili MA, Agha-Rahimi A, Nabi A, Findikli N. Comparison of the efficiency of magnetic-activated cell sorting (MACS) and physiological intracytoplasmic sperm injection (PICSI) for sperm selection in cases with unexplained infertility. J Reprod Infertil. 2022;23:184.

141. Xi Y, Zhang C, Feng Y, Zhao S, Zhang Y, Duan G, et al. Genetically predicted the causal relationship between gut microbiota and infertility: bidirectional Mendelian randomization analysis in the framework of predictive, preventive, and personalized medicine. EPMA J. 2023;14:405–16.
142. Bruno C, Basile U, Vergani E, Napodano C, Oliva A, Gulli F, et al. Inflammation and oxidative stress in seminal plasma: search for biomarkers in diagnostic approach to male infertility. J Pers Med. 2022;12:857.
143. Santacroce L, Imbimbo C, Ballini A, Crocetto F, Scacco S, Cantore S, et al. Testicular immunity and its connection with the microbiota physiological and clinical implications in the light of personalized medicine. J Pers Med. 2022;12:1335.
144. Zamani-Badi T, Karimian M, Azami-Tameh A, Nikzad H. Association of C3953T transition in interleukin 1β gene with idiopathic male infertility in an Iranian population. Hum Fertil (Camb). 2017;22(2):111–7.
145. Aras-Tosun D. Genetic alterations in azoospermia patients may reveal potential biomarkers for male infertility: a bioinformatic study. J Surg Med. 2023;7(3):239–44.

Chapter 3
Genetic Testing in Nonobstructive Azoospermia and Idiopathic Male Infertility

Tan V. Le, Asli Metin Mahmutoglu, and Hussein Kandil

Introduction

Infertility refers to the inability to achieve pregnancy after engaging in regular intercourse without contraception for at least 1 year. Approximately 8–12% of couples of reproductive age face infertility issues, with male factors contributing to about 50% of these cases [1]. Azoospermia, a condition characterized by the absence of sperm in the ejaculate, affects roughly 1% of all men and is prevalent in 10–15% of infertile men [2]. Given these prevalence rates, male infertility and azoospermia can be considered relatively common conditions. However, a significant portion of male infertility cases, around 50%, are classified as idiopathic, meaning their causes remain unknown [3]. In instances of nonobstructive azoospermia (NOA) and severe oligo-astheno-teratozoospermia, chromosomal or genetic abnormalities are identified in 15–20% of patients [4].

Spermatogenesis is an intricate process involving successive mitotic, meiotic, and postmeiotic phases, governed by numerous molecular pathways. In humans, it

T. V. Le (✉)
Science Research and Training Department, Binh Dan Hospital, Ho Chi Minh City, Vietnam

Department of Surgery, Pham Ngoc Thach University of Medicine, Ho Chi Minh City, Vietnam

A. Metin Mahmutoglu
Department of Medical Biology, Faculty of Medicine, Yozgat Bozok University, Yozgat, Turkey

H. Kandil
Fakih IVF Fertility Center, Abu Dhabi, UAE

Global Andrology Forum (GAF), Moreland Hills, OH, USA

E. Chung et al. (eds.), *Advances in Andrology*,
https://doi.org/10.1007/978-3-032-29112-7_3

necessitates the orchestrated expression of over 4000 genes across various germ cell subtypes [5]. Given this complexity, male infertility exhibits highly heterogeneous phenotype presentations among affected individuals. Current estimates attribute known genetic factors such as chromosomal abnormalities, aneuploidies, Y chromosome microdeletions, and single-gene defects to approximately 15–30% of male infertility cases [3, 5]. Over the past two decades, several studies have identified additional genetic factors, both single-gene and multiple-gene defects, associated with male infertility. Nevertheless, the etiology remains obscure in a significant proportion of infertile men (40%), highlighting the critical need to uncover novel genetic factors linked with idiopathic male infertility [3].

Hence, it is imperative for physicians and researchers in reproductive medicine to categorize idiopathic male infertility according to its underlying causes and elucidate the pathogenic mechanisms involved.

Genetic Testing in NOA

Genetic testing is indicated in some of the subpopulation of infertile men in the workup of male infertility. Nonobstructive azoospermic and severe oligozoospermic men are involved in them. Currently, karyotyping and Y chromosome microdeletion testing are recommended in the clinical practice for the diagnosis and prognosis of these men [6–8].

Karyotype Analysis

Karyotype analysis is a cytogenetic method enabling the determination of numerical and structural anomalies of human chromosomes. Various chromosome banding techniques including giemsa-, quinacrine-, and reverse-banding are used for the evaluation of individual chromosomes and the identification of the particular segments of them according to the cytogenetic nomenclature—The International System for Human Cytogenomic Nomenclature (ISCN)—in karyotyping [9–11]. Chromosomes can be extracted from various cell types and tissues including amniocytes, blood lymphocytes and tumor tissues [12]. The most commonly used cell types and banding techniques for karyotype analysis in infertile men with NOA and severe oligozoospermia are peripheral blood lymphocytes and giemsa (G)-banding, respectively [13, 14]. Chromosomes are examined at one of the stages of mitosis, metaphase, in which their condensation and visibility are optimum for the analysis. To arrest the chromosomes at metaphase stage is provided via deterioration of spindle fibers by treating with colcemid. During the G-banding process (also known as GTG banding), giemsa stain and trypsin are implemented to these cells, resulting in unique light and dark bands on individual chromosomes [12]. Besides G-banding, other banding techniques such as centromere (C-banding) and telomere banding

(T-banding) are also utilized in the karyotype analysis of infertile men but in a relatively less manner [7]. The C-banding is preferred to identify chromosomes with heterochromatin such as Y chromosome which has a heterochromatin structure on the long arm [10]. A pericentric inversion between the centromere and heterochromatin region of the Y chromosome has been revealed in a man without fertility problem by the C-banding, which is caused a dicentric Y, and the abnormality transmitted to his son [15]. Karyotype analysis can detect large structural abnormalities including Robertsonian and reciprocal translocations as well as inversions, even though it has limited resolution only 5–10 Mb. Nevertheless, nucleotide variants, mosaicism with less than 10% and uniparental disomy cannot be detected by karyotyping [16].

Infertile males represent by high incidence of chromosomal abnormalities which is adversely linked with the severity of spermatogenic failure. The frequency of cytogenic abnormalities in almost 9800 oligozoospermic and azoospermic men is 5.8%. Azoospermic males demonstrate a predominance in sex chromosomal aneuploidy risk (4.2%), while autosomal chromosome abnormalities are more common in oligozoospermic cases (1.5%). These incidences are also higher than those of newborn males with normal phenotype, in whom sex and autosomal chromosome anomalies are 0.14% and 0.25%, respectively [17]. Similarly, a study evaluating the cytogenetic data from five studies of oligozoospermia cases with <20 million spermatozoa/mL and six studies of azoospermic ones has indicated that the sex chromosome abnormalities is more common than autosomal abnormalities in azoospermic infertile men (12.6% vs. 1.1%), whereas oligozoospermic individuals are commonly represented by autosomal chromosome abnormalities rather than sex chromosome ones (3% vs. 1.6%). Klinefelter syndrome (47,XXY) and its mosaic form (47,XXY/46,XY) are the predominant cause of azoospermia with an incidence of 10.8% [14]. Structural chromosomal abnormalities including Robertsonian and reciprocal translocations, and inversions have been also detected by karyotyping in infertile men especially with oligozoospermia [3]. Despite the rareness, 46,XX testicular disorder may involve in the pathogenesis of NOA, caused by a translocation of the chromosome part containing sex determining region of Y (*SRY*) gene from Y to X chromosome during paternal meiosis [18–20]. Therefore, karyotyping is recommended by several association—The American Society for Reproductive Medicine (ASRM), The American Urological Association (AUA), and The European Association of Urology (EUA)—for nonobstructive azoospermia cases and oligozoospermic men with 5 or ten million sperm per milliliter (mL). The ASRM/AUA guideline advocates the karyotype analysis for nonobstructive azoospermic men and severe oligozoospermic individuals with five million sperm/mL and high level of follicle stimulating hormone (FSH) or testicular atrophy, whereas the EAU guideline proposes a karyotype analysis for oligozoospermic cases with ten million spermatozoa/mL as well as azoospermic ones. The EAU and ASRM/AUA guidelines also suggest a karyotype analysis for couples with recurrent pregnancy loss (RPL) regardless of spermatogenic failure. Besides RPL, in the presence of malformations and mental retardation, a karyotype testing is moderately recommended by the EAU guideline [6, 8, 21]. Sperm concentration threshold seems an indicator for karyotype testing in men with fertility problems in the current guidelines, a validation study by Ventimiglia and colleagues has revealed that the sensitivity, specificity and discrimination of the EAU guideline are only 80%, 37%, and 59%, respectively. They have developed a nomogram depended upon not only sperm concentration but also the level of luteinizing hormone and mean testis volume, resulting in more sensitivity (94%) than the EAU criteria for karyotype analysis [22]. In conclusion, current guidelines may be improved and updated according to the related articles and validation studies.

Fluorescence in situ hybridization (FISH) is another technique utilized in karyotype analysis, which is based on the hybridization between the specific DNA sequences labeled with a hapten or a fluorochrome (DNA probe) and the genomic regions of the target DNA. In this technique, visualization is performed by fluorescence microscopy [23]. However, FISH technique is not usually preferred for routine karyotype analysis of infertile male patients, which is generally utilized as a supplement for the characterization of particular cytogenetic anomalies. Evaluation of the sperm chromosomal aneuploidy and the determination of the presence or absence of the *SRY* gene in cases with 46,XX testicular disorder are involved in the usage fields of FISH [24, 25]. Multicolor FISH analysis has shown that NOA cases have an increased risk of YY disomy—presence of an extra Y chromosome in a haploid state—in their testicular spermatozoa [26]. Sperm chromosomal abnormalities may cause a risk of recurrent abortion due to trisomy, monosomy or triploidy [27]. Therefore, sperm FISH has been commonly suggested as a screening tool for the couples with repeated assisted reproduction techniques (ART) failure or RPL [28].

Y Chromosome Microdeletion Testing

Structure of the Male-Specific Region of the Y Chromosome

The human Y chromosome with ~62.5 Mb length is one of the smallest chromosomes, and hosts 147 protein-coding genes that are vital for the male sex determination and spermatogenesis [29]. The male-specific region of Y (MSY) encompasses the 95% of the Y chromosome, which was revealed by using 220 bacterial artificial chromosome (BAC) clones in the sequence analysis. Each of the DNA clones included portions of the MSY from one man in order to avoid the variation between different individuals. The MSY involves three different classes of euchromatic sequences (i) X-transposed classes display relatively high similarity (99%) to the X chromosome, (ii) X-degenerate sequences originated from ancient autosomes during the evolutionary process of sex chromosomes encompasses single-copy genes or pseudogenes, and (iii) ampliconic sequences cover nearly 30% of the euchromatin sequences in the MSY, and are characterized by large duplicated sequences organized into eight palindromes (named as P1-P8) [30]. These amliconic/palindromic sequences undergo arm-to-arm gene conversion to maintain their sequence integrity as well as non-allelic homologous recombination (NAHR) owing to their highly repetitive content [31, 32]. Furthermore, this peculiar sequence organization in the MSY, amplicons/palindromes, has the potential to generate certain structural chromosomal abnormalities including deletions, duplications and inversions [33]. The NAHR, a recombination between non-allelic repeats, is known to be an actual mechanism taking part in the generation of azoospermia factor (AZF) deletions of the Y chromosome [32].

Y Chromosome Microdeletion Types

The AZF region is located on the long arm of the Y chromosome, and consists mainly of spermatogenesis-related genes [29]. This unique region has been mapped to three subregions on the Y chromosome—AZFa, AZFb, and AZFc—followed by the first description in 1970's [34, 35]. The AZFb and AZFc subregions are partially overlap [36]. Microdeletions in these subregions are characterized by various spermatogenesis impairments (e.g., Sertoli cell only syndrome and maturation arrest) [35].

The AZFa region is almost 795 kb length and includes single copy of ubiquitin specific peptidase 9 (*USP9Y*), DEAD-box helicase 3 Y-linked (*DDX3Y*), and ubiquitous transcribed Y (*UTY*) genes [37]. The complete deletion of AZFa region has been attributed to the NAHR mechanism [33]. The breakpoints of the AZFa deletion mapped to the Yq11; the proximal breakpoint is located in the human endogenous retrovirus 15 1 (HERV15yq1), whereas the distal breakpoint is in HERV15yq2 sequence. The HERV15yq1 and HERV15yq2 are homologues sequences, and intrachromosomal recombination between these two identical retroviral sequences has eventuated in complete AZFa deletion via removing *USP9Y* and *DDX3Y* genes [38]. A deletion of the entire AZFb causes the removal of 32 genes and transcription units encompassing 6.2 Mb length. Nonobstructive azoospermic men have been characterized by a deletion between P5 and proximal P1 (P5/proximal P1) in the AZFb region due to NAHR mechanism [39]. The complete AZFb deletion has been associated with maturation arrest [39, 40]. The AZFc mapped in the region with 3.5 Mb hosting 42 genes and transcripts. The complete deletion of that, also referred as b2/b4, occurs between breakpoints in P3 and P1, which gives rise to various phenotypic presentation ranging from oligozoospermia to azoospermia [39, 41]. The complete AZFbc deletion is represented by SCOS and MA due to the removal of 38 genes and transcripts by NAHR mechanism [33, 39]. Moreover, AZF deletions are related with not only testicular phenotypes but also with the outcome of sperm retrieval techniques. Individuals with complete deletion of AZFa, and AZFb are characterized by the complete absence of spermatogenesis. As for AZFc carriers, the likelihood of sperm retrieval is 50–60%. The chance of cases with partial deletions in AZF regions may vary according to the result of extension deletion analysis [40].

The AZFc microdeletion is the most common Y chromosome microdeletion type with nearly 70–80% incidence. That is followed by AZFa (0.5–9%), AZFb (1–7%), and AZFbc (1–20%). The frequency of the complete AZF deletions is 1:4000 in the general male population, while it reaches to 5–10% in idiopathic infertile men with NOA [41, 42]. In conclusion, complete microdeletion of AZFa, AZFb (P5/proximal P1), AZFc (b2/b4), and AZFbc (P5/distal P1 or P4/distal P1) are clinically relevant as a cause of azoospermia and severe oligozoospermia [33]. Moreover, normozoospermic men have never carried AZF deletions, stating a clear association between Y chromosome microdeletions and spermatogenic disturbances [43]. Based on these, current guidelines for male infertility advocates the Y chromosome microdeletion testing for infertile men who have fewer than five million spermatozoa in per milliliter of semen [6, 8].

Genetic Testing for Y Chromosome Microdeletion

The ASRM/AUA and the EUA guidelines have recommended the Y chromosome microdeletion (YCMD) testing for severe oligozoospermic (sperm concentration <5 million/mL) and azoospermic cases with elevated FSH or testicular atrophy [6, 8, 21]. However, the exact cut-off value for sperm concentration for the indication of YMCD testing in infertile patients continues to be controversial. A systematic review and meta-analysis of European and North American studies by Kohn et al., evaluated the prevalence of YCMD in 10.866 oligozoospermic men. They have stated the highest frequency of YCMD in infertile men with 0–1 million spermatozooa/mL, and proposed that YCMD testing should be recommended for infertile men with less than one million/mL sperm concentration rather than five million/mL [44]. Furthermore, Johnson et al. have also suggested lowering the cut-off value for sperm concentration to 0.5 million/mL to increase the sensitivity to 100%, as they did not detect any AZF microdeletion in men with more than 0.5 million sperm/mL [17].

The YCMD testing is depended on whether the amplification of specific sequence tagged sites (STSs) by polymerase chain reaction (PCR) or not [13]. The STSs are short (200–500 bp) and single-copy DNA sequences that may be easily detected by two primers in the PCR assay [45]. For YCMD testing, STSs are located in and near the spermatogenesis-related genes on the MSY [13]. The EAA/EMQN association releases the best practice guidelines for molecular diagnosis of YCMDs at regular intervals, and the last one has been published recently. This guideline enables the quality of the clinical diagnostic assay through offering external quality control trials. sY84 and sY86 are recommended primers for AZFa region; while sY127 and sY134 for AZFb, and sY254 and sY255 for AZFc by this association [33]. The sY84 and sY86 are identified upstream of the genes in AZFa region, *USP9Y* and *DBY* genes. In case of the AZFa deletion, amplification is not occurred with these primers in the PCR reaction [46]. It is same for other primers and AZF region deletions. The reverse primer sequence of sY84 has been updated in the recent guideline. Since a single nucleotide polymorphism in this reverse primer sequence are commonly seen in Asian population [33].

Two-step multiplex PCR reaction assay is commonly preferred for microdeletion testing of Y chromosome in the clinical setting, and conducted according to the EAA/EMQN guideline. In this multiplex PCR assay, an internal control is used to eliminate negative result(s) derived from technical problems. An SRY gene marker (sY14) for the SRY gene on Yp, and *ZFX/ZFY* genes for the determination of male and female DNA serve as internal controls involving in the multiplex PCR. Once any deletion in AZF regions are detected, deletion extension analysis must be done by suggested primers. For example: sY105 and sY121/sY1224 for proximal breakpoint of AZFb and sY1192 and sY153 for distal breakpoint of AZFb; and sY160 for AZFc deletion [33]. The amplification of a specific distal STS with sY1192 primers in cases of AZFb deletion may indicate a sperm retrieval chance in TESE [40].

Besides multiplex PCR, alternative methods have been used for the detection of AZF deletions including capillary electrophoresis, real-time PCR, multiplex ligation dependent probe amplification (MLPA), array-based comparative genomic hybridization (aCGH), and next-generation sequencing (NGS). The capillary electrophoresis in which primers tagged with fluorescence to detection of the submicroscopic deletion has been used by some laboratories [33, 47–50]. Real-time PCR enables the identification of the AZF deletions according to differences in their melting points. It has certain advantages over multiplex PCR system such as time saving and no need for gel electrophoresis [48]. With the genomic microarray technology, the integrity of Y chromosome may be detected in only one assay, and a number of different loci can be interrogated at the same time. Yuen and colleagues have reported copy number variations of the Y chromosome as well as YCMD with this technique [51]. Recently, advancement in the NGS technology and in its application—targeted sequencing, and whole exome and genome sequencing—allows identification of new candidate genes related to male infertility [3, 52]. NGS-based approaches ensure more rapid and accurate results but necessitated advanced equipment, high cost and expertise person as compared to PCR-based techniques [7] (Table 3.1).

Table 3.1 Genetic testing recommended by urological association/society in nonobstructive azoospermia [6, 8, 21]

Genetic test	Genetic abnormality of interest	Strength rating	Commonly used technique(s)	Alternative genetic testing
Karyotype analysis	Numerical and structural chromosomal abnormalities of sex and autosomal chromosomes (e.g., Klinefelter syndrome, translocations)	Strong	G-banding	C-banding R-banding Q-banding FISH
Y chromosome microdeletion	Microdeletion in AZF subregions	Strong	Multiplex PCR	Real-time PCR Capillary electrophoresis MLPA aCGH NGS

Abbreviations: *G-banding* Giemsa-banding, *C-banding* centromere-banding, *R-banding* reverse-banding, *Q-banding* quinacrine banding, *FISH* fluorescence in situ hybridization, *MLPA* multiplex ligation dependent probe amplification, *aCGH* array-based comparative genomic hybridization, *NGS* next-generation sequencing

The result of YCMD testing provides not only valuable information for genetic counseling, but also offering a prognostic value, once TESE-ICSI is a treatment option for these patients. Individuals with YCMD should be informed by genetic counselor about the transmission of this deletion to their son [33].

Genetic Testing and Sperm Retrieval Success in NOA Patient

Nonobstructive azoospermia patients are evaluated by karyotyping and YCMD analysis in the workup of male infertility [8]. Klinefelter syndrome (KS) is the well-known karyotypic abnormality causing NOA [53]. The probability of sperm retrieval in non-mosaic KS cases is 20–44% by TESE, and the pregnancy and live birth rates are >40%, once using these retrieved testicular spermatozoa [54–58]. An increased risk of karyotypic abnormalities has not been suggested in biological children of KS males [59].

The YCMD testing has a paramount importance in the diagnosis and the prognosis of severe oligozoospermic and nonobstructive azoospermic males [33]. TESE in not contraindicated in individuals with complete AZFa, AZFb, and AZFbc microdeletions, since no report has stated the presence of spermatozoa in these patients. Nevertheless, a discrimination between complete or partial deletions in the AZF subregions by deletion extension analysis is essential in the case of any deletion(s) [33, 40]. Residual spermatogenesis has been reported in two NOA men without STSs specific to AZFb region (sY127 and sY137). However, the deletion extension analysis in these patients has demonstrated the existence of sY1192, suggesting the retention of certain genes related to spermatogenesis, and the prognostic value of sY1192 in men with partial AZFb deletion [60]. The AZFc deletion carriers have a good probability in the sperm retrieval success via mTESE (50–60%) [61]. Nevertheless, mosaicism (45,X/46,XY) may have an adverse impact on the severity of spermatogenic failure in nonobstructive azoospermic patients with AZFc deletion [62]. An association of AZF deletion with Y chromosome instability may also culminate in the formation of cell lines with 45,X karyotype, which is a negative predictor in the success rate of TESE [43, 62–64].

Genetic Testing in Idiopathic Male Infertility

The Challenges of Diagnosing Idiopathic Male Infertility

The process of diagnosing idiopathic male infertility is fraught with difficulties due to its multifaceted nature, encompassing a wide array of potential genetic irregularities and the current diagnostic methods' inadequacies in pinpointing these anomalies. The intricate genetic landscape of spermatogenesis, featuring over two thousand genes, coupled with the diverse clinical presentations of infertility, underscores the complexity of establishing accurate diagnoses. The utilization of advanced genetic diagnostics like next-generation sequencing (NGS) has illuminated some of these genetic underpinnings, yet the sheer genetic diversity and the subtleties of sperm and testicular pathologies remain challenging hurdles to overcome in fully elucidating idiopathic male infertility's etiology [65].

The Potential Role of Genetic Factors in Iidiopathic Male Infertility

The potential role of genetic factors in idiopathic male infertility has been increasingly recognized due to the complexity of genetic contributions to reproductive capabilities. Infertility affects a significant portion of the population globally, with male factors contributing to nearly half of all cases. Despite advancements, about 40% of male infertility remains idiopathic, suggesting that unknown genetic factors may play a role. Literature reviews underscores the advancements in genetic research over the last two decades, highlighting the identification of single-gene and multiple-gene defects associated with male infertility. However, the etiology for a majority of cases remains unclear, pointing to the necessity for further genetic exploration [66].

The development and application of comprehensive genetic tools, including NGS and microarray technologies, have been crucial in identifying these genetic factors. These methods allow for the detailed analysis of the male genome, offering insights into the complex processes of spermatogenesis and the various genetic anomalies that can impair fertility. Over 4000 genes are involved in various stages of germ cell development, with known genetic factors accounting for 15–30% of infertility cases. This suggests a vast landscape of genetic influence yet to be fully understood, necessitating broad and inclusive genome-wide studies to uncover these hidden genetic causes [66].

Genetic Tools Applied for Idiopathic Male Infertility

The application of genetic tools in the study of idiopathic male infertility has significantly advanced our understanding of the condition, highlighting the intricate role genetic factors play. Advances in genomic technologies, particularly NGS, have paved the way for the identification of a multitude of genetic anomalies that contribute to male infertility. These technologies have enabled researchers to delve deeper into the genetic architecture of idiopathic male infertility, identifying specific genes associated with NOA due to maturation/meiotic arrest, among other conditions [65].

The narrative review by Sudhakar et al. emphasizes that despite considerable progress in identifying genetic factors associated with male infertility, the etiology remains obscure for a significant portion of infertile men. The authors also highlighted the utility of advanced genomic technologies in uncovering monogenic causes of male infertility with diagnostic implications. It underscores the need for a swift implementation of genomic analysis in clinical practice, which could enhance genetic counseling and contribute to the development of tailored treatment plans [66]. By employing these advanced genetic tools, researchers can identify novel genes and genetic pathways that contribute to male infertility, thereby enhancing our understanding of the condition and improving diagnostic and therapeutic strategies [66].

The investigation into idiopathic male infertility has been significantly enhanced by the evolution of genetic analysis methodologies, notably through microarray techniques and NGS [7].

Microarray Techniques

Employing microarray methods, such as Comparative Genomic Hybridization (CGH) and Single Nucleotide Polymorphism (SNP) arrays, has offered a deeper insight into the genetic landscapes affecting male fertility. CGH arrays, utilized within some fertility clinics, are adept at identifying copy number variations and specific syndromes related to microdeletions or duplications, although they fall short in detecting balanced chromosomal alterations. Conversely, SNP arrays have become a staple in fertility research, enabling the examination of vast numbers of polymorphisms across the genome to discern differences in SNP frequencies between infertile men and control groups, thereby contributing to a broader understanding of infertility's genetic foundations [67].

Advances in NGS

The advent and reduced cost of NGS have marked a transformative leap in genetic research related to male infertility, making whole exome and genome sequencing increasingly preferred for discovering genetic anomalies linked to this condition. While Whole Genome Sequencing (WGS) aims to catalog the entirety of the genome, focusing on about 95–96% due to technical limitations in sequencing certain regions, Whole Exome Sequencing (WES) concentrates on the exonic regions, which represent a smaller but highly significant portion of the genome. Although these methods offer a more cost-effective approach to sequencing, they also introduce analytical challenges, necessitating the validation of identified variants through additional techniques such as Sanger sequencing [67].

These advanced genetic analysis tools have propelled forward our comprehension of the intricate genetic factors contributing to idiopathic male infertility. By delineating novel genes and pathways involved in fertility, these methodologies not only deepen our understanding of the condition but also pave the way for enhanced diagnostic and treatment modalities (Table 3.2) [67].

Table 3.2 Genetic testing in idiopathic male infertility [68, 69]

Test type	Description	Clinical relevance
CGH array	Allows for the analysis of CNVs across the entire genome	Identifies CNVs that may lead to infertility, offering a broader genetic understanding beyond single-gene defects
SNP array	Detects SNPs across the genome, which can be associated with diseases or conditions like male infertility	Facilitates the study of genetic variants that may contribute to idiopathic infertility through association studies
Whole Exome Sequencing (WES)	Sequences all the protein-coding regions in the genome. This can uncover genetic variants that affect protein function and lead to infertility	Provides a focused yet comprehensive insight into genetic defects affecting sperm production or function
Whole Genome Sequencing (WGS)	Involves sequencing the entire genome. It can identify both known and novel genetic variants contributing to idiopathic male infertility	Offers the most comprehensive genetic analysis, allowing for the identification of all potential genetic causes of infertility, including non-coding regions

Abbreviations: *CGH* Comparative Genomic Hybridization, *CNV* copy number variations, *SNP* single nucleotide polymorphisms, *WES* Whole Exome Sequencing, *WGS* Whole Genome Sequencing

Epigenetic Factors in NOA and Idiopathic Male Infertility

Gene mutations and chromosomal abnormalities are not the only factors involving in the etiopathology of male infertility, but also epigenetic factors are also playing a crucial role in the pathogenesis of the disease [70]. There is emerging evidence that epigenetic modifications including DNA methylation, histone modifications, chromatin remodeling and non-coding RNAs are associated with NOA and idiopathic male infertility [71–74].

DNA methylation is a prevalent epigenetic modification. This is fulfilled by DNA methyltransferases (DNMTs) especially in cytosine-phosphate-guanine (CpG) islands, eventuating in gene silencing [75]. Methylation of DNA is essential for genomic imprinting, X-chromosome inactivation, silencing of transposons and regulation of gene expression in certain developmental stages or tissues [76]. During germ cell development, genome-wide methylation reprogramming occurs via methylation and demethylation [77, 78]. Aberration(s) in the methylation profile of the whole genome, and imprinted and non-imprinted genes has been reported in testicular tissues, germ line cells or mature spermatozoa of men with various subtypes of infertility [79–82]. Nonobstructive azoospermic males have been identified by decreased expression of DNMT1, resulting in altered global DNA methylation in correlation with the severity of the testicular phenotype. The expression level of DNMT1 enzyme gradually reduced from hypospermatogenesis to SCOS group [83]. Genetic variants or expression changes of de novo methyltransferase enzymes—DNMT3A,

DNMT3B, and DNMT3L—have been also correlated with various testicular phenotypes in NOA men, and genome-wide DNA methylation defects [84, 85]. Single nucleotide polymorphisms of *DNMT3L* have been suggested to increase the risk of idiopathic male infertility in Chinese population [86]. Imprinted genes, *H19* and *MEST/PEG1*, represented by hypo- or unmethylated states in testicular spermatozoa of men with anejaculation, obstructive azoospermia or hypospermatogenesis. This hypomethylation status affected CTCF-binding site 6, which presents in the H19 differentially methylated region and regulates IGF2 expression [87]. Complete or incomplete maturation arrest has also identified by aberrant methylation of *H19* and *MEST* gene in azoospermic males [88]. A recent systematic review of ten studies indicated that methylation defects of *H19/IGF2* and *KCNQ1* genes could be associated with ART outcomes and sperm DNA fragmentation [89]. Besides imprinted genes, the methylation changes of single genes including methylenetetrahydrofolate reductase (*MTHFR*), discoidin domain receptor 1 *(DDR1)*, and glutathione s-transferase mu 1 (*GSTM1*) might have an adverse impact on fertility, culminating in NOA or male infertility with unknown causes [90–92]. Moreover, Tang et al. reported that m^6A expression (N6-methyadenosine), the most common mRNA modification, was downregulated in testicular tissue of idiopathic NOA cases, suggesting the critical role of m^6A as an epigenetic regulator in spermatogenesis [93].

Histone modifications and chromatin remodeling are other epigenetic modifications required for successful spermatogenesis. These modifications occur in spermiogenesis, and necessitate several factors and mechanisms including histone variants (e.g., H1T, H2AL1, H3T, and H3.5) and post-translational modifications of histones (PTMs) (e.g., acetylation, methylation, phosphorylation) [94–96]. Histone variants act as a regulator in the chromatin remodeling process. The H3T is expressed in male spermatogenic cells but not in mature sperm, and plays a role in the generation of open chromatin structure. A mutation in the *H3t* gene resulted in azoospermia in mice [97]. NOA cases showed decreased expression level of H3.5 in their testicular tissue as compared to OA patients [98]. The PTMs of histones have presented differential profiles in NOA men. Hyperacetylation of histone 4 (H4) is one of the PTM controlling chromatin condensation and interaction of chromatin fiber with non-histone proteins [99]. The H4 hyperacetylation (H4K12Ac) defect gives rise to abnormalities in spermatogenesis. The H4K12Ac level was reported to be low in NOA men with mixed atrophy than men with complete spermatogenesis [100]. Hashemi et al. proposed that testicular expression of *ZMYND15*, function of which is depended on histone deacetylase enzyme, decreased in men with NOA [101]. The expression level of *ZMYND15* and *JMJD1A* (histone demethylase), targeting transition protein 1 and protamine 1 genes, is a predictor for sperm retrieval rate in these cases [101, 102].

Non-coding RNAs (ncRNAs) are divided into small (<200 nucleotides) and long non-coding RNAs (>200 nucleotides) according to its length. ncRNAs have a function in the reproductive system via regulation of essential events in male gametogenesis [103]. microRNAs (miRNAs), PIWI-interacting RNAs (piRNAs), and transfer RNA derived small RNAs (tsRNAs) are included in small non-coding RNAs. miRNAs play a role in the cleavage or translational repression of target mRNA transcripts [103, 104]. NOA males exhibit distinct miRNA profiles in their seminal plasma and testicular tissues [105–110]. Lian et al. reported that 173 miRNAs including miR302a, miR-491-3p, miR-383 were differentially expressed in testicular tissue of NOA cases [106]. Down- or upregulated miRNAs in NOA testis target genes involving in spermatogenesis, cell cycle, mitotic division particularly prometaphase, and sex determination [106, 110]. SCOS, mixed atrophy and germ cell arrest have been characterized by 197, 68 and 46 differentially expressed miRNAs as compared to normal spermatogenesis [111]. Furthermore, 86 miRNAs have been found to be exclusively expressed in testicular tissue of men with successfully sperm retrieval [112]. Seminal level of various miRNAs such as hsa-miR-3653, hsa-miR-6752-5p, hsa-miR-424-5p, and hsa-miR-1181 has been indicated as a predictor for the presence of spermatogonia in NOA testis [109]. Besides miRNAs, tsRNAs (tRF-Gly-GCC-002 and tRF-Glu-CTC-005) have been suggested to be a biomarker candidate for sperm retrieval via mTESE [104].

lncRNAs possess a regulator function in spermatogenesis transcriptionally, post-transcriptionally and translationally [113, 114]. LncRNAs, HOX antisense intergenic RNA (HOTAIR) and AK015322 maintain spermatogonial stem cell population in mice [113, 115]. The inhibition of HOTAIR caused to repressing of proliferation and induction of apoptosis through competing endogenous RNAs (ceRNAs) [113]. Bo et al. have stated that lncRNAs could participate in the spermatogenesis process via ceRNA mechanism. CeRNA mechanism is a molecular mechanism in which ceRNAs regulate the gene expression due to "sponge" role of lncRNAs for miRNAs, suggesting the importance of interactions between miRNA-lncRNA and miRNA-mRNA in target gene expression [116]. In NOA cases, ~175 lncRNAs including SPATA42, ZNF295-AS1, and LINC00467 were downregulated in their testis [116]. Idiopathic NOA patients have been characterized by dysregulated mRNA-miRNA-lncRNA interactions, as well [117]. Certain extracellular vesicles lncRNAs (e.g., LOC100505685, LOC440934, and LINC00343) derived from seminal plasma of NOA men has been indicated to be a biomarker for predicting testicular spermatozoa [118].

Currently, epigenetic factors are not used for routine assessment of male infertility, although the significance of epigenomic studies in elucidating the unknown causes of male infertility is undeniable. By the advancement in molecular techniques and further research, epigenomic profiling can pave the way for personalized management strategies of male infertility and prevent the transmission risk of epigenetic pattern.

Genetic Counseling Before IVF—ICSI in Patients with Genetic Abnormalities

With the advancements in Assisted Reproductive Technologies (ART), individuals grappling with infertility now have the opportunity to conceive biological offspring through in vitro fertilization (IVF) and Intracytoplasmic Sperm Injection (ICSI). However, such procedures may entail implications for the offspring of these individuals.

Male Infertility Linked to Anomalies in the Chromosome

In instances where infertility stems from the deletion or microdeletion of the long arm of chromosome Y, as observed in isodicentric Yp, this genetic aberration is likely to be inherited by subsequent male offspring, resulting in infertility. The repercussions of such conditions may extend beyond male infertility, potentially leading to heightened risks for future offspring [61, 119]. For example, if infertility arises from a balanced translocation, there's an increased likelihood of passing on an unbalanced chromosome translocation to offspring, regardless of gender, which could manifest as medical or intellectual disabilities [3, 61, 120]. Males diagnosed with Klinefelter syndrome, characterized by 47,XXY or 47,XXY/46,XY chromosomal configurations, typically experience gonadal failure impacting both sperm production and testosterone synthesis, leading to azoospermia and hypomasculinization [3, 61, 120]. Nevertheless, documented cases exist where sperm retrieval from some 47,XXY males has been successful for subsequent ICSI procedures. Literature on the subject presents conflicting findings regarding the risk of aneuploidy in offspring conceived through ICSI from males with 47,XXY chromosomal composition, although existing case reports suggest a generally low risk [121]. Couples facing such circumstances should undergo genetic counseling to thoroughly explore available information, including the potential risk of fetal aneuploidy, along with options for preimplantation and prenatal diagnosis, supplemented with appropriate support and reassurance as needed [119, 121, 122].

Preimplantation and Prenatal Genetic Diagnosis

To mitigate the risk of conceiving an affected offspring, such as in the case of cystic fibrosis (CF), preimplantation genetic testing (PGT) may be considered. The use of PGT for detecting chromosome abnormalities (PGT-A) or single-gene disorders (PGT-D) has sparked significant discourse concerning its implications, including issues of sex selection, the safety of embryonic manipulation, and should be integral to genetic counseling sessions [121].

PGT typically involves several sequential steps: (I) undergoing in vitro fertilization (IVF) or Intracytoplasmic Sperm Injection (ICSI), followed by (II) the biopsy of embryonic cells—typically trophectoderm cells—for testing, and (III) conducting PGT (A or D) to selectively transfer an unaffected embryo. Over the past 25 years, PGT has been utilized, resulting in the birth of thousands of "PGD-babies." Although the reliability of genetic tests utilized in PGT is generally high, concerns persist regarding safety and accuracy, particularly concerning embryos with chromosome mosaicism [123].

Current knowledge suggests that while PGT may slightly decrease pregnancy rates, it does not correlate with an increased incidence of congenital abnormalities or developmental delays in resulting children [121, 123, 124]. However, the potential for diagnostic inaccuracies, especially concerning PGT-A's reduced chromosome resolution compared to microarray analysis from chorionic villus sampling (CVS) and amniocentesis, should be discussed during counseling sessions. Additionally, the option of CVS/amniocentesis, along with the minimal risk of miscarriage associated with these procedures, must be carefully explained, weighing the benefits against the risks.

The possibility of no unaffected embryo being available for transplantation should be addressed upfront to manage expectations. In cases where female sex selection through PGT-A is deemed justifiable, especially for Y-linked genetic abnormalities, this option should be discussed with the patient or couple.

Through genetic counseling, clients or couples are empowered to make informed decisions aligned with their cultural, ethical values, and religious beliefs. This discussion should maintain a non-judgmental approach, fostering shared decision-making [125].

Moreover, the option of prenatal diagnosis via CVS and amniocentesis should be explored, alongside discussions regarding the timing and associated risk of miscarriage with each procedure.

Effects on Other Family Members

When a genetic diagnosis carries implications for other family members, genetic counseling offers guidance to the client or couple on how they might inform other at-risk individuals in the family. However, obstacles to communication with these at-risk family members may arise, such as loss of contact or feelings of stigma and guilt associated with harboring an underlying genetic condition, compounded by a desire to keep their reproductive issues private and avoid discussing them with other family members [126]. Genetic counseling aims to foster discussion regarding the importance of communicating the results to other family members and to assist in facilitating their decision-making process. Should the client or couple opt not to disclose this information, their privacy and autonomy remain prioritized over any obligation to disclose to at-risk relatives [126, 127].

Conclusion

Recent advancements in the understanding of NOA and idiopathic male infertility have been significantly driven by genetic research. Key genetic tests include karyotyping and screening for Y chromosome microdeletions as first-line tests, followed by microarray techniques and advances in NGS for more comprehensive insights. The potential benefits of an advanced genetic understanding includes early detection, diagnosis, and treatment. Early genetic testing can lead to the identification of the specific causes of infertility, enabling healthcare providers to tailor treatments more effectively. This approach not only increases the efficiency and efficacy of treatments but also potentially reduces costs by avoiding unnecessary procedures. Moreover, the impact on family planning and reproductive choices is significant. Genetic testing offers insights that can guide individuals and couples in making informed decisions about their reproductive futures. For instance, identifying genetic causes could facilitate a tailored decision-making between attempting sperm extraction, using donor gametes, or considering adoption. It also opens the door to the use of assisted reproductive technologies, such as preimplantation genetic diagnosis, to ensure the health and well-being of offspring. As research continues to unravel the genetic complexities of NOA and idiopathic male infertility, the horizon looks promising for early detection, precise diagnoses, and innovative treatments, ultimately enhancing the possibilities for family planning and the realization of reproductive goals.

References

1. Vander Borght M, Wyns C. Fertility and infertility: definition and epidemiology. Clin Biochem. 2018;62:2–10. https://doi.org/10.1016/j.clinbiochem.2018.03.012.
2. Cocuzza M, Alvarenga C, Pagani R. The epidemiology and etiology of azoospermia. Clinics (Sao Paulo). 2013;68((Suppl 1)):15–26. https://doi.org/10.6061/clinics/2013(sup01)03.
3. Krausz C, Riera-Escamilla A. Genetics of male infertility. Nat Rev Urol. 2018;15(6):369–84. https://doi.org/10.1038/s41585-018-0003-3.
4. de Kretser DM. Male infertility. Lancet. 1997;349(9054):787–90. https://doi.org/10.1016/s0140-6736(96)08341-9.
5. Neto FTL, Bach PV, Najari BB, Li PS, Goldstein M. Genetics of male infertility. Curr Urol Rep. 2016;17(10):70. https://doi.org/10.1007/s11934-016-0627-x.
6. Minhas S, Bettocchi C, Boeri L, et al. European Association of urology guidelines on male sexual and reproductive health: 2021 update on male infertility. Eur Urol. 2021;80(5):603–20. https://doi.org/10.1016/j.eururo.2021.08.014.
7. Pelzman DL, Hwang K. Genetic testing for men with infertility: techniques and indications. Transl Androl Urol. 2021;10(3):1354–64. https://doi.org/10.21037/tau-19-725.
8. Schlegel PN, Sigman M, Collura B, et al. Diagnosis and treatment of infertility in men: AUA/ASRM guideline part I. J Urol. 2021;205(1):36–43. https://doi.org/10.1097/ju.0000000000001521.
9. ISCN 2020. An international system for human cytogenomic nomenclature (2020). S.Karger AG; 2020.
10. Huang H, Chen J. Chromosome bandings. In: Cancer cytogenetics: methods and protocols; 2017. p. 59–66.
11. Schreck RR, Distèche CM. Chromosome banding techniques. Curr Protoc Hum Genet. 1994;4.2(1):1–4.2. 36.
12. Howe B, Umrigar A, Tsien F. Chromosome preparation from cultured cells. J Vis Exp. 2014;83:e50203. https://doi.org/10.3791/50203.
13. Foresta C, Ferlin A, Gianaroli L, Dallapiccola B. Guidelines for the appropriate use of genetic tests in infertile couples. Eur J Hum Genet. 2002;10(5):303–12. https://doi.org/10.1038/sj.ejhg.5200805.
14. Van Assche E, Bonduelle M, Tournaye H, et al. Cytogenetics of infertile men. Hum Reprod. 1996;11(Suppl 4):1–24; discussion 25–6. https://doi.org/10.1093/humrep/11.suppl_4.1.

15. Kuan LC, Su MT, Chen M, Kuo PL, Kuo TC. A dicentric Y chromosome resulting from pericentric inversion between the centromere and Yq heterochromatin. Taiwan J Obstet Gynecol. 2013;52(3):443–5. https://doi.org/10.1016/j.tjog.2013.06.006.
16. Silva M, de Leeuw N, Mann K, et al. European guidelines for constitutional cytogenomic analysis. Eur J Hum Genet. 2019;27(1):1–16. https://doi.org/10.1038/s41431-018-0244-x.
17. Johnson M, Raheem A, De Luca F, et al. An analysis of the frequency of Y-chromosome microdeletions and the determination of a threshold sperm concentration for genetic testing in infertile men. BJU Int. 2019;123(2):367–72. https://doi.org/10.1111/bju.14521.
18. de la Chapelle A. The etiology of maleness in XX men. Hum Genet. 1981;58(1):105–16. https://doi.org/10.1007/bf00284157.
19. Majzoub A, Arafa M, Starks C, Elbardisi H, Al Said S, Sabanegh E. 46 XX karyotype during male fertility evaluation; case series and literature review. Asian J Androl. 2017;19(2):168–72. https://doi.org/10.4103/1008-682x.181224.
20. Vorona E, Zitzmann M, Gromoll J, Schüring AN, Nieschlag E. Clinical, endocrinological, and epigenetic features of the 46,XX male syndrome, compared with 47,XXY Klinefelter patients. J Clin Endocrinol Metab. 2007;92(9):3458–65. https://doi.org/10.1210/jc.2007-0447.
21. Jungwirth A, Giwercman A, Tournaye H, et al. European Association of Urology guidelines on male infertility: the 2012 update. Eur Urol. 2012;62(2):324–32. https://doi.org/10.1016/j.eururo.2012.04.048.
22. Ventimiglia E, Capogrosso P, Boeri L, et al. When to perform karyotype analysis in infertile men? validation of the European Association of urology guidelines with the proposal of a new predictive model. Eur Urol. 2016;70(6):920–3. https://doi.org/10.1016/j.eururo.2016.06.015.
23. Bayani J, Squire JA. Fluorescence in situ Hybridization (FISH). Curr Protoc Cell Biol. 2004;Chapter 22:Unit 22.4. https://doi.org/10.1002/0471143030.cb2204s23.
24. Ioannou D, Fortun J, Tempest HG. Meiotic nondisjunction and sperm aneuploidy in humans. Reproduction. 2019;157(1):R15–r31. https://doi.org/10.1530/rep-18-0318.
25. Rawal L, Prabhash S, Kumar R, et al. 46,XX males with SRY gene translocation: cytogenetics and molecular characterization. J Rare Dis. 2024;3(1):1. https://doi.org/10.1007/s44162-023-00025-8.
26. Martin RH, Greene C, Rademaker AW, Ko E, Chernos J. Analysis of aneuploidy in spermatozoa from testicular biopsies from men with nonobstructive azoospermia. J Androl. 2003;24(1):100–3.
27. Egozcue S, Blanco J, Vendrell JM, et al. Human male infertility: chromosome anomalies, meiotic disorders, abnormal spermatozoa and recurrent abortion. Hum Reprod Update. 2000;6(1):93–105. https://doi.org/10.1093/humupd/6.1.93.
28. Hwang K, Weedin JW, Lamb DJ. The use of fluorescent in situ hybridization in male infertility. Ther Adv Urol. 2010;2(4):157–69. https://doi.org/10.1177/1756287210373758.
29. Rhie A, Nurk S, Cechova M, et al. The complete sequence of a human Y chromosome. Nature. 2023;621(7978):344–54. https://doi.org/10.1038/s41586-023-06457-y.
30. Skaletsky H, Kuroda-Kawaguchi T, Minx PJ, et al. The male-specific region of the human Y chromosome is a mosaic of discrete sequence classes. Nature. 2003;423(6942):825–37. https://doi.org/10.1038/nature01722.
31. Bonito M, D'Atanasio E, Ravasini F, et al. New insights into the evolution of human Y chromosome palindromes through mutation and gene conversion. Hum Mol Genet. 2021;30(23):2272–85. https://doi.org/10.1093/hmg/ddab189.
32. Navarro-Costa P, Gonçalves J, Plancha CE. The AZFc region of the Y chromosome: at the crossroads between genetic diversity and male infertility. Hum Reprod Update. 2010;16(5):525–42. https://doi.org/10.1093/humupd/dmq005.
33. Krausz C, Navarro-Costa P, Wilke M, Tüttelmann F. EAA/EMQN best practice guidelines for molecular diagnosis of Y-chromosomal microdeletions: State of the art 2023. Andrology. 2024;12(3):487–504. https://doi.org/10.1111/andr.13514.

34. Tiepolo L, Zuffardi O. Localization of factors controlling spermatogenesis in the nonfluorescent portion of the human Y chromosome long arm. Hum Genet. 1976;34(2):119–24. https://doi.org/10.1007/bf00278879.
35. Vogt PH, Edelmann A, Kirsch S, et al. Human Y chromosome azoospermia factors (AZF) mapped to different subregions in Yq11. Hum Mol Genet. 1996;5(7):933–43. https://doi.org/10.1093/hmg/5.7.933.
36. Kuroda-Kawaguchi T, Skaletsky H, Brown LG, et al. The AZFc region of the Y chromosome features massive palindromes and uniform recurrent deletions in infertile men. Nat Genet. 2001;29(3):279–86. https://doi.org/10.1038/ng757.
37. Vogt PH, Zimmer J, Bender U, Strowitzki T. AZFa candidate gene UTY and its X homologue UTX are expressed in human germ cells. Reprod Fertil. 2021;2(2):151–60. https://doi.org/10.1530/raf-20-0049.
38. Kamp C, Hirschmann P, Voss H, Huellen K, Vogt PH. Two long homologous retroviral sequence blocks in proximal Yq11 cause AZFa microdeletions as a result of intrachromosomal recombination events. Hum Mol Genet. 2000;9(17):2563–72. https://doi.org/10.1093/hmg/9.17.2563.
39. Repping S, Skaletsky H, Lange J, et al. Recombination between palindromes P5 and P1 on the human Y chromosome causes massive deletions and spermatogenic failure. Am J Hum Genet. 2002;71(4):906–22. https://doi.org/10.1086/342928.
40. Cioppi F, Rosta V, Krausz C. Genetics of azoospermia. Int J Mol Sci. 2021;22:6. https://doi.org/10.3390/ijms22063264.
41. Lo Giacco D, Chianese C, Sánchez-Curbelo J, et al. Clinical relevance of Y-linked CNV screening in male infertility: new insights based on the 8-year experience of a diagnostic genetic laboratory. Eur J Hum Genet. 2014;22(6):754–61. https://doi.org/10.1038/ejhg.2013.253.
42. Krausz C, Casamonti E. Spermatogenic failure and the Y chromosome. Hum Genet. 2017;136(5):637–55. https://doi.org/10.1007/s00439-017-1793-8.
43. Krausz C, Degl'Innocenti S. Y chromosome and male infertility: update, 2006. Front Biosci. 2006;11:3049–61. https://doi.org/10.2741/2032.
44. Kohn TP, Kohn JR, Owen RC, Coward RM. The prevalence of Y-chromosome microdeletions in oligozoospermic men: a systematic review and meta-analysis of European and North American studies. Eur Urol. 2019;76(5):626–36.
45. Olson M, Hood L, Cantor C, Botstein D. A common language for physical mapping of the human genome. Science. 1989;245(4925):1434–5. https://doi.org/10.1126/science.2781285.
46. Ghorbian S. Routine diagnostic testing of Y chromosome deletions in male infertile and subfertile. Gene. 2012;503(1):160–4. https://doi.org/10.1016/j.gene.2012.04.079.
47. Guo Q, Lan F, Xu L, et al. Quadruplex real-time polymerase chain reaction assay for molecular diagnosis of Y-chromosomal microdeletions. Fertil Steril. 2012;97(4):864–9. https://doi.org/10.1016/j.fertnstert.2012.01.088.
48. Kozina V, Cappallo-Obermann H, Gromoll J, Spiess AN. A one-step real-time multiplex PCR for screening Y-chromosomal microdeletions without downstream amplicon size analysis. PLoS One. 2011;6(8):e23174. https://doi.org/10.1371/journal.pone.0023174.
49. Osborne EC, Lynch M, McLachlan R, Trounson AO, Cram DS. Microarray detection of Y chromosome deletions associated with male infertility. Reprod Biomed Online. 2007;15(6):673–80. https://doi.org/10.1016/s1472-6483(10)60534-2.
50. Segat L, Padovan L, Doc D, et al. A real-time polymerase chain reaction-based protocol for low/medium-throughput Y-chromosome microdeletions analysis. Genet Test Mol Biomarkers. 2012;16(12):1349–55. https://doi.org/10.1089/gtmb.2012.0220.
51. Yuen RK, Merkoulovitch A, MacDonald JR, et al. Development of a high-resolution Y-chromosome microarray for improved male infertility diagnosis. Fertil Steril. 2014;101(4):1079–1085.e3. https://doi.org/10.1016/j.fertnstert.2013.12.027.

52. Okutman O, Muller J, Baert Y, et al. Exome sequencing reveals a nonsense mutation in TEX15 causing spermatogenic failure in a Turkish family. Hum Mol Genet. 2015;24(19):5581–8. https://doi.org/10.1093/hmg/ddv290.
53. Ghorbel M, Gargouri Baklouti S, Ben Abdallah F, et al. Chromosomal defects in infertile men with poor semen quality. J Assist Reprod Genet. 2012;29(5):451–6. https://doi.org/10.1007/s10815-012-9737-7.
54. Corona G, Pizzocaro A, Lanfranco F, et al. Sperm recovery and ICSI outcomes in Klinefelter syndrome: a systematic review and meta-analysis. Hum Reprod Update. 2017;23(3):265–75. https://doi.org/10.1093/humupd/dmx008.
55. Fullerton G, Hamilton M, Maheshwari A. Should non-mosaic Klinefelter syndrome men be labelled as infertile in 2009? Hum Reprod. 2010;25(3):588–97. https://doi.org/10.1093/humrep/dep431.
56. Levron J, Aviram-Goldring A, Madgar I, Raviv G, Barkai G, Dor J. Sperm chromosome analysis and outcome of IVF in patients with non-mosaic Klinefelter's syndrome. Fertil Steril. 2000;74(5):925–9. https://doi.org/10.1016/s0015-0282(00)01556-9.
57. Ozer C, Caglar Aytac P, Goren MR, Toksoz S, Gul U, Turunc T. Sperm retrieval by microdissection testicular sperm extraction and intracytoplasmic sperm injection outcomes in nonobstructive azoospermic patients with Klinefelter syndrome. Andrologia. 2018;50:3. https://doi.org/10.1111/and.12983.
58. Vloeberghs V, Verheyen G, Santos-Ribeiro S, et al. Is genetic fatherhood within reach for all azoospermic Klinefelter men? PLoS One. 2018;13(7):e0200300. https://doi.org/10.1371/journal.pone.0200300.
59. Greco E, Scarselli F, Minasi MG, et al. Birth of 16 healthy children after ICSI in cases of nonmosaic Klinefelter syndrome. Hum Reprod. 2013;28(5):1155–60. https://doi.org/10.1093/humrep/det046.
60. Stouffs K, Vloeberghs V, Gheldof A, Tournaye H, Seneca S. Are AZFb deletions always incompatible with sperm production? Andrology. 2017;5(4):691–4. https://doi.org/10.1111/andr.12350.
61. Flannigan R, Schlegel PN. Genetic diagnostics of male infertility in clinical practice. Best Pract Res Clin Obstet Gynaecol. 2017;44:26–37. https://doi.org/10.1016/j.bpobgyn.2017.05.002.
62. Jaruzelska J, Korcz A, Wojda A, et al. Mosaicism for 45,X cell line may accentuate the severity of spermatogenic defects in men with AZFc deletion. J Med Genet. 2001;38(11):798–802. https://doi.org/10.1136/jmg.38.11.798.
63. Le Bourhis C, Siffroi JP, McElreavey K, Dadoune JP. Y chromosome microdeletions and germinal mosaicism in infertile males. Mol Hum Reprod. 2000;6(8):688–93. https://doi.org/10.1093/molehr/6.8.688.
64. Patsalis PC, Skordis N, Sismani C, et al. Identification of high frequency of Y chromosome deletions in patients with sex chromosome mosaicism and correlation with the clinical phenotype and Y-chromosome instability. Am J Med Genet A. 2005;135(2):145–9. https://doi.org/10.1002/ajmg.a.30712.
65. Precone V, Cannarella R, Paolacci S, et al. Male infertility diagnosis: improvement of genetic analysis performance by the introduction of pre-diagnostic genes in a next-generation sequencing custom-made panel. Front Endocrinol (Lausanne). 2020;11:605237. https://doi.org/10.3389/fendo.2020.605237.
66. Sudhakar DVS, Shah R, Gajbhiye RK. Genetics of male infertility-present and future: a narrative review. J Hum Reprod Sci. 2021;14(3):217–27. https://doi.org/10.4103/jhrs.jhrs_115_21.
67. Salas-Huetos A, Aston KI. Defining new genetic etiologies of male infertility: progress and future prospects. Transl Androl Urol. 2021;10(3):1486–98. https://doi.org/10.21037/tau.2020.03.43.
68. Tüttelmann F, Ruckert C, Röpke A. Disorders of spermatogenesis: perspectives for novel genetic diagnostics after 20 years of unchanged routine. Med Genet. 2018;30(1):12–20. https://doi.org/10.1007/s11825-018-0181-7.

69. Oud MS, Volozonoka L, Smits RM, Vissers L, Ramos L, Veltman JA. A systematic review and standardized clinical validity assessment of male infertility genes. Hum Reprod. 2019;34(5):932–41. https://doi.org/10.1093/humrep/dez022.
70. Dada R, Kumar M, Jesudasan R, Fernández JL, Gosálvez J, Agarwal A. Epigenetics and its role in male infertility. J Assist Reprod Genet. 2012;29(3):213–23. https://doi.org/10.1007/s10815-012-9715-0.
71. Gunes S, Esteves SC. Role of genetics and epigenetics in male infertility. Andrologia. 2021;53(1):e13586. https://doi.org/10.1111/and.13586.
72. Han F, Jiang X, Li ZM, et al. Epigenetic inactivation of SOX30 is associated with male infertility and offers a therapy target for non-obstructive azoospermia. Mol Ther Nucleic Acids. 2020;19:72–83. https://doi.org/10.1016/j.omtn.2019.10.038.
73. Li Z, Huang Y, Li H, et al. Excess of rare variants in genes that are key epigenetic regulators of spermatogenesis in the patients with non-obstructive azoospermia. Sci Rep. 2015;5:8785. https://doi.org/10.1038/srep08785.
74. Rajender S, Avery K, Agarwal A. Epigenetics, spermatogenesis and male infertility. Mutat Res. 2011;727(3):62–71. https://doi.org/10.1016/j.mrrev.2011.04.002.
75. Rotondo JC, Lanzillotti C, Mazziotta C, Tognon M, Martini F. Epigenetics of male infertility: the role of DNA methylation. Front Cell Dev Biol. 2021;9:689624. https://doi.org/10.3389/fcell.2021.689624.
76. Moore LD, Le T, Fan G. DNA methylation and its basic function. Neuropsychopharmacology. 2013;38(1):23–38. https://doi.org/10.1038/npp.2012.112.
77. Gkountela S, Zhang Kelvin X, Shafiq Tiasha A, et al. DNA demethylation dynamics in the human prenatal germline. Cell. 2015;161(6):1425–36. https://doi.org/10.1016/j.cell.2015.05.012.
78. Hajkova P, Erhardt S, Lane N, et al. Epigenetic reprogramming in mouse primordial germ cells. Mech Dev. 2002;117(1–2):15–23. https://doi.org/10.1016/s0925-4773(02)00181-8.
79. Di Persio S, Leitão E, Wöste M, et al. Whole-genome methylation analysis of testicular germ cells from cryptozoospermic men points to recurrent and functionally relevant DNA methylation changes. Clin Epigenetics. 2021;13(1):160. https://doi.org/10.1186/s13148-021-01144-z.
80. Ferfouri F, Boitrelle F, Ghout I, et al. A genome-wide DNA methylation study in azoospermia. Andrology. 2013;1(6):815–21. https://doi.org/10.1111/j.2047-2927.2013.00117.x.
81. Poplinski A, Tüttelmann F, Kanber D, Horsthemke B, Gromoll J. Idiopathic male infertility is strongly associated with aberrant methylation of MEST and IGF2/H19 ICR1. Int J Androl. 2010;33(4):642–9. https://doi.org/10.1111/j.1365-2605.2009.01000.x.
82. Tang Q, Pan F, Yang J, et al. Idiopathic male infertility is strongly associated with aberrant DNA methylation of imprinted loci in sperm: a case-control study. Clin Epigenetics. 2018;10(1):134. https://doi.org/10.1186/s13148-018-0568-y.
83. Uysal F, Akkoyunlu G, Ozturk S. Decreased expression of DNA methyltransferases in the testes of patients with non-obstructive azoospermia leads to changes in global DNA methylation levels. Reprod Fertil Dev. 2019;31(8):1386–94. https://doi.org/10.1071/rd18246.
84. Araujo TF, Friedrich C, Grangeiro CHP, et al. Sequence analysis of 37 candidate genes for male infertility: challenges in variant assessment and validating genes. Andrology. 2020;8(2):434–41. https://doi.org/10.1111/andr.12704.
85. Uysal F, Sukur G, Cinar O. DNMT enzymes differentially alter global DNA methylation in a stage-dependent manner during spermatogenesis. Andrologia. 2022;54(4):e14357. https://doi.org/10.1111/and.14357.
86. Huang JX, Scott MB, Pu XY, Zhou-Cun A. Association between single-nucleotide polymorphisms of DNMT3L and infertility with azoospermia in Chinese men. Reprod Biomed Online. 2012;24(1):66–71. https://doi.org/10.1016/j.rbmo.2011.09.004.
87. Marques CJ, Francisco T, Sousa S, Carvalho F, Barros A, Sousa M. Methylation defects of imprinted genes in human testicular spermatozoa. Fertil Steril. 2010;94(2):585–94. https://doi.org/10.1016/j.fertnstert.2009.02.051.

88. Marques PI, Fernandes S, Carvalho F, Barros A, Sousa M, Marques CJ. DNA methylation imprinting errors in spermatogenic cells from maturation arrest azoospermic patients. Andrology. 2017;5(3):451–9. https://doi.org/10.1111/andr.12329.
89. Cannarella R, Crafa A, Condorelli RA, Mongioì LM, La Vignera S, Calogero AE. Relevance of sperm imprinted gene methylation on assisted reproductive technique outcomes and pregnancy loss: a systematic review. Syst Biol Reprod Med. 2021;67(4):251–9. https://doi.org/10.1080/19396368.2021.1909667.
90. Dhillon VS, Shahid M, Husain SA. Associations of MTHFR DNMT3b 4977 bp deletion in mtDNA and GSTM1 deletion, and aberrant CpG Island hypermethylation of GSTM1 in non-obstructive infertility in Indian men. Mol Hum Reprod. 2007;13(4):213–22. https://doi.org/10.1093/molehr/gal118.
91. Ramasamy R, Ridgeway A, Lipshultz LI, Lamb DJ. Integrative DNA methylation and gene expression analysis identifies discoidin domain receptor 1 association with idiopathic nonobstructive azoospermia. Fertil Steril. 2014;102(4):968–973.e3. https://doi.org/10.1016/j.fertnstert.2014.06.028.
92. Wu W, Shen O, Qin Y, et al. Idiopathic male infertility is strongly associated with aberrant promoter methylation of methylenetetrahydrofolate reductase (MTHFR). PLoS One. 2010;5(11):e13884. https://doi.org/10.1371/journal.pone.0013884.
93. Tang Q, Wu W, Lu Y, et al. Joint analysis of m(6)A and mRNA expression profiles in the testes of idiopathic nonobstructive azoospermia patients. Front Endocrinol (Lausanne). 2022;13:1063929. https://doi.org/10.3389/fendo.2022.1063929.
94. Govin J, Caron C, Lestrat C, Rousseaux S, Khochbin S. The role of histones in chromatin remodelling during mammalian spermiogenesis. Eur J Biochem. 2004;271(17):3459–69. https://doi.org/10.1111/j.1432-1033.2004.04266.x.
95. Luense LJ, Wang X, Schon SB, et al. Comprehensive analysis of histone post-translational modifications in mouse and human male germ cells. Epigenetics Chromatin. 2016;9:24. https://doi.org/10.1186/s13072-016-0072-6.
96. Wang T, Gao H, Li W, Liu C. Essential role of histone replacement and modifications in male fertility. Front Genet. 2019;10:962. https://doi.org/10.3389/fgene.2019.00962.
97. Ueda J, Harada A, Urahama T, et al. Testis-specific histone variant H3t gene is essential for entry into spermatogenesis. Cell Rep. 2017;18(3):593–600. https://doi.org/10.1016/j.celrep.2016.12.065.
98. Shiraishi K, Shindo A, Harada A, et al. Roles of histone H3.5 in human spermatogenesis and spermatogenic disorders. Andrology. 2018;6(1):158–65. https://doi.org/10.1111/andr.12438.
99. Shogren-Knaak M, Ishii H, Sun JM, Pazin MJ, Davie JR, Peterson CL. Histone H4-K16 acetylation controls chromatin structure and protein interactions. Science. 2006;311(5762):844–7. https://doi.org/10.1126/science.1124000.
100. Kleiman SE, Bar-Shira Maymon B, Hauser R, et al. Histone H4 acetylation and AZFc involvement in germ cells of specimens of impaired spermatogenesis. Fertil Steril. 2008;89(6):1728–36. https://doi.org/10.1016/j.fertnstert.2007.05.068.
101. Hashemi MS, Mozdarani H, Ghaedi K, Nasr-Esfahani MH. Expression of ZMYND15 in testes of azoospermic men and association with sperm retrieval. Urology. 2018;114:99–104. https://doi.org/10.1016/j.urology.2017.12.023.
102. Eelaminejad Z, Favaedi R, Modarresi T, Sabbaghian M, Sadighi Gilani MA, Shahhoseini M. Association between JMJD1A expression and sperm retrieval in non-obstructive azoospermic patients. Cell J. 2018;19(4):660–5. https://doi.org/10.22074/cellj.2018.4409.
103. He C, Wang K, Gao Y, et al. Roles of noncoding RNA in reproduction. Front Genet. 2021;12:777510. https://doi.org/10.3389/fgene.2021.777510.
104. Zhang Q, Liu Z, Han X, et al. Circulatory exosomal tRF-Glu-CTC-005 and tRF-Gly-GCC-002 serve as predictive factors of successful microdissection testicular sperm extraction in patients with nonobstructive azoospermia. Fertil Steril. 2022;117(3):512–21. https://doi.org/10.1016/j.fertnstert.2021.11.010.

105. Finocchi F, Pelloni M, Balercia G, et al. Seminal plasma miRNAs in Klinefelter syndrome and in obstructive and non-obstructive azoospermia. Mol Biol Rep. 2020;47(6):4373–82. https://doi.org/10.1007/s11033-020-05552-x.
106. Lian J, Zhang X, Tian H, et al. Altered microRNA expression in patients with non-obstructive azoospermia. Reprod Biol Endocrinol. 2009;7:13. https://doi.org/10.1186/1477-7827-7-13.
107. Piryaei F, Mozdarani H, Sadighi Gilani MA, et al. Global analysis in nonobstructive azoospermic testis identifies miRNAs critical to spermatogenesis. Andrologia. 2023;2023:1–13.
108. Tang D, Huang Z, He X, et al. Altered miRNA profile in testis of post-cryptorchidopexy patients with non-obstructive azoospermia. Reprod Biol Endocrinol. 2018;16(1):78. https://doi.org/10.1186/s12958-018-0393-3.
109. Willems M, Devriendt C, Olsen C, et al. Micro RNA in semen/urine from non-obstructive azoospermia patients as biomarkers to predict the presence of testicular spermatozoa and spermatogonia. Life (Basel). 2023;13(3):616. https://doi.org/10.3390/life13030616.
110. Zhang HT, Zhang Z, Hong K, et al. Altered microRNA profiles of testicular biopsies from patients with nonobstructive azoospermia. Asian J Androl. 2020;22(1):100–5. https://doi.org/10.4103/aja.aja_35_19.
111. Abu-Halima M, Backes C, Leidinger P, et al. MicroRNA expression profiles in human testicular tissues of infertile men with different histopathologic patterns. Fertil Steril. 2014;101(1):78–86.e2. https://doi.org/10.1016/j.fertnstert.2013.09.009.
112. Fang N, Cao C, Wen Y, Wang X, Yuan S, Huang X. MicroRNA profile comparison of testicular tissues derived from successful and unsuccessful microdissection testicular sperm extraction retrieval in non-obstructive azoospermia patients. Reprod Fertil Dev. 2019;31(4):671–82. https://doi.org/10.1071/rd17423.
113. Kong X, Fei Q, Pan C, et al. LncRNA HOTAIR promotes proliferation and suppresses apoptosis of mouse spermatogonium GC-1 cells by sponging miR-761 to modulate NANOS2 expression. In Vitro Cell Dev Biol Anim. 2022;58(4):295–306. https://doi.org/10.1007/s11626-022-00657-y.
114. Statello L, Guo CJ, Chen LL, Huarte M. Gene regulation by long non-coding RNAs and its biological functions. Nat Rev Mol Cell Biol. 2021;22(2):96–118. https://doi.org/10.1038/s41580-020-00315-9.
115. Hu K, Li L, Liao Y, Liang M. LncRNA Gm2044 highly expresses in spermatocyte and inhibits Utf1 translation by interacting with Utf1 mRNA. Genes Genomics. 2018;40(7):781–7. https://doi.org/10.1007/s13258-018-0690-4.
116. Bo H, Liu Z, Tang R, et al. Testicular biopsies microarray analysis reveals circRNAs are involved in the pathogenesis of non-obstructive azoospermia. Aging (Albany NY). 2020;12(3):2610–25. https://doi.org/10.18632/aging.102765.
117. Sabetian S, Zarei M, Jahromi BN, Morowvat MH, Tabei SMB, Cava C. Exploring the dysregulated mRNAs-miRNAs-lncRNAs interactions associated to idiopathic non-obstructive azoospermia. J Biomol Struct Dyn. 2022;40(13):5956–64. https://doi.org/10.1080/07391102.2021.1875879.
118. Xie Y, Yao J, Zhang X, et al. A panel of extracellular vesicle long noncoding RNAs in seminal plasma for predicting testicular spermatozoa in nonobstructive azoospermia patients. Hum Reprod. 2020;35(11):2413–27. https://doi.org/10.1093/humrep/deaa184.
119. Wilkes S, Chinn DJ, Murdoch A, Rubin G. Epidemiology and management of infertility: a population-based study in UK primary care. Fam Pract. 2009;26(4):269–74. https://doi.org/10.1093/fampra/cmp029.
120. Feng HL. Molecular biology of male infertility. Arch Androl. 2003;49(1):19–27. https://doi.org/10.1080/01485010290031556-1.
121. Geraedts JP, De Wert GM. Preimplantation genetic diagnosis. Clin Genet. 2009;76(4):315–25. https://doi.org/10.1111/j.1399-0004.2009.01273.x.
122. Resta R, Biesecker BB, Bennett RL, et al. A new definition of genetic counseling: National Society of Genetic Counselors' Task Force report. J Genet Couns. 2006;15(2):77–83. https://doi.org/10.1007/s10897-005-9014-3.

123. Liebaers I, Desmyttere S, Verpoest W, et al. Report on a consecutive series of 581 children born after blastomere biopsy for preimplantation genetic diagnosis. Hum Reprod. 2010;25(1):275–82. https://doi.org/10.1093/humrep/dep298.
124. De Wert G, Dondorp W, Shenfield F, et al. ESHRE task force on ethics and Law22: preimplantation genetic diagnosis. Hum Reprod. 2014;29(8):1610–7. https://doi.org/10.1093/humrep/deu132.
125. Helmes AW, Bowen DJ, Bengel J. Patient preferences of decision-making in the context of genetic testing for breast cancer risk. Genet Med. 2002;4(3):150–7. https://doi.org/10.1097/00125817-200205000-00009.
126. ASHG statement. Professional disclosure of familial genetic information. The American Society of Human Genetics Social Issues Subcommittee on Familial Disclosure. Am J Hum Genet. 1998;62(2):474–83.
127. Lacroix M, Nycum G, Godard B, Knoppers BM. Should physicians warn patients' relatives of genetic risks? CMAJ. 2008;178(5):593–5. https://doi.org/10.1503/cmaj.070956.

Chapter 4
Advances in the Diagnosis of Obstructive Azoospermia

Matthew Chabot, Ana Puigvert, and Amarnath Rambhatla

Introduction

Infertility, defined as a couple's inability to achieve pregnancy after >12 months of regular unprotected intercourse, affects approximately 17.5% of couples worldwide, with male factor contributing in up to 30–50% of those cases [1]. Among men presenting for infertility evaluation, azoospermia is present in 5–15% of cases and can be due to either obstructive (OA) or non-obstructive (NOA) causes [2, 3]. Azoospermia is defined as the absence of sperm in the pellet of a centrifuged ejaculated sample [4]. Obstructive Azoospermia (OA) accounts for approximately 40% of infertile men with azoospermia, and it can be caused by congenital and acquired conditions [3]. In this chapter, we will review both genetic and acquired causes of obstructive azoospermia, patient presentation, and associated work-up including recent advances, as well as treatment options.

All images provided by Dr. Ana Puigvert, who provided permission for their use in this chapter.

M. Chabot (✉) ·
University of Massachusetts Chan Medical School, Worcester, MA, USA
e-mail: matthew.chabot3@umassmemorial.org

A. Puigvert
Quiron Hospital, Barcelona, Spain

A. Rambhatla
Vattikuti Urology Institute, Henry Ford Health, Detroit, MI, USA
e-mail: arambha1@hfhs.org

E. Chung et al. (eds.), *Advances in Andrology*,
https://doi.org/10.1007/978-3-032-29112-7_4

Clinical Presentation/Work-Up

The work-up of any male patient with azoospermia should include a detailed history and physical examination. It is imperative to determine if azoospermia is due to an obstructive or non-obstructive etiology. Key factors differentiating OA from NOA are listed in Table 4.1 [5].

Important details in the history include prior medical conditions or surgeries that could cause a subsequent obstruction along the male genitourinary tract. Important history items include a prior history of vasectomy, prior scrotal surgery including hydrocelectomy, scrotal trauma, prior inguinal/hernia surgery, a history of prior epididymal/testicular infection, and chronic pulmonary infection. History should also focus on sexual and reproductive history, including any prior pregnancies, changes to the quantity of ejaculate, as well as any pain with ejaculation, as this may point to an Ejaculatory Duct Obstruction (EDO).

Physical exam should include a detailed examination of the scrotum and testicles with particular focus on testicular size, presence of epididymal fullness/induration, presence of bilateral vasa, as well as any vasal gaps or irregularities to indicate prior vasectomy, presence of varicocele, and a detailed examination of the scrotal and abdominal skin for prior surgical scars. Penile examination should include assessment of the meatus to ensure an orthotopic position, as well as assessment of the foreskin to rule out the presence of phimosis. A prostate examination should be considered in suspected cases of EDO.

Table 4.1 Features of obstructive azoospermia and non-obstructive azoospermia

	Obstructive azoospermia	Non-obstructive azoospermia
Physical exam	Normal testicular volume	Small volume testicle <16 mL
	Dilated epididymis	Testicular length <4.6 cm
	Absent or atretic vas	
	Dilated seminal vesical	
Laboratory evaluation	Normal FSH/LH	Elevated FSH (testicular failure)
	Normal testosterone	Low FSH (hypogonadotropic hypogonadism)
	Normal prolactin	Low testosterone
		Normal or elevated prolactin
Semen analysis	Low ejaculate volume <1.4 mL	Normal ejaculate volume >1.4 mL
	Azoospermia	Azoospermia
	Acidic pH	Normal pH >7

Adapted from Hubbard et al. [5]
Abbreviations: *FSH* follicle-stimulating hormone, *LH* luteinizing hormone

Causes of Obstructive Azoospermia

During work-up of the patient with a diagnosis of obstructive azoospermia, it is important to distinguish between congenital causes of OA and acquired causes of OA.

Acquired Causes of OA

The most common cause of acquired obstructive azoospermia is prior vasectomy [3]. A total of 500,000 vasectomies are performed in the United States each years [6] and the rate of vasectomy has been rising in recent years [7, 8]. Up to 6% of men who undergo a vasectomy will ultimately seek a vasectomy reversal [3]. Other common iatrogenic causes include vasal obstruction secondary to inguinal hernia repair with mesh in both the pediatric and adult population [9] and hydrocelectomy [10].

Infectious causes of obstructive azoospermia include recurrent epididymitis or epididymoorchitis, as well as prostatitis. Chronic inflammation from recurrent infection may lead to scarring of the epididymis or vas deferens, thus causing obstruction and subsequent azoospermia. An infectious etiology may be found in up to 6–44% of patients with azoospermia due to obstruction [11].

EDO is present in 5% of azoospermic men [3]. This may be caused by prior catheterization or transurethral procedures, trauma, infections, or compression from congenital prostatic or seminal vesicle cysts. Semen analysis in cases of EDO typically reveals low-volume semen (<1.5 mL), with acidic pH, and absent fructose due to absence of seminal fluid contribution, with patients at times experiencing hematospermia or pain with ejaculation [12].

Other important etiologies of acquired OA include prior genitourinary tract trauma and idiopathic OA.

Congenital Causes of OA

Congenital causes of OA include congenital unilateral (CUAVD) or bilateral absence (CBAVD) of the vas deferens, with CBAVD present in 1–2% of men presenting with subfertility [13]. ~75% of men with CBAVD are found to be carriers for Cystic Fibrosis Transmembrane Conductance Regulator (CFTR) gene mutations, while >95% of men with Cystic Fibrosis (CF) have CBAVD [3].

Cystic Fibrosis (CF) is an autosomal recessive disease affecting approximately 1:2000 newborns, most frequently in those of European descent [13]. Clinical manifestations include chronic airway disease, male infertility, pancreatic insufficiency, and high chloride concentration of sweat [14, 15].

The CFTR gene contains 27 exons and is located on chromosome 7q31.2; it encodes for a transmembrane protein which acts as a chloride channel [13, 16]. This is expressed in exocrine glands including the pancreas, lungs, sweat glands, and vas deferens [16]. Over 2000 mutations of the CFTR gene have been reported [17]. The most common mutations include the F508del, the 5T, 7T, and 9T variants [3].

CF genetic testing should be performed when the physical exam identifies either a unilateral or bilateral absence of the vas to determine if the patient is a carrier of CFTR gene mutations. In addition, the female partner should be tested and undergo genetic counseling prior to Assisted Reproductive Technology (ART), as CF gene mutations may be passed on to future offspring.

In cases of CUAVD, renal imaging with ultrasound is indicated as there is an association with ipsilateral renal agenesis in 20–40% of men with CUAVD [18].

Young's syndrome is a rare, inherited genetic disorder causing chronic rhinosinusitis, bronchiectasis, and obstructive azoospermia. Patients with this syndrome tend to produce thick, viscous mucus. While the clinical picture is similar to Kartagener Syndrome (KS), patients with Young's syndrome have normal spermatogenesis but with an obstructive azoospermia due to epididymal obstruction from thick secretions. Diagnosis is based on clinical evaluation, along with the exclusion of CF and KS. While the exact cause of Young's syndrome is not known, there is an association with mercury exposure [19].

Semen, Hormonal, and Genetic Testing

Laboratory evaluation includes at least 2 separate semen analysis with confirmation of azoospermia on centrifuged specimen [4]. Based on the location of the obstruction, total semen volume may be normal (for a bilateral proximal obstruction) or may be reduced <1.5 mL for a more distal obstruction at the level of the ejaculatory ducts, for example.

Additional semen testing on semen analysis includes semen pH and fructose. In cases of ejaculatory duct obstruction, semen analysis will reveal acidic pH and negative fructose due to obstruction of seminal vesicle fluid.

Hormonal evaluation includes FSH and testosterone to confirm normal testicular function, which is expected in cases of obstructive azoospermia. If FSH >7.6 and testicular size is less than 4.6 cm in the long axis, then NOA should be considered. In some instances, primary testicular failure is observed, and in these cases, testosterone is usually less than 300 ng/dL. In equivocal cases when the diagnosis of NOA versus OA is not clear, a testicular biopsy may be considered to assess for presence of normal spermatogenesis.

Genetic testing in cases of OA is typically only indicated when a unilateral or bilateral absence of the vas deferens is identified on physical exam. In these cases, evaluation for possible CFTR gene mutations should be completed to determine if the patient is a carrier of CF. If the patient is positive for this mutation, the female partner should then be tested and undergo genetic counseling prior to ART, as these gene mutations may be passed on to potential offspring causing cystic fibrosis. Further genetic testing, including karyotype and Y-chromosome microdeletion testing, is reserved for suspected cases of NOA.

Imaging

Certain imaging modalities may be utilized to confirm findings in cases of suspected obstructive azoospermia.

Scrotal ultrasound is not typically utilized in the work-up of patients with OA. It may be used to confirm physical exam findings, such as atresia or absence of epididymal segments or the vas deferens, in select cases.

Transrectal ultrasound is an effective method to evaluate for ejaculatory duct obstruction. Findings to indicate obstruction may include dilated seminal vesicles with diameter >1.5 cm or ejaculatory duct diameter >2.3 mm [12]. Other findings on TRUS to indicate an obstructive process include the presence of prostatic cysts, seminal vesicle cysts, or ejaculatory duct stones/calcification. At the time of TRUS, the seminal vesicle may be aspirated under imaging guidance; the presence of sperm in a dilated seminal vesicle (but oligo or azoospermia in the ejaculate) may confirm a diagnosis of ejaculatory duct obstruction.

Ejaculatory duct obstruction may be due to cysts, ductal atresia or stenosis, or from acquired conditions including inflammation, infection, iatrogenic causes such as prior surgical procedures or catheterization, or even ejaculatory stones. Ejaculatory duct cysts will present as cystic lesions within the prostate with low signal intensity on T1 and high signal intensity on T2-weighted imaging [20].

Pelvic MRI may also be utilized in cases of suspected obstructive azoospermia, particularly in patients who are unable to tolerate or wish to avoid transrectal ultrasound. Findings on MRI may include seminal vesicle dilation or cyst, seminal vesicle agenesis, or prostatic cyst.

Unilateral congenital SV cysts may be associated with ipsilateral renal agenesis in Zinner's Syndrome, while bilateral SV cysts may be associated with ADPKD.

Other findings on MRI causing obstructive azoospermia may include mullerian duct cysts located near the verumontanum, and prostatic utricle cysts located in the midline and communicating with the posterior urethra or ejaculatory duct (Fig. 4.1) [20].

Diagnostic vasography and vesiculography had previously been utilized to assess vasal or SV obstruction. These imaging studies are useful to identify the exact location of obstruction if a reconstructive surgery is being considered. The procedure includes isolation of the vas deferens typically through a small scrotal incision, catheterization of the vas with a small angiocath, and injection of contrast media [21]. With the availability of MRI, however, this imaging modality has largely fallen out of favor given its invasiveness. Vasography may be utilized, however, during reconstructive surgery procedures to assess for vasal patency at the time of vasovasostomy or vasoepididymostomy (Figs. 4.2, 4.3, 4.4, and 4.5).

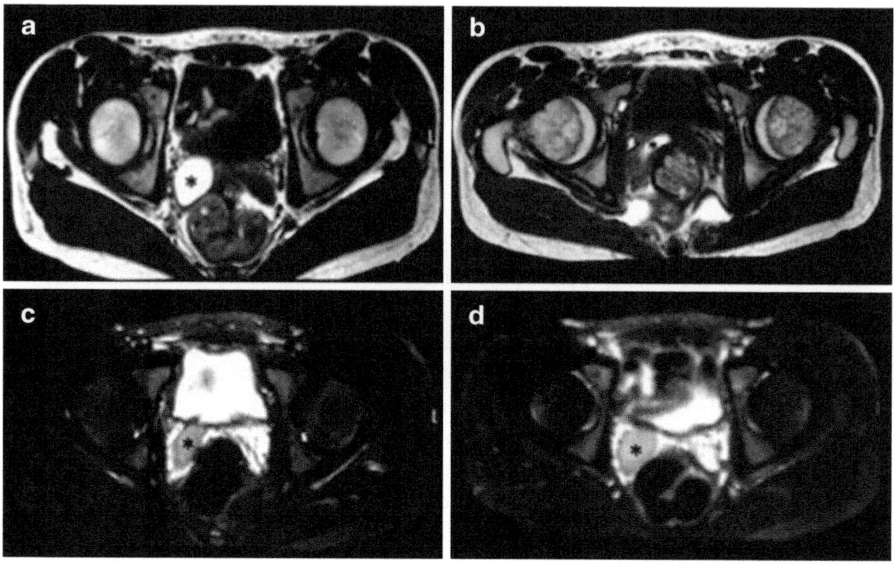

Fig. 4.1 MRI demonstrating large SV cyst

Fig. 4.2 Vasography demonstrating distal vasal obstruction

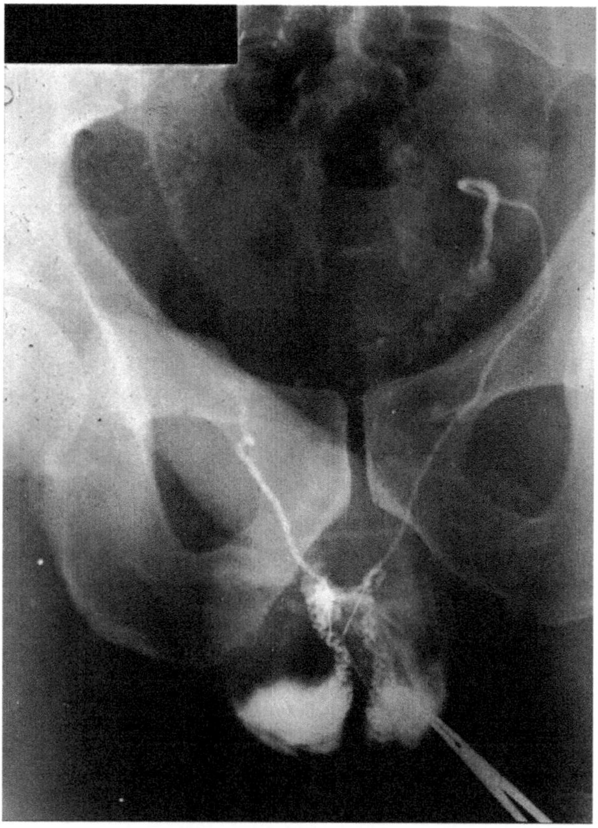

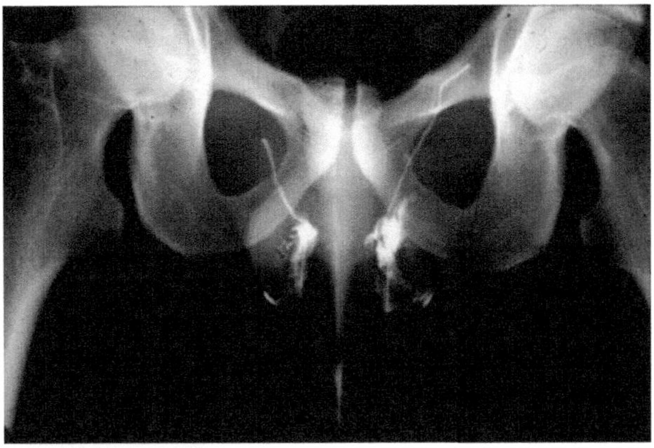

Fig. 4.3 Vasography demonstrating bilateral vasal obstruction after herniorrhaphy

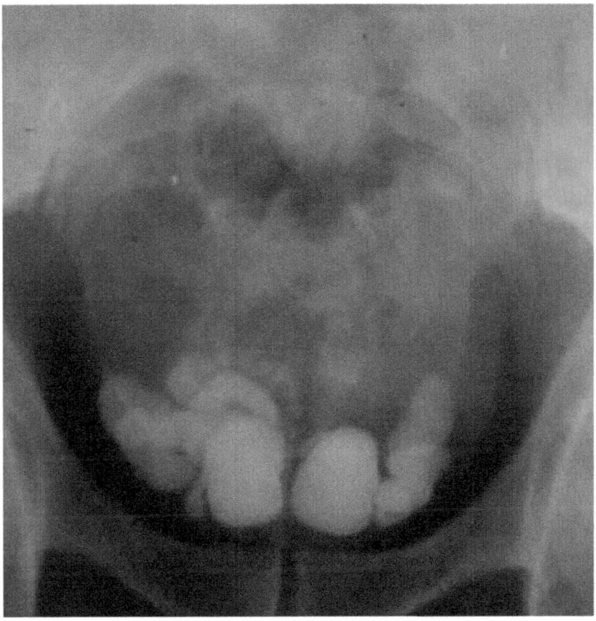

Fig. 4.4 Ejaculatory duct obstruction

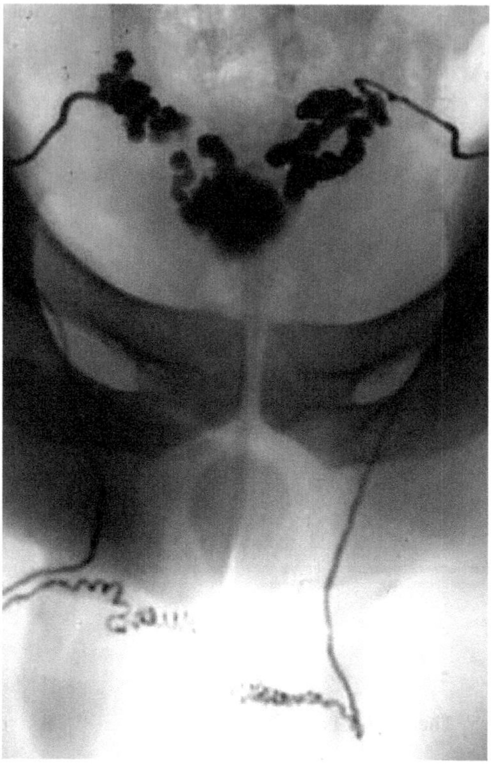

Fig. 4.5 Large prostatic cyst causing bilateral obstruction

Advances in OA Diagnosis

Proteomic Biomarkers

There have been recent developments in the discovery of Seminal Plasma (SP) proteins which can serve as biomarkers in the work-up of infertile patients. The testis-specific protein TEX101 and the epididymis-specific ECM1 have specifically been identified and validated as specific biomarkers for the diagnosis of OA versus NOA [22, 23].

A study by Korbakis et al. compared SP samples from healthy men pre-vasectomy, post-vasectomy, and men referred for unexplained infertility. Levels of TEX101 protein were calculated in 805 SP samples. Levels were found to be elevated in all samples in the pre-vasectomy cohort ($N = 64$), but they were undetectable in the post-vasectomy cohort ($N = 57$) [24]; a cutoff value of TEX101 >0.9 ng/mL predicted pre- and post-vasectomy samples with 100% sensitivity and 100% specificity (95% CI 1.00–1.00).

When focusing on NOA versus OA/post-vasectomy samples, however, the use of TEX101 as a biomarker only demonstrated 32% sensitivity with 99% specificity. The authors therefore combined TEX101 with ECM1 and were able to improve the diagnostic sensitivity to 81% with 100% specificity at diagnosing NOA from OA/post-vasectomy samples [24]. While additional studies are needed, this development shows promise as a potential non-invasive means to diagnose OA from NOA without the need for testicular biopsy.

Circulating Extracellular Vesicle microRNAs

Extracellular Vesicles (EVs) are small spherical structures composed of a lipid bilayer membrane and play critical roles in regulating biologic and cellular-specific functions, including in spermatogenesis and sperm maturation [25]. MicroRNAs, small non-coding RNA segments, help to regulate gene expression via downregulation of signaling pathways [26], with altered miRNA expression found in infertile men.

A recent study by Qi et al. compared the isolated EV miRNA of men with NOA, OA, and normal fertility. Two specific miRNAs, that is, miR-513c-5p and miR-202-5p, were found to be upregulated in the EV miRNA of NOA patients as compared to OA patients [25]. Plasma expression of these 2 miRNAs were then compared among NOA and OA patients to determine predictive accuracy for diagnosis of NOA; miR-513c-5p demonstrated sensitivity 92.31% and specificity 95.24% ($p < 0.0001$), and miR-202-5p with sensitivity 92.31% and 100% specificity ($p < 0.0001$) [25]. Combining these factors with FSH levels, utilizing a binomial regression equation, was able to predict a diagnosis of OA versus NOA. While more research is needed in the utility of these EV miRNAs in diagnosis of OA versus NOA, they do show promise as a potential future non-invasive means of distinguishing causes of azoospermia without the need for more invasive testing or testicular biopsy.

Ultrasound Localization Microscopy

Ultrasound Localization Microscopy (ULM) provides detailed assessment of microvascular structure, including blood vessel diameter and blood velocity [27]. Though its use in other fields has been well established, thus far, its potential role in determining testicular microvasculature in cases of NOA and OA has not been well understood. A recent study by Li et al. aimed to better characterize testicular microvasculature using ULM in 94 infertile patients, including 36 patients with NOA and 58 patients with OA. Comparing ULM, there were significantly higher values in the OA group in terms of mean vessel diameter, vessel density, and fractal number. No significant difference was observed in mean velocity or mean tortuosity among the two groups [27]. When combining the mean diameter value calculated on ULM with serum FSH, the model yielded a sensitivity of 96.6% and specificity of 86.1%, with an overall accuracy of 92.6% for predicting either NOA or OA [27]. The detail of ULM may provide key insights into the vascular pressure and distribution within the testicles of azoospermic patients, and in combination with serum hormonal testing may provide additional non-invasive means for characterizing OA from NOA.

Imaging Techniques

MRI can be a useful tool in the evaluation of patients with azoospermia, and the use of Diffusion-Weighted Imaging (DWI) sequence in MRI can provide important functional information. The Apparent Diffusion Coefficient (ADC) has been calculated for other organs/body tissues, but new research is utilizing this important factor in evaluating both normal and abnormal testes.

Han et al. recently compared ADC values among 30 infertile men, 16 with OA and 14 with NOA who had all undergone prior testis biopsy during their infertility work-up. In examining testicular volumes, the median testis volume was 16.9 mL in the OA group and 8.1 mL in the NOA group ($p < 0.001$) [28], an expected difference given that testicular volume can generally reflect spermatogenesis and is expected to be higher in OA rather than NOA. Both ADC ($p = 0.0094$) and normalized ADC ($p < 0.001$) were significantly lower in the OA group of patients, and they were correlated with histopathologic grade of the biopsy specimen. In particular, a normalized ADC cutoff value of >0.425 predicted NOA from OA with sensitivity 78.57% and specificity 93.75% [28]. This demonstrates the utility of incorporating MRI into the work-up of patients with azoospermia, as calculated testicular volume, ADC, and normalized ADC may aid in distinguishing OA from NOA.

Treatment

Treatment options for patients with obstructive azoospermia are largely based on the etiology of their obstruction, as well as fertility potential and goals. Decisions should include consideration of the possibility of natural conception, female age and fertility potential, and cost.

For patients with iatrogenic obstruction after a vasectomy or with epididymal obstruction, reconstruction with a microsurgical Vasovasostomy (VV) or Vasoepididymostomy (VE) may be performed to restore vasal patency. At the time of vasal transection of the vasectomy site, expressed vasal fluid should be assessed both macroscopically and microscopically to determine which procedure (VV or VE) should be performed. Success rates of restoring sperm to the ejaculate after VV range from 70% to 99%, while success rates after VE range from 30% to 90% [29]. A saline vasogram should also be performed on the abdominal end to rule out possible distal obstruction prior to reconstruction.

For those patients with OA and normal spermatogenesis who are pursuing ART, either a Percutaneous Epidydymal Sperm Aspiration (PESA), Microsurgical Epididymal Sperm Aspiration (MESA), a Testicular Sperm Aspiration (TESA), or a Testicular Sperm Extraction (TESE) may be considered to extract viable sperm for use in IVF/ICSI.

These procedures may be performed under local anesthetic or under sedation based on patient and provider preference and anesthesia availability and cost. The scrotal skin is shaved and cleansed, then the area is draped with sterile drapes. Local anesthetic is then administered, including both a cord block in the ipsilateral spermatic cord and a skin block overlying the incision site.

If planning for a PESA, then testicle is stabilized by either the surgeon or an assistant. A 25-g butterfly needle attached to a 1-mL tuberculin syringe is then inserted into the caput of the epididymis. Negative pressure is applied to the needle until flow of epididymal fluid into the syringe is visualized, at which point the needle is slowly withdrawn. Care is taken to maintain negative pressure on the syringe as the needle is withdrawn, so as not to spill epididymal fluid. Aspirated fluid is then washed in IVF medium and may be examined microscopically for the presence of motile sperm. The procedure may be repeated until an adequate sample has been collected [30].

During a TESE procedure, a similar scrotal preparation and spermatic cord block is performed. The testicle is again stabilized, and local anesthetic is applied to the scrotal skin at the incision site. A small skin incision is then made in the scrotal skin. Dissection is carried down through the dartos until the tunica vaginalis is opened and the testicle is visualized. A small incision is then made in the tunica albuginea and seminiferous tubules are extruded. Samples of seminiferous tubules may then be collected, prepared in IVF medium, and microscopically examined for presence of sperm. Additional samples may then be collected until sufficient sperm has been collected. The testicle, tunica, dartos, and skin are then closed, ensuring adequate hemostasis. A scrotal supporter/dressing may then be applied to aid with post-operative pain or swelling.

Prior to any sperm extraction procedure, the serum FSH level should be checked to ensure adequate spermatogenesis. If serum FSH is >7.4, failure of spermatogenesis should be considered and may dictate further testing and/or extraction procedures.

Ejaculatory Duct Obstruction (EDO) is another cause of obstructive azoospermia. In cases of ejaculatory duct obstruction, a Transurethral Resection of the Ejaculatory Duct (TURED) may be performed to relieve obstruction and restore antegrade flow of semen.

At the time of TURED, a transrectal ultrasound probe is placed to assess for dilation of the SV. EDO is suspected if seminal vesicle width on TRUS is >1.5 cm, or the ejaculatory duct diameter is >2.3 mm [12]. Fluid is aspirated from the dilated SV and assessed under the microscope for the presence of motile sperm. Once sperm have been found, methylene blue is instilled into the dilated SV while concurrent cystoscopy at the level of the verumontanum is performed. Resection or dilation is then performed to relieve the obstruction until free flow of methylene blue is observed [12].

Success rates of TURED with improvement in sperm concentration and variables have been shown to be high, though they can be variable depending on the type of obstruction (94% improvement in partial obstruction and 59% improvement with complete obstruction) [31]. Spontaneous pregnancy rates are variable, with some studies showing only a 13% spontaneous pregnancy rate after the procedure [31].

Conclusion

In the work-up of the patient with azoospermia, it is important to distinguish obstructive from non-obstructive causes of azoospermia. Among men with OA, a stepwise approach can help delineate the cause of obstruction (either congenital or acquired), as well as the site of obstruction. Treatment options depend on the etiology and site of obstruction, as well as the patient/couple's ultimate fertility goals. Recent advancements in proteomic biomarker identification, circulating mRNA identification, and imaging techniques may help distinguish OA from NOA and may change the diagnostic algorithm in the future.

Bibliography

1. World Health Organization. Infertility prevalence estimates, 1990–2021. Geneva: World Health Organization; 2023.
2. AUA. The management of obstructive azoospermia: AUA best practice statement. Linthicum: American Urological Association Education and Research, Inc; 2010.
3. Wosnitzer M, Goldstein M. Obstructive azoospermia. Urol Clin N Am. 2014;41(1):83–95.
4. World Health Organization. WHO laboratory manual for the examination and processing of human semen. 6th ed. Geneva: World Health Organization; 2021.
5. Hubbard L, Rambhatla A, Colpi G. Differentiation between nonobstructive azoospermia and obstructive azoospermia: then and now. Asian J Androl. 2024;26:1–9.
6. Barone MA, Hutchinson PL, Johnson CH, et al. Vasectomy in the United States, 2002. J Urol. 2006;176:232.
7. Huang Z, Hyman M, Raheem O. Trends in the vasectomy rate among privately insured men aged 18–64 in the United States between 2014 and 2021. Urology. 2023;179:80–6.
8. Bole R, Lundy SD, Pei E, et al. Rising vasectomy volume following reversal of federal protections for abortion rights in the United States. Int J Impot Res. 2024;36:265–8.
9. Sheynkin Y, Hendin B, Schlegel P, Goldestein M. Microsurgical repair of iatrogenic injury to the vas deferens. J Urol. 1998;159(1):139–41.
10. Hopps C, Goldstein M. Microsurigcal reconstruction of iatrogenic injuries to the epididymis from hydrocelectomy. J Urol. 2006;176:2077–9.
11. Pilatz A, Kilb J, Kaplan H, et al. High prevalence of urogenital infection/inflammation in patients with azoospermia does not impede surgical sperm retrieval. Andrologia. 2019;51:10.

12. Avellino G, Lipshultz L, Sigman M, Hwang K. Transurethral resection of the ejaculatory ducts: etiology and surgical treatment options. Fertil Steril. 2019;111(3):427–43.
13. de Souza DAS, Faucz FR, Pereira-Ferrari L, Sotomaior VS, Raskin S. Congenital bilateral absence of the vas deferens as an atypical form of cystic fibrosis: reproductive implications and genetic counseling. Andrology. 2018;6(1):127–35.
14. White R, Woodward S, Leppert M, O'connell P, Hoff M, Herbst J, Lalouel JM, Dean M, Woude GV. A closely linked genetic marker for cystic fibrosis. Nature. 1985;318:382–4.
15. Welsh M, Smith E. Molecular mechanisms of CFTR chloride channel dysfunction in cystic fibrosis. Cell. 1993;73:1251–4.
16. Radpour R, Gourabi H, et al. Genetic investigations of CFTR mutations in congenital absence of vas deferns, uterus, and vagina as a cause of infertility. J Androl. 2008;29(5):506–13.
17. Cioppi F, Rosta V, Krausz C. Genetics of azoospermia. Int J Mol Sci. 2021;22(6):3264.
18. Bieth E, Hamdi S, Mieusset R. Genetics of the congenital absence of the vas deferns. Urology. 2021;140:59–76.
19. Mohammed SK, Jan A. Young syndrome. In: StatPearls. Treasure Island: StatPearls Publishing; 2025.
20. Wang H, Peng Y, Fu W, et al. MRI findings of obstructive azoospermia: lesion in and out of pelvic cavity. Abdom Radiol. 2020;45:851–64.
21. Payne SR, Pryor JP, Parks CM. Vasography, its indications and complications. Br J Urol. 1985;2:215–7.
22. Drabovich A, Jarvi K, Diamandis E. Verification of male infertility biomarkers in seminal plasma by multiplex selected reaction monitoring assay. Mol Cell Proteomics. 2011;10:12.
23. Drabovich AP, Dimitromanolakis A, Saraon P, Soosaipillai A, Batruch I, Mullen B, Jarvi K, Diamandis EP. Differential diagnosis of azoospermia with proteomic biomarkers ECM1 and TEX101 quantified in seminal plasma. Sci Transl Med. 2013;5(212):212ra160.
24. Korbakis D, Schiza C, Brinc D, et al. Preclinical evaluation of a TEX101 protein ELISA test for the differential diagnosis of male infertility. BMC Med. 2017;15:60.
25. Qi Y, Wu Y, Pang K, Cao Y, Li H, Qiao Y, Yuan D, Liu X, Li Z, Hu F, Yang W, Han C, Zhu Z. Profiling of circulating extracellular vesicle microRNAs reveals diagnostic potential and pathways in non-obstructive and obstructive azoospermia†. Biol Reprod. 2024;111(6):1297–310.
26. Moreno-Moya JM, Vilella F, Simon C. MicroRNA: key gene expression regulators. Fertil Steril. 2014;101(6):1516–23.
27. Li M, Zhang X, Yan J, Shu H, Li Z, Ye C, Chen L, Feng C, Zheng Y. Non-invasive ultrasound localization microscopy (ULM) in azoospermia: connecting testicular microcirculation to spermatogenic functions. Theranostics. 2024;14(13):4967–82.
28. Han BH, Park SB, Seo JT, Chun YK. Usefulness of testicular volume, apparent diffusion coefficient, and normalized apparent diffusion coefficient in the MRI evaluation of infertile men with azoospermia. AJR Am J Roentgenol. 2018;210(3):543–8.
29. Goldstein M, Shihua P, Matthews G. Microsurgical vasovasostomy: the microdot technique of precision suture placement. J Urol. 1998;159):1:188–90.
30. Shrivastav P, Nadkarni P, Wensvoort S, Craft I. Percutaneous epididymal sperm aspiration for obstructive azoospermia. Hum Reprod. 1994;9(11):2058–61.
31. Kadioglu A, Cayan S, et al. Does response to treatment of ejaculatory duct obstruction in infertile men vary with pathology? Fertil Steril. 2001;76(1):138–42.

Chapter 5
Novel Predictors of Successful Surgical Sperm Retrieval in Non-obstructive Azoospermia

Omer Raheem and Marwan Alkassis

Introduction

Surgical Sperm Retrieval (SSR) procedures play a critical role in male infertility treatment, particularly for men with azoospermia. The success of SSR depends on various factors, and recent research has focused on identifying novel predictors that can enhance the outcomes of these procedures. This chapter explores emerging predictors and contemporary advancement of successful SSR, such as molecular and imaging evaluations, and their implications in clinical practice. Patients undergoing sperm retrieval nurture hope of having their own biological children and would have undergone multiple investigations before retrieval. Success rates of sperm retrieval in non-obstructive azoospermia patients are about 50%. Hence, these predictors help in pre-procedure counseling and provide information for such couples, which helps set realistic expectations of treatment.

Traditional Predictors and Limitations

Historically, predictors such as patient age, testicular volume, serum hormone levels (e.g., FSH and Inhibin-B), and testicular histology have been used to assess the likelihood of successful sperm retrieval at the time of various Assisted Reproductive

O. Raheem (✉)
Cleveland Clinic Abu Dhabi, Abu Dhabi, UAE

Cleveland Clinic Lerner College of Medicine, Cleveland, OH, USA

M. Alkassis
Department of Urology, Hotel-Dieu De France University Hospital, Faculty of Medicine, Saint Joseph University of Beirut, Beirut, Lebanon

E. Chung et al. (eds.), *Advances in Andrology*,
https://doi.org/10.1007/978-3-032-29112-7_5

Treatments (ARTs) (AUA/ASRM guidelines 2011; [1, 3]). It has been found that young patients with high FSH values have lower chances of successful sperm retrieval. Testicular biopsies have been said to be the strongest predictors of successful retrieval. The presence of associated conditions like undescended testis could affect sperm retrieval chances. However, these traditional predictors have limitations in accurately predicting outcomes and guiding clinical decision-making for future ART. As a result, recent studies have focused on exploring novel avenues to identify more robust predictors of SSR.

Emerging and Novel Predictors of SSR Success

Genetic Markers

Genetic abnormalities, particularly Y-chromosome microdeletions, have been associated with impaired spermatogenesis and reduced SSR success rates. Specific deletions in the AZF (Azoospermia Factor) regions of the Y chromosome have been linked to non-obstructive azoospermia and poor sperm retrieval outcomes. Additional and more specific genetic abnormalities like Klinefelter Syndrome with its molecular variations have also been linked to poor SSR outcomes, guiding clinicians in patient selection and future treatment planning and offerings [4]. Comprehensive genetic screening panels can identify mutations in genes critical for spermatogenesis. Mutations in genes such as CFTR (Cystic Fibrosis Transmembrane Conductance Regulator) and SYCP3 (Synaptonemal Complex Protein 3) have been associated with impaired sperm production and reduced SSR success rates [5].

Given the association of azoospermia and severe oligospermia (<5 million) with genetic abnormalities, including mutations in the CFTR gene, Klinefelter syndrome (47,XXY), and the prevalence of microdeletions in the Azoospermic Factor (AZF) region of the long arm of the Y-chromosome (YCMD), genetic testing is strongly indicated for patients with azoospermia/severe oligospermia. Karyotyping and Y-chromosome microdeletion analysis can play a key role in the diagnostic workup and management of these patients. Specific to Y Chromosome Microdeletion (YCMD), there are three microdeletions (AZFa, AZFb, AZFc) on the long arm of the Y-chromosome that account for about 7% of cases of severe oligospermia/azoospermia in infertile male patients [14]. If an AZFc microdeletion is detected, microscopic Testicular Sperm Extraction (TESE) (micro-TESE) might be indicated, as micro-TESE yields a sperm retrieval rate of up to 70% in patients with AZFc microdeletions for future ART such as IVF and/or IVF/ICSI. However, for patients with AZFa or AZFb microdeletions or combination, the chances of surgical sperm retrieval through micro-TESE are virtually nonexistent and donor sperm is highly recommended as per AUA/ASRM guidelines. Given the close association of mutations in the CFTR gene and possible etiologies of obstructive azoospermia (CBAVD, CUAVD, and idiopathic epididymal obstruction), clinicians should consider referring patients with these conditions for genetic counseling. The AUA and ASRM recommend genetic testing to provide information on possible offspring transmission, which warrants the use of gene sequencing and carrier screening, including testing for the 5-thymidine (5T) allele of CFTR. If CFTR mutations are identified, preconception counseling should be offered to the patient and their partner to outline the risks of having a child with cystic fibrosis given the carrier status of the couple. Karyotyping should be considered during genetic evaluation given the association of chromosomal abnormalities in patients with male infertility. In particular, Klinefelter syndrome (47,XXY) is the most common chromosomal abnormality seen in infertile men, accounting for approximately 15% of non-obstructive azoospermia. Klinefelter syndrome has an incidence of 1 in 600 phenotypic males and presents clinically with small, firm testicles [15].

Other Mutations

NOA patients are assessed with karyotyping, Y-chromosome AZF region microdeletions, and in a few cases, gene sequencing to identify possible monogenic conditions. Identifying genetic alterations helps understand the effect on offspring. The possible outcomes of such changes, viz. infertility and miscarriages, should be discussed with the couple before starting assisted reproduction techniques.

M1AP gene (Meiosis 1-Associated Protein, OMIM: 619098) dysfunction results in primary testicular failure. Variations can cause cryptozoospermia and oligozoospermia. Biallelic variants in *TDRD9* (Tudor Domain-Containing Protein 9, OMIM: 617963) can cause maturation arrest in azoospermic males.

KASH5 mutations (Coiled-Coil Domain-Containing 155, OMIM: 618125) involve the LINC complex. It has been reported in consanguineous marriages.

The presence of Wilms Tumor 1 (*WT1*) gene, Kallmann syndrome (OMIM: 308700), and Fanconi anemia (OMIM: 227650) can all have azoospermia.

Hence, along with karyotyping, AZF microdeletion analysis, targeted gene assays must be the minimum required for genetic assessment. Whole-Exome Sequencing (WES) can comprehensively identify variations in genetic makeup more efficiently in the target genome. This could help predict the likelihood of successful sperm retrieval. Added to this is the advantage of informing the parents about possible genetic defects in children and options for prenatal testing through well-planned counseling. A thorough family history can be elicited and inheritance patterns understood.

Cell-free DNA (cfDNA) in semen can predict successful sperm retrieval better than cfRNA. High levels of cfDNA denote abnormal spermatogenesis and lower chances of retrieval. The use of cfDNA in practice is limited due to lack of validation and standardization, wide variation in cfDNA levels in multiple conditions, cost, and accessibility. In addition, sensitivity, specificity, and underlying biological mechanisms need to be completely understood. Proteonomics to identify testosterone, LH, FSH, LDHC (L Lactate Dehydrogenase C), PGK2 (Phosphoglycerate

Kinase 2), TKTL1 (Transketolase like protein 1), TEX101 (Testis expressed 101), ECM1 (Extracellular Matrix protein 1) need further research before they can be brought into practice. Use of microRNAs (miRNAs), messenger RNAs (mRNAs), circular RNAs (circRNAs), long non-coding RNAs (lncRNAs) through transcriptonomics is similarly limited in practice.

Hormonal Profiles

Recent studies have explored the role of hormonal markers beyond FSH in predicting SSR success. Inhibin-B and Anti-Müllerian Hormone (AMH) levels have been investigated as indicators of testicular function. Lower levels of inhibin-B and AMH are associated with compromised spermatogenesis and may predict poorer SSR outcomes [9]. AUA/ASRM guideline indicates that a higher FSH level than 7.6 may indicate lower SSR (AUA/ASRM 2011). Serum testosterone, prolactin, Luteinizing Hormone (LH) have not proven to be useful in predicting successful sperm retrieval. Testosterone to LH ratio needs more investigation. Among inflammatory markers, the Neutrophil to Lymphocyte Ratio (NLR) and systemic immune inflammation index were found to be better predictors than platelet to lymphocyte ratio for sperm retrieval in multiple studies.

Clinical Characteristics

The etiologies of azoospermia are characterized as obstructive/post-testicular non-obstructive/testicular. In obstructive azoospermia, there is adequate testicular sperm production in the setting of ductal obstruction. In non-obstructive azoospermia, sperm production is absent. The history, physical examination, hormonal studies, and imaging can help to differentiate between obstructive and non-obstructive azoospermia. It is worthwhile mentioning that semen volume, semen pH (alkaline vs acidic), and presence of fructose also aid in diagnosing azoospermia. The type of azoospermia (obstructive vs. non-obstructive) significantly influences SSR success rates. Obstructive azoospermia generally presents with higher success rates due to the presence of normal sperm production within the testes, whereas non-obstructive cases pose greater challenges [10]. Testicular non-obstructive azoospermia, which will present with endocrine abnormalities suggestive of hypergonadotropic hypogonadism, involves impaired spermatogenesis (as is the case in the genetic disorder Klinefelter syndrome [47,XXY]), undescended testes and/or testicular torsion, varicoceles, testicular cancer, and gonadotoxins. Although pre- and post-testicular azoospermia is often treatable, testicular causes currently lack effective reversible management options.

Most studies have shown that the age of the male is not important for SSR except in cases where orchidopexy was done. In such cases, orchidopexy done before the age of 10 years had higher chances of SSR. Only one study which conducted multiple logistic regression analysis concluded that age was a significant factor predicting SSR. In Klinefelter's syndrome, the highest sperm retrieval was found in the age group between 20 and 29 years. Obesity had no effect on SSR but had lower levels of clinical pregnancy rates. In patients with a history of cryptorchidism, higher retrieval rates were found in those who had orchidopexy before the age of 10 years, testicular volume greater than 13.75 mL, testosterone more than 300.5 ng/dL, and FSH less than 17.25 mIU/mL.

Semen Parameters

Although SSR is typically performed in cases of azoospermia, specific semen parameters such as ejaculated sperm count, motility, and morphology may provide insights into testicular function. Higher baseline semen parameters may indicate better sperm production within the testes, improving the likelihood of successful SSR [8].

Imaging Studies

Advanced imaging modalities like Magnetic Resonance Imaging (MRI) and ultrasound elastography offer detailed assessments of testicular architecture and tissue composition. These imaging techniques can aid in preoperative planning and predicting the presence of retrievable sperm [6].

Scrotal diffusion-weighted Magnetic Resonance Imaging (MRI) with normalized Apparent Diffusion Coefficients (ADCs) and proton magnetic resonance spectroscopy help differentiate non-obstructive and obstructive azoospermia, predict successful sperm retrieval, and other histological alterations in non-obstructive azoospermia. ADCs were higher in non-obstructive azoospermia, whereas choline and lipids were lower, with cutoff values being 0.353, 0.31, and 0.725. Lower normalized diffusion coefficient values predicted successful sperm retrieval. A study also revealed that testicular volumes below 7.2 mL on scrotal MRI suggested absence of sperms on mTESE. Lower ADC values of 1.12×10^{-3} mm^2/s and low Magnetic Transfer Ratio (MTR) of 46.5% may indicate spermatozoa after mTESE. Using the ADC histogram analysis, median ADC was the most useful to predict successful sperm retrieval. In addition to the above, Fractional Anisotropy (FA) and Normalized Metabolite Concentrations (NMCs) can be used to differentiate non-obstructive and obstructive azoospermia; however, they are not predictive for successful sperm retrieval. Diffusion tensor imaging sequence on MRI has not directly been found to be a predictor for sperm retrieval. It traditionally does qualitative and quantitative analysis by estimating direction and extent of water diffusion and derives parameters such as Mean Diffusivity (MD) and Fractional

Anisotropy (FA). Among the two, mean diffusivity was lower in those with unsuccessful sperm retrieval.

Traditionally, scrotal ultrasound is typically not recommended in the initial evaluation of male infertility as per AUA/ASRM guidelines. This is because a thorough history and physical examination can typically identify the most common scrotal pathologies accounting for an infertility factor, including the presence of varicoceles, absent vasa deferens, and testicular masses. Scrotal ultrasound might be indicated in patients who are difficult to examine because of body habitus, undescended testis, testicular pain, or for patients with risk factors for malignancy, and lately, with the emergence of telehealth. Scrotal ultrasound can be helpful in examining spermatic cord vasculature. However, scrotal ultrasound should not be routinely used to identify subclinical varicoceles as treatment of such varicoceles has little clinical utility. Traditionally, varicoceles are graded by size. Grade 0 varicoceles are subclinical and visible only via imaging; grade 1 varicoceles are palpable when patients perform the Valsalva maneuver; grade 2 varicoceles are palpable without the Valsalva maneuver; and grade 3 varicoceles are visible at rest. Transrectal Ultrasound (TRUS) is also not typically recommended as part of the initial workup for male infertility. However, in patients with possible ejaculatory duct, 772 Rama et al. obstruction per SA (with low semen volume, azoospermia, acidic SA, and fructose-negative), dilated seminal vesicles (>2.5 cm), and/or midline prostatic cysts can be identified by TRUS. In addition, cystoscopy evaluation of the lower urinary tract, including midline utricle cysts, ejaculatory duct obstruction, strictures or stones, and urethral or prostate scarring or strictures, can also be documented. Pelvic and renal ultrasound and/or cross-sectional abdominal imaging with CT/MRI can be particularly helpful in patients with suspected pelvic cystic abnormalities or vasal agenesis, given the high association of renal agenesis in disorders of vasal agenesis [13].

Doppler ultrasound studies assessing testicular blood flow have emerged as potential predictors of SSR success. Poor testicular perfusion, indicated by decreased blood flow, correlates with impaired spermatogenesis and lower chances of finding sperm during SSR procedures [7]. Testicular microlithiasis on ultrasound predicts low chances of sperm retrieval and has been proven in multiple studies.

ORBEYE is a new, 4K three-dimensional surgical exoscope or camera system that helps increase accuracy in surgical sperm retrieval. When placed over the surgical field, the operative image is projected on two 55-inch screens to be viewed using lightweight passive light 3D glasses. This eliminates the need to frequently reposition the scope when compared to the traditional microscopes due to wider field of view and longer depth of field. It is ergonomically better for surgeons since they do not have to stare at the eyepieces for long at awkward postures. Other team members can also view the procedure comfortably and learn at training centers.

Testis Mapping and Biopsy

Traditionally, a testicular biopsy is considered to differentiate between obstructive and NOA, albeit the recent AUA/ASRM guidelines do not recommend a diagnostic testicular biopsy [12] owing to heterogeneity of spermatogenesis in men with azoospermia. On the contrary, Fine-Needle Aspiration (FNA) testicular mapping has been popularized as an alternative diagnostic tool to stratify spermatogenesis in men with azoospermia based on the amount of sperm present or absent, early maturation arrest, and Sertoli cell-only syndrome finding. FNA testis mapping consists of 12–18 (depending on testis size) fine-needle aspiration sites to extract the seminiferous tubules. These are then analyzed by a cytopathologist to assess the presence or absence of sperm and other findings as above. Mapping can aid in localizing sperm for future sperm retrieval techniques by identifying spermatogenesis loci for successful sperm retrieval and thus minimizing invasiveness and long-term sequelae, such as hypogonadism. These digital "heat maps" created after FNAC have been found to be useful in patients who have failed mTESE in the past. Peripheral areas in the testis were more likely to harbor sperm than the central areas.

Sperm Retrieval Technique

The choice of SSR technique also influences success rates. Microdissection Testicular Sperm Extraction (Micro-TESE) has gained popularity for its ability to identify and extract sperm-containing tubules with higher precision compared to conventional TESE, resulting in improved SSR outcomes [11, 16–23].

Artificial Intelligence and Machine Learning

Artificial intelligence (AI) has gained importance in the recent past and has found a role in multiple fields. It is defined as "capability of an engineered system to acquire, process, and apply knowledge and skills." It utilizes algorithms from healthcare data analysis to improve outcomes. The interplay and advancements in medical information technology, computer science, robotics, and the demand for personalized medicine have brought AI into the forefront today. Machine Learning (ML), Deep Learning (DL), and Artificial Neural Networks (ANNs) are various AI applications that can be used in semen analysis, oocyte and embryo selection, decision systems and sperm selection. AI systems could predict fertility potential and sperm retrieval. Robotic-assisted micro-TESE has been performed safely in few centers. Using leptin and ANN, AI can increase the precision of sperm retrieval. ANN could use both clinical and imaging data to help improve sperm retrieval. These systems will only improve with time since they mature with use, taking in more data inputs and analysis. However, ethical and privacy considerations with incorporation of AI into andrology practice should be dealt with appropriately since such a framework is still to mature in most countries [24–35].

Clinical Implications and Future Directions

Understanding these emerging predictors of SSR success is crucial for optimizing patient selection and counseling. Tailoring SSR approaches based on individual patient characteristics and predictive markers can improve outcomes and reduce unnecessary procedures. Future research should focus on validating these predictors in larger cohorts and exploring additional biomarkers and imaging techniques to enhance SSR success rates further.

Conclusion

In conclusion, the identification of new predictors of successful surgical sperm retrieval represents a significant advancement in the field of male infertility treatment. Genetic markers, hormonal profiles, testicular blood flow assessments, and advanced imaging studies offer valuable insights into testicular function and aid in predicting SSR outcomes. Integrating these predictors into clinical practice can refine patient management strategies and ultimately improve the success rates of SSR procedures.

References

1. Schlegel PN, Sigman M, Collura B, De Jonge CJ, Eisenberg ML, Lamb DJ, et al. Diagnosis and treatment of infertility in men: AUA/ASRM guideline part I. Fertil Steril. 2021;115(1):54–61.
2. Schlegel PN, Sigman M, Collura B, De Jonge CJ, Eisenberg ML, Lamb DJ, Mulhall JP, Niederberger C, Sandlow JI, Sokol RZ, Spandorfer SD, Tanrikut C, Treadwell JR, Oristaglio JT, Zini A. Diagnosis and treatment of infertility in men: AUA/ASRM guideline PART II. J Urol. 2021;205(1):44–51.
3. Negri F, Boeri L, Cilio S, Pozzi E, Belladelli F, Corsini C, Raffo M, Fallara G, Ventimiglia E, Candela L, d'Arma A, Montorsi F, Salonia A. The importance of discordant follicle stimulating hormone and Inhibin B levels in primary infertile men: findings from a cross-sectional study. World J Mens Health. 2024;43(1):134–41.
4. Krausz C, Casamonti E. Y chromosome microdeletions: history, discovery, clinical significance and spermatogenesis. In: Krausz C, Casamonti E, editors. Genetic damage in human spermatozoa. Berlin/Heidelberg: Springer; 2014. p. 45–54.

5. Esteves SC, Agarwal A. Genetic testing in male infertility: insights into the clinical utility. In: Esteves SC, Agarwal A, editors. Clinical management of male infertility. Cham: Springer; 2016. p. 95–106.
6. Schurich M, Aigner F. Diagnostic imaging of the scrotum: ultrasound, MRI and CT. In: Schurich M, Aigner F, editors. Radiology of the male reproductive system. Berlin/Heidelberg: Springer; 2015. p. 91–105.
7. Cocci A, Capogrosso P. Ultrasonographic evaluation of testicular blood flow in infertile men. In: Sforza S, Colpi GM, editors. Testicular autoimmunity: a cause of male infertility. Cham: Springer; 2016. p. 143–53.
8. Esteves SC, Agarwal A. Insights into sperm retrieval techniques for Azoospermic males. In: Agarwal A, Esteves SC, Majzoub A, editors. Advances in assisted reproductive technologies. Cham: Springer; 2018. p. 141–60.
9. Foresta C, Ferlin A. The genetic basis of male infertility. In: Foresta C, Ferlin A, editors. Male infertility: understanding, causes and treatment. Cham: Springer; 2018. p. 53–66.
10. Ramasamy R, Schlegel PN. Obstructive azoospermia: role of microsurgery. In: Ramasamy R, Schlegel PN, editors. Microsurgery for male infertility. New York: Springer; 2013. p. 71–80.
11. Schlegel PN. Microdissection testicular sperm extraction: an overview. In: Schlegel PN, editor. Microsurgical treatment of male infertility. New York: Springer; 2012. p. 123–36.
12. Kapadia AA, Walsh TJ. Testicular mapping: a roadmap to sperm retrieval in nonobstructive azoospermia? Male Infertil. 2020;47(2):157–64.
13. Schlegel PN, Shin D, Goldstein M. Urogenital anomalies in men with congenital absence of the vas deferens. J Urol. 1996;155(5):1644–8.
14. Stahl PJ, Masson P, Mielnik A, et al. A decade of experience emphasizes that testing for Y microdeletions is essential in American men with azoospermia and severe oligozoospermia. Fertil Steril. 2010;94(5):1753–6. 47.
15. Ward WS. Function of sperm chromatin structural elements in fertilization and development. Mol Hum Reprod. 2010;16(1):30–6.
16. Aljubran A, Safar O, Elatreisy A, Alwadai R, Shalkamy O, Assiri HM, Eskander M, Arezki A, Ibrahim A. Factors predicting successful sperm retrieval in men with nonobstructive azoospermia: a single center perspective. Health Sci Rep. 2022;5(4):e727. https://doi.org/10.1002/hsr2.727. PMID: 35899179; PMCID: PMC9304940.
17. Qi L, Liu YP, Zhang NN, Su YC. Predictors of testicular sperm retrieval in patients with non-obstructive azoospermia: a review. J Int Med Res. 2021;49(4):3000605211002703. https://doi.org/10.1177/03000605211002703. PMID: 33794677; PMCID: PMC8020245.
18. Fontana L, Sirchia SM, Pesenti C, Colpi GM, Miozzo MR. Non-invasive biomarkers for sperm retrieval in non-obstructive patients: a comprehensive review. Front Endocrinol (Lausanne). 2024;15:1349000. https://doi.org/10.3389/fendo.2024.1349000. PMID: 38689732; PMCID: PMC11058837.
19. Yucel C, Keskin MZ, Cakmak O, Ergani B, Kose C, Celik O, Islamoglu E, Ucar M, Koc G, Kozacioglu Z. Predictive value of pre-operative inflammation-based prognostic scores (neutrophil-to-lymphocyte ratio, platelet-to-lymphocyte ratio, and monocyte-to-eosinophil ratio) in testicular sperm extraction: a pilot study. Andrology. 2017;5(6):1100–4. https://doi.org/10.1111/andr.12417. Epub 2017 Oct 9. PMID: 28992369.
20. Yavuz B, Emre T, Nesrin B, Ilker A, Cagatay T, Halime SC, Serdar A, Systemic immune-inflammation index, neutrophil-lymphocyte ratio and platelet-lymphocyte ratio are predictors of sperm presence in microdissection testicular sperm extraction. Andrologia. https://doi.org/10.1111/and.14419.
21. Althakafi SA, Mustafa OM, Seyam RM, et al. Serum testosterone levels and other determinants of sperm retrieval in microdissection testicular sperm extraction. Transl Androl Urol. 2017;6:282–7.
22. Kang C, Punjani N, Kashanian JA, Schlegel PN. Age, sperm retrieval, and testicular histology in Klinefelter syndrome. J Urol. 2024;211(1):163–9. https://doi.org/10.1097/JU.0000000000003737. Epub 2023 Oct 24. PMID: 37873937.

23. Çayan S, Orhan İ, Altay B, et al. Fertility outcomes and predictors for successful sperm-retrieval and pregnancy in 327 azoospermic men with a historyof cryptorchidism who underwent microdissection testicularsperm extraction. Andrology. 2021;9:253–9. https://doi.org/10.1111/andr.12910.
24. Hesham Said A, Ragab A, Zohdy W, Ibrahim AS, Abd El Basset AS. Diffusion-weighted magnetic resonance imaging and magnetic resonance spectroscopy for non-invasive characterization of azoospermia: a prospective comparative single-center study. Andrology. 2023;11:1096–106.
25. Ntorkou A, et al. Testicular apparent diffusion coefficient and magnetization transfer ratio: can these MRI parameters be used to predict successful sperm retrieval in nonobstructive azoospermia? AJR Am J Roentgenol. 2019;213:610–8.
26. Tsili AC, et al. A magnetic resonance imaging study in etiology of nonobstructive azoospermia. Andrology. 2022;10:241–53.
27. Tsili AC, Astrakas LG, Goussia AC, Sofikitis N, Argyropoulou MI. Volumetric apparent diffusion coefficient histogram analysis of the testes in nonobstructive azoospermia: a noninvasive fingerprint of impaired spermatogenesis? Eur Radiol. 2022;32:7522–31.
28. Tsili AC, et al. Diffusion tensor imaging parameters in testes with nonobstructive azoospermia. J Magn Reson Imaging. 2018;48:1318–25.
29. Gao S, et al. Noninvasive prediction of sperm retrieval using diffusion tensor imaging in patients with nonobstructive azoospermia. J Imaging. 2023;9:182.
30. Rassam Y, Gromoll J, Kliesch S, Schubert M. Testicular Microlithiasis is associated with impaired spermatogenesis in patients with unexplained infertility. Urol Int. 2020;104(7–8):610–6. https://doi.org/10.1159/000508584. Epub 2020 Jun 26. PMID: 32594086.
31. Barda S, Hauser R, Mano R, Savin Z, Molad-Hayo Y, Lehavi O, Kleiman SE, Azem F, Yossepowitch O, Dekalo S. Testicular microlithiasis defines a subgroup of azoospermic men with low rates of sperm retrieval. Int J Urol. 2022;29(1):65–8. https://doi.org/10.1111/iju.14717. Epub 2021 Oct 4. PMID: 34605564.
32. Jarvis S, Yee HK, Thomas N, Cha I, Prasad KC, Ramsay A, JW, Turek PJ. Sperm fine-needle aspiration (FNA) mapping after failed microdissection testicular sperm extraction (TESE): location and patterns of found sperm. Asian J Androl. 2018;21(1):50–5. https://doi.org/10.4103/aja.aja_68_18. Epub ahead of print. PMID: 30178775; PMCID: PMC6337941.
33. Kresch E, Efimenko I, Gonzalez D, Rizk PJ, Ramasamy R. Novel methods to enhance surgical sperm retrieval: a systematic review. Arab J Urol. 2021;19(3):227–37. https://doi.org/10.1080/2090598X.2021.1926752. PMID: 34552774; PMCID: PMC8451700.
34. Ghayda RA, Cannarella R, Calogero AE, et al. Global andrology forum. Artificial intelligence in andrology: from semen analysis to image diagnostics. World J Mens Health. 2024;42(1):39–61. https://doi.org/10.5534/wjmh.230050. Epub 2023 Jun 15. PMID: 37382282; PMCID: PMC10782130.
35. Cherouveim P, Velmahos C, Bormann CL. Artificial intelligence for sperm selection-a systematic review. Fertil Steril. 2023;120(1):24–31. https://doi.org/10.1016/j.fertnstert.2023.05.157. Epub 2023 May 24. PMID: 3723641.

Chapter 6
Oxidative Stress and Sperm DNA Fragmentation: What Is New?

Ayad Palani, Chirag Gupta, and Ramadan Saleh

Introduction

Male factor infertility has been reported by the World Health Organization as a main factor in half of the 15% infertility cases affecting couples around the world [128, 181]. Male infertility has received a global concern in recent years, as a temporal decline in sperm quality, and male fertility rates has been reported in different studies [51, 85, 172, 184].

Although male infertility is diagnosed as a decline in sperm function, the etiological factor has not been identified in almost one half of all cases and considered idiopathic [31].

Despite various environmental and nutritional factors that have been suggested to contribute to the decline in sperm quality, the particular reason for the increased incidence of male infertility remains unknown [31]. Over the past years, oxidative stress (OS) has received a global concern as the time-related decline in male fertility was observed concurrently with increasing physiological and environmental production of reactive oxygen species (ROS). Many studies suggested OS as a new emerging factor in cases diagnosed as unexplained and idiopathic male infertility

A. Palani (✉)
College of Medicine, University of Garmian, Kalar, Iraq
e-mail: ayad.palani@garmian.edu.krd

C. Gupta
Matratva Fertility and Andrology Clinic, Jaipur, Rajasthan, India

R. Saleh
Department of Dermatology, Venereology and Andrology, Faculty of Medicine, Sohag University, Sohag, Egypt

Ajyal IVF Center, Ajyal Hospital, Sohag, Egypt

E. Chung et al. (eds.), *Advances in Andrology*,
https://doi.org/10.1007/978-3-032-29112-7_6

[11, 22, 110, 135, 159]. High levels of ROS were observed in the ejaculates of 30–80% of patients with male infertility [191, 201, 218].

The clinical significance of OS is evident in its association with both natural and assisted conception rates [164]. Oxidative stress leads to a reduction in natural fertility rates [166], and a poor-assisted reproductive technology (ART) outcomes, such as lower fertilization rates, inhibition of embryonic development, unsuccessful of implantation, recurrent pregnancy loss, and lower live birth rates [17, 23].

The mechanism by which OS impacts sperm function is complex and multifunctional. When the harmful ROS molecules overcome the antioxidant defense, a cascade of unfavorable reactions occurs, resulting in significant damage to vital biomolecules such as lipids, proteins, and nucleic acids (Fig. 6.1) [16].

Oxidative stress can cause sperm DNA fragmentation (SDF) through different mechanisms, including formation of modified bases, creating abasic sites, DNA-protein cross-linking [71], DNA strand breaks (both single and double), chromosomal aberrations [102], and epigenetic modifications by disruption of the normal DNA methylation patterns [206].

There is emerging evidence supporting various approaches to reduce SDF and increase the likelihood of successful natural and assisted conception [71]. Antioxidant-rich foods and antioxidant supplementation have shown positive results in reducing oxidative damage [34]. Additionally, lifestyle modifications, such as

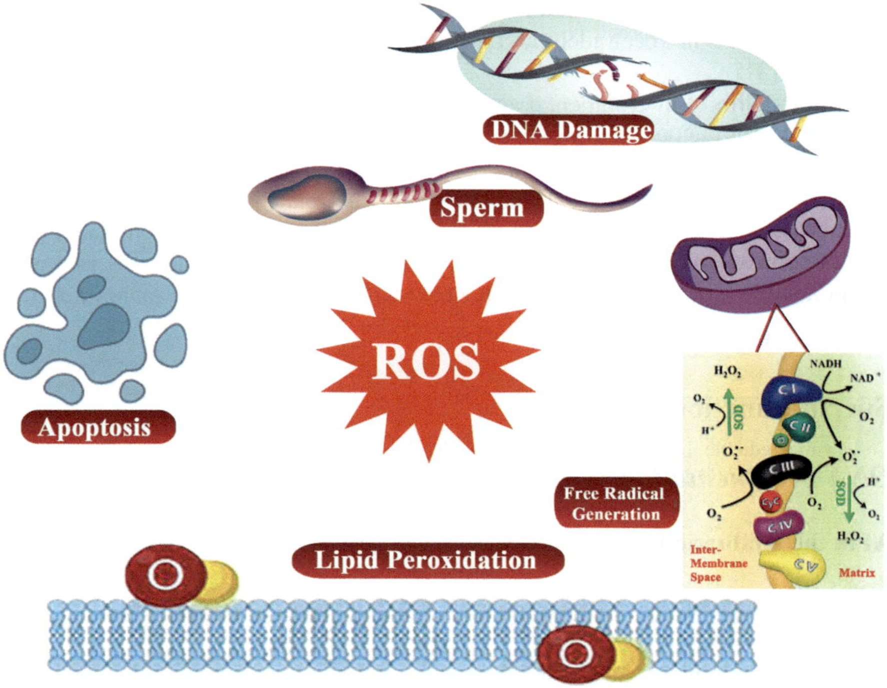

Fig. 6.1 Pathological effects of Reactive Oxygen Species (ROS) on sperm

avoiding smoking, excessive alcohol consumption, and exposure to environmental toxins, play a significant role in minimizing OS. Moreover, addressing underlying factors like varicoceles, hormonal imbalances, and infections through medical interventions can help in alleviating OS in semen, reducing SDF and ultimately improving male fertility potential [210]. The aims of this chapter are as follows:

- Review the pathogenesis of seminal OS and sperm DNA damage, and highlight the underlying mechanisms beyond these conditions in the male reproductive system.
- Illustrate the implications of seminal OS and SDF on both natural fertility and ART outcomes highlighting how these factors can affect male fertility and the success rates of ART.
- Furthermore, this chapter will explore the current strategies for reducing seminal oxidative OS and SDF, offering therapeutic approaches to enhance male fertility and improve outcomes in ARTs. It will also cover the latest updates from professional societies and expert recommendations on the indications for SDF testing.

Pathogenesis of Seminal Oxidative Stress

Spermatozoal production of ROS is associated with both normal and pathophysiological conditions. The critical determinant between these conditions lies in maintaining the balance between ROS production and the antioxidant defense capability. Excessive ROS production by endogenous or exogenous factors can overwhelm the antioxidant capacity, leading to OS, the key factor in various pathological conditions [151].

Endogenous Factors

Naturally, sperm cell produces small amount of ROS for various cellular functions, including energy metabolism. Sperm requires a high and rapid energy supply to meet the energetic demands of its journey toward the egg. In addition, ROS have a critical role in different physiological functions such as sperm hyperactivation, capacitation, and acrosome reaction [62, 63, 65, 92]. Like other mammalian cells, spermatozoa produce energy in the mitochondria through the process of cellular respiration. Mitochondria is the primary sources of ROS in spermatozoa [62]. The key product of the electron transport chain (ETC) is the superoxide radical ($O_2^{\bullet-}$), which is produced as a byproduct along with ATP synthesis in the oxidative phosphorylation pathway. Superoxide ion could trigger a series of unfavorable reactions, resulting in generation of additional reactive species such as hydrogen peroxide (H_2O_2), hydroxyl ion radical ($OH^{\bullet-}$), peroxyl, and others reactive molecules [56].

Another endogenous ROS generation pathway is the NADPH oxidase system, which is located on spermatozoa plasma membrane [39]. NADPH oxidase catalyzes the transfer of electrons from NADPH to oxygen resulting in the generation of reactive oxygen molecules to promote normal sperm functions such as maturation, activation, and acrosome reaction. Furthermore, immature spermatozoa with excess residual cytoplasm (cytoplasmic droplet) are correlated with high ROS generation [18]. Abnormal spermatozoa retaining residual cytoplasm contain high level of glucose-6-phosphate dehydrogenase (G6PDH), a key enzyme in the pentose phosphate pathway (PPP) which generates excessive amounts of NADPH. This surplus NADPH undergoes oxidation through two different pathways, (I) NADPH oxidase (NOX2) located in sperm plasma membrane and (II) NADPH oxidoreductase catalysis redox reactions at the mitochondrial level [18, 118].

Exogenous Factors

In addition to endogenous sources of ROS, many exogenous factors contribute in inducing of OS in the male reproductive system. These external factors include various pathological and environmental factors such as varicocele, infection, smoking and alcohol intake, testicular overheat, radiation, and pollution [64, 187].

The fundamental mechanism underlying these various factors is the inflammatory pathway [13, 44]. Inflammation within the male reproductive system intricately connects with OS. This relationship forms a cycle wherein inflammation and OS mutually exacerbate each other's effects, leading to synergistic effect [120, 140, 204]. This mechanism was evidenced by the observation of a positive correlation between ROS and pro-inflammatory seminal plasma cytokines, including IL-6, IL-8, and TNFα [108, 163].

ROS-regulated transcription factors such as nuclear factor kappa B (NF-κB) are localized in the cytoplasm of sperm cell and bound to the cytosolic proteins like IκB (inactive form). ROS modifies IκB proteins via phosphorylation by a serine kinase, inhibitor of NF-κB kinase (IKK), leading to its degradation and releasing free NF-κB, that can then translocate to the cell nucleus where it induces expression of numerous genes that express inflammatory proteins [52].

NF-κB and other transcription factors, such as the activator protein-1 (AP-1), the hypoxia-inducible factor (HIF-1α), and nuclear factor like 2 (Nrf-2), can regulate numerous genes that induce expression of pro-inflammatory cytokines [207]. Seminal cytokines promote the peroxidation process, resulting in increasing ROS generation in situ [32, 108]. An overview of exogenous sources of excess seminal ROS production is provided in this section:

Varicocele

Varicocele is a leading factor of male infertility, with reports indicating its presence in 35–40% of men experiencing fertility issues [73]. Due to varicocele, excessive ROS is produced in the testes, which can lead to SDF [6]. In males with high grades of varicocele, chances of elevated SDF increases. Normozoospermic men with clinical varicocele often have elevated OS markers and high SDF indices [6, 70, 171, 219]. Approximately 50% of individuals with clinical varicoceles have elevated SDF.

The exact mechanism by which varicocele affects sperm function is not fully established. Possible mechanisms underlying varicocele-mediated infertility include OS, inflammation, testicular hyperthermia, hormonal disorders, testicular hypoxia, Leydig cell dysfunction, and retrograde flow of toxic metabolites [15, 193, 196]. However, current evidences support OS and inflammation pathways as central mediator of testicular damage in varicocele [14, 38, 79, 125, 209]. High level of ROS and pro-inflammatory cytokines has been observed in semen of varicocele patients compared to fertile men with no varicocele, supporting the central role of these two pathways in varicocele [12, 214].

Infection

Acute or chronic, male genital tract infection may cause overproduction of ROS which results in OS [96, 188]. It may induce an apoptotic-like response or may directly damage sperm DNA that results in SDF [21, 142].

During the male genital tract infection, inflammatory process involves mainly the accumulation and activation of leukocytes, mostly phagocytes [81]. Leukocytes can generate up to 1000 times ROS more than spermatozoa [65]. Activated neutrophils and macrophages are recruited to the site of damage, which leads to a "oxidative burst" due to an increased uptake of oxygen and, thus, an increased release of large amounts of ROS through the activation of NOX2 [165, 182]. Additionally, the chlamydial lipopolysaccharide may induce excessive ROS production by the spermatozoa, thus enhancing the OS and SDF [68].

Smoking

Smoking has long been recognized as a risk factor for male infertility. It can lead to testicular damage, deterioration of semen parameters, and SDF by initiating OS and inflammation in semen [64, 98]. Increased OS is the main mechanism through which smoking damages spermatozoa and induces male infertility. Smoking significantly increases ROS level in semen by 107%. Additionally, it disrupts the balance between ROS and total antioxidant capacity [13].

Cigarette smoke contains many toxic chemicals such as cadmium and nicotine, which are capable of increasing generation of free radicals and reducing antioxidant defense capability [112]. The role of OS in smokers is supported by the overexpression of certain proteins that have been found overexpressed in patients with an increased ROS production [48].

Alcohol Intake

The implication of alcohol intake in deterioration of male infertility has been studied widely. A study indicated that about 42% of men with infertility reported alcohol consumption [55]. Excessive chronic alcohol intake is linked to numerous deleterious effects on the male reproductive tract including disturbance of gonadotropin level, decrease in testosterone secretion, impaired spermatogenesis, and increased leukocyte concentrations in semen [42]. The association between alcohol excessive consumption and poor semen quality occurs mainly due to the development of OS, as well as the genotoxic impact on sperm DNA integrity, affecting the embryo health [80, 154, 199]. A meta-analysis showed that alcohol intake is associated with a reduction in semen antioxidant levels, leading to the induction of OS [146].

Obesity

Alongside the observed global decline in male fertility, overweightness has been significantly increasing over recent decades [122]. Obesity impacts male fertility through decreasing spermatogenesis, sperm concentration, motility, viability, normal morphology, and increasing SDF [19]. Various factors have been shown to influence fertility in obese individuals such as factors altering endocrine system, inflammation response, stimulation of OS, and genetic or epigenetic expression affecting spermatogenesis and sperm function [53, 87].

Among the several proposed mechanisms contributing to sperm dysfunction in obese males, inflammation and OS play a pivotal role [37]. Oxidative stress may alter testicular functions and negatively affecting sperm parameters [69, 99].

Chemical Toxins

The claim of global trend of declining sperm count has been re-evaluated by numerous studies, resulting in a conclusion that in certain geographical regions, this decline may be attributed to exposure to chemicals that disrupt male reproductive system [160, 183]. Nowadays, humans are exposed to different types of pollutants, including air pollutant, bisphenol A, phthalate, heavy metals, pesticides, and insecticides. These pollutants are able to minimize male fertility by exhibiting oestrogenic properties [183] or inducing OS [35]. These factors induce OS either by increasing free radical generation or by triggering the inflammatory response cascade [28].

Metabolic Syndrome

Metabolic syndrome, which is a set of conditions that increase the risk of diabetes mellitus type II and vascular complications, is closely associated with OS [134].

Advanced glycation end products (AGEs) are a family of unfavorable byproducts formed through a series of non-enzymatic reactions between reducing sugars and amino groups of other compounds. These harmful compounds are associated with hyperglycemic and/or OS conditions [211].

AGEs accumulation has been shown to play a crucial role in pathogenesis of infertility-related diseases.

Iatrogenic Causes

Oxidative stress can also occur due to medical treatment, which is referred to as iatrogenic. Sperm preparation techniques employed in ART, such as centrifugation, resuspension, and vortexing, have been shown to cause excessive generation of ROS in the isolated sperm of the washed specimen [7].

Centrifugation causes a sudden burst of ROS production in isolated motile sperm, affecting both motility and fertilizing capacity [20]. ROS levels due to mechanical stress induced by repeated centrifugation-resuspension cycles increase by more than 20-fold [105].

Cryopreservation of spermatozoa is also associated with an increase in ROS generation [40]. Oxidative stress during cryopreservation may be generated through different mechanisms, such as osmotic stress and alteration in oxidative metabolisms [203]. Although ROS formation occurs throughout the entire cryopreservation process, it is the excessive production of ROS during the freeze-thaw cycle that primarily causes OS [117].

Accumulating evidence suggests that the addition of antioxidants may reduce the impact of ROS-induced OS and cold-shock injuries [26, 33].

Other Sources of Exogenous ROS

Several other factors were reported to be associated with increased OS in semen, including chemotherapy [200], certain medications, chronic diseases, heat, radiation, lack of exercise, stress ([86, 166], and aging [143].

Table 6.1 outlines the major factors contributing to OS in the male reproductive system, along with their effects on semen parameters and sperm genomic integrity.

Table 6.1 Impact of common OS-inducing factors on semen characteristics and sperm genetic materials

OS-inducing factor	Effect on basic semen parameters	Effect on the genetic materials
Varicocele	Negative impact on spermatogenesis, basic semen parameters, and sperm function [95]	Increases SDF [215]
Infection	Different bacteria negatively affecting spermatogenesis and sperm functions ([74]; [77])	Increases SDF ([74]; [77])
Smoking	Impairers spermatogenesis, sperm maturation, spermatozoa function, and hormone system dysfunction [61]	Induces sperm DNA strand fragmentation, genome instability, mutations, alterations in microRNA expression in sperm, and causes DNA methylation [152]
Alcohol	Negatively affects sperm concentration, motility, and morphology, and induces hormonal imbalance [121]	Induces protamine deficiency and DNA damage [27]
Obesity	Decreases semen volume, sperm count and concentration, vitality, motility and normal morphology [179]	Increases DNA fragmentation [47]
Environmental toxins	Associated with abnormal semen parameters. Decreases sperm counts, motility, viability, and normal morphology [115]	Increases DNA damage [115]
Heat	Decreases semen volume, sperm concentration, total and progressive motility, and normal morphology [101]	Induces an increase in DNA damage [94]

Mechanisms of Sperm DNA Fragmentation

During the process of spermatogenesis, structural and chemical changes in the germ cell DNA take place. DNA is the important genetic material present in spermatozoa. In order to avoid damage, it is highly condensed and compactly packed in spermatozoa. Usually, DNA is wrapped around the histone proteins, and for effective condensation of the sperm DNA [83, 162], they are replaced by highly basic protamines gradually, which make the spermatozoa transcriptionally and translationally inactive [97]. Extensive chromatin remodeling subjects double-stranded DNA (dsDNA) to torsional stress, resulting in the formation of transient DNA strand breaks. These breaks are normally repaired to enable efficient histone replacement, chromatin condensation, and proper sperm nuclear packaging [129]. Reduced protamination leads to failure of repair of the nicks, and its accumulative effect results in DNA damage. ROS generated by immature spermatozoa can cause SDF [29]. During epididymal transit, ROS attacks the spermatozoa and activates the endonuclease or sperm caspases which cause SDF. ROS targets the spermatozoa with poor chromatin packing or with high

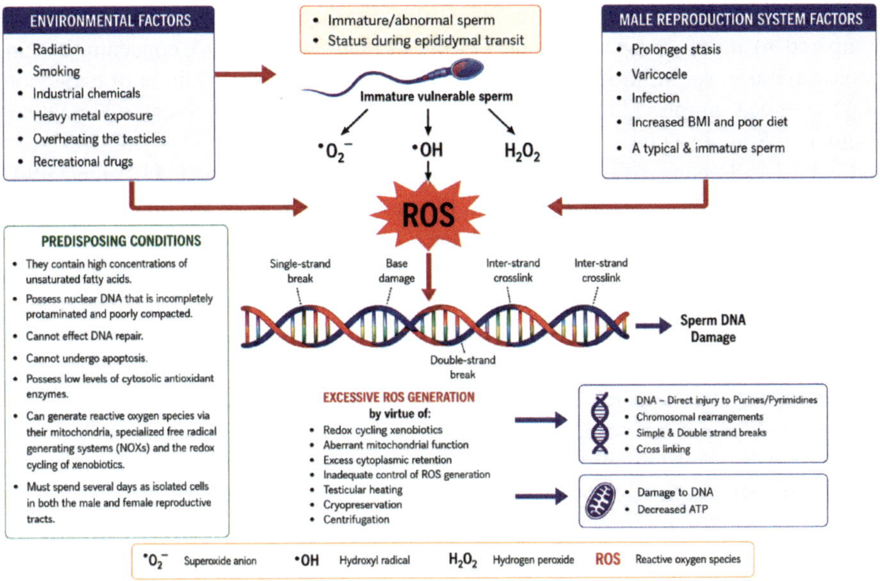

Fig. 6.2 DNA damage in sperm induced by reactive oxygen species (ROS)

protamination, as they are more susceptible [176]. Poor disulphide cross-links in the mature spermatozoa represents another cause of SDF due to altered chromatin packaging. That's why epididymal sperms are more susceptible to DNA damage [90, 194]. High levels of ROS and reactive nitrogen species resulting from various endogenous and exogenous factors can activate multiple harmful pathways (Fig. 6.2).

ROS can initiate both intrinsic and extrinsic apoptosis pathways. Leakage of cytochrome C from the mitochondrial membrane occurs as a result of activation of pro-apoptotic factors by ROS and leads to activation of intrinsic caspase cascade causing SDF [93, 185, 194]. Activation of pro-apoptotic proteins by binding of leucocytes expressing ligands FasL to Fas protein receptors on the spermatozoa initiates extrinsic pathway of apoptosis which leads to disturbance in the mitochondrial pathways resulting in DNA damage [14]. It has been reported that 10% of normozoospermic and 50% of oligozoospermic men express Fas protein receptors on spermatozoa [177]. Activation of both the intrinsic and extrinsic apoptotic pathways is associated with the highest levels of SDF [93, 131]. Fragmentation of single-strand DNA (ssDNA) and dsDNA is detrimental for DNA and makes it unstable; however, irreversible damage is caused by dsDNA fragmentation which affects fertilization and embryo development. DNA repair mechanisms, such as nucleotide excision repair, mismatch repair, ssDNA and dsDNA break repair, help in maintaining DNA integrity and thus counteract the DNA damage process. If the DNA repair mechanism is defective, then it leads to abnormal sperm with a high degree of DNA damage [93].

Excess ROS has been found in the seminiferous tubules and seminal plasma of most patients with idiopathic male infertility [8, 105, 198, 212]. In asthenospermic and oligo-asthenospermic patients, the concentration of malondialdehyde (MDA), a marker of lipid peroxidation, was found to be almost twice as high in sperm pellet suspensions compared to normozoospermic males [198]. A decrease in MDA concentration and improvement in sperm motility was demonstrated with in vitro addition of exogenous SOD to semen samples [113]. An increase in SDF and apoptosis was caused by vulnerability to OS in vitro due to zinc deficiency [153]. The levels of pro-apoptotic p53, p21, and bcl 2 family gene expression and caspase-3 activity are modulated by intracellular zinc. Bcl-2 functions as an antioxidant at the outer membrane of the mitochondria and has a role in regulating programmed cell death [82, 150]. Omu et al., demonstrated that as compared to oligozoospermic and asthenozoospermic men, the antiapoptotic protein Bcl-2 was more highly expressed in normozoospermic men, whereas in men with oligozoospermia and asthenozoospermia, the pro-apoptotic Bax was greatly expressed [153]. Sperm motility, morphology, vitality, and concentration [192] are inversely correlated with apoptosis and markers of programmed cell death. Increased severity of idiopathic male infertility is seen in individuals with decreased expression of survivin, a programmed cell death inhibitor. It was noted in that hormonal dysregulation infertility [100], anti-sperm antibody-associated infertility, varicocele, testicular torsion [175], and inflammation [186] are associated with oligoasthenoteratozoospermia (OAT), which is caused by increased apoptosis. Hence, for idiopathic OAT, accentuated programmed cell death is not pathognomonic. It was demonstrated in various studies that spermatozoa from OAT patients often exhibit chromosomal aneuploidy and mitochondrial dysfunction, in addition to an increased susceptibility to apoptosis and SDF [123]. In asthenozoospermic infertile men, mitochondrial DNA oxidative damage has been observed and confirmed in experimental models, which are similar to the mitochondrial modifications in apoptotic sperm cells [158, 190]. These alterations are very similar to the mitochondrial modifications seen in apoptotic sperm cells [43, 208].

Impact of Sperm DNA Fragmentation on Male Fertility

Sperm DNA fragmentation is now recognized as a valuable tool for evaluating male fertility due to its negative impact on reproductive outcomes in both natural and assisted conception [178]. Sperm DNA damage, either single- or double-strand breaks, occurs either during sperm production, maturation, or transport through the male genital tract [11].

Impact of SDF on Natural Pregnancy Outcomes

An increasing number of couples fail to achieve pregnancy despite the absence of an identifiable male or female factor of infertility. This condition is classified under the name "unexplained infertility." It is probable that many of these couples may possess a male genomic defect, which may include sperm DNA damage. The integrity of sperm DNA is crucial for initiating and maintaining a viable pregnancy [176]. After fertilization, paternal genome is transcriptionally inactive for approximately 48 h. However, once the damaged genome is active, it results in poor blastocyst development, unequal cleavage, implantation failure, or early fetal loss [45]. If the DNA damage is low, the oocyte can use its repair mechanism to repair the injury and maintain the development of the embryo.

A small number of studies explored the effect of DNA damage on natural pregnancy. Vončina et al. [127, 216] have showed that sperm DNA damage is associated with a prolonged time to pregnancy and a low possibility of achieving a natural pregnancy [127, 216]. However, the data on the impact of SDF on natural pregnancy are still scarce.

Impact of SDF on ART Outcomes

The impact of SDF on assisted pregnancy outcome has been studied widely. However, due to the presence of conflicting findings in reported results, the evidence concerning the role of SDF in the success of ART remains inconclusive. Three recent meta-analyses by Sugihara et al. [197], Ribas-Maynou et al. [167], and Chen et al. [54] have been conducted to investigate the impact of SDF on ART outcomes.

For intrauterine insemination (IUI) outcomes, Sugiharaa et al. have analyzed date of 917 IUI cycles. The association between low SDF and clinical pregnancy was having risk ratio (RR) of 3.30 (95% CI: 1.16; 9.39, I^2 = 38%). The results showed that couples with low levels of SDF are three times more likely to conceive after performing IUI procedure.

By analyzing a total of 12,380 IVF/ICSI cycles, Ribas-Maynou et al. showed that for IVF and ICSI procedures, the implantation rate (RR = 0.74; 95% CI = 0.61–0.91; I^2 = 69%, P = 0.01) and pregnancy rate (RR = 0.83; 0.73–0.94; I^2 = 58%, P = 0.01) are negatively influenced by sperm DNA damage, while live birth rate (RR = 0.78; 0.58–1.06; I^2 = 72%, P = 0.12) was not affected by SDF. For IVF outcomes, data showed a significant impact of SDF on implantation rates (RR = 0.68; 0.52–0.89; I^2 = 50%, P = 0.01) and pregnancy rates (RR = 0.72; 0.55–0.95; I^2 = 72%, P = 0.02), while no significant difference was found in the live birth rate (RR = 0.48; 0.22–1.02; I^2 = 79%, 0.06). Additionally, for ICSI outcomes, a non-significant difference was observed for implantation (RR = 0.79; 0.60–1.04; I^2 = 72%, P = 0.09), pregnancy rates (RR = 0.89; 0.78–1.02; I^2 = 44%, P = 0.09), and live birth rate (RR = 0.92; 0.67–1.27; I^2 = 70%, P = 0.62).

Conversely, Chen et al. illustrated that following IVF, there was no influence of SDF on fertilization rate (RR = 0.94, 95% CI: 0.77–1.14, P = 0.61), pregnancy rate (RR = 0.83, 95% CI: 0.57–1.21, P = 0.32), and live birth rate (RR = 0.53, 95% CI: 0.16–1.80, P = 0.31) in men with high SDF level.

Although it has been shown that SDF provides promise as a predictor of natural and ART outcomes, the available evidence remains scarce. Further investigation is needed to fully understand its implication in natural and assisted pregnancies.

Methods of SDF Assessment

SDF can be measured by several different methods (Table 6.2). These tests can measure sperm DNA integrity either directly or indirectly. TUNEL (Terminal deoxynucleotidyl transferase dUTP Nick End Labeling) and COMET (single-cell

Table 6.2 Laboratory methods for sperm DNA fragmentation assessment

Test	Principle	Method	Interpretation	Specimen required	Male infertility diagnosis threshold
Terminal deoxynucleotidyl Transferase mediated dUTP biotin Nick End Labeling (TUNEL)	Terminal deoxynucleotidyl transferase (TdTA) enzyme adds labeled nucleotides to free DNA ends, Template independent, Labels SS and DS breaks, With the aid of optical fluorescence microscopy and flow cytometry, sites of breaks can be identified	Visualization of sperm DNA damage using terminal deoxynucleotidyl Transferase dUTP Nick End Labeling (TUNEL) Digoxigenin-dUTP is incorporated to DNA breaks using a terminal transferase; anti-digoxigenin FITC is used to label the sites where digoxigenin-dUTP is present (green color)	% Cells with labeled DNA	Whole ejaculate 2.0–2.5 × 106 Spermatozoa for flow cytometry	>17% by flow cytometry
Single-cell gel electrophoresis assay (Comet)	Electrophoresis of single sperm cells leads to migration of fragments of single- and double-stranded DNA toward the anode, DNA fragments form tail, Intact DNA stays in head	Assay relies on DNA decompaction and protein depletion Alkaline or neutral pH conditions allow the uncoil of double-stranded DNA Immerse the slides in the buffer for 20 minutes and start the electrophoresis by applying current at 25 V (0.714 V/cm) adjusted to 300 mA	The relative fluorescence in the tail compared with It's head reflects the level of SDF; spermatozoa with increased fluorescence intensity in the comet tails have high levels of chromatin damage	A minimum of 100 µl volume of neat semen containing a minimum of 5000 spermatozoa	>20%–25%6 (DFI)

Sperm chromatin structure assay (SCSA)	Nicked DNA denatures more easily than double-stranded DNA Acridine Orange (AO) is used for staining; Intact DNA—green light single- or double-strand breaks—red light	Acid denaturation of the DNA at the sites of existing single- or double-strand breaks Acridine Orange (AO) is used for staining. The fluorescence patterns emitted by spermatozoa are captured using a flow cytometer	The ratio of red to total (green + red) fluorescence intensity is used to calculate the percentage of spermatozoa with DNA fragmentation	>0.5 million sperm/ml raw semen for direct measurement If <0.5 million/ ml, specimens should be concentrated by centrifugation and resuspended	>26%
Sperm Chromatin Dispersion (SCD)	Spermatozoa with DNA fragmentation fail to produce the characteristic halo of dispersed DNA loops that are observed in spermatozoa with non-fragmented DNA	(1) Acid denaturation and removal of nuclear proteins (2) Sperm suspensions are embedded in agarose gel on slides and treated with an acid denaturation solution (HCl). (3) Spermatozoa are exposed to a lysing solution based on DTT, sodium dodecyl sulfate, and NaCl to remove the sperm membrane and nuclear proteins Then, slides are stained with DAPI (4′,6-diamidino-2-phenylindole) or DiffQuik, and spermatozoa with non-dispersed and dispersed chromatin loops are identified by fluorescence or bright-field microscopy examination, respectively	The halos correspond to relaxed DNA loops attached to the residual nuclear structure as seen in spermatozoa with low or no SDF Spermatozoa with very small or no halos correspond to those exhibiting SD	The test can be performed in a single to several hundred spermatozoa, both in fresh and frozen/ thawed specimens The recommended sperm concentration is 1–3 million per ml, but it can be performed using less concentrated samples	<20%

gel electrophoresis) assays directly assess the presence of single- and/or double-strand breaks in the DNA, whereas AO FCM (Acridine Orange Flow Cytometry) and SCD (Sperm Chromatin Dispersion) assays detect the susceptibility of chromatin to treatment by acid. These tests have varying characteristics and cutoff values, and currently, there is no universally recommended "gold standard" test for assessing SDF. However, a global survey conducted by Global Andrology Forum (GAF) among reproductive clinicians revealed that the TUNEL assay is the most commonly used method, followed by the sperm chromatin structure assay (SCSA) and the SCD test [5].

Indications of Sperm DNA Fragmentation (SDF) Testing

Although sperm DNA damage has been shown to have significant adverse effects on reproductive outcomes, such as reduced pregnancy rates and an increased risk of miscarriage (Level I evidence), there remains limited evidence on the optimal methods for performing and interpreting SDF testing in clinical practice [130]. Additionally, SDF testing was not included in previous editions of the World Health Organization's (WHO) *Manual of Semen Analysis* [67]. However, in its latest edition, the WHO manual has classified SDF as an extended semen test that can be requested under specific conditions [155]. Despite this update, the manual does not provide detailed indications for testing, nor does it offer clear diagnostic thresholds.

It is speculated that SDF testing could be beneficial for infertile men in cases of unexplained or idiopathic male infertility, those with risk factors such as clinical varicocele, or couples experiencing recurrent pregnancy loss (RPL) [4]. In this section, we expanded on the updated indications for SDF testing within the context of infertility management.

Varicocele

Experts recommend SDF testing for patients with grade II-III varicocele and with borderline abnormal or normal basic semen parameters (grade C recommendation) [3].

This recommendation is based on evidence form numerous studies that reported the increase of SDF in varicocele. Over the decades, numerous studies have investigated the intricate mechanisms of varicocele's impact on male reproductive health [144]. Recently, SDF has emerged as a significant player in varicocele pathophysiology. A meta-analysis by Zhang et al. analyzed a total of 12 studies with a total of 845 patients diagnosed with varicocele and 2377 healthy controls. The analysis revealed that infertile men diagnosed with grade I varicocele had higher DNA damage than healthy controls [215].

Concerning the treatment of varicocele, studies showed that varicocele repair (VR) may improve sperm basic parameters and fertility outcomes. Several meta-analyses have explored the efficacy of VR as an effective strategy in treating high SDF. The most recent study by Canarella et al. analyzed 29 studies involving 1491 infertile men [49]. Their findings demonstrated a significant decrease in sperm DNA damage following VR, thus highlighting the potential benefits of utilizing SDF as a clinical diagnostic tool in varicocele-associated male infertility.

Idiopathic and Unexplained Infertility

Experts recommend undergoing SDF testing in couples with idiopathic and unexplained infertility and RPL (grade C recommendation) [10, 58]. This recommendation is raised based on evidence linking elevated SDF levels to the infertility conditions [104]. DNA damage is linked to male infertility and may be increased in conditions that are classified as unexplained or idiopathic infertility and can also lead to RPL [76]. The global survey conducted by GAF showed that more than half of the participants would recommend SDF testing in couples experiencing unexplained infertility, while only a small fraction (7%) of the participants expressed the belief that the results of SDF testing would not influence treatment decisions. Their findings revealed that SDF testing should be regarded as a valuable tool for all couples with unexplained infertility, especially following exclusion of known causes of male infertility [4]. Additionally, the European Association of Urology guidelines recommend SDF assessment in diagnosis of men with unexplained infertility [139].

Recurrent Pregnancy Loss

High SDF level is linked with RPL and negatively impacts outcomes of different ARTs. A meta-analysis by Tan et al. indicated that SDF is strongly associated with RPL, and paternally derived genetic is possibly potential factor in unexplained RPL [202]. Sperm DNA damage has also been linked to lower pregnancy rate following IUI procedure [46]. Therefore, SDF testing is indicated in couples with recurrent miscarriage or IUI failure (grade C recommendation) [3].

Early IVF or ICSI may be an alternative in case of RPL or failed IUI. SDF testing is also indicated in couples with recurrent failure of assisted pregnancy by IVF or ICSI [3]. Although high SDF value may not significantly affect ICSI pregnancy rates, two meta-analyses have reported an increased risk of miscarriage rate following ICSI [217, 220].

Modifiable Lifestyle Risk Factors

Men with modifiable lifestyle risk factors may undergo SDF testing (grade C recommendation) [3]. Life style such as obesity, smoking, alcohol intake, and pollution have been implicated in increased SDF. This recommendation is based on the evidence involving these factors in high sperm DNA damage [157]. Recommending the SDF assay in the above-mentioned cases aim to offer a relevant treatment strategy for reducing SDF level. Antioxidant therapy may be considered as a first-line treatment for this purpose (grade C recommendation) [88].

Strategies to Overcome the Oxidative Stress-Induced Sperm DNA Fragmentation

Treating the causes of high SDF is essential for alleviating reproductive challenges and enhancing fertility outcomes. Factors associated with SDF are modifiable and could be adverse by the use of specific treatments, lifestyle changes, and averting exposure to environmental/occupational toxicants [71].

Various strategies have demonstrated effectiveness in significantly reducing OS and SDF, including oral antioxidant supplementation, infection control, VR, and lifestyle modifications [57].

Antioxidant Therapy

Treatment with antioxidants is the first line of defense against OS-mediated male reproductive defect. Oral antioxidants is often used as a key therapeutic strategy to improve male fertility [1]. Several clinical studies have investigated the correlation between antioxidant levels and sperm DNA damage and have reported conflicting results [195, 221]. Among the concurring findings, various antioxidant types like vitamins E and C, coenzyme-Q10, glutathione, carnitines, zinc, selenium, N-acetylcysteine, carotenoids, and pentoxifylline, whether used alone or in combination, have demonstrated benefits in reducing OS-induced sperm DNA damage [41]. However, few studies have reported no effects [156, 195]. Moreover, attention is rising regarding the potential disruption of spermatozoal redox balance due to uncontrolled and high-antioxidant doses, which may lead to "reductive stress," known to be associated with adverse effects on basic sperm parameters [66, 137].

Despite numerous studies supporting the use of antioxidants in treatment of sperm DNA damage, the available data remain uncertain and more investigation are required [169]. This uncertainty arises due to factors such as lack of standard SDF test, lack of control groups, and poor study design [195], as well as the use of different antioxidants in different combinations and doses [124].

Despite these limitations, antioxidant therapy is still an accepted strategy for treatment of male infertility due to high SDF, with recommendation of using antioxidant that readily penetrates the blood-testis and blood-epididymis barriers [9, 133]. Results of different studies on the use of antioxidant therapy for treatment of men with high SDF are shown in Table 6.3.

Varicocele Repair

Varicocele represents the most frequent correctable cause of male infertility [139]. A systematic review including 21 studies and 1270 infertile men showed that VR decreases SDF by 7.23% (95% CI, −8.86 to −5.59) [171].

In general, there is a concurrent decline in SDF after VR [219]. A recent systematic review and meta-analysis of 19 varicocele studies including more than 1000 men demonstrated that the mean difference (MD) in SDF values after VR repair (versus preoperative levels) was −8.3% (95% CI −10.3%, −6.4%; $p < 0.0001$; [170]. Higher grades of clinical varicocele are reported with elevated SDF rates [2, 114, 148, 149, 173, 213]. It is advisable to test SDF before VR, to detect and/or confirm a detrimental effect of varicocele on sperm quality and fertility, thus reinforcing the need for interventional therapy to reduce SDF and improve fertility.

Information provided by SDF tests can be distinctly valuable when the decision to recommend VR is doubtful, in particular, for infertile men with (a) low-grade (e.g., grade 1) varicocele and borderline to normal semen parameters (e.g., count, motility, morphology) and (b) moderate (grade 2) or large (grade 3) varicocele and semen parameters within normal ranges [59].

SDF retesting after VR may be useful for monitoring the intervention's outcome and guiding further management. The persistence of abnormal postoperative SDF values usually leads to poor outcomes in both natural and assisted conception. In contrast, the reduction of SDF correlates with good chances of conception, both naturally and by ART [170]; the decision to pursue expectant management of ART will be based mainly on female factors. The association between subclinical varicocele (i.e., nonpalpable on physical exam but vein dilation and reflux detected by color Doppler ultrasound) and SDF, on the other hand, remains controversial. After repair of subclinical varicoceles, a controlled study involving 337 men reported a remarkable improvement in semen parameters and increased clinical pregnancy rates [50]. To the contrary, a systematic review and meta-analysis compiling the data of seven randomized-controlled trials demonstrated no improvement in pregnancy rates (OR 1.29, 95% CI: 0.99–1.67 [111]. Thus, more evidence is needed to allow any recommendation concerning the clinical value of SDF testing in men with subclinical varicocele [72].

Table 6.3 Oral antioxidants in treatment of sperm DNA fragmentation

Study	Antioxidant	Patients	Comparison	Dosage and duration	Result
Lahimer et al. [119]	Fertilis homme®	Couples consulting for male infertility	Treatment group and placebo group	Twice daily for 3 months	Increased in sperm motility and decreased DFI, in addition to a significant improvement in clinical pregnancy rate and life birth rate
Micic et al. [138]	Proxeed Plus®	Idiopathic oligoasthenozoospermia infertile men	Treatment group and placebo group	Twice daily for 6 months	Improved, volume, progressive motility, vitality and decreased sperm DFI
Nazari et al. [145]	400 IU synthetic vitamin E in combination with 10 mg zinc	Couples with recurrent pregnancy loss	Before and after	Once daily for 3 months	Improved in sperm concentration, motility, progressive motility, and normal morphology and decreased SDF
Rochdi et al. [168]	A combination of 40 Vitamin C, 0.1 Vitamin B9, 25 Selenium, 50 Zinc 200 Arginine, 200 L-carnitine, and 15 Q10	Men with infertility and idiopathic OAT	Before and after	Twice daily for 6 months	Improved sperm concentration, total motility, progressive motility, and total motile sperm count and decreased SDF
Patki et al. [161]	A combination of essential amino acids, antioxidants, vitamins, ginseng extract, lycopene, folic acid along with elemental zinc, iron, copper selenium, manganese	Sub-fertile males	Treatment group and placebo group	Once daily for 3 months	Improved sperm count in severe oligospermia subjects and improved DNA integrity in high-extremely higher baseline DFI
Jannatifar et al. [106]	600 mg N-acetyl-cysteine	Asthenoteratozoospermic infertile men	Before and after	Once daily for 3 months	Improved sperm count, motility and normal morphology, and increased hormone levels. Also decreased DNA fragmentation and protamine deficiency

Martínez-Soto et al. [132]	500 mg docosahexaenoic acid (DHA)	Infertile men	Treatment group and placebo group	Three capsules of oil per day for 10 weeks	Significant decrease in SDF
Humaidan et al. [103]	CoQ10 100 mg, Omega-3 1 g, and one multivitamin tablet	Infertile males with a history of failed IVF/ICSI	Healthy control	Once daily for 3 months	Significant decrease in SDF
Moskovtsev et al. [141]	Empirical oral antioxidant	Infertile patients	Before and after	Once daily for 3 months	Significant decrease in SDF
Salehi et al. [180]	Antioxidant supplementation contained the following active ingredients: 50 mg Vitamin E, 500 mg Vitamin C, and 100 mg Coenzyme Q10	Infertile men	Before and after	Once daily for 3 months	Improved sperm concentration motility, progressive motility and morphology, and decreased sperm DNA fragmentation
Alahmar et al. [25]	200 mg CoQ10	Idiopathic	Before and after treatment	Once daily for 3 months	Increased motility and decreased SDF
Greco et al. [88]	1 g Vitamin C and 1 g Vitamin E	Men with unexplained infertility	Treatment group and placebo group	Once daily for 2 months	Decreased SDF
Abad et al. [1]	Androferti®	Infertile men with known asthenoteratozoospermia	Before and after treatment	Once daily for 3 months	Improved sperm concentration, motility and normal morphology and decreased SDF
Greco et al. [88]	500 mg vitamin C and 500 mg vitamin E	Infertile men	Treatment group and placebo group	Twice daily for 2 months	Decreased SDF
Alahmar [24]	200 µg Selenium	Infertile patients with idiopathic oligoasthenoteratospermia	Before and after treatment	Once daily for 6 months	Increased TAC, sperm concentration, progressive motility and total motility, and decreased SDF

(continued)

Table 6.3 (continued)

Study	Antioxidant	Patients	Comparison	Dosage and duration	Result
Nguyen et al. [147]	A combination of 60 mg Vitamin E, 400 µg folic acid, 30 mg selenium, 125 mg L-arginine, 220 mg L-carnitine, 7.5 mg coenzyme Q10, 40 mg L-glutathione, and 20 mg zinc citrate	Men from infertile couples	Before and after treatment	Twice daily for 3 months	Increased sperm concentration, a total number of spermatozoa, and sperm vitality, and decreased SDF
Gual-Frau et al. [91]	Formula: 1500 mg L-carnitine, 60 mg vitamin C, 20 mg coenzyme Q10, 10 mg Vitamin E, 200 µg Vitamin B9, 1 µg Vitamin B12, 10 mg zinc, 50 µg selenium	Infertile patients with grade I varicocele	Before and after treatment	Once daily for 3 months	Improved total numbers of sperm and decreased SDF
Arafa et al. [30]	FH PRO®	Infertile men of unknown etiology	Before and after treatment	Three capsules, twice a day for 3 months	Improved sperm concentration, total and progressive motility, normal morphology, and seminal ORP and reduced SDF
Tunc et al. [205]	Menevit®	Infertile men	Before and after	Once daily for 3 months	Reduced seminal ROS and improved sperm DNA integrity
Greco et al. [89]	1 g Vitamin C and 1 g Vitamin E	Couples with failed ICSI attempt	Before and after	Once daily for 2 months	Reduced SDF and improved clinical pregnancy and implantation rates

DFI DNA Fragmentation Index, *SDF* Sperm DNA Fragmentation, *OAT* Oligoasthenozoospermia, *TAC* Total Antioxidant Capacity, *ICSI* Intracytoplasmic Sperm Injection, *IVF* In vitro Fertilization, *OPR* Oxidation Reduction Potential, *ROS*: Reactive Oxygen Species

Lifestyle Modifications

Testicular function improves on avoidance of exposure to toxicants. These measures may improve the genetic and epigenetic constitution of spermatozoa. The measures include avoidance of exposure to environmental and occupational toxicants, smoking cessation, dietary and lifestyle changes, and weight loss. A meta-analysis which included 20 studies with 5865 participants has shown exposure to cigarette smoking was associated with reduced sperm count (MD: −9.72 × 106/ml; 95% CI, −13.32 to −6.12), motility (MD: −3.48%; 95% CI, −5.53 to −1.44), and morphology (MD: −1.37%; 95% CI, −2.63 to −0.11). Further analyses indicated that reduction of sperm parameters was higher in infertile men than in the general population and in moderate/heavy smokers than in mild smokers [189]. In another study, high levels of DNA damages in spermatozoa of smokers were observed compared with non-smokers, but this difference was not statistically significant [189].

In an observational study, 336 infertile men with normal sperm parameters were interviewed regarding their diet. Three groups, namely Western, Mixed, or Prudent dietary patterns were formed [109]. The Prudent diet consist of high intakes of fish, chicken, fruit, vegetables, and whole grains, whereas the Western diet included high intakes of red and processed meat, butter, high-fat dairy, refined grains, fast-food, high-energy drinks, and sweets.

After controlling for variables like ejaculatory abstinence, age, smoking, previous diseases, and alcohol consumption, the results have shown that the Prudent diet was associated with increased sperm counts, higher testosterone serum levels, and decreased SDF rates compared with the Western diet (SDF: 15.2% ± 10.4% vs. 17.9% ± 8.1, $P < 0.05$). Similarly a study from India suggested that improvement in SDF could be obtained by adopting meditation and yoga-based lifestyle [60]. Levels of ROS were reduced in alcohol users ($P < 0.05$) as well as in tobacco users ($P < 0.05$) after the adoption of meditation and yoga-based lifestyle modification. After six months of yoga and meditation practice, SDF values decreased ($P < 0.05$), whereas a decrease in the levels of 8-Hydroxyguanosine was evident from the third month of practice. Another important factor is obesity. A small cohort study involving six obese men was published to date [78]. All participants were individuals with unexplained infertility and SDF values—by TUNEL—of 25% or higher. In this latter study, reduction in an intra-abdominal fat over a 3- to 8-month period was achieved in a nutritionist-led individualized dietary program coupled with exercise. The DNA quality improved ($P = 0.01$) in all patients who had their semen specimens analyzed both before and after the intervention, and their partners achieved pregnancy and full-term deliveries, either naturally or assisted.

Infection Control

Antibiotic therapy reduces the percentage of spermatozoa with fragmented DNA and was shown to improve pregnancy rates in a small group study [84]. The authors of this study suggested that the improvement in sperm DNA integrity due to antibiotic therapy could be a significant factor in achieving pregnancy.

Innovative Strategies Targeting DNA Damage

Although no specific treatment strategy for sperm DNA damage in infertile couples is universally recommended, lifestyle modifications and the administration of empiric antioxidants are the most commonly used approaches among clinicians. However, several interventions including the use of sperm with short ejaculatory abstinence, advanced sperm selection techniques, and the use of testicular sperm have shown their efficacy in obtaining sperm with low DNA damage [75].

A meta-analysis of 19 studies concluded that collecting sperm from a second ejaculation shortly after the first could be a simple and effective method for obtaining sperm with lower DNA damage, benefiting both natural conception and ART pregnancies [36]. While this strategy offers a less invasive and more cost-effective alternative to surgical testicular sperm extraction, testicular sperm is better than ejaculated sperm in reducing sperm DNA damage in infertility treatments [116].

Additionally, improvements in sperm DNA integrity have been achieved through advanced sperm selection techniques, including: (i) electrostatic charge (electrophoresis and zeta method), (ii) apoptosis-based techniques (magnetic activated sperm cell sorting and glass wool filtration), (iii) membrane maturity assessments (hyaluronic acid binding), and (iv) ultrastructural characteristics (high-magnification imaging) [174].

SDF Testing in Male Infertility: Updated Guidelines and Expert Recommendations

The significance of SDF in male infertility has been acknowledged by the international societies, the American Society of Reproductive Medicine (ASRM), the American Urological Association (AUA), and the EAU guidelines. Although, SDF assay is not recommended in the initial evaluation of the infertile couple, the EAU (2021) recommends its assessment in cases of RPL in both natural and assisted pregnancies, in the context of unexplained infertility. The ASRM indicated that SDF values may be clinically informative in IUI or IVF and ICSI procedures. However, the AUA notes insufficient evidence regarding the use of SDF in diagnosis of male infertility [107, 136, 139].

The Global Andrology Forum survey identified that the most common reasons for the delay in incorporating SDF testing into clinical practice are the lack of clear recommendations from professional society guidelines and the absence of globally accepted reference range [5].

However, despite several key barriers and limitations to incorporating SDF testing into clinical practice—such as cost, test availability, the lack of standardized methods, and the absence of universally accepted cutoff values—fertility experts have increasingly recognized the clinical utility of assessing SDF. This recognition is supported by accumulating evidence and emerging clinical practice recommendations [5].

Conclusion

Currently, evaluation and diagnosis of male infertility mainly rely on traditional semen analysis, including the volume, concentration, vitality, and morphology of the semen. However, approximately 15–20% of men with a normal semen analysis are diagnosed as infertile. Additional proportion of infertile men presented with abnormal basic semen parameters in the absence of an identifiable cause and are thus diagnosed as idiopathic male infertility. High seminal OS and SDF have been incriminated to play significance role in the pathogenesis of idiopathic and unexplained male infertility. The common causes of sperm DNA damage are often linked to factors that induce high seminal OS, such as smoking, infections, varicocele, and poor dietary habits. These factors have been shown to be treatable, potentially reducing SDF and improving sperm fertility potential. Reduction of SDF has been suggested after correction of causal factor. However, optimal SDF test, with widespread availability, low inter-laboratory variation, and clear-cut reference values, is still lacking. More research is needed to foster SDF testing in routine clinical practice.

References

1. Abad C, Amengual M, Gosálvez J, Coward K, Hannaoui N, Benet J, et al. Effects of oral antioxidant treatment upon the dynamics of human sperm DNA fragmentation and subpopulations of sperm with highly degraded DNA. Andrologia. 2013;45(3):211–6.
2. Abdelbaki SA, Sabry JH, Al-Adl AM, Sabry HH. The impact of coexisting sperm DNA fragmentation and seminal oxidative stress on the outcome of varicocelectomy in infertile patients: a prospective controlled study. Arab J Urol. 2017;15(2):131–9.
3. Agarwal A, Cho C-L, Majzoub A, Esteves SC. The Society for Translational Medicine: clinical practice guidelines for sperm DNA fragmentation testing in male infertility. Transl Androl Urol. 2017;6(Suppl 4):S720.
4. Agarwal A, Farkouh A, Saleh R, Hamoda TA-AA-M, Harraz AM, Kavoussi P, et al. Controversy and consensus on indications for sperm DNA fragmentation testing in male infertility: a global survey, current guidelines, and expert recommendations. World J Mens Health. 2023;41(3):575.

5. Agarwal A, Farkouh A, Saleh R, Hamoda TA-AA-M, Salvio G, Boitrelle F, et al. Technical aspects and clinical limitations of sperm DNA fragmentation testing in male infertility: a global survey, current guidelines, and expert recommendations. World J Mens Health. 2024;42(1):202.
6. Agarwal A, Hamada A, Esteves SC. Insight into oxidative stress in varicocele-associated male infertility: part 1. Nat Rev Urol. 2012;9(12):678–90.
7. Agarwal A, Ikemoto I, Loughlin K. Effect of sperm washing on levels of reactive oxygen species in semen. Arch Androl. 1994a;33(3):157–62.
8. Agarwal A, Ikemoto I, Loughlin KR. Relationship of sperm parameters with levels of reactive oxygen species in semen specimens. J Urol. 1994b;152(1):107–10.
9. Agarwal A, Leisegang K, Majzoub A, Henkel R, Finelli R, Selvam MKP, et al. Utility of antioxidants in the treatment of male infertility: clinical guidelines based on a systematic review and analysis of evidence. World J Mens Health. 2021;39(2):233.
10. Agarwal A, Majzoub A, Baskaran S, Selvam MKP, Cho CL, Henkel R, et al. Sperm DNA fragmentation: a new guideline for clinicians. World J Mens Health. 2020;38(4):412.
11. Agarwal A, Panner Selvam MK, Baskaran S, Cho C-L. Sperm DNA damage and its impact on male reproductive health: a critical review for clinicians, reproductive professionals and researchers. Expert Rev Mol Diagn. 2019;19(6):443–57.
12. Agarwal A, Prabakaran S, Allamaneni SS. Relationship between oxidative stress, varicocele and infertility: a meta-analysis. Reprod Biomed Online. 2006;12(5):630–3.
13. Agarwal A, Rana M, Qiu E, AlBunni H, Bui AD, Henkel R. Role of oxidative stress, infection and inflammation in male infertility. Andrologia. 2018;50(11):e13126.
14. Agarwal A, Said TM. Role of sperm chromatin abnormalities and DNA damage in male infertility. Hum Reprod Update. 2003;9(4):331–45.
15. Agarwal A, Sharma RK, Desai NR, Prabakaran S, Tavares A, Sabanegh E. Role of oxidative stress in pathogenesis of varicocele and infertility. Urology. 2009;73(3):461–9.
16. Agarwal A, Virk G, Ong C, Du Plessis SS. Effect of oxidative stress on male reproduction. World J Mens Health. 2014;32(1):1.
17. Ahelik A, Mändar R, Korrovits P, Karits P, Talving E, Rosenstein K, et al. Systemic oxidative stress could predict assisted reproductive technique outcome. J Assist Reprod Genet. 2015;32:699–704.
18. Ahmad G, Almasry M, Dhillon AS, Abuayyash MM, Kothandaraman N, Cakar Z. Overview and sources of reactive oxygen species (ROS) in the reproductive system. In: Oxidative stress in human reproduction: shedding light on a complicated phenomenon; 2017. p. 1–16.
19. Ahmad R, Haque M. Obesity: a doorway to a molecular path leading to infertility. Cureus. 2022;14(10):e30770.
20. Aitken RJ, Clarkson JS. Significance of reactive oxygen species and antioxidants in defining the efficacy of sperm preparation techniques. J Androl. 1988;9(6):367–76.
21. Aitken RJ, Gordon E, Harkiss D, Twigg JP, Milne P, Jennings Z, Irvine DS. Relative impact of oxidative stress on the functional competence and genomic integrity of human spermatozoa. Biol Reprod. 1998;59(5):1037–46.
22. Aktan G, Doğru-Abbasoğlu S, Küçükgergin C, Kadıoğlu A, Özdemirler-Erata G, Koçak-Toker N. Mystery of idiopathic male infertility: is oxidative stress an actual risk? Fertil Steril. 2013;99(5):1211–5.
23. Alahmar AT. Role of oxidative stress in male infertility: an updated review. J Human Reprod Sci. 2019;12(1):4–18.
24. Alahmar AT. The effect of selenium therapy on semen parameters, antioxidant capacity, and sperm DNA fragmentation in men with idiopathic oligoasthenoteratospermia. Biol Trace Elem Res. 2023;201(12):5671–6.
25. Alahmar AT, Sengupta P, Dutta S, Calogero AE. Coenzyme Q10, oxidative stress markers, and sperm DNA damage in men with idiopathic oligoasthenoteratospermia. Clin Exp Reprod Med. 2021;48(2):150.

26. Amidi F, Pazhohan A, Shabani Nashtaei M, Khodarahmian M, Nekoonam S. The role of antioxidants in sperm freezing: a review. Cell Tissue Bank. 2016;17:745–56.
27. Amor H, Hammadeh ME, Mohd I, Jankowski PM. Impact of heavy alcohol consumption and cigarette smoking on sperm DNA integrity. Andrologia. 2022;54(7):e14434.
28. Anyanwu BO, Orisakwe OE. Current mechanistic perspectives on male reproductive toxicity induced by heavy metals. J Environ Sci Health C. 2020;38(3):204–44.
29. Aoki VW, Liu L, Carrell DT. Identification and evaluation of a novel sperm protamine abnormality in a population of infertile males. Hum Reprod. 2005;20(5):1298–306.
30. Arafa M, Agarwal A, Majzoub A, Panner Selvam MK, Baskaran S, Henkel R, Elbardisi H. Efficacy of antioxidant supplementation on conventional and advanced sperm function tests in patients with idiopathic male infertility. Antioxidants. 2020;9(3):219.
31. Ayad B, Omolaoye TS, Louw N, Ramsunder Y, Skosana BT, Oyeipo PI, Du Plessis SS. Oxidative stress and male infertility: evidence from a research perspective. Front Reprod Health. 2022;4:822257.
32. Azenabor A, Ekun AO, Akinloye O. Impact of inflammation on male reproductive tract. J Reprod Infertil. 2015;16(3):123.
33. Bahmyari R, Zare M, Sharma R, Agarwal A, Halvaei I. The efficacy of antioxidants in sperm parameters and production of reactive oxygen species levels during the freeze-thaw process: A systematic review and meta-analysis. Andrologia. 2020;52(3):e13514.
34. Bansal AK, Bilaspuri G. Impacts of oxidative stress and antioxidants on semen functions. Veterinary Medicine International; 2011.
35. Barati E, Nikzad H, Karimian M. Oxidative stress and male infertility: current knowledge of pathophysiology and role of antioxidant therapy in disease management. Cell Mol Life Sci. 2020;77:93–113.
36. Barbagallo F, Cannarella R, Crafa A, Manna C, La Vignera S, Condorelli RA, Calogero AE. The impact of a very short abstinence period on conventional sperm parameters and sperm DNA fragmentation: a systematic review and meta-analysis. J Clin Med. 2022;11(24):7303.
37. Barbagallo F, Condorelli RA, Mongioì LM, Cannarella R, Cimino L, Magagnini MC, et al. Molecular mechanisms underlying the relationship between obesity and male infertility. Metabolites. 2021;11(12):840.
38. Barbieri ER, Hidalgo ME, Venegas A, Smith R, Lissi EA. Varicocele-associated decrease in antioxidant defenses. J Androl. 1999;20(6):713–7.
39. Baskaran S, Finelli R, Agarwal A, Henkel R. Reactive oxygen species in male reproduction: a boon or a bane? Andrologia. 2021;53(1):e13577.
40. Baumber J, Ball BA, Linfor JJ, Meyers SA. Reactive oxygen species and cryopreservation promote DNA fragmentation in equine spermatozoa. J Androl. 2003;24(4):621–8.
41. Beygi Z, Forouhari S, Mahmoudi E, Hayat SM, Nourimand F. Role of oxidative stress and antioxidant supplementation in male fertility. Curr Mol Med. 2021;21(4):265–82.
42. Bisht S, Faiq M, Tolahunase M, Dada R. Oxidative stress and male infertility. Nat Rev Urol. 2017;14(8):470–85.
43. Boekelheide K, Fleming SL, Johnson KJ, Patel SR, Schoenfeld HA. Role of Sertoli cells in injury-associated testicular germ cell apoptosis. Proc Soc Exp Biol Med: Minirev. 2000;225(2):105–15.
44. Borchers A, Pieler T. Programming pluripotent precursor cells derived from Xenopus embryos to generate specific tissues and organs. Genes (Basel). 2010;1(3):413–26. https://doi.org/10.3390/genes1030413.
45. Brahem S, Mehdi M, Landolsi H, Mougou S, Elghezal H, Saad A. Semen parameters and sperm DNA fragmentation as causes of recurrent pregnancy loss. Urology. 2011;78(4):792–6. https://doi.org/10.1016/j.urology.2011.05.049.
46. Bungum M, Humaidan P, Axmon A, Spano M, Bungum L, Erenpreiss J, Giwercman A. Sperm DNA integrity assessment in prediction of assisted reproduction technology outcome. Hum Reprod. 2007;22(1):174–9.

47. Campbell JM, Lane M, Owens JA, Bakos HW. Paternal obesity negatively affects male fertility and assisted reproduction outcomes: a systematic review and meta-analysis. Reprod Biomed Online. 2015;31(5):593–604.
48. Cannarella R, Crafa A, Barbagallo F, Mongioì LM, Condorelli RA, Aversa A, et al. Seminal plasma proteomic biomarkers of oxidative stress. Int J Mol Sci. 2020;21(23):9113.
49. Cannarella R, Shah R, Saleh R, Boitrelle F, Hamoda TA-AA-M, Singh R, et al. Effects of Varicocele repair on sperm DNA fragmentation and seminal malondialdehyde levels in infertile men with clinical Varicocele: a systematic review and meta-analysis. World J Mens Health. 2024;42(2):321.
50. Cantoro U, Polito M, Muzzonigro G. Reassessing the role of subclinical varicocele in infertile men with impaired semen quality: a prospective study. Urology. 2015;85(4):826–30.
51. Carlsen E, Giwercman A, Keiding N, Skakkebæk NE. Evidence for decreasing quality of semen during past 50 years. Br Med J. 1992;305(6854):609–13.
52. Chatterjee S. Oxidative stress, inflammation, and disease Oxidative stress and biomaterials. Elsevier; 2016. p. 35–58.
53. Chaudhuri GR, Das A, Kesh SB, Bhattacharya K, Dutta S, Sengupta P, Syamal AK. Obesity and male infertility: multifaceted reproductive disruption. Middle East Fertility Soc J. 2022;27(1):8.
54. Chen Y, Li W, Chen X. The association of sperm DNA fragment and assisted reproductive outcomes: a meta-analysis computational and mathematical methods in medicine. Comput Math Methods Med. 2022;2022:1126616.
55. Chia SE, Lim STA, Tay SK, Lim ST. Factors associated with male infertility: a case-control study of 218 infertile and 240 fertile men. BJOG Int J Obstet Gynaecol. 2000;107(1):55–61.
56. Chianese R, Pierantoni R. Mitochondrial reactive oxygen species (ROS) production alters sperm quality. Antioxidants. 2021;10(1):92.
57. Cho C-L. The role of interventions to reduce oxidative stress and improve sperm DNA integrity before ICSI. In: Male infertility: contemporary clinical approaches, andrology, art and antioxidants; 2020. p. 605–19.
58. Cho C-L, Agarwal A. Role of sperm DNA fragmentation in male factor infertility: a systematic review. Arab J Urol. 2018;16(1):21–34.
59. Cho C-L, Agarwal A, Majzoub A, Esteves SC. Clinical utility of sperm DNA fragmentation testing: concise practice recommendations. Transl Androl Urol. 2017;6(Suppl 4):S366.
60. Dada R, Basant Kumar S, Chawla B, Bisht S, Khan S. Oxidative stress induced damage to paternal genome and impact of meditation and yoga-can it reduce incidence of childhood cancer? Asian Pac J Cancer Prev. 2016;17(9):4517–25.
61. Dai J-B, Wang Z-X, Qiao Z-D. The hazardous effects of tobacco smoking on male fertility. Asian J Androl. 2015;17(6):954–60.
62. Drevet JR, Hallak J, Nasr-Esfahani M-H, Aitken RJ. Reactive oxygen species and their consequences on the structure and function of mammalian spermatozoa. Antioxid Redox Signal. 2022;37(7–9):481–500.
63. Du Plessis SS, Agarwal A, Halabi J, Tvrda E. Contemporary evidence on the physiological role of reactive oxygen species in human sperm function. J Assist Reprod Genet. 2015;32:509–20.
64. Durairajanayagam D. Lifestyle causes of male infertility. Arab J Urol. 2018;16(1):10–20.
65. Dutta S, Majzoub A, Agarwal A. Oxidative stress and sperm function: a systematic review on evaluation and management. Arab J Urol. 2019;17(2):87–97.
66. Dutta S, Sengupta P, Roychoudhury S, Chakravarthi S, Wang CW, Slama P. Antioxidant paradox in male infertility: 'a blind eye' on inflammation. Antioxidants. 2022;11(1):167.
67. Edition F. Examination and processing of human semen. World Health; 2010.
68. Eley A, Pacey AA, Galdiero M, Galdiero M, Galdiero F. Can Chlamydia trachomatis directly damage your sperm? Lancet Infect Dis. 2005;5(1):53–7.

69. Erdemir F, Atilgan D, Markoc F, Boztepe O, Suha-Parlaktas B, Sahin S. The effect of diet induced obesity on testicular tissue and serum oxidative stress parameters. Actas Urológicas Españolas (English Edition). 2012;36(3):153–9.
70. Esteves SC, Gosálvez J, López-Fernández C, Núñez-Calonge R, Caballero P, Agarwal A, Fernández JL. Diagnostic accuracy of sperm DNA degradation index (DDSi) as a potential noninvasive biomarker to identify men with varicocele-associated infertility. Int Urol Nephrol. 2015;47:1471–7.
71. Esteves SC, Santi D, Simoni M. An update on clinical and surgical interventions to reduce sperm DNA fragmentation in infertile men. Andrology. 2020;8(1):53–81.
72. Esteves SC, Zini A, Coward RM, Evenson DP, Gosálvez J, Lewis SE, et al. Sperm DNA fragmentation testing: summary evidence and clinical practice recommendations. Andrologia. 2021;53(2):e13874.
73. Fang Y, Su Y, Xu J, Hu Z, Zhao K, Liu C. Varicocele-mediated male infertility: from the perspective of testicular immunity and inflammation. Front Immunol. 2021;12:729539.
74. Farahani L, Tharakan T, Yap T, Ramsay JW, Jayasena CN, Minhas S. The semen microbiome and its impact on sperm function and male fertility: a systematic review and meta-analysis. Andrology. 2021;9(1):115–44.
75. Farkouh A, Agarwal A, Hamoda TA-A, Arafa M, Kavoussi P, Saleh R, Zini A, et al. Controversy and consensus on the management of elevated sperm DNA fragmentation in male infertility: a global survey, current guidelines, and expert recommendations. World J Mens Health. 2023;41(4):809.
76. Farkouh A, Finelli R, Agarwal A. Beyond conventional sperm parameters: the role of sperm DNA fragmentation in male infertility. Minerva Endocrinol. 2021;47(1):23–37.
77. Farsimadan M, Motamedifar M. Bacterial infection of the male reproductive system causing infertility. J Reprod Immunol. 2020;142:103183.
78. Faure C, Dupont C, Baraibar MA, Ladouce R, Cedrin-Durnerin I, Wolf JP, Levy R. In subfertile couple, abdominal fat loss in men is associated with improvement of sperm quality and pregnancy: a case-series. PLoS One. 2014;9(2):e86300.
79. Finelli R, Leisegang K, Kandil H, Agarwal A. Oxidative stress: a comprehensive review of biochemical, molecular, and genetic aspects in the pathogenesis and management of varicocele. World J Mens Health. 2022;40(1):87.
80. Finelli R, Mottola F, Agarwal A. Impact of alcohol consumption on male fertility potential: a narrative review. Int J Environ Res Public Health. 2021;19(1):328.
81. Fraczek M, Kurpisz M. Inflammatory mediators exert toxic effects of oxidative stress on human spermatozoa. J Androl. 2007;28(2):325–33. https://doi.org/10.2164/jandrol.106.001149.
82. Fraker PJ. Roles for cell death in zinc deficiency. J Nutr. 2005;135(3):359–62.
83. Fuentes-Mascorro G, Serrano H, Rosado A. Sperm chromatin archives of andrology. Arch Androl. 2000;45(3):215–25.
84. Gallegos G, Ramos B, Santiso R, Goyanes V, Gosálvez J, Fernández JL. Sperm DNA fragmentation in infertile men with genitourinary infection by Chlamydia trachomatis and Mycoplasma. Fertil Steril. 2008;90(2):328–34.
85. Garcia-Grau E, Lleberia J, Costa L, Guitart M, Yeste M, Benet J, et al. Decline of sperm quality over the last two decades in the south of Europe: a retrospective study in infertile patients. Biology. 2022;12(1):70.
86. García-Sánchez A, Miranda-Díaz AG, Cardona-Muñoz EG. The role of oxidative stress in physiopathology and pharmacological treatment with pro-and antioxidant properties in chronic diseases. Oxidative Med Cell Longev. 2020;2020:2082145.
87. George BT, Jhancy M, Dube R, Kar SS, Annamma LM. The molecular basis of male infertility in obesity: a literature review. Int J Mol Sci. 2023;25(1):179.
88. Greco E, Iacobelli M, Rienzi L, Ubaldi F, Ferrero S, Tesarik J. Reduction of the incidence of sperm DNA fragmentation by oral antioxidant treatment. J Androl. 2005a;26(3):349–53.

89. Greco E, Romano S, Iacobelli M, Ferrero S, Baroni E, Minasi MG, et al. ICSI in cases of sperm DNA damage: beneficial effect of oral antioxidant treatment. Hum Reprod. 2005b;20(9):2590–4.
90. Greco E, Scarselli F, Iacobelli M, Rienzi L, Ubaldi F, Ferrero S, et al. Efficient treatment of infertility due to sperm DNA damage by ICSI with testicular spermatozoa. Hum Reprod. 2005c;20(1):226–30.
91. Gual-Frau J, Abad C, Amengual MJ, Hannaoui N, Checa MA, Ribas-Maynou J, et al. Oral antioxidant treatment partly improves integrity of human sperm DNA in infertile grade I varicocele patients. Hum Fertil. 2015;18(3):225–9.
92. Gualtieri R, Kalthur G, Barbato V, Longobardi S, Di Rella F, Adiga SK, Talevi R. Sperm oxidative stress during in vitro manipulation and its effects on sperm function and embryo development. Antioxidants. 2021;10(7):1025.
93. Gunes S, Al-Sadaan M, Agarwal A. Spermatogenesis, DNA damage and DNA repair mechanisms in male infertility. Reprod Biomed Online. 2015;31(3):309–19.
94. Habibi P, Ostad SN, Heydari A, Aliebrahimi S, Montazeri V, Foroushani AR, et al. Effect of heat stress on DNA damage: a systematic literature review. Int J Biometeorol. 2022;66(11):2147–58.
95. Hassanin A, Ahmed H, Kaddah A. A global view of the pathophysiology of varicocele. Andrology. 2018;6(5):654–61.
96. Henkel R, Offor U, Fisher D. The role of infections and leukocytes in male infertility. Andrologia. 2021;53(1):e13743.
97. Henkel RR, Franken DR. Sperm DNA fragmentation: origin and impact on human reproduction. J Reprod Stem Cell Biotechnol. 2011;2(2):88–108.
98. Henriques MC, Santiago J, Patrício A, Herdeiro MT, Loureiro S, Fardilha M. Smoking induces a decline in semen quality and the activation of stress response pathways in sperm. Antioxidants. 2023;12(10):1828.
99. Heydari H, Ghiasi R, Ghaderpour S, Keyhanmanesh R. The mechanisms involved in obesity-induced male infertility. Curr Diabetes Rev. 2021;17(3):259–67.
100. Hikim AS, Swerdloff RS. Hormonal and genetic control of germ cell apoptosis in the testis. Rev Reprod. 1999;4(1):38–47.
101. Hoang-Thi A-P, Dang-Thi A-T, Phan-Van S, Nguyen-Ba T, Truong-Thi P-L, Le-Minh T, et al. The impact of high ambient temperature on human sperm parameters: a meta-analysis. Iran J Public Health. 2022;51(4):710.
102. Hosen MB, Islam MR, Begum F, Kabir Y, Howlader MZH. Oxidative stress induced sperm DNA damage, a possible reason for male infertility. Iran J Reprod Med. 2015;13(9):525.
103. Humaidan P, Haahr T, Povlsen BB, Kofod L, Laursen RJ, Alsbjerg B, et al. The combined effect of lifestyle intervention and antioxidant therapy on sperm DNA fragmentation and seminal oxidative stress in IVF patients: a pilot study. Int Braz J Urol. 2022;48:131–56.
104. Inversetti A, Bossi A, Cristodoro M, Larcher A, Busnelli A, Grande G, et al. Recurrent pregnancy loss: a male crucial factor—a systematic review and meta-analysis. Andrology. 2023; https://doi.org/10.1111/andr.13540.
105. Iwasaki A, Gagnon C. Formation of reactive oxygen species in spermatozoa of infertile patients. Fertil Steril. 1992;57(2):409–16.
106. Jannatifar R, Parivar K, Roodbari NH, Nasr-Esfahani MH. Effects of N-acetyl-cysteine supplementation on sperm quality, chromatin integrity and level of oxidative stress in infertile men. Reprod Biol Endocrinol. 2019;17:1–9.
107. Jarow, J., Sigman, M., Kolettis, P., Lipshultz, L., McClure, D., Nangia, A., … Schlegel, P. The optimal evaluation of the infertile male: best practice statement reviewed and validity confirmed 2011. (2011).
108. Jiang L, Zheng T, Huang J, Mo J, Zhou H, Liu M, et al. Association of semen cytokines with reactive oxygen species and histone transition abnormalities. J Assist Reprod Genet. 2016;33:1239–46.

109. Jurewicz J, Radwan M, Sobala W, Radwan P, Bochenek M, Hanke W. Dietary patterns and their relationship with semen quality. Am J Mens Health. 2018;12(3):575–83.
110. Khalil AA, Hussien HM, Sarhan EM. Oxidative stress induces idiopathic infertility in Egyptian males. Afr J Biotechnol. 2012;11(6):1516–22.
111. Kim H, Seo J, Kim K, Ahn H, Jeong J, Kim J, et al. Clinical significance of subclinical varicocelectomy in male infertility: systematic review and meta-analysis. Andrologia. 2016;48(6):654–61.
112. Kiziler AR, Aydemir B, Onaran I, Alici B, Ozkara H, Gulyasar T, Akyolcu MC. High levels of cadmium and lead in seminal fluid and blood of smoking men are associated with high oxidative stress and damage in infertile subjects. Biol Trace Elem Res. 2007;120:82–91.
113. Kobayashi T, Miyazaki T, Natori M, Nozawa S. Protective role of superoxide dismutase in human sperm motifity: superoxide dismutase activity and lipid peroxide in human seminal plasma and spermatozoa. Hum Reprod. 1991;6(7):987–91.
114. Krishna Reddy S, Basha Shaik A, Sailaja S, Venkataramanaiah M. Outcome of varicocelectomy with different degrees of clinical varicocele in infertile male. Adv Androl. 2015;2015:1–9.
115. Krzastek SC, Farhi J, Gray M, Smith RP. Impact of environmental toxin exposure on male fertility potential. Transl Androl Urol. 2020;9(6):2797.
116. Kugelman N, Hochberg A, Dahan MH. Impact of short abstinence versus testicular sperm on sperm DNA fragmentation: a systematic review and meta-analysis. Arch Gynecol Obstet. 2024;310:1–13.
117. Kumar A, Prasad J, Srivastava N, Ghosh S. Strategies to minimize various stress-related freeze–thaw damages during conventional cryopreservation of mammalian spermatozoa. Biopreserv Biobank. 2019;17(6):603–12.
118. Kumar N, Singh AK. Reactive oxygen species in seminal plasma as a cause of male infertility. J Gynecol Obstet Hum Reprod. 2018;47(10):565–72.
119. Lahimer M, Gherissi O, Ben Salem N, Ben Mustapha H, Bach V, Khorsi-Cauet H, et al. Effect of micronutrients and L-Carnitine as antioxidant on sperm parameters, genome integrity, and ICSI outcomes: randomized, Double-blind, and Placebo-controlled clinical trial. Antioxidants. 2023;12(11):1937.
120. Lazaros LA, Xita NV, Chatzikyriakidou AL, Kaponis AI, Grigoriadis NG, Hatzi EG, et al. Association of TNFα, TNFR1, and TNFR2 polymorphisms with sperm concentration and motility. J Androl. 2012;33(1):74–80.
121. Leisegang K, Dutta S. Do lifestyle practices impede male fertility? Andrologia. 2021;53(1):e13595.
122. Leisegang K, Sengupta P, Agarwal A, Henkel R. Obesity and male infertility: mechanisms and management. Andrologia. 2021;53(1):e13617.
123. Liu C-H, Tsao H-M, Cheng T-C, Wu H-M, Huang C-C, Chen C-I, et al. DNA fragmentation, mitochondrial dysfunction and chromosomal aneuploidy in the spermatozoa of oligoasthenoteratozoospermic males. J Assist Reprod Genet. 2004;21:119–26.
124. Lombardo F, Sansone A, Romanelli F, Paoli D, Gandini L, Lenzi A. The role of antioxidant therapy in the treatment of male infertility: an overview. Asian J Androl. 2011;13(5):690.
125. Lorian K, Kadkhodaee M, Kianian F, Abdi A, Sadeghipour H, Seifi B. Oxidative stress, nitric oxide and inflammation in the pathophysiology of varicocele and the effect of hydrogen sulfide as a potential treatment. Physiol Pharmacol. 2019;23(4):249–60.
126. Mahfouz R, Sharma R, Thiyagarajan A, Kale V, Gupta S, Sabanegh E, Agarwal A. Semen characteristics and sperm DNA fragmentation in infertile men with low and high levels of seminal reactive oxygen species. Fertil Steril. 2010;94(6):2141–6.
127. Malić Vončina S, Ihan AGB, Kopitar AN, Kolbezen M, Zorn B. Sperm DNA fragmentation and mitochondrial membrane potential combined are better for predicting natural conception than standard sperm parameters. Fertil Steril. 2016;105(3):637–644.e1. https://doi.org/10.1016/j.fertnstert.2015.11.037. Epub 2015 Dec 13. PMID: 26696300

128. Mannucci A, Argento FR, Fini E, Coccia ME, Taddei N, Becatti M, Fiorillo C. The impact of oxidative stress in male infertility. Front Mol Biosci. 2022;8:799294.
129. Marcon L, Boissonneault G. Transient DNA strand breaks during mouse and human spermiogenesis: new insights in stage specificity and link to chromatin remodeling. Biol Reprod. 2004;70(4):910–8.
130. Marinaro JA, Schlegel PN. Sperm DNA damage and its relevance in fertility treatment: a review of recent literature and current practice guidelines. Int J Mol Sci. 2023;24(2):1446.
131. Martin S, Reutelingsperger C, McGahon AJ, Rader JA, Van Schie R, LaFace DM, Green DR. Early redistribution of plasma membrane phosphatidylserine is a general feature of apoptosis regardless of the initiating stimulus: inhibition by overexpression of Bcl-2 and Abl. J Exp Med. 1995;182(5):1545–56.
132. Martínez-Soto JC, Domingo JC, Cordobilla B, Nicolás M, Fernández L, Albero P, et al. Dietary supplementation with docosahexaenoic acid (DHA) improves seminal antioxidant status and decreases sperm DNA fragmentation. Syst Biol Reprod Med. 2016;62(6):387–95.
133. Martinez MP, Majzoub A, Agarwal A. Antioxidants use and sperm DNA damage. In: Male infertility: contemporary clinical approaches, andrology, art and antioxidants; 2020. p. 577–92.
134. Masenga SK, Kabwe LS, Chakulya M, Kirabo A. Mechanisms of oxidative stress in metabolic syndrome. Int J Mol Sci. 2023;24(9):7898.
135. Mayorga-Torres B, Camargo M, Cadavid A, Du Plessis S, Cardona Maya W. Are oxidative stress markers associated with unexplained male infertility? Andrologia. 2017;49(5):e12659.
136. Practice Committee of American Society for Reproductive Medicine. Diagnostic evaluation of the infertile male: a committee opinion. Fertil Steril. 2012;98(2):294–301.
137. Ménézo YJ, Hazout A, Panteix G, Robert F, Rollet J, Cohen-Bacrie P, et al. Antioxidants to reduce sperm DNA fragmentation: an unexpected adverse effect. Reprod Biomed Online. 2007;14(4):418–21.
138. Micic S, Lalic N, Djordjevic D, Bojanic N, Bogavac-Stanojevic N, Busetto GM, et al. Double-blind, randomised, placebo-controlled trial on the effect of L-carnitine and L-acetylcarnitine on sperm parameters in men with idiopathic oligoasthenozoospermia. Andrologia. 2019;51(6):e13267.
139. Minhas S, Bettocchi C, Boeri L, Capogrosso P, Carvalho J, Cilesiz NC, et al. European association of urology guidelines on male sexual and reproductive health: 2021 update on male infertility. Eur Urol. 2021;80(5):603–20.
140. Moretti E, Collodel G, Mazzi L, Campagna M, Iacoponi F, Figura N. Resistin, interleukin-6, tumor necrosis factor-alpha, and human semen parameters in the presence of leukocytospermia, smoking habit, and varicocele. Fertil Steril. 2014;102(2):354–60.
141. Moskovtsev SI, Lecker I, Mullen JBM, Jarvi K, Willis J, White J, Lo KC. Cause-specific treatment in patients with high sperm DNA damage resulted in significant DNA improvement. Syst Biol Reprod Med. 2009;55(2–3):109–15.
142. Moustafa MH, Sharma RK, Thornton J, Mascha E, Abdel-Hafez MA, Thomas AJ, Agarwal A. Relationship between ROS production, apoptosis and DNA denaturation in spermatozoa from patients examined for infertility. Hum Reprod. 2004;19(1):129–38.
143. Nago M, Arichi A, Omura N, Iwashita Y, Kawamura T, Yumura Y. Aging increases oxidative stress in semen. Investig Clin Urol. 2021;62(2):233.
144. Naughton CK, Nangia AK, Agarwal A. Varicocele and male infertility: part II: pathophysiology of varicoceles in male infertility. Hum Reprod Update. 2001;7(5):473–81.
145. Nazari A, Sabeti P, Pourmasumi S. Comparison between sperm parameters and chromatin in recurrent pregnancy loss couples after antioxidant therapy. J Family Med Prim Care. 2020;9(2):597–601.
146. Nguyen-Thanh T, Hoang-Thi A-P, Thu DTA. Investigating the association between alcohol intake and male reproductive function: a current meta-analysis. Heliyon. 2023;9(5):e15723.

147. Nguyen ND, Le MT, Tran NQT, Nguyen QHV, Cao TN. Micronutrient supplements as antioxidants in improving sperm quality and reducing DNA fragmentation. Basic Clin Androl. 2023;33(1):23.
148. Ni K, Steger K, Yang H, Wang H, Hu K, Chen B. Sperm protamine mRNA ratio and DNA fragmentation index represent reliable clinical biomarkers for men with varicocele after microsurgical varicocele ligation. J Urol. 2014;192(1):170–6.
149. Ni K, Steger K, Yang H, Wang H, Hu K, Zhang T, Chen B. A comprehensive investigation of sperm DNA damage and oxidative stress injury in infertile patients with subclinical, normozoospermic, and astheno/oligozoospermic clinical varicocoele. Andrology. 2016;4(5):816–24.
150. Niki E. Action of ascorbic acid as a scavenger of active and stable oxygen radicals. Am J Clin Nutr. 1991;54(6):1119S–24S.
151. Nowicka-Bauer K, Nixon B. Molecular changes induced by oxidative stress that impair human sperm motility. Antioxidants. 2020;9(2):134.
152. Omolaoye TS, El Shahawy O, Skosana BT, Boillat T, Loney T, Du Plessis SS. The mutagenic effect of tobacco smoke on male fertility. Environ Sci Pollut Res. 2022;29(41):62055–66.
153. Omu A, Al-Azemi M, Kehinde E, Anim J, Oriowo M, Mathew T. Indications of the mechanisms involved in improved sperm parameters by zinc therapy. Med Princ Pract. 2008;17(2):108–16.
154. Oremosu A, Akang E. Impact of alcohol on male reproductive hormones, oxidative stress and semen parameters in Sprague–Dawley rats. Middle East Fertil Soc J. 2015;20(2):114–8.
155. Organization, W. H. WHO laboratory manual for the examination and processing of human semen. World Health Organization; 2021.
156. Ozer C. Antioxidant treatment of increased sperm DNA fragmentation: complex combinations are not more successful. Arch Ital Urol Androl. 2020;92(4) https://doi.org/10.4081/aiua.2020.4.362.
157. Pacey A. Environmental and lifestyle factors associated with sperm DNA damage. Hum Fertil. 2010;13(4):189–93.
158. Paisley D, Banks S, Selfridge J, McLennan NF, Ritchie A-M, McEwan C, et al. Male infertility and DNA damage in Doppel knockout and prion protein/Doppel double-knockout mice. Am J Pathol. 2004;164(6):2279–88.
159. Palani A, Alahmar A. Impact of oxidative stress on semen parameters in normozoospermic infertile men: a case–control study. Afr J Urol. 2020;26(1):50.
160. Palani A, Sengupta P, Agarwal A, Henkel R. Geographical differences in semen characteristics: comparing semen parameters of infertile men of the United States and Iraq. Andrologia. 2020;52(3):e13519.
161. Patki A, Shelatkar R, Singh M, Agarwal S, Venugopal M, Umbardand S, et al. Impact of antioxidants in improving semen parameters like count, motility and DNA fragmentation in sub-fertile males: a randomized, double-blind, placebo-controlled clinical trial. Trans Clin Pharmacol. 2023;31(1):28.
162. Poccia D. Remodeling of nucleoproteins during gametogenesis, fertilization, and early development. Int Rev Cytol. 1986;105:1–65.
163. Potts J, Pasqualotto F. Seminal oxidative stress in patients with chronic prostatitis. Andrologia. 2003;35(5):304–8.
164. Radwan M, Jurewicz J, Merecz-Kot D, Sobala W, Radwan P, Bochenek M, Hanke W. Sperm DNA damage—the effect of stress and everyday life factors. Int J Impot Res. 2016;28(4):148–54.
165. Reuter S, Gupta SC, Chaturvedi MM, Aggarwal BB. Oxidative stress, inflammation, and cancer: how are they linked? Free Radic Biol Med. 2010;49(11):1603–16.
166. Ribas-Maynou J, Yeste M. Oxidative stress in male infertility: causes, effects in assisted reproductive techniques, and protective support of antioxidants. Biology. 2020;9(4):77.

167. Ribas-Maynou J, Yeste M, Becerra-Tomás N, Aston KI, James ER, Salas-Huetos A. Clinical implications of sperm DNA damage in IVF and ICSI: updated systematic review and meta-analysis. Biol Rev. 2021;96(4):1284–300.
168. Rochdi C, Ouadrhiri M, Allai L, Bellajdel I, Mamri S, Taheri H, et al. Beneficial effects of oral antioxidant supplementation on semen quality parameters, reproductive hormones, and sperm DNA integrity in men with idiopathic oligoasthenoteratozoospermia alternative title (right-running-head): multi-antioxidant therapy in men with idiopathic oligoasthenoteratozoospermia. Metabolism. 2024;9:10.
169. Romano M, Cirillo F, Spadaro D, Busnelli A, Castellano S, Albani E, Levi-Setti PE. High sperm DNA fragmentation: do we have robust evidence to support antioxidants and testicular sperm extraction to improve fertility outcomes? a narrative review. Front Endocrinol. 2023;14:1150951.
170. Roque M, Bedoschi G, Esteves S. Effect of varicocele repair on sperm DNA fragmentation: a systematic review and meta-analysis. Fertil Steril. 2018;110(4):e162.
171. Roque M, Esteves SC. Effect of varicocele repair on sperm DNA fragmentation: a review. Int Urol Nephrol. 2018;50(4):583–603.
172. Rosa-Villagrán L, Barrera N, Montes J, Riso C, Sapiro R. Decline of semen quality over the last 30 years in Uruguay. Basic Clin Androl. 2021;31:1–10.
173. Sadek A, Almohamdy ASA, Zaki A, Aref M, Ibrahim SM, Mostafa T. Sperm chromatin condensation in infertile men with varicocele before and after surgical repair. Fertil Steril. 2011;95(5):1705–8.
174. Said TM, Land JA. Effects of advanced selection methods on sperm quality and ART outcome: a systematic review. Hum Reprod Update. 2011;17(6):719–33.
175. Said TM, Paasch U, Glander HJ, Agarwal A. Role of caspases in male infertility. Hum Reprod Update. 2004;10(1):39–51.
176. Sakkas D, Alvarez JG. Sperm DNA fragmentation: mechanisms of origin, impact on reproductive outcome, and analysis. Fertil Steril. 2010;93(4):1027–36.
177. Sakkas D, Mariethoz E, John JCS. Abnormal sperm parameters in humans are indicative of an abortive apoptotic mechanism linked to the fas-mediated pathway. Exp Cell Res. 1999;251(2):350–5.
178. Salas-Huetos A, Babio N, Carrell DT, Bulló M, Salas-Salvadó J. Adherence to the Mediterranean diet is positively associated with sperm motility: a cross-sectional analysis. Sci Rep. 2019;9(1):3389.
179. Salas-Huetos A, Maghsoumi-Norouzabad L, James ER, Carrell DT, Aston KI, Jenkins TG, et al. Male adiposity, sperm parameters and reproductive hormones: An updated systematic review and collaborative meta-analysis. Obes Rev. 2021;22(1):e13082.
180. Salehi P, Shahrokhi SZ, Kamran T, Ajami A, Taghiyar S, Deemeh MR. Effect of antioxidant therapy on the sperm DNA integrity improvement; a longitudinal cohort study. Int J Reprod BioMed. 2019;17(2):99.
181. Sanità OMD. WHO laboratory manual for the examination and processing of human semen. World Health Organization; 2010.
182. Segal BH, Grimm MJ, Khan ANH, Han W, Blackwell TS. Regulation of innate immunity by NADPH oxidase. Free Radic Biol Med. 2012;53(1):72–80.
183. Selvaraju V, Baskaran S, Agarwal A, Henkel R. Environmental contaminants and male infertility: Effects and mechanisms. Andrologia. 2021;53(1):e13646.
184. Sengupta P, Dutta S, Krajewska-Kulak E. The disappearing sperms: analysis of reports published between 1980 and 2015. Am J Mens Health. 2017;11(4):1279–304.
185. Shaha C, Tripathi R, Mishra DP. Male germ cell apoptosis: regulation and biology. Philos Trans R Soc B. 2010;365(1546):1501–15.
186. Shang X, Huang Y, Xiong C, Xu J, Yin L, Wan C. Ureaplasma urealyticum infection and apoptosis of spermatogenic cells. Asian J Androl. 1999;1(3):127–9.

187. Sharifi-Rad M, Anil Kumar NV, Varoni EM, Dini L, Panzarini E, Rajkovic J, et al. Lifestyle, oxidative stress, and antioxidants: back and forth in the pathophysiology of chronic diseases. Front Physiol. 2020;11:552535.
188. Sharma R, Gupta S, Agarwal A, Henkel R, Finelli R, Parekh N, et al. Relevance of leukocytospermia and semen culture and its true place in diagnosing and treating male infertility. World J Mens Health. 2022;40(2):191.
189. Sharma R, Harlev A, Agarwal A, Esteves SC. Cigarette smoking and semen quality: a new meta-analysis examining the effect of the 2010 World Health Organization laboratory methods for the examination of human semen. Eur Urol. 2016;70(4):635–45.
190. Sharma R, Said T, Agarwal A. Sperm DNA damage and its clinical relevance in assessing reproductive outcome. Asian J Androl. 2004;6(2):139–48.
191. Shekarriz M, Thomas A Jr, Agarwal A. Incidence and level of seminal reactive oxygen species in normal men. Urology. 1995;45(1):103–7.
192. Shen H-M, Dai J, Chia S-E, Lim A, Ong C-N. Detection of apoptotic alterations in sperm in subfertile patients and their correlations with sperm quality. Hum Reprod. 2002;17(5):1266–73.
193. Smith R, Kaune H, Parodi D, Madariaga M, Ríos R, Morales I, Castro A. Increased sperm DNA damage in patients with varicocele: relationship with seminal oxidative stress. Hum Reprod. 2006;21(4):986–93.
194. Steele EK, McClure N, Maxwell RJ, Lewis SE. A comparison of DNA damage in testicular and proximal epididymal spermatozoa in obstructive azoospermia. Mol Hum Reprod. 1999;5(9):831–5.
195. Stenqvist A, Oleszczuk K, Leijonhufvud I, Giwercman A. Impact of antioxidant treatment on DNA fragmentation index: a double-blind placebo-controlled randomized trial. Andrology. 2018;6(6):811–6.
196. Su JS, Farber NJ, Vij SC. Pathophysiology and treatment options of varicocele: an overview. Andrologia. 2021;53(1):e13576.
197. Sugihara A, Van Avermaete F, Roelant E, Punjabi U, De Neubourg D. The role of sperm DNA fragmentation testing in predicting intra-uterine insemination outcome: a systematic review and meta-analysis. Eur J Obstet Gynecol Reprod Biol. 2020;244:8–15.
198. Suleiman SA, Ali ME, Zaki Z, El-Malik E, Nasr M. Lipid peroxidation and human sperm motility: protective role of vitamin E. J Androl. 1996;17(5):530–7.
199. Sun AY, Ingelman-Sundberg M, Neve E, Matsumoto H, Nishitani Y, Minowa Y, et al. Ethanol and oxidative stress. Alcohol Clin Exp Res. 2001;25:237S–43S.
200. Takeshima T, Kuroda S, Yumura Y. Cancer chemotherapy and chemiluminescence detection of reactive oxygen species in human semen. Antioxidants. 2019;8(10):449.
201. Takeshima T, Usui K, Mori K, Asai T, Yasuda K, Kuroda S, Yumura Y. Oxidative stress and male infertility. Reprod Med Biol. 2021;20(1):41–52.
202. Tan J, Taskin O, Albert A, Bedaiwy MA. Association between sperm DNA fragmentation and idiopathic recurrent pregnancy loss: a systematic review and meta-analysis. Reprod Biomed Online. 2019;38(6):951–60.
203. Tatone C, Di Emidio G, Vento M, Ciriminna R, Artini PG. Cryopreservation and oxidative stress in reproductive cells. Gynecol Endocrinol. 2010;26(8):563–7.
204. Tremellen K. Oxidative stress and male infertility—a clinical perspective. Hum Reprod Update. 2008;14(3):243–58.
205. Tunc O, Thompson J, Tremellen K. Improvement in sperm DNA quality using an oral antioxidant therapy. Reprod Biomed Online. 2009;18(6):761–8.
206. Tunc O, Tremellen K. Oxidative DNA damage impairs global sperm DNA methylation in infertile men. J Assist Reprod Genet. 2009;26:537–44.
207. Verstrepen L, Beyaert R. Receptor proximal kinases in NF-κB signaling as potential therapeutic targets in cancer and inflammation. Biochem Pharmacol. 2014;92(4):519–29.
208. Villegas J, Schulz M, Soto L, Iglesias T, Miska W, Sánchez R. Influence of reactive oxygen species produced by activated leukocytes at the level of apoptosis in mature human spermatozoa. Fertil Steril. 2005;83(3):808–10.

209. Wang K, Gao Y, Wang C, Liang M, Liao Y, Hu K. Role of oxidative stress in varicocele. Front Genet. 2022;13:850114.
210. Wright C, Milne S, Leeson H. Sperm DNA damage caused by oxidative stress: modifiable clinical, lifestyle and nutritional factors in male infertility. Reprod Biomed Online. 2014;28(6):684–703.
211. Yamagishi SI, Maeda S, Matsui T, Ueda S, Fukami K, Okuda S. Role of advanced glycation end products (AGEs) and oxidative stress in vascular complications in diabetes. Biochim Biophys Acta Gen Subj. 2012;1820(5):663–71.
212. Yeung C-H, de Geyter C, de Geyter M, Nieschlag E. Production of reactive oxygen species by and hydrogen peroxide scavenging activity of spermatozoa in an IVF program. J Assist Reprod Genet. 1996;13:495–500.
213. Zaazaa A, Adel A, Fahmy I, Elkhiat Y, Awaad AA, Mostafa T. Effect of varicocelectomy and/ or mast cells stabilizer on sperm DNA fragmentation in infertile patients with varicocele. Andrology. 2018;6(1):146–50.
214. Zeinali M, Hadian Amree A, Khorramdelazad H, Karami H, Abedinzadeh M. Inflammatory and anti-inflammatory cytokines in the seminal plasma of infertile men suffering from varicocele. Andrologia. 2017;49(6):e12685.
215. Zhang Y, Zhang W, Wu X, Liu G, Dai Y, Jiang H, Zhang X. Effect of varicocele on sperm DNA damage: a systematic review and meta-analysis. Andrologia. 2022;54(1):e14275.
216. Zini A. Are sperm chromatin and DNA defects relevant in the clinic? Syst Biol Reprod Med. 2011;57(1–2):78–85.
217. Zini A, Boman JM, Belzile E, Ciampi A. Sperm DNA damage is associated with an increased risk of pregnancy loss after IVF and ICSI: systematic review and meta-analysis. Hum Reprod. 2008;23(12):2663–8.
218. Zini A, De Lamirande E, Gagnon C. Reactive oxygen species in semen of infertile patients: levels of superoxide dismutase-and catalase-like activities in seminal plasma and spermatozoa. Int J Androl. 1993;16(3):183–8.
219. Zini A, Dohle G. Are varicoceles associated with increased deoxyribonucleic acid fragmentation? Fertil Steril. 2011;96(6):1283–7.
220. Zini A, Meriano J, Kader K, Jarvi K, Laskin CA, Cadesky K. Potential adverse effect of sperm DNA damage on embryo quality after ICSI. Hum Reprod. 2005;20(12):3476–80.
221. Zini A, San Gabriel M, Baazeem A. Antioxidants and sperm DNA damage: a clinical perspective. J Assist Reprod Genet. 2009;26:427–32.

Chapter 7
Antioxidants and Male Infertility: State of Current Evidence

Imad Ziouziou, Fahmi Bahar, and Taymour Mostafa

Key Points

- Oxidative stress is a known cause of male infertility, which underscores the rationale for using antioxidants (AOX).
- Recent data from systematic reviews and meta-analyses support the improvement of semen quality following AOX treatment.
- The recommended duration of AOX treatment is typically 3–6 months, although the optimal duration remains uncertain.
- No comparative data are available regarding the efficacy of different types or combinations of AOX.
- There is evidence of an improvement in pregnancy rates; however, no significant improvement in live birth rates has been observed.

Introduction

Infertility and problems of impaired fecundity have been a concern through ages and are also a significant clinical problem today, which affects 8–12% of couples worldwide. Of all infertility cases, approximately 40–50% are due to "male factor"

I. Ziouziou (✉)
Department of Urology and Andrology, Mohammed VI University Hospital, College of Medicine and Pharmacy, Ibn Zohr University, Agadir, Morocco

F. Bahar
Faculty of Medicine, Muhammadiyah Palembang University, Palembang, Indonesia

Siloam Sriwijaya Palembang Hospital, Palembang, Indonesia

T. Mostafa
Department of Andrology, Sexology & STIs, Faculty of Medicine, Cairo University, Giza, Egypt

E. Chung et al. (eds.), *Advances in Andrology*,
https://doi.org/10.1007/978-3-032-29112-7_7

infertility [1]. Oxidative stress (OS), one of the primary contributors to male infertility, refers to an imbalance between the production of reactive oxygen species (ROS) and antioxidant defense mechanisms of the body. ROS, such as superoxide anions, hydrogen peroxide, and hydroxyl radicals, are formed as by-products of normal cellular metabolism, especially during the mitochondrial electron transport process [2]. However, when produced in excess, especially under conditions of environmental stress, infections, or exposure to toxins, they can cause significant cellular damage [3, 4]. The plasma membrane of spermatozoa contains high amounts of polyunsaturated fatty acids, making them vulnerable to lipid peroxidation and ROS-induced damage [5, 6]. OS may also affect the integrity of DNA, resulting in high levels of sperm DNA fragmentation (SDF) [7]. Furthermore, OS is associated with increased apoptosis [8].

These pathological pathways are correlated with a range of negative clinical outcomes like damaged germ cells, impaired fertilization, increased miscarriages, and enhanced risk of disease in the next generation [9, 10]. Studies show that 30–80% of infertile men exhibit elevated ROS levels, which attack and damage deoxyribonucleic acid (DNA) and the proteins and lipids of sperm, leading to compromised functionality, including interference with capacitation processes needed for successful fertilization (Kaltasas 2023) [11].

Antioxidant AOX treatments are a controversial subject in male infertility. They can be used as a treatment strategy to lower ROS and enhance semen quality. Besides, AOX are appealing since they are freely obtainable over-the-counter, are considered all-natural, and are thus healthful [12].

Although the mechanisms by which OS leads to impaired male fertility are well established, the evidence evaluating AOX in infertile male patients is still discordant with the heterogeneity of molecules, dosages, and combinations. Despite the low quality, it does not mean the absence of evidence.

In this chapter, we revisit the question of AOX in male infertility: Does it help improve sperm quality and reproductive outcomes? Does it matter to prescribe this treatment? Which patient will benefit more from AOX?

Oxidative Stress and Male Infertility

OS is defined as the imbalance between the antioxidant defense system and reactive oxygen species (ROS) [13]. ROS play a physiological role in smaller quantities without overwhelming the antioxidant capacity. This role is crucial for the maturation of spermatozoa and the capacity of fertilization. However, an increase in ROS, overwhelming the antioxidant capacity, triggers various mechanisms that result in male infertility [14, 15]. These mechanisms include DNA damage both in the nucleus and the mitochondria, lipid peroxidation, mitochondrial dysfunction, and apoptosis. Consequently, sperm count, as well as mobility, viability, and morphology, are negatively impacted. OS can influence the development of spermatozoa during intratesticular spermatogenesis and during transit through the epididymis and the genital tract. OS interferes in the setting of assisted reproductive technologies (ART), in particular, during cryopreservation. Many studies have demonstrated the impact of OS on fertility, pregnancy rates, and ART outcomes [16]. Besides, OS is considered a potential contributing factor in idiopathic male infertility (IMI), which consists of normal findings on physical examination, and on genetic and hormonal assessment, with abnormal semen parameters [17, 18]. Interestingly, Agarwal et al. [19] suggested a new term, "Male Oxidative Stress Infertility" (MOSI), for patients who were previously classified as having IMI.

Rationale for Antioxidants' Use

The rationale behind using antioxidant supplementation in male infertility is based on the effect of counteracting the increased ROS. Mechanisms of action are scavenging of ROS, neutralization, and contribution in maintaining the sperm DNA integrity and preserving the mitochondrial function [20]. There are two principal types of antioxidants, AOX: enzymatic and non-enzymatic (Table 7.1). Enzymatic AOXs encompass superoxide dismutase, catalase, glutathione peroxidase, and glutathione reductase. Non-enzymatic AOXs consist of glutathione, cysteine, N-acetylcysteine (NAC), vitamin C, vitamin E, carotenoids, carnitine, coenzyme Q10 (CoQ10), ferritin, L-arginine, transferrin, myo-inositol, lycopene, zinc, selenium, and folate [20].

Table 7.1 Antioxidant system

Enzymatic factors	Non-enzymatic factors
Superoxide dismutase Catalase Glutathione peroxidase Glutathione reductase	Glutathione Cysteine N-acetylcysteine Carotenoids Vitamin C Vitamin E Carnitine Ferritin L-arginine Transferrin Coenzyme Q10 Myo-inositol Lycopene Selenium Zinc Folate

Impact of Antioxidants on Infertile Men

Semen Parameters

Several studies have demonstrated the improvement of semen quality and reproductive outcomes after treatment by AOXs. Along with their meta-analysis, Zhang et al. [21] included 7 randomized controlled trials and 693 patients. The authors reported that the treatment by L-Carnitine and L-Acetyl-Carnitine significantly improved progressive sperm motility, total sperm motility, and the number of pregnancies. Wei et al. [22] published a meta-analysis, including 7 studies and 621 patients. They reported an improvement in sperm motility and normal morphology in patients who received L-Carnitine/L-Acetyl-Carnitine and N-Acetyl-Cysteine compared to the placebo group. Moreover, N-acetyl-cysteine has been demonstrated to increase sperm concentration and ejaculate volume. A recent SRMA published by Agarwal et al. [20] included 45 RCTs with 4332 infertile patients. This study addressed significantly higher semen parameters, including sperm concentration, sperm progressive motility, sperm total motility, and normal sperm morphology percentage in patients who were treated by AOX compared to controls. The common limits of these meta-analyses include the heterogeneity of AOX used, with different dosages and combinations. Also, the majority of included studies were observational.

Sperm DNA Fragmentation (SDF)

Bahmyari et al. (2019) [24] published a meta-analysis that included 23 studies reporting a reduction in SDF when AOXs were used in patients undergoing sperm freezing and thawing. In the meta-analysis of Agarwal et al. [20], three studies were eligible for analyzing the effect of AOX on SDF, but no improvement was observed.

OS Markers

Singh et al. [23] studied the efficacy of antioxidant therapy on oxidative stress parameters in the seminal plasma of infertile males in 40 infertile patients. The first semen sample was collected at the time of enrollment in the study, and the second semen sample was collected 3 months after combined antioxidant therapy. After 3 months of treatment with combined antioxidants, semen parameters like count and motility were significantly increased. The seminal level of MDA as a marker of OS was significantly lower, whereas the seminal level of antioxidant glutathione peroxidase was significantly increased after the 3 months of therapy antioxidants.

Alahmar et al. [25] investigated the effect of CoQ10 on OS markers and sperm DNA damage in infertile patients with idiopathic oligoasthenoteratospermia (OAT) in a prospective controlled study. Patients and controls received 200 mg of oral CoQ10 once daily for 3 months. The administration of CoQ10 to patients with idiopathic OAT significantly improved sperm quality and seminal antioxidant status and significantly reduced total ROS and SDF levels compared to pre-treatment values.

The SRMA by Agarwal et al. [20] found significantly higher seminal levels of total antioxidant capacity and lower seminal malondialdehyde acid in patients who received AOX. The authors reported that the results did not change after the exclusion of studies performed following varicocele repair.

Reproductive Outcomes

Pregnancy Rates

The Cochrane review, published in 2019, evaluated the effect of different AOXs on the reproductive outcomes: pregnancy, live birth, and miscarriage rates. The quality of evidence was low. However, this Cochrane review reported the efficacy of AOXs in improving the pregnancy rate (Odds ratio 2.97, 95% confidence interval 1.91–4.63) [26]. Lately, Agarwal et al. [20] published a new systematic review and meta-analysis including 45 RCTs and 4332 infertile patients. The authors reported a significantly higher pregnancy rate in patients who received AOX compared to those who received placebo or no treatment. A double-blind, placebo-controlled clinical trial has evaluated an oral antioxidant treatment containing L-carnitine and some micronutrients in terms of improvement of conventional sperm parameters, sperm DNA integrity, and IVF/ICSI outcomes. This study included a total of 263 patients who were randomly divided into two groups: The first group received the AOX treatment ($n = 131$), and the second received a placebo ($n = 132$). The duration of treatment was 3 months. Interestingly, the study revealed a significant improvement in the clinical pregnancy rate ($p = 0.01$) in addition to a significant decrease in the DFI and a significant increase in sperm motility [27].

Live Birth Rates

The 2019 Cochrane review failed to show evidence of improvement of live birth rates with AOX treatment [26]. Furthermore, the meta-analysis of Agarwal et al. [20] did not report an effect of AOX treatment on the live birth or miscarriage rates. A multicenter, double-blind, randomized, placebo-controlled trial involving nine fertility centers in the United States from December 2015 to December 2018 had the

Table 7.2 Impact of AOX on male infertility

Impact of AOX on male infertility	Type of benefit	Limitations	Type of studies	Level of evidence	References
Semen parameters	Improved semen parameters (concentration, motility, and morphology)	Heterogeneity in AOX types/ dosages, many non-RCTs	Meta-analyses, RCTs, observational	Low–moderate	[20, 21]
SDF	SDF was reported to be reduced by AOX treatment	Inconsistent findings few RCTs on SDF	Meta-analyses, limited RCTs	Low–moderate	Bahmyari et al. (2019) and Agarwal et al. [20]
OS biomarkers	Reduced MDA, increased glutathione peroxidase	Small sample sizes of the prospective studies, short durations	Prospective controlled studies, meta-analysis	Low	[23, 25]
Pregnancy rates	Improved pregnancy rates in several RCTs and meta-analyses	Not correlated with live birth	Cochrane review, meta-analyses	Moderate	[20, 26, 27]
Live birth rates	No significant effect	Large RCTs show null results	RCTs	Moderate	[20, 28]

live birth rate as a primary outcome. Males were randomly assigned into two groups. The first group ($n = 85$) received an antioxidant formulation ($n = 85$) containing 500 mg of vitamin C, 400 mg of vitamin E, 0.20 mg of selenium, 1000 mg of l-carnitine, 20 mg of zinc, 1000 μg of folic acid, 10 mg of lycopene daily, and the second received placebo ($n = 86$). The minimal duration of AOX treatment was 3 months and the maximum 6 months. Couples attempted to conceive naturally during the first 3 months of AOX treatment, and with clomiphene citrate with intrauterine insemination in months 4–6. Cumulative live birth did not differ at 6 months between the AOX and placebo groups: 15% versus 24% [28]. Given that live birth following natural pregnancy or ART is of paramount importance, these findings highlight the need for more selection of patients who will benefit from AOX treatment. More research is needed to define which AOX treatment would improve the live birth rate (Table 7.2).

Impact on Idiopathic Male Infertility Cases

Idiopathic male infertility (IMI) refers to the condition where semen quality declines, occurring in almost 30–40% of infertile men, but their exact causes are not identified. Traditional semen analyses are extensively used to determine semen quality, but these bear critical shortcomings such as poor reproducibility, subjectivity, and reduced fertility prediction. OS has been identified as the core common mechanism by which various endogenous and exogenous factors may induce IMI. For its treatment, antioxidants are mostly used to counteract OS and improve sperm parameters with appropriate combinations, dosage, and duration [17, 18]. Previously, Alahmar et al. [29] explored the evidence provided by several studies published from 2002 to 2017 on the impact of different oral antioxidants (vitamin C, vitamin E, L-carnitine, coenzyme Q10, zinc, selenium, and pentoxifylline) on semen parameters in men with idiopathic oligoasthenoteratozoospermia. Most of these studies were randomized controlled studies investigating the effect of single or combined antioxidants and reported improvements in at least one semen parameter. The most notable effect was that the use of multiple antioxidants increased sperm motility and concentration, but there was a lack of agreement on the dose, the duration of treatment, and whether individual or combined oral antioxidants should be used.

Along with their systematic review on antioxidants and male infertility, Agarwal et al. [30] showed that antioxidant supplementation improves semen parameters. In addition, it provides indications for antioxidant treatment in specific clinical conditions, including varicocele and unexplained and idiopathic male infertility, as well as in cases of altered semen quality. Also, in their scientometric analysis, Agarwal et al. [30] recognized the top 100 cited articles on "Male infertility and Antioxidants" and analyzed their publication characteristics. The articles were published in 56 journals between 1995 and 2019 with a median (interquartile range) citation score of 17 [5–61]. Antioxidant therapy was mostly investigated in male cohorts with sperm abnormalities such as asthenozoospermia (28%) and clinical conditions such as idiopathic male infertility (20%), varicocele/varicocelectomy (17%), and general male infertility (16%).

In their study, Li et al. [40] network meta-analysis studied the effects of different antioxidants on the sperm quality and pregnancy rate of idiopathic male infertility in a total of 23 RCTs with 1917 patients and 10 kinds of antioxidants. L-carnitine, l-carnitine+l-acetylcarnitine, coenzyme-Q10, ω-3 fatty acid, and selenium were more efficacious than placebo in sperm quality parameters. L-Carnitine was ranked first in sperm motility and sperm morphology, and ω-3 fatty acid was ranked first in sperm concentration.

Lately, Rochdi et al. [41] evaluated the effects of treatment with vitamin C, vitamin E, selenium, zinc, arginine, L-carnitine, and coenzyme Q10 on sperm quality parameters, DNA integrity, reproductive hormones, and pregnancy rates in 420 men with infertility and idiopathic oligoasthenoteratozoospermia (OAT) twice daily for 6 months. Significant improvement in sperm concentration was observed after supplementation at baseline, 3, and 6 months, respectively. The total sperm motility, progressive motility, and total motile sperm count also increased significantly, whereas the sperm DNA fragmentation index decreased after 6 months. There was also an increase in normal serum FSH levels and testosterone levels after 6 months of supplementation, but these differences were not statistically significant.

However, Alfaro Gómez et al. [42] pointed out that no evidence-based antioxidant treatments directly improve seminal parameters or birth ratio. While certain scientists argue against their use due to the lack of results, others support it because of their safety profile and low cost. Some uncertainties related to using antioxidants for treating MI are their questionable efficacy or the difficulties in knowing their correct dosage. In addition, the lack of quality methods for OS detection can lead to excessive antioxidant supplementation, resulting in "reductive stress." Another important problem is that, although the inflammatory process is interdependent and closely linked to OS, it is usually ignored. To solve these uncertainties, new trends have recently emerged. These include the use of molecules with anti-inflammatory and antioxidant potential, which are also able to target the reproductive tissue specifically; as well as the use of new methods that allow for reliable quantification of OS and a quality diagnosis. Also, Avila et al. [43] pointed out that despite an increased understanding of the role of OS in the pathophysiology of male infertility, therapeutic interventions based on antioxidants have not yet provided a consistent benefit for it.

On the other hand, Sengupta et al. [17, 18] pointed out that strong research evidence underpinned the concepts of OS-mediated male reproductive disruptions, which bear answers to several cases of IMI. Although antioxidant treatment held the prime solution for OS-mediated male infertility, reductive stress challenges its excess use and also predisposes men to male infertility, resolutely instituting that any biological extremes of the redox spectrum are deleterious to male fertility. The superfluity of the reducing agents may hinder essential oxidation mechanisms, affecting physiological homeostasis, looking for the fine thread between OS-mediated male infertility treatment and induction of reductive stress. In line, Dutta et al. [44] pointed out that due to the lack of proper detection of OS in male infertility, the use of antioxidant(s) in some cases may be arbitrary or lead to overuse and induction of "reductive stress." Moreover, inflammation is closely linked to OS and may establish a vicious loop that is capable of disrupting male reproductive tissues. The result is the exaggeration of cellular damage and disruption of male reproductive tissues. Therefore, the limitations of antioxidant therapy in treating male infertility are the failure in the selection of specific treatments targeting inflammation and OS simultaneously, two of the core mechanisms of male infertility.

Infertile Men Associated with Genital Tract Infection

Male infertility is a multifactorial condition influenced by epigenetic regulation, OS, and mitochondrial dysfunction. OS-induced damage leads to epigenetic modifications, disrupting gene expression crucial for spermatogenesis. Mitochondrial dysfunction impairs sperm function, while leukocytospermia exacerbates OS-related sperm dysfunction [32]. Among numerous other causes, the prevalence of male genital tract infections reportedly ranges between 10% and 35%. Leukocytospermia is found in 30% of infertile men and up to 20% in fertile men. Bacterial infections cause an inflammatory response attracting leukocytes, which produce ROS and release cytokines, rendering sperm dysfunction. The pathogenic mechanisms leading to sperm dysfunction include direct interaction of bacteria with the male germ cells, bacterial release of spermatotoxic substances, and induction of pro-inflammatory cytokines and ROS, all of which lead to OS [32].

Previously, Omu et al. [33] investigated the effect of antibiotic therapy on seminal infection along with 50 men who were divided into three groups: men with seminal infection, men with leukocytospermia only, and [3] fertile men. These authors demonstrated that antibiotic therapy improves sperm parameters by increasing antioxidant activity and IL-4 and by reducing IL-2 and IL-8. Along with their study, Yadav et al. [34] suggested that supplementary treatment with antioxidants and antibiotics for leukocytospermic infertile male patients may improve sperm membrane integrity. Besides, Gambera et al. [35] suggested that a combined immunomodulating and antioxidant treatment protects spermatozoa during maturation and migration through the male genital tract, resulting in a functional rescue demonstrated by improved semen quality.

Piomboni et al. [36] studied the immune-modulating and antioxidant effects of beta-glucan, papaya, lactoferrin, and vitamins C and E on sperm parameters of 51 infertile patients with asthenoteratozoospermia associated with leukocytosis. After 90 days of treatment, an increase in the percentage of morphologically normal spermatozoa and total progressive sperm motility was detected. Structural sperm characteristics, as well as chromatin integrity, were also improved after treatment. A significant reduction of the leukocyte concentration in seminal fluid was reported. These authors concluded that treating this inflammatory process by the synergic action of immune modulators and antioxidants could protect sperm during maturation and migration, leading to improved sperm function.

Gill et al. [37] assessed the relationship between male infertility, basic semen characteristics, SDF, oxidation-reduction potential in semen, and leukocytospermia. The results showed that [1] there is a relationship between male infertility, SDF, and OS in semen [2]; in infertile men, there is a significant risk of SDF and OS irrespective of leukocytopenia; and [3] the assessment of SDF and OS should be independent of leukocytopenia. Additionally, Henkel [38] addressed that those seminal bacterial infections, including "silent" infections, are treatable, with antibiotics being the treatment of choice. Yet, antioxidants should also be considered to alleviate the inflammatory process and improve semen quality [38].

While co-administration of antioxidants with antimicrobial therapy may enhance outcomes, optimal protocols, treatment duration, and patient selection criteria are yet to be defined. More research is needed to identify effective strategies in managing infection-related male infertility.

Impact of Adjuvant AOX Therapy on Non-operated Varicocele

Varicocele-associated male infertility has been classically managed using surgery or ART. With increasing evidence of OS as a pathophysiological factor in varicocele-associated infertility, medical therapy, especially antioxidants, might become a treatment option due to its theoretical benefit, data from preclinical studies, and lack of major side effects. Along with their study, Garg and Kumar [45] reviewed the existing literature on the role of various medical agents in managing male infertility associated with varicoceles. Medical therapy was evaluated in three different situations such as (a) a comparison of two drugs or one drug with a placebo, (b) a comparison of drugs versus surgery, and (c) a comparison of drugs as adjuvant therapy with surgery versus drug therapy alone. Due to the heterogeneity of data and lack of well-conducted studies, there is insufficient data to recommend routine use of medical therapy for men with varicocele-associated infertility, and surgery remains the treatment of choice.

Later on, Pyrgidis et al. [46] performed a systematic review and meta-analysis to explore the role of antioxidant supplementation in patients with operated or non-operated varicocele, including 14 studies (980 individuals). Of the 14 studies, 2 explored the effect of antioxidant supplementation in patients with non-operated varicocele, 1 compared antioxidants versus surgical repair of varicocele, and 11 explored antioxidants after surgical varicocele repair. Regarding pregnancy rates, no significant differences were demonstrated after treatment with antioxidants versus no treatment at 3 (OR: 2.28, 95% CI: 0.7–7.48) and 6 months (OR: 1.88, 95% CI: 0.62–5.72). Accordingly, contradictory findings were reported in sperm concentration, morphology, motility, and DNA fragmentation. These authors indicated that antioxidant supplementation does not improve pregnancy rates and semen parameters in patients with varicocele-associated infertility in the absence of previous screening for oxidative stress.

In their study, Arab et al. [47] collected scientific evidence from both basic and clinical studies which support the use of dietary supplements, such as minerals, vitamins, and antioxidants, have an essential role in the treatment of varicocele by increasing the levels of antioxidant enzymes (e.g., peroxidase, superoxide dismutase, and catalase) and decreasing the levels of inflammatory markers (e.g., tumor necrosis factor-α, interleukin-6, and interleukin-1) in the testis.

In their systematic review on antioxidants and male infertility, Agarwal et al. [30] provided the indications for antioxidant treatment in specific clinical conditions, including varicocele, unexplained and idiopathic male infertility, as well as in cases of altered semen quality.

Lately, along with their study, Szymański et al. [48] investigated a total of 85 men with varicocele-related infertility group. All patients received treatment with a male fertility supplement containing a combination of 1725 mg of L-carnitine fumarate, 500 mg of acetyl-L-carnitine, 90 mg of vitamin C, 20 mg of coenzyme Q10, 10 mg of zinc, 200 μg of folic acid, 50 μg of selenium, and 1.5 μg of vitamin B12 (Proxeed® Plus, Sigma-Tau, Italy) twice/day for 6 months. The treatment resulted in significant improvement in semen parameters, particularly sperm count, sperm concentration, total motility, and progressive motility, with a marked therapeutic benefit in patients with Grade III varicocele, having a greater improvement in progressive motility than in men with less severe or no varicocele. These authors concluded that the use of the antioxidant preparations seems reasonable as an adjuvant in those with varicocele-related infertility, particularly in patients with Grade III varicocele who do not wish to undergo surgical treatment or in whom such a treatment is not possible for various reasons.

Impact of Adjuvant AOX Therapy After Varicocelectomy

Nematollahi-Mahani et al. [49] evaluated serum hormonal levels (inhibin B, FSH, and testosterone) and seminal plasma antioxidant defense levels after folic acid and zinc sulfate administration in varicocelectomy patients that were randomly allocated to 4 groups: zinc sulfate/folic acid, folic acid, zinc sulfate, and placebo. Patients in different groups took one capsule per day after dinner following varicocelectomy for 6 months. A significant rise in peripheral blood inhibin B and seminal plasma activity was detected in the zinc sulfate/folic acid group after 6 months, indicating a change in the hormonal status of post-varicocelectomy patients following long-term administration of zinc sulfate and folic acid.

Pourmand et al. [50] concluded that the addition of 750 mg of L-carnitine orally daily to standard inguinal varicocelectomy does not add any extra benefit in terms of improvement in semen analysis parameters or DNA damage.

Barekat et al. [51] evaluated the outcome of N-acetyl-L-cysteine (NAC) on semen quality, protamine content, DNA damage, OS, and fertility following varicocelectomy in 35 infertile men with varicocele, randomly divided into control ($n = 20$) and NAC ($n = 15$) groups. The percentages of abnormal semen parameters, protamine deficiency, SDF, and OS were significantly decreased in both groups compared to before surgery. The results revealed that NAC improved chromatin integrity and pregnancy rate when administered as adjunct therapy post-varicocelectomy.

Ener et al. [52] showed that vitamin E supplementation might improve sperm parameters after varicocelectomy.

Chen et al. [53] performed a systematic review and meta-analysis to assess the efficacy of adjuvant drug therapy after varicocelectomy along 10 randomized controlled trials containing 533 patients with adjuvant drug therapy after varicocelectomy and 368 patients with no medical treatment after varicocelectomy. It had been revealed that the improvement in pregnancy rate after adjuvant drug therapy was insignificant but resulted in significant improvements in sperm concentration and motility at 3 months, sperm DNA integrity, and serum FSH level. Therefore, compared to no medical treatment, adjuvant drug therapy, especially the use of antioxidants, seems to be associated with better fertility outcomes.

Wang et al. (2019) [64] carried out a systematic review and a meta-analysis to evaluate the efficacy of antioxidant therapy in sperm parameters' quality after varicocelectomy during 3 or 6 months treatment cycle in six studies including 576 patients. Significant improvements in sperm concentration, sperm motility, progressive sperm motility, and sperm morphology existed in the antioxidant group 3 months after varicocelectomy. With regard to the 6 months' outcomes, sperm parameters were improved as well, except sperm motility and progressive sperm motility. Referring to pregnancy rate, no significant difference existed between the two groups, and the FSH level of the antioxidant group was lower than that of the placebo group 3 or 6 months after varicocelectomy. These authors concluded that, compared with the placebo, the antioxidant therapy after varicocelectomy can improve the quality of sperm parameters and construct a favorable living condition for spermatozoa by reducing FSH levels.

Ardestani Zadeh et al. [54] evaluated the effects of antioxidants, including Vitamin E-Selenium-Folic acid (Vit E-Se-FA), on semen parameters following varicocelectomy (VCT).

Sixty patients out of 64 infertile male patients diagnosed with varicocele (VC) who underwent sub-inguinal VCT were included in the study. Following sub-inguinal VCT, the patients were randomized into two groups: 30 receiving Vit E-Se-FA supplementation for 6 months and 30 as the control group with supplemental treatment. The postoperative semen parameters of the Vit E-Se-FA group were compared with those of the control group. There were significant differences in terms of count and motility of sperm after 6 months of receiving Vit E-Se-FA supplementation compared with the control group. It was concluded that E-Se-FA supplementation could improve sperm parameters (count and motility of sperm) after VCT.

In their study, Kızılay et al. (2019) [55] evaluated the effect of oral antioxidant treatment on semen parameters and pregnancy rates in infertile men who underwent varicocelectomy in 90 patients. They were divided into two groups; the first group received antioxidant treatment for 6 months after the operation, and the second group did not receive treatment after the operation. The improvement in total sperm count (+45.9% vs +26.8%), total motile sperm count (+50.6% vs +29.7%), sperm concentration (+71.4% vs +54.5%), sperm count in normal morphology (+75.7% vs +39.9%), and total (+28.6% vs +18.3%) and progressive motile sperm count (+60.4% vs +38.9%) were significantly higher in the treated group than in the untreated group ($p = 0.011$, $p < 0.001$, $p = 0.008$, $p < 0.001$, $p = 0.024$ and $p < 0.001$, respectively). The clinical pregnancy rate in the first group was significantly higher than that in the second group (29% vs 17.9%) ($p = 0.029$). These authors concluded that the antioxidant treatment provides an important contribution to varicocelectomy outcomes and improves pregnancy rates.

Along with their systematic review and meta-analysis, Pyrgidis et al. [46] explored the role of antioxidants in patients with operated varicocele in 11 studies. Their findings indicated that antioxidant supplementation does not improve pregnancy rates and semen parameters in patients with varicocele-associated infertility in the absence of previous screening for OS.

Table 7.3 Current guidelines regarding antioxidant use for male infertility

	Year	Guideline
ESHRE	2023	Adjunct oral antioxidant therapy to males undergoing fertility treatment is probably not recommended [56]
AUA/ ASRM	2024	« Clinicians should counsel patients that the benefits of supplements (eg, antioxidants, vitamins) are of questionable clinical utility in treating male infertility. Existing data are inadequate to provide recommendation for specific agents to use for this purpose. (Mod erate Recommendation; Evidence Level: Grade B) » [57]
EAA	2018	No recommendation for using antioxidant [58]
EAU	2025	"No conclusive data are available regarding the beneficial treatment with antioxidants in men with idiopathic infertility, although they may improve semen parameters" (EAU 2025)

- *Current Guideline Statements on Antioxidants*

Several associations involved in the field of male infertility provide their respective views in the form of guidelines that can be seen in Table 7.3. Interestingly, all of these guidelines unanimously agree not to recommend the use of antioxidant therapy in cases of male infertility. This contrasts with the latest SRMA results from Agarwal et al. [20], which concluded that antioxidants could improve sperm parameters and are beneficial for specific clinical indications such as idiopathic male infertility, unexplained male infertility, and varicocele.

- *Practical Points*

When Would AOX Be Useful?

There is actually no definitive guideline yet on when antioxidant therapy will truly be beneficial, as research on this matter still yields conflicting results. Some studies claim that antioxidants are very beneficial, while others say the opposite. To prove the efficacy of antioxidants in treating male infertility, there is still limited availability of RCTs and numerous biases in the subject selection process [31, 60].

AOX Use Before ART?

Is antioxidant therapy necessary for men undergoing ART? Questions like this will never find a definitive answer. This is reflected in the research conducted so far, where the results of these studies do not align. Some studies support it, while others state that antioxidant therapy before ART is futile [61]. A prospective randomized double-blind placebo-controlled trial involving 60 couples with severe male infertility issues was conducted. Some were given antioxidants, while others received a placebo for 3 months before undergoing IVF. It was found that the pregnancy rate was significantly higher in the treatment group compared to the control group (38.5% vs. 16%) [62]. In 2021, a retrospective cohort study was conducted with the same antioxidants and placebos involving 657 men. The live birth rate in the antioxidant group was significantly higher (odds ratio of 1.57, 95% confidence interval of 1.01 to 2.45, $P = 0.046$) [63]. One of the contributing factors is believed to be the effect of antioxidants in reducing SDF levels and improving the zona binding assay.

AOX Use in NOA?

The benefits of antioxidant therapy in cases of mild male infertility with oligozoospermia, asthenozoospermia, teratozoospermia, or oligoasthenoteratozoospermia are perceived to be quite powerful in improving sperm parameters and increasing the chances of natural pregnancy, as outlined in the above sub-section. However, this does not apply to cases of azoospermia, especially NOA. In such cases, clinicians typically recommend surgical sperm retrieval (SSR) directly. If treatment is administered before this procedure, pharmacotherapy usually includes drugs such as GnRH, SERM, and aromatase inhibitors [65, 66].

However, only one study was found that examined the benefits of multivitamin combination therapy (Coenzyme Q10, vitamin A, vitamin B1, B2, B6, B12, Nicotinamide, d-panthenol, folic acid, vitamin C, vitamin D3, vitamin E, potassium iodide, calcium, magnesium, ferrous fumarate, copper sulfate, manganese sulfate, and zinc sulfate) at a dose of 3× daily for 10 months and compared with placebo in men with NOA. In the treatment group, the appearance of sperm with a concentration of four million/ml was obtained at the first-month follow-up [67]. Unfortunately, this study, according to Kumar [65], was not accompanied by a well-documented methodology.

Conclusions

There is more evidence supporting that antioxidants improve sperm quality and reproductive outcomes, particularly in cases of idiopathic male infertility and patients undergoing varicocelectomy. Despite the positive reported findings, the quality of available evidence remains low. Moreover, there is an issue of heterogeneity in the studies in terms of AOX formulations, dosages, and duration of the treatment. More robust, high-quality, randomized controlled trials are needed to clearly establish more precise clinical indications. Furthermore, it is important to note that the excessive AOX treatment could be detrimental. Indeed, over-supplementation can lead to a state of reductive stress.

References

1. Kumar N, Singh AK. Trends of male factor infertility, an important cause of infertility: a review of literature. J Hum Reprod Sci. 2015;8(4):191–6. https://doi.org/10.4103/0974-1208.170370.
2. Schieber M, Chandel NS. ROS function in redox signaling and oxidative stress. Curr Biol. 2014;24(10):R453–62.
3. Pizzino G, Irrera N, Cucinotta M, Pallio G, Mannino F, Arcoraci V, Squadrito F, Altavilla D, Bitto A. Oxidative stress: harms and benefits for human health. Oxidative Med Cell Longev. 2017;2017:8416763.
4. Andersson KE. Oxidative stress and its possible relation to lower urinary tract functional pathology. BJU Int. 2018;121(4):527–33.
5. Koppers AJ, Garg ML, Aitken RJ. Stimulation of mitochondrial reactive oxygen species production by unesterified, unsaturated fatty acids in defective human spermatozoa. Free Radic Biol Med. 2010;48(1):112–9.
6. Alahmar AT. Role of oxidative stress in male infertility: an updated review. J Hum Reprod Sci. 2019;12(1):4–18.
7. Wang Y, Su M, Chen Y, Huang X, Ruan L, Lv Q, Li L. Research progress on the role and mechanism of DNA damage repair in germ cell development. Front Endocrinol (Lausanne). 2023;14:1234280.
8. Sharma P, Kaushal N, Saleth LR, Ghavami S, Dhingra S, Kaur P. Oxidative stress-induced apoptosis and autophagy: balancing the contrary forces in spermatogenesis. Biochim Biophys Acta Mol basis Dis. 2023;1869(6):166742.
9. Castleton PE, Deluao JC, Sharkey DJ, McPherson NO. Measuring reactive oxygen species in semen for male preconception care: a scientist perspective. Antioxidants. 2022;11(2):264.
10. Ojo OA, Nwafor-Ezeh PI, Rotimi DE, Iyobhebhe M, Ogunlakin AD, Ojo AB. Apoptosis, inflammation, and oxidative stress in infertility: a mini review. Toxicol Rep. 2023;10:448–62.
11. Kaltsas A. Oxidative Stress and Male Infertility: The Protective Role of Antioxidants. Medicina (Kaunas). 2023;59(10):1769.
12. Ali M, Martinez M, Parekh N. Are antioxidants a viable treatment option for male infertility? Andrologia. 2021;53(1):e13644.
13. Houldsworth A. Role of oxidative stress in neurodegenerative disorders: a review of reactive oxygen species and prevention by antioxidants. Brain Commun. 2024;6(1):fcad356.
14. Dutta S, Majzoub A, Agarwal A. Oxidative stress and sperm function: a systematic review on evaluation and management. Arab J Urol. 2019;17(2):87–97.
15. Sengupta P, Pinggera GM, Calogero AE, Agarwal A. Oxidative stress affects sperm health and fertility-time to apply facts learned at the bench to help the patient: lessons for busy clinicians. Reprod Med Biol. 2024;23(1):e12598.
16. Takalani NB, Monageng EM, Mohlala K, Monsees TK, Henkel R, Opuwari CS. Role of oxidative stress in male infertility. Reprod Fertil. 2023;4(3):e230024.
17. Sengupta P, Roychoudhury S, Nath M, Dutta S. Oxidative Stress and Idiopathic Male Infertility. In: Kesari KK, Roychoudhury S (eds) Oxidative Stress and Toxicity in Reproductive Biology and Medicine. Advances in Experimental Medicine and Biology, vol.1358, Springer, Cham, 2022. https://doi.org/10.1007/978-3-030-89340-8_9.
18. Sengupta P, Dutta S, Alahmar AT. Reductive Stress and Male Infertility. In: Roychoudhury S, Kesari, KK (eds) Oxidative Stress and Toxicity in Reproductive Biology and Medicine. Advances in Experimental Medicine and Biology, vol.1391, Springer, Cham, 2022. https://doi.org/10.1007/978-3-031-12966-7_17.
19. Agarwal A, Parekh N, Panner Selvam MK, Henkel R, Shah R, Homa ST, Ramasamy R, Ko E, Tremellen K, Esteves S, Majzoub A, Alvarez JG, Gardner DK, Jayasena CN, Ramsay JW, Cho CL, Saleh R, Sakkas D, Hotaling JM, Lundy SD, Vij S, Marmar J, Gosalvez J, Sabanegh E, Park HJ, Zini A, Kavoussi P, Micic S, Smith R, Busetto GM, Bakırcıoğlu ME, Haidl G, Balercia G, Puchalt NG, Ben-Khalifa M, Tadros N, Kirkman-Browne J, Moskovtsev S, Huang

X, Borges E, Franken D, Bar-Chama N, Morimoto Y, Tomita K, Srini VS, Ombelet W, Baldi E, Muratori M, Yumura Y, La Vignera S, Kosgi R, Martinez MP, Evenson DP, Zylbersztejn DS, Roque M, Cocuzza M, Vieira M, Ben-Meir A, Orvieto R, Levitas E, Wiser A, Arafa M, Malhotra V, Parekattil SJ, Elbardisi H, Carvalho L, Dada R, Sifer C, Talwar P, Gudeloglu A, Mahmoud AMA, Terras K, Yazbeck C, Nebojsa B, Durairajanayagam D, Mounir A, Kahn LG, Baskaran S, Pai RD, Paoli D, Leisegang K, Moein MR, Malik S, Yaman O, Samanta L, Bayane F, Jindal SK, Kendirci M, Altay B, Perovic D, Harlev A. Male oxidative stress infertility (MOSI): proposed terminology and clinical practice guidelines for management of idiopathic male infertility. World J Mens Health. 2019;37(3):296–312.
20. Agarwal A, Cannarella R, Saleh R, Harraz AM, Kandil H, Salvio G, Boitrelle F, Kuroda S, Farkouh A, Rambhatla A, Zini A, Colpi G, Gül M, Kavoussi P, Hamoda TAA, Ko E, Calik G, Toprak T, Pinggera GM, Park HJ, Ghayda RA, Minhas S, Busetto GM, Bakırcıoğlu ME, Kadioglu A, Chung E, Russo GI, Calogero AE, Ambar RF, Jayasena CN, Shah R. Impact of antioxidant therapy on natural pregnancy outcomes and semen parameters in infertile men: a systematic review and meta-analysis of randomized controlled trials. World J Mens Health. 2023;41(1):14–48.
21. Zhang X, Cui Y, Dong L, Sun M, Zhang Y. The efficacy of combined l-carnitine and l-acetyl carnitine in men with idiopathic oligoasthenoteratozoospermia: a systematic review and meta-analysis. Andrologia. 2020;52(2):e13470.
22. Wei G, Zhou Z, Cui Y, Huang Y, Wan Z, Che X, Chai Y, Zhang Y. A meta-analysis of the efficacy of L-carnitine/l-acetyl-carnitine or N-acetyl-cysteine in men with idiopathic asthenozoospermia. Am J Mens Health. 2021;15(2):15579883211011371.
23. Singh A, Jahan N, Radhakrishnan G, Banerjee BD. To evaluate the efficacy of combination antioxidant therapy on oxidative stress parameters in seminal plasma in the male infertility. Clin Diagn Res. 2016;10(7):QC14–7.
24. Bahmyari R, Zare M, Sharma R, Agarwal A, Halvaei I. The efficacy of antioxidants in sperm parameters and production of reactive oxygen species levels during the freeze-thaw process: A systematic review and metaanalysis. Andrologia. 2020;52(3):e13514. https://doi.org/10.1111/and.13514.
25. Alahmar AT, Sengupta P, Dutta S, Calogero AE. Coenzyme Q10, oxidative stress markers, and sperm DNA damage in men with idiopathic oligoasthenoteratospermia. Clin Exp Reprod Med. 2021;48(2):150–5.
26. Smits RM, Mackenzie-Proctor R, Yazdani A, Stankiewicz MT, Jordan V, Showell MG. Antioxidants for male subfertility. Cochrane Database Syst Rev. 2019;3(3):CD007411.
27. Lahimer M, Gherissi O, Ben Salem N, Ben Mustapha H, Bach V, Khorsi-Cauet H, Khairi H, Ben Ali H, BenKhalifa M, Ajina M. Effect of micronutrients and L-carnitine as antioxidant on sperm parameters, genome integrity, and ICSI outcomes: randomized, double-blind, and placebo-controlled clinical trial. Antioxidants. 2023;12(11):1937.
28. Steiner AZ, Hansen KR, Barnhart KT, Cedars MI, Legro RS, Diamond MP, Krawetz SA, Usadi R, Baker VL, Coward RM, Huang H, Wild R, Masson P, Smith JF, Santoro N, Eisenberg E, Zhang H, Reproductive Medicine Network. The effect of antioxidants on male factor infertility: the males, antioxidants, and infertility (MOXI) randomized clinical trial. Fertil Steril. 2020;113(3):552–560.e3.
29. Alahmar AT. The effects of oral antioxidants on the semen of men with idiopathic oligoasthenoteratozoospermia. Clin Exp Reprod Med. 2018;45:57–66.
30. Agarwal A, Leisegang K, Majzoub A, Henkel R, Finelli R, Panner Selvam MK, Tadros N, Parekh N, Ko EY, Cho CL, Arafa M, Alves MG, Oliveira PF, Alvarez JG, Shah R. Utility of antioxidants in the treatment of male infertility: clinical guidelines based on a systematic review and analysis of evidence. World J Mens Health. 2021;39(2):233–90.
31. Kaltsas A. Oxidative stress and male infertility: the protective role of antioxidants. Medicina (Kaunas). 2023;59(10):1769.
32. Sudhakaran G, Kesavan D, Kandaswamy K, Guru A, Arockiaraj J. Unravelling the epigenetic impact: oxidative stress and its role in male infertility-associated sperm dysfunction. Reprod Toxicol. 2024;124:108531.

33. Omu AE, al-Othman S, Mohamad AS, al-Kaluwby NM, Fernandes S. Antibiotic therapy for seminal infection. Effect on antioxidant activity and T-helper cytokines. J Reprod Med. 1998;43(10):857–64.
34. Yadav SB, Suryakar AN, Huddedar AD, Shukla PS. Effect of antioxidants and antibiotics on levels of seminal oxidative stress in leukocytospermic infertile men. Indian J Clin Biochem. 2006;21(1):152–6.
35. Gambera L, Campanella G, Piomboni P, Serafini F, Morgante G, De Leo V. Association of antioxidants and natural immune activators in the treatment of astheno-teratospermia and abacterial leukocytosis. Minerva Ginecol. 2007;59(5):473–9.
36. Piomboni P, Gambera L, Serafini F, Campanella G, Morgante G, De Leo V. Sperm quality improvement after natural anti-oxidant treatment of asthenoteratospermic men with leukocytospermia. Asian J Androl. 2008;10(2):201–6.
37. Gill K, Machalowski T, Harasny P, Kups M, Grabowska M, Duchnik E, Sipak O, Fraczek M, Kurpisz M, Kurzawa R, Piasecka M. Male infertility coexists with decreased sperm genomic integrity and oxidative stress in semen irrespective of leukocytospermia. Antioxidants. 2022;11(10):1987.
38. Henkel R. Leukocytospermia and/or bacteriospermia: impact on male infertility. J Clin Med. 2024;13(10):2841.
39. Agarwal A, Selvam MKP, Baskaran S, Finelli R, Leisegang K, Barbăroşie C, Pushparaj PN, Robert KA, Ambar RF, Iovine C, Durairajanayagam D, Henkel R. Highly cited articles in the field of male infertility and antioxidants: a scientometric analysis. World J Mens Health. 2021;39(4):760–75.
40. Li KP, Yang XS, Wu T. The effect of antioxidants on sperm quality parameters and pregnancy rates for idiopathic male infertility: a network meta-analysis of randomized controlled trials. Front Endocrinol (Lausanne). 2022;13:810242.
41. Rochdi C, Ouadrhiri M, Allai L, Bellajdel I, Mamri S, Taheri H, Saadi H, Mimouni A, Choukri M. Beneficial effects of oral antioxidant supplementation on semen quality parameters, reproductive hormones, and sperm DNA integrity in men with idiopathic oligoasthenoteratozoospermia. Clin Exp Reprod Med. 2024;51(2):135–41.
42. Alfaro Gómez M, Fernández-Santos MDR, Jurado-Campos A, Soria-Meneses PJ, Montoro Angulo V, Soler AJ, Garde JJ, Rodríguez-Robledo V. On males, antioxidants and infertility (MOXI): certitudes, uncertainties and trends. Antioxidants. 2023;12(8):1626.
43. Ávila C, Vinay JI, Arese M, Saso L, Rodrigo R. Antioxidant intervention against male infertility: time to design novel strategies. Biomedicine. 2022;10(12):3058.
44. Dutta S, Sengupta P, Roychoudhury S, Chakravarthi S, Wang CW, Slama P. Antioxidant paradox in male infertility: 'a blind eye' on inflammation. Antioxidants. 2022;11(1):167.
45. Garg H, Kumar R. An update on the role of medical treatment including antioxidant therapy in varicocele. Asian J Androl. 2016;18(2):222–8.
46. Pyrgidis N, Sokolakis I, Palapelas V, Tishukov M, Mykoniatis I, Symeonidis N, Zachariou A, Kaltsas A, Sofikitis N, Hatzichristodoulou G, Tsiampali C, Dimitriadis F. The effect of antioxidant supplementation on operated or non-operated varicocele-associated infertility: a systematic review and meta-analysis. Antioxidants. 2021;10(7):1067.
47. Arab D, Doustmohammadi H, Ardestani ZA. Dietary supplements in the management of varicocele-induced infertility: a review of potential mechanisms. Andrologia. 2021;53(1):e13879.
48. Szymański M, Domaracki P, Szymańska A, Wandtke T, Szyca R, Brycht Ł, Wasilow K, Skorupski WJ. The role and place of antioxidants in the treatment of male infertility caused by varicocele. J Clin Med. 2022;11(21):6391.
49. Nematollahi-Mahani SN, Azizollahi GH, Baneshi MR, Safari Z, Azizollahi S. Effect of folic acid and zinc sulphate on endocrine parameters and seminal antioxidant level after varicocelectomy. Andrologia. 2014;46(3):240–5.
50. Pourmand G, Movahedin M, Dehghani S, Mehrsai A, Ahmadi A, Pourhosein M, Hoseini M, Ziloochi M, Heidari F, Beladi L, Noori M. Does L-carnitine therapy add any extra benefit to

standard inguinal varicocelectomy in terms of deoxyribonucleic acid damage or sperm quality factor indices: a randomized study. Urology. 2014;84(4):821–5.
51. Barekat F, Tavalaee M, Deemeh MR, Bahreinian M, Azadi L, Abbasi H, Rozbahani S, Nasr-Esfahani MH. A preliminary study: N-acetyl-L-cysteine improves semen quality following varicocelectomy. Int J Fertil Steril. 2016;10(1):120–6.
52. Ener K, Aldemir M, Işık E, Okulu E, Özcan MF, Uğurlu M, Tangal S, Özayar A. The impact of vitamin E supplementation on semen parameters and pregnancy rates after varicocelectomy: a randomised controlled study. Andrologia. 2016;48(7):829–34.
53. Chen YW, Niu YH, Wang DQ, Li H, Pokhrel G, Xu WT, Wang SG, Liu JH. Effect of adjuvant drug therapy after varicocelectomy on fertility outcome in males with varicocele-associated infertility: systematic review and meta-analysis. Andrologia. 2018;50(8):e13070.
54. Ardestani Zadeh A, Arab D, Kia NS, Heshmati S, Amirkhalili SN. The role of vitamin E - selenium - folic acid supplementation in improving sperm parameters after varicocelectomy: a randomized clinical trial. Urol J. 2019;16(5):495–500.
55. Kızılay F, Altay B. Evaluation of the effects of antioxidant treatment on sperm parameters and pregnancy rates in infertile patients after varicocelectomy: a randomized controlled trial. Int J Impot Res. 2019;31(6):424–31.
56. Guideline Group on Unexplained Infertility, Romualdi D, Ata B, Bhattacharya S, Bosch E, Costello M, Gersak K, Homburg R, Mincheva M, Norman RJ, Piltonen T, Dos Santos-Ribeiro S, Scicluna D, Somers S, Sunkara SK, Verhoeve HR, Le Clef N. Evidence-based guideline: unexplained infertility. Hum Reprod. 2023;38(10):1881–90.
57. Brannigan RE, Hermanson L, Kaczmarek J, Kim SK, Kirkby E, Tanrikut C. Updates to male infertility: AUA/ASRM guideline. J Urol. Published online August. 2024;15:2024.
58. Colpi GM, Francavilla S, Haidl G, Link K, Behre HM, Goulis DG, Krausz C, Giwercman A. European academy of andrology guideline management of oligo-astheno-teratozoospermia. Andrology. 2018;6(4):513–24.
59. European Association of Urology. EAU Guidelines. Arnhem, The Netherlands: EAU Guidelines Office; 2022. Edn. presented at the EAU Annual Congress Amsterdam, the Netherlands. ISBN 978-94-92671-16-5.
60. Lanzafame FM, La Vignera S, Vicari E, Calogero AE. Oxidative stress and medical antioxidant treatment in male infertility. Reprod Biomed Online. 2009;19(5):638–59.
61. de Ligny W, Smits RM, Mackenzie-Proctor R, Jordan V, Fleischer K, de Bruin JP, Showell MG. Antioxidants for male subfertility. Cochrane Database Syst Rev. 2022;5(5):CD007411.
62. Tremellen K, Miari G, Froiland D, Thompson J. A randomised control trial examining the effect of an antioxidant (Menevit) on pregnancy outcome during IVF-ICSI treatment. Aust N Z J Obstet Gynaecol. 2007;47(3):216–21.
63. Tremellen K, Woodman R, Hill A, Shehadeh H, Lane M, Zander-Fox D. Use of a male antioxidant nutraceutical is associated with superior live birth rates during IVF treatment. Asian J Androl. 2021;23(1):16–23.
64. Wang J, Wang T, Ding W, et al. Efficacy of antioxidant therapy on sperm quality measurements after varicocelectomy: A systematic review and meta-analysis. Andrologia. 2019;51(10):e13396. https://doi.org/10.1111/and.13396.
65. Kumar R. Medical management of non-obstructive azoospermia. Clinics. 2013;68(Suppl 1):75–9.
66. Ring JD, Lwin AA, Köhler TS. Current medical management of endocrine-related male infertility. Asian J Androl. 2016;18(3):357–63.
67. Singh AK, Tiwari AK, Singh PB, Dwivedi US, Trivedi S, Singh SK, Agrawal NK, Deshpande SB. Multivitamin and micronutrient treatment improves semen parameters of azoospermic patients with maturation arrest. Indian J Physiol Pharmacol. 2010;54(2):157–63.

Chapter 8
Controversies in Varicocele Diagnosis and Management

Naveen Kumar, Fahmi Bahar, and Taymour Mostafa

Introduction

Varicocele is an abnormal dilatation of the internal spermatic vein and veins in the pampiniform plexus in the scrotum, which drain blood from both testes [1]. In De Medicina, written during the first century AD, Celsus credits the Greeks with the first description of a varicocele, and he recorded his own acute observation: "The veins are swollen and twisted over the testicle, which becomes smaller" [2]. Many epidemiological studies have shown that varicoceles develop at puberty and its prevalence in adult men increases with age [3, 4]. Generally, varicocele is more common on the left side; however, up to half of the patients have bilateral varicoceles [5]. Varicoceles are usually present in about 15% of males, in 35% of males affected with primary infertility, and in up to 80% of men having secondary infertility [6, 7].

Several mechanisms explaining varicocele leading to male infertility have been proposed; however, the exact pathophysiology has not yet been proven. An increase in the local scrotal temperature due to varicocele has been postulated to be the primary mechanism affecting the decline in the hormonal as well as the reproductive function of the testes [8, 9]. The reflux of the adrenal and renal metabolites into the testes through the dilated veins has also been proposed as another mechanism for

N. Kumar (✉)
Department of Urology, All India Institute of Medical Sciences, Patna, India

F. Bahar
Faculty of Medicine, Muhammadiyah Palembang University, Palembang, Indonesia

Siloam Sriwijaya Palembang Hospital, Palembang, Indonesia

T. Mostafa
Department of Andrology, Sexology & STIs, Faculty of Medicine, Cairo University, Cairo, Egypt

E. Chung et al. (eds.), *Advances in Andrology*,
https://doi.org/10.1007/978-3-032-29112-7_8

varicocele-associated male infertility [10, 11]. Varicocele has also been linked with its negative impact on the endocrine function of the testis, leading to decreased testosterone (T) synthesis [12]. Experimental studies in animals have shown impairment in Leydig cell function due to varicocele [13]. Testicular hyperthermia related to varicocele may lead to impairment in the androgen synthesis pathway by interfering with the function of the enzymes involved in the pathway, like defecting 17α-hydroxylase and 17,20-lyase enzyme inhibition, leading to increased reactive oxygen species (ROS). Ando et al. also performed clinical studies to prove this and reported decreased serum T levels in the patients with varicocele compared to controls [14]. However, the effect of varicocele repair on serum T levels has not been proven conclusively. Li et al. performed a meta-analysis consisting of 9 studies with 814 patients concluding improved testicular Leydig cell function and an increase in serum T level after surgical varicocele repair [15].

Physical examination is an important step in the diagnosis and grading of varicocele, but there have been multiple proposed grading systems leading to variability in treatment decisions and thus standardization of physical examination findings is looked for. Similar controversies exist in its ultrasound (US) classifications. Additionally, the indication of endocrine evaluation in these patients has not been clearly defined and the role of varicocele repair in male infertility has no conclusive evidence due to the lack of well-conducted studies, variation of population as well as treatment practices.

The aim of this chapter is to address and discuss the various controversies regarding diagnosis and management of varicocele.

Controversies in the Diagnosis of Varicocele

Grading of Varicocele—Different Classifications [Clinical and US Diagnosis (Cut-Off Values)]

Evaluation of varicocele starts with a detailed history and physical examination. Physical examination helps in dividing varicocele into large, moderate, and small, based on the classification given by Dubin [16]. Large varicoceles are easily visible and are historically correlated with the pathognomonic "bag of worms" appearance. On palpation, the bulk of venous channels is >2 cm in diameter on Valsalva maneuver. Moderate varicoceles are usually palpable without Valsalva pressure, with the bulk of veins estimated to have a diameter of 1–2 cm with Valsalva pressure. Small varicoceles are detectable only by palpation during Valsalva maneuver and the size of veins is <1 cm in diameter. However, most studies now address small, moderate, and large varicoceles as grades I, II, and III, respectively [17].

Physical examination detects only half of varicoceles identifiable on venography and falsely detects about 23% of varicoceles not present on venography [18]. Also, grading of varicocele by physical examination can have inter-observer and intra-observer variation, even if performed by experienced andrologists [19]. In this context, scrotal skin thickness, contractile state of the scrotum, and scrotal temperature may affect the physical examination findings. Stahl and Schlegel provided recommendations to standardize physical examination as scrotal warming should be done with a heating pad to relax the cremaster before examination [20]. Also, initial examination should be performed with the patient in supine position and it should then be repeated in standing position, with and without the Valsalva maneuver [11].

Assessment of varicoceles with color Doppler ultrasound (CDUS) is more reliable with high sensitivity and specificity (94% and 97%, respectively) [21]. The initial part of US examination is B-mode gray-scale sonography which detects the enlarged veins and measures their diameter. Adding the color doppler mode detects the blood flow and colorimetric changes. However, no consensus has been reached regarding the diameter of veins on CDUS to define varicocele. Many studies diagnose varicocele at a venous diameter of ≥3 mm with a reversal of flow on Valsalva maneuver [22]. Some studies propose no minimum threshold value due to reversal of flow present in veins below diameter of 2 mm, while others have suggested variable minimum diameter of 1–5 mm to detect varicocele [23–26]. This variability makes it difficult to compare the various diagnostic and treatment modalities. Recently, Pilatz et al. utilized receiver-operator curve analysis in 217 men and determined the optimal cut-off points of venous diameter for diagnosing clinical varicocele in the supine position at rest and during Valsalva maneuver to be >2.45 mm [sensitivity 84%, specificity 81%, area under the curve (AUC) 0.88] and >2.95 mm (sensitivity 84%, specificity 84%, AUC 0.90), respectively [27].

Ultrasound may detect varicocele not identifiable on physical examination, termed "subclinical varicocele," which is not correlated with male infertility and is found in 35–60% of fertile and asymptomatic men [28, 29]. No consensus has been built at present regarding assessment of varicoceles with CDUS in terms of the position of the patient (supine, standing, or both), the location along the spermatic cord or testis to image and measure the veins of the pampiniform plexus, the indication and method of eliciting a Valsalva maneuver, and the indication and technique to quantify reversal of blood flow during Valsalva maneuver [20]. The inter- and intra-observer variability in performing Doppler US has also not been well studied, but it is indicated only when physical examination is indeterminate, e.g., in a small scrotum, an obese patient, or a history of prior scrotal surgery [21].

Varicocele classification according to the US findings has been proposed by many authors, but most of them vary in examination techniques as well as severity of grading. One of the commonest classifications on the basis of CDUS findings proposed by Sarteschi et al. described five grades of varicocele, based on the presence of dilated veins in upright or supine position and their relation with the testis and characteristics of the reflux [30] (Table 8.1). Due to these specifications, it is the most widely used classification.

Chiou et al. proposed varicocele diagnosis at a minimum score of 4 out of 9 comprising the maximum venous diameter (scores 0–3), the presence of venous plexuses (scores 0–3), and the change of flow on Valsalva man oeuvre (scores 0–3), with all parameters evaluated in supine position [31] (Table 8.2).

Table 8.1 Sarteschi Grading of Varicocele Based on Ultrasound

Grade 1	Inguinal reflux only during Valsalva in not enlarged vessels
Grade 2	Supra-testicular varicosities with reflux only during Valsalva
Grade 3	Peri-testicular reflux only during Valsalva in enlarged vessels. Visible but not dilated vessels when supine. Enlarged when standing
Grade 4	Enlarged vessels in supine and standing position, with increasing caliber during Valsalva. Reflux at rest, increasing during Valsalva. Possible testicular hypotrophy
Grade 5	Enlarged vessels in supine and standing position, with caliber not increasing with Valsalva. Reflux at rest, not increasing during Valsalva. Testicular hypotrophy. Intratesticular varices may be present

Source: Adapted from the book "Varicocele and Male Infertility: A Complete Guide" edited by Sandro C Esteves, Chak-Lam Cho, Ahmad Majzoub, Ashok Agarwal, https://doi.org/10.1007/978-3-319-79102-9

Table 8.2 Chiou's scoring system for color doppler ultrasound diagnosis of varicocele

Maximum vein diameter (mm)	
<2.5	0
2.5–2.9	1
3.0–3.9	2
≥4.0	3
Plexus/sum of diameter of veins	
No plexus identified	0
Plexus (+) with sum diameter <3 mm	1
Plexus (+) with sum diameter 3–5.9 mm	2
Plexus (+) with sum diameter ≥6 mm	3
Change of flow velocity on Valsalva maneuver	
<2 cm/s or duration <1 s	0
2–4.9	1
5–9.9	2
≥10	3

Source: Adapted from the book "Varicocele and Male Infertility: A Complete Guide" edited by Sandro C Esteves, Chak-Lam Cho, Ahmad Majzoub, Ashok Agarwal, https://doi.org/10.1007/978-3-319-79102-9

Other classification systems have been proposed on the basis of CDUS findings in patients with varicocele; however, the variability in standardization has led to heterogeneous reporting in the literature [32].

Recently, the European Society of Urogenital Radiology Scrotal and Penile Imaging Working Group (ESUR-SPIWG) attempted to establish comprehensive guidelines for examination, interpretation, and classification of varicocele by US [33].

The key recommendations by the group are as follows:

1. Both gray-scale and Doppler US modes should be utilized for evaluating varicoceles due to their non-invasive nature and ability to assess venous reflux.

2. Standardized Examination Technique: Patients should be evaluated in both supine and standing positions to assess the size and flow characteristics of the veins accurately, during spontaneous breathing, and the Valsalva maneuver should also be utilized during the examination to provoke venous reflux, which is critical for diagnosis.
3. Measurement Parameters: The maximum venous diameter should be measured, with a threshold of ≥3 mm is considered diagnostic for a varicocele. The presence and duration of venous reflux should be documented; a reflux lasting more than 2 s during the Valsalva maneuver is deemed abnormal and indicative of varicocele severity.
4. Testicular Volume Assessment: Testicular volume correlates with testicular function, so it must be routinely measured in all cases, using Lambert's formula (length × width × height × 0.71) to evaluate the potential testicular atrophy associated with varicoceles.
5. Documentation Requirements: Reports should include details on the location (inguinal, supratesticular, peritesticular) and diameter of the largest vein, as well as the level and duration of venous reflux. Any testicular abnormalities or extratesticular varices observed during the examination should also be documented.
6. Preferred Classification System: While there is no universally accepted classification system, if a classification system is used, the use of the Sarteschi/Liguori classification is recommended due to its comprehensive nature and widespread acceptance.
7. Quality Assurance Measures: To ensure adherence to these guidelines, regular audits of US practices are recommended. This includes publicizing standards within departments and creating standardized reporting templates.
8. Training and Education: Continuous education for sonographers and radiologists regarding these guidelines is essential for improving compliance and enhancing diagnostic accuracy.

Role of Hormonal Profile

Several literature sources stated that varicocele affects the function of Leydig cells in their activity to produce T hormone, thus varicocele can lower T levels and ultimately affect the quality and quantity of spermatozoa as reflected in semen analysis results [34]. This is consistent with a meta-analysis study in 2012 involving 814 research subjects, reporting that varicocelectomy significantly improves Leydig cell function, leading to increased T hormone levels compared to before the surgical procedure (Fig. 8.1) [15].

From the perspective of serum FSH (follicle-stimulating hormone) and LH (luteinizing hormone) hormones, it is observed that varicocele tends to increase the levels of both hormones. This correlates with the decrease in T levels, leading to reduced negative feedback to the anterior pituitary, resulting in increased LH. In line with this, Inhibin B produced by Sertoli cells also decreases, leading to an increase

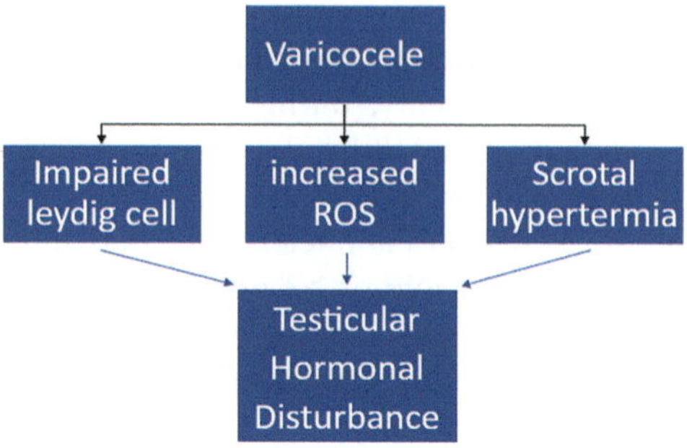

Fig. 8.1 Pathophysiology of hormonal disturbance due to varicocele

Table 8.3 Effect of varicocele on hormones

Type of hormones	The effect due to varicocele
FSH	↑
LH	↑
Testosterone	↓
Inhibin B	↓

in FSH [34]. After varicocelectomy, there is a significant decrease in FSH and LH levels, which is believed to support a higher quality of spermatogenesis. The effects of varicocele on the male hormonal profile are summarized in Table 8.3.

Controversies in Varicocele Treatment in Adults

Indications of Management of Varicocele in Infertile Men

One of the biggest dilemmas in the management of male infertility is determining the appropriate indications for the treatment of varicocele, particularly concerning surgical treatment. There are at least five indications where invasive intervention is necessary in the management of varicocele cases:

I. any palpable varicocele;
II. a significant difference in the volume between the two testes with a volume difference of >20%;
III. abnormal results from semen analysis;
IV. subjective complaints such as discomfort; and
V. testicular Doppler US findings showing spontaneous reflux or peak retrograde flow >30 cm/s [35].

According to the American Society for Reproductive Medicine (ASRM), the indications for treatment in varicocele cases can be divided into four categories:

I. couples struggling to conceive, confirmed infertility in the couple;
II. a varicocele that is palpable during a physical examination;
III. the wife is presumed not to have infertility or only has mild infertility issues;
IV. abnormalities are found in the semen analysis parameters [36].

Role of Varicocelectomy in Non-obstructive Azoospermia

The role of varicocelectomy in cases of non-obstructive azoospermia (NOA) is still debated among experts. The guidelines from the European Association of Urology (EAU) explain that post-varicocelectomy, around 20–55% of NOA cases associated with varicocele may show sperm's presence in the semen, and even if sperm are not present, there is an increased success rate of surgical sperm retrieval (SSR). However, this does not mean that varicocelectomy should be performed routinely in all NOA cases. Diagnosis confirmation still needs to begin with a thorough medical history, physical examination, and other supporting tests such as hormonal tests, US, and genetic testing. It is important to determine whether varicocele is indeed the sole cause or just an incidental finding unrelated to the occurrence of NOA. If all other possible causes can be excluded, then the patient can experience significant benefits after undergoing varicocelectomy. Even if spermatozoa do not appear in the semen after varicocelectomy (still azoospermia), at least the chance of obtaining sperm through SSR is considered higher compared to cases of NOA that do not undergo varicocelectomy [37].

Varicocele Treatment or ART?

When faced with a couple planning to undergo IVF/ICSI while the husband has a varicocele, what steps should be taken? Should they proceed directly with IVF/ICSI, or is it better to perform varicocelectomy first? This question is not easy to answer, as the presence of varicocele often poses a dilemma for the clinicians.

For consideration, several conditions need attention:

- NOA
  - In cases of NOA not caused by genetic factors, where varicocele is suspected to be the cause of azoospermia, varicocelectomy might be considered before proceeding with ART. The expectation is that following this procedure, spermatozoa may be obtained from semen, allowing the patient to avoid more

invasive procedures (such as biopsy, TESE, or microTESE) [38]. Even if, after varicocelectomy, the semen analysis still shows azoospermia, necessitating TESE; the success rate of obtaining spermatozoa in men who have undergone varicocelectomy has been demonstrated to be higher compared to those who have not undergone varicocele repair [39]. Takeshima et al. suggested that varicocele repair could be considered in men with NOA who have clinical varicoceles and that its repair seemed to improve SSR rate during microTESE for those in the non-responder group [40]. Along with their systemic review, Esteves et al. investigated 18 studies accounting for 468 patients who were diagnosed with NOA and varicocele. They concluded that varicocelectomy in patients with NOA and clinical varicocele is associated with improved SRR (OR: 2.65; 95% CI: 1.69–4.14; $P < 0.001$) [41]. Lately, Birowo et al. study investigated 104 patients (age range: 26–54 years), 42 of whom had undergone varicocele repair before the SSR procedure and 62 who had not. Motile spermatozoa were found in 29 (69.1%) and 17 (27.4%) patients who had undergone varicocele repair before the sperm retrieval procedure and those who had not undergone the repair, respectively (relative risk: 2.51; 95% CI: 1.60–3.96; $P < 0.001$). A predicted probabilities graph showed consistently higher sperm retrieval rates for patients with varicocele repair, regardless of their serum FSH levels [42].

- High DNA Fragmentation Index (DFI)
  - An increase in DFI >30% negatively correlates with implantation success in ART, and varicocele is suspected to be one of the factors responsible for the increase in DFI. Therefore, it is advisable to consider performing varicocelectomy before ART in cases with high DFI [43].
- Maternal Age
  - The improvement in sperm quality after varicocele surgery is estimated to take 3–6 months, and this does not guarantee that all patients undergoing varicocelectomy will achieve these desired results. Special attention is needed for patients whose wives are of advanced reproductive age (>35 years) by a thorough discussion involving all clinicians to determine the best course of action [43].
- Cost Effectiveness
  - Cost considerations should also be taken into account. In cases of infertility caused by varicocele, performing a varicocelectomy is generally more cost-effective than proceeding directly with ART. It is estimated that treatment with varicocelectomy is more economical [38, 44].

Timing of Varicocele Repair After Diagnosis

Establishing a diagnosis of varicocele is not particularly difficult. In some cases of high-grade varicocele (clinically palpable varicocele), the diagnosis can even be confirmed simply through inspection and palpation of the testes. The challenge lies in determining the appropriate time to initiate comprehensive management of the varicocele. Should treatment begin immediately after the diagnosis is made? Or is it better to wait for a certain moment?

According to Machen and Sandlow, three key moments should be considered as guidelines for performing varicocele repair [45], as follows:

(i) *NOA*

Based on the systematic review and meta-analysis (SRMA) by Esteves et al. (2016), it is stated that approximately 43.9% of NOA patients will show the presence of sperm in their semen after undergoing varicocelectomy [41]. In that case, varicocelectomy can minimize the need for more invasive procedures for a man to achieve parenthood (such as TESE or microTESE).

(ii) *Hypogonadism*

Varicocele is believed to affect the testes' overall function, including the testes' role in steroidogenesis, which is carried out by Leydig cells. The factors underlying this include hypoxia, increased scrotal temperature, oxidative stress, testicular cell death, and alteration of the testicular microenvironment, all of which contribute to a decrease in Leydig cell activity and consequently testosterone synthesis. Hypogonadism resulting from this phenomenon can serve as one of the predictors for performing varicocele repair [46].

Men with varicocele may exhibit hypogonadism symptoms such as tiredness, erectile dysfunction, low libido, and diminished muscle mass. Varicocelectomy has been demonstrated in certain trials to boost testosterone levels in males with varicocele-related hypogonadism.

The specific mechanism underlying the increase in testosterone following varicocelectomy is unknown, although it is thought that treating the varicocele improves the testicular microenvironment by lowering scrotal temperature, reducing oxidative stress and enhancing oxygenation. This increases the function of Leydig cells, which produce testosterone.

Tanrikut et al. (2011) found that testosterone levels improved dramatically following varicocelectomy. In their study of males with varicoceles and low testosterone, 70% had a boost in testosterone following varicocelectomy [47]. While varicocele repair increases testosterone levels in some men, it does not benefit all men with varicocele and hypogonadism. The extent of improvement may vary depending on the size and length of the varicocele, the patient's age, and his baseline testosterone levels. Zohdy et al. (2011) found that males with clinically severe varicoceles and low testosterone levels saw a substantial increase in testosterone following varicocele repair. According to their findings, males with bigger varicoceles and more severe testosterone shortage before surgery showed the greatest improvements [48].

Repairing varicoceles may be beneficial for men with clinically significant varicoceles who exhibit symptoms of hypogonadism or low testosterone. Surgical correction may also enhance energy, sexual function, and general well-being linked to regulated testosterone levels, in addition to its benefits for fertility.

(iii) *Increase in SDF*
One factor that can increase sperm DNA fragmentation (SDF) is varicocele, where varicocelectomy, according to a study by Zini and Dohle, is believed to reduce SDF and increase the chances of achieving pregnancy [49].

In addition to the above indications, subjective discomfort experienced by the patients with varicocele can also indicate varicocelectomy. This is particularly true if conservative or medical management has been attempted but proves insufficient, with the patient's discomfort progressively increasing, thereby disrupting daily activities and reducing quality of life. If this occurs, it can also be used as a guideline for the timing of surgical intervention [50].

Recent Techniques of Varicocele Repair

The management of varicocele has significantly evolved over the years, with recent techniques offering improved efficacy, reduced complications, and earlier recovery. Traditionally, open surgical approaches through the inguinal or subinguinal route have been most commonly employed for varicocele repair. They are quite effective in preventing recurrence of varicocele although they may lead to postoperative pain, longer hospital stays, and complications such as hydrocele and testicular atrophy later on. Adult varicoceles may benefit from laparoscopic management due to the laparoscope's excellent visibility of the extraperitoneal structures, which may help in preserving lymphatics and the genital branches of the genitofemoral nerve that travel along the spermatic veins, thus preventing recurrence of varicocele and ischemic damage to the testis [51]. However, it may lead to complications like air embolism, inadvertent arterial division, genitofemoral nerve injury, hydrocele, intestinal injury, and peritonitis occurring in 8–12% of cases [52]. High cost and the need for general anaesthesia preclude this technique to be performed widely.

Microsurgical subinguinal varicocelectomy is considered the procedure of choice by many professionals, in which an operating microscope is used for better visualization of the veins, arteries, and lymphatic vessels. It results in decreased rates of complications and recurrences as well as better reproductive outcomes [53].

A less invasive method for repair of varicocele is the endovascular approach, in which the dilated veins are embolized using a variety of materials, including glue, sclerosants, and coils, or occluded with a balloon [54]. The benefits of this approach include quick recovery and reduced scarring with the ability to perform the procedure under local anaesthesia. The process of percutaneous embolization entails guiding a catheter to the impacted veins after inserting it through a vein in the neck or groin. Embolic agents like sclerosants which cause the veins to collapse, and coils, which physically occlude the veins, are then injected into the impacted veins [55]. According to several studies, percutaneous embolization has a success rate that is similar to microsurgical varicocelectomy and a 10% recurrence rate [56]. However, there are risks like the possibility of coil migration and radiation exposure during fluoroscopy. The radiation exposure can be avoided by performing glue embolization in which an adhesive agent, typically N-butyl cyanoacrylate, is used to occlude the varicocele under US guidance. It is easier to treat collateral veins with glue, which are frequently responsible for varicocele recurrence [57]. This technique is a promising alternative to the conventional embolization procedures, with a good success rate and fewer complications.

The dilated veins can also be occluded by inserting a balloon catheter into the afflicted vein and then inflating the balloon to block the vein and stop blood flow. Even though less popular than coil embolization, balloon occlusion has advantages over coil embolization with respect to success rates and recovery times [58]. This method can be combined with sclerosant injection to increase its efficacy. This approach is especially helpful in the case of individuals with complicated venous anatomy.

Lately, multiple robotic platforms have been developed leading to better visualization and accuracy during varicocele repair, making robotic-assisted varicocelectomy a noteworthy option [59]. Corcione and associates were the first to describe the robotic-assisted microsurgical subinguinal varicocelectomy in 2008 with notably good outcomes [60], in which the accuracy and dexterity of robotic technology are combined with the advantages of traditional microsurgery. The robotic platform leads to precise, tremor-free movements by the surgeon with third-arm retraction while viewing the operative field in high definition and three dimensions. This is very helpful in dissecting small arteries which must be preserved during varicocelectomy to prevent testicular atrophy [61]. Also, improved ergonomics during robotic surgery help surgeons perform long surgeries with less fatigue. All these factors have led to improvement in results in terms of success rates, patient satisfaction, and complications after varicocelectomy [62, 63]. However, high procedural cost and the requirement for specialized training have been obstacles to the widespread use of robotic surgery for varicocele repair.

Robotic extraperitoneal varicocelectomy is another approach for varicocele repair utilizing robotic technology, especially in cases of recurrent varicocele or when conventional methods are not feasible. Robotic arms are used to access the dilated veins through the extraperitoneal space. It has been demonstrated to have a lower recurrence rate than open retroperitoneal varicocele repair. But a robotic extraperitoneal approach may not be feasible for handling external spermatic perforators/gubernacular veins [64].

Role of Oral Antioxidant in the Management of Varicocele

The pathophysiology of varicocele-related infertility is multifactorial, with oxidative stress (OS) playing a significant role. Oral antioxidants have been investigated as a therapeutic option to mitigate oxidative damage and improve fertility outcomes in men with varicocele. OS occurs when there is an imbalance between ROS production and the body's ability to neutralize these reactive molecules with antioxidants. In varicocele, increased temperature in the testicular region due to increased blood flow causes a decrease in the activities of the antioxidant enzymes superoxide dismutase and catalase in the spermatozoa. This in turn results in an increased hydrogen peroxide concentration, reflux of renal and adrenal toxic metabolites, reduced blood supply to the testes and associated hypoxia and subsequent tissue damage, and the production of oxygen free radicals, leading to sperm DNA damage, reduced sperm motility, altered sperm morphology, and decreased sperm concentration [65]. These factors collectively impair male fertility, making the management of OS crucial in treating varicocele-associated infertility.

Oral antioxidants aim to restore the balance between ROS and antioxidant defenses by preventing the peroxidation of membrane lipids, and DNA, thereby protecting sperm from oxidative damage [66]. The use of antioxidants in varicocele management may improve the sperm parameters like sperm motility, sperm concentration, and sperm morphology, and reduce SDF [67], but the conclusive evidence regarding their efficacy in improving natural conception rates and better outcomes with ART is lacking [68]. The nature of oral antioxidants along with their dose and duration has also been variable in multiple studies [68].

The potential role of common individual antioxidants in men with varicocele:

- *Carnitine:* L-carnitine is the bioactive form which carries the activated long-chain fatty acids into the mitochondria of the spermatozoa where they provide energy to mature spermatozoa (with positive effects on sperm motility) during their maturation and the spermatogenic process [69]. Multiple studies have shown the positive effect of oral L-carnitine in variable doses and combinations on various sperm parameters [70, 71], however these effects have not been consistent [72].
- *Vitamin E (Tocopherol):* Vitamin E has been used as a lipid-soluble antioxidant due to its property of stabilizing cell membranes and reducing lipid peroxidation, exerting positive effects on sperm functions, such as sperm concentration and motility [73]. Its effect on improvement in fertility rates has been suggested but not proven inconclusively [74].
- *Selenium:* Selenium is a constituent of sperm capsule selenoprotein which maintain the sperm structure integrity [75]. Selenium also increases activity of antioxidant enzyme glutathione peroxidase [76]. Selenium deficiency has been shown to lead to impaired spermatogenesis, reduced sperm motility, and altered

sperm morphology [72]. In men with fertility issues, studies have reported improvements in sperm quality parameters such as count, motility, and morphology following selenium supplementation [77, 78].

Various other oral antioxidants like zinc, lycopene, vitamin C, and coenzyme Q10 have also been studied individually as well as in multiple combinations in infertile men with variable results. In their study, Greco et al. found that infertile men treated with a combination of vitamins C and E for 2 months had a significant reduction in sperm DNA fragmentation [79]. A Cochrane review of 48 randomized controlled trials (RCTs) by Showell et al. evaluated the role of oral antioxidants in infertile men, and only four low-quality studies in the review reported on clinical pregnancy rate which improved with oral antioxidant therapy [80]. Another recent meta-analysis in 2023 included 45 RCTs and favored using oral antioxidants in infertile men to improve conventional sperm parameters and spontaneous pregnancy rate; however, it was not specific to patients with varicocele and the fertility parameters improved even in patients who had previously undergone varicocele repair, thus it recommended oral antioxidants in patients with idiopathic male infertility with varicocele even after varicocele repair [81].

Clinical Varicocele with Contralateral Subclinical Varicocele

Varicocele does not typically happen on both sides (bilaterally). Approximately 85–90% of varicocele cases happen only on the left side, while right-sided varicocele is usually found in cases of bilateral varicocele. If a right-sided varicocele happens alone, it is quite rare, and clinicians should be cautious about the possibility of a retroperitoneal mass if the varicocele is present only on the right side [35, 82, 83].

Although several guidelines clearly do not recommend intervention for subclinical varicocele and only suggest varicocelectomy for varicocele of at least grade II, this does not mean there is no evidence supporting varicocelectomy in cases of subclinical varicocele. For example, Yamamoto et al. demonstrated a significant increase in sperm density after treating subclinical varicocele cases [37, 84].

Should Bilateral Varicoceles be Repaired Simultaneously?

In cases where bilateral varicocele happens, even if the varicocele on the right side is subclinical, performing simultaneous varicocelectomy on both sides is believed to provide better outcomes compared to treating only one side. This belief is based on evaluations of improvements in sperm parameters and pregnancy rates after varicocelectomy [85].

Pediatric and Adolescent Varicocele—Should it be Actively Treated and When?

Varicocele can appear starting from childhood or adolescence with a prevalence reaching 15.7% in European adolescents with a median age of 19 years [86]. Meanwhile, in a study conducted in Turkey that divided subjects by age, a prevalence of 0.8% was found in boys aged 2–6 years, 1% in children aged 7–10 years, 7.8% in those aged 11–14 years, and reaching 14.1% in individuals aged 15–19 years [3]. This indicates an increased varicocele risk with advancing age [87].

Varicoceles appearing in children/adolescents have effects similar to those in adults and fertile men, causing discomfort (pain), testicular hypotrophy, abnormalities in semen analysis, and hormonal disorders [83]. These cases are usually self-diagnosed or based on routine genital examinations for educational purposes, which then need to be confirmed by scrotal Doppler US to determine their degree, typically classified according to Dubin or Sarteschi, and measuring the maximum vein diameter during peak retrograde flow (PRF) [88].

Managing varicocele cases in this age range is still controversial, much like the dilemma faced when dealing with varicocele in adults. Generally, varicocele management in these cases can be divided into two categories: conservative and surgical. In cases where the patients do not complain of testicular pain accompanied by normal testicular volume, conservative therapy is usually considered the primary option. Additionally, a difference in testicular volume between the left and right sides of <20% still allows for conservative therapy. The use of Doppler US is not only important as a supporting examination for diagnosing varicocele but also plays a role in determining treatment options. In cases where PRF is <30 cm, strict monitoring is usually sufficient, unless PRF continues to increase to >38 cm, in which case surgical treatment may be considered. Abnormalities in spermatozoa can also be an indicator for surgery, but this examination can only be performed on adolescents who have already gone through puberty [87]. Optional treatment for pediatric varicocele is illustrated in Table 8.4.

Table 8.4 Optional treatment for pediatric varicocele

Indicator	Conservative	Surgical
Testicular asymmetry	<20%	>20%
PRF	<38 cm	>38 cm
Pain	No or mild	Severe
Sperm abnormalities (after puberty)	Absent	Present

Varicocele Repair and ART Outcome

In their recent systematic review and meta-analysis, Palani et al. [89] investigated ART success in infertile men with clinical varicocele and abnormal semen parameters who underwent varicocele repair before the ART procedure compared to those who did not. Men with varicocele repair showed a significant improvement in fertilization rate (mean difference 10.9, 95% CI: 5.94, 15.89; $p < 0.01$), clinical pregnancy rate (OR 1.38, 95% CI: 1.07, 1.78; $p = 0.01$), and live-birth rate (OR 2.07, 95% CI: 1.45, 2.97; $p < 0.01$), compared to men who did not undergo varicocele repair.

Varicocele in Fertile Men

In their study, Mostafa et al. [90] assessed the seminal ROS-antioxidants relationship in fertile and infertile men with/without varicocele including fertile healthy volunteers, fertile men with varicocele, infertile oligoasthenozoospermia without varicocele, and infertile OA with varicocele. Compared with the fertile healthy men, in fertile males with varicocele, the estimated seminal ROS were significantly higher and the estimated seminal antioxidants were significantly lower. These authors concluded that patients with varicocele have an OS even in fertile normozoospermic bearing conditions. This may allow us to understand that, in men with varicocele, there is a threshold value of oxidative stress over which male fertility may be impaired.

Approach to Persistent/Recurrent Varicocele after Treatment

Clinical or radiological presence of varicocele on first follow-up within a year of any form of treatment is considered varicocele persistence, whereas appearance of varicocele on follow-up after a confirmed absence following treatment may indicate recurrence of varicocele [91]. Open retroperitoneal approach has the highest recurrence rate between 7% and 35%, which reduces to 2.2–7.1% with laparoscopic retroperitoneal approach. Percutaneous embolization has a comparable recurrence rate of 2–25%, as reported in several studies. Least recurrence of varicocele occurs with microscopic subinguinal approach (0–3.57%), while it's much higher with the macroscopic approach (0–37%). This may be due to individual ligation of all the venous tributaries due to enhanced magnification [92]. The recurrence rates differ greatly in studies because of differences in the severity of varicocele, age group being studied (children, adolescents or adults), type of technique (radiological, microsurgical ligation, open or laparoscopic), follow-up duration, and definition of persistence or recurrence [93]. The major cause of recurrence may be missing any tributary of spermatic vein during initial treatment [93, 94].

The optimal management of recurrent varicocele is a matter of debate due to low-quality evidence on the matter [92, 93]. Till now, four studies have reported on surgical treatment for recurrent varicocele with three of them employing a microsurgical subinguinal approach and one utilizing a transumbilical single-port laparoscopic approach. Most of them had <20% recurrence and an acceptable pregnancy rate of >40%. Two studies have reported on embolization for recurrent varicoceles with significant success rate; however, none of them showed the fertility parameters after intervention. The best approach and the target population which will benefit the most from intervention is not clear from these studies, due to lack of randomization and variable results. According to Chen et al., the predictive factors of improvement in semen parameters following the repeat varicocelectomy were lower follicle-stimulating hormone levels, reduced peak retrograde flow on Doppler ultrasound, delayed recurrence of varicocele, larger testicular volume preoperatively, and higher number of ligated veins during redo varicocelectomy [95].

There are no current guidelines to advise the ideal treatment for recurrent varicocele, and further randomized studies are required to make strong recommendations. Till then, clinicians should treat recurrent varicocele based on individual patient characteristics and the available resources.

Conclusions

Varicocele-associated male infertility is still considered a matter of controversy between different professionals as its exact pathophysiology of varicocele leading to male infertility is debated. Several contentious points regarding varicocele have been discussed extensively in the current chapter: the clinical as well as radiological grading due to the discrepancies in clinical examination methods and protocols reporting sonographic findings, the role of hormonal profile in its evaluation, lack of precise indications and timing for its management in infertile men, its unclear role in NOA cases, performing varicocele repair or directly proceeding for ART, role of oral antioxidants, role of the endovascular and robotic approaches in its management, decision of bilateral varicocele repair especially in patients with contralateral subclinical varicocele and lack of consensus on when to initiate treatment or which surgical technique to employ. Therefore, continuous research and clinical trials are crucial to refine the diagnosis and treatment of varicocele, ensuring they meet diverse patient needs and pave the way for more effective, personalized, and patient-friendly solutions for managing male infertility.

References

1. Leslie SW, Sajjad H, Siref LE. Varicocele. [Updated 2023 Nov 13]. In: StatPearls [Internet]. Treasure Island: StatPearls Publishing; 2023. Available from: https://www.ncbi.nlm.nih.gov/books/NBK448113/.
2. Marte A. The history of varicocele: from antiquity to the modern ERA. Int Braz J Urol. 2018;44(3):563–76. https://doi.org/10.1590/S1677-5538.IBJU.2017.0386.
3. Akbay E, Cayan S, Doruk E, Duce MN, Bozlu M. The prevalence of varicocele and varicocele-related testicular atrophy in Turkish children and adolescents. BJU Int. 2000;86(4):490–3. https://doi.org/10.1046/j.1464-410x.2000.00735.x. PMID: 10971279.
4. Levinger U, Gornish M, Gat Y, Bachar GN. Is varicocele prevalence increasing with age? Andrologia. 2007;39(3):77–80. https://doi.org/10.1111/j.1439-0272.2007.00766.x. PMID: 17683466.
5. Abdulmaaboud MR, Shokeir AA, Farage Y, Abd El-Rahman A, El-Rakhawy MM, Mutabagani H. Treatment of varicocele: a comparative study of conventional open surgery, percutaneous retrograde sclerotherapy, and laparoscopy. Urology. 1998;52(2):294–300. https://doi.org/10.1016/s0090-4295(98)00178-2. PMID: 9697798.
6. Clarke BG. Incidence of varicocele in normal men and among men of different ages. JAMA. 1966;198(10):1121–2. PMID: 5953394.
7. Gorelick JI, Goldstein M. Loss of fertility in men with varicocele. Fertil Steril. 1993;59(3):613–6. PMID: 8458466.
8. Zorgniotti AW, Macleod J. Studies in temperature, human semen quality, and varicocele. Fertil Steril. 1973;24(11):854–63. PMID: 4742006.
9. Ali JI, Weaver DJ, Weinstein SH, Grimes EM. Scrotal temperature and semen quality in men with and without varicocele. Arch Androl. 1990;24(2):215–9. https://doi.org/10.3109/01485019008986882. PMID: 2327832.
10. Cohen MS, Plaine L, Brown JS. The role of internal spermatic vein plasma catecholamine determinations in subfertile men with varicoceles. Fertil Steril. 1975;26(12):1243–9. https://doi.org/10.1016/s0015-0282(16)41541-4. PMID: 803040.0.
11. Ito H, Fuse H, Minagawa H, Kawamura K, Murakami M, Shimazaki J. Internal spermatic vein prostaglandins in varicocele patients. Fertil Steril. 1982;37(2):218–22. https://doi.org/10.1016/s0015-0282(16)46043-7. PMID: 7060770.
12. Çayan S, Akbay E, Saylam B, Kadıoğlu A. Effect of varicocele and its treatment on testosterone in hypogonadal men with varicocele: review of the literature. Balkan Med J. 2020;37(3):121–4. https://doi.org/10.4274/balkanmedj.galenos.2020.2020.1.85. Epub 2020 Feb 19. PMID: 32070086; PMCID: PMC7161614.
13. Zheng YQ, Zhang XB, Zhou JQ, Cheng F, Rao T, Yao Y. The effects of artery-ligating and artery-preserving varicocelectomy on the ipsilateral testes in rats. Urology. 2008;72(5):1179–84. https://doi.org/10.1016/j.urology.2008.03.035. Epub 2008 Jun 2. PMID: 18514768.
14. Andò S, Giacchetto C, Colpi G, Beraldi E, Panno ML, Lombardi A, Sposato G. Physiopathologic aspects of Leydig cell function in varicocele patients. J Androl. 1984;5(3):163–70. https://doi.org/10.1002/j.1939-4640.1984.tb02388.x. PMID: 6430851
15. Li F, Yue H, Yamaguchi K, Okada K, Matsushita K, Ando M, Chiba K, Fujisawa M. Effect of surgical repair on testosterone production in infertile men with varicocele: a meta-analysis. Int J Urol. 2012;19(2):149–54. https://doi.org/10.1111/j.1442-2042.2011.02890.x. Epub 2011 Nov 8. PMID: 22059526.
16. Dubin L, Amelar RD. Varicocele size and results of varicocelectomy in selected subfertile men with varicocele. Fertil Steril. 1970;21(8):606–9. https://doi.org/10.1016/s0015-0282(16)37684-1. PMID: 5433164.
17. Choi WS, Kim SW. Current issues in varicocele management: a review. World J Mens Health. 2013;31(1):12–20. https://doi.org/10.5534/wjmh.2013.31.1.12. Epub 2013 Apr 23. PMID: 23658861; PMCID: PMC3640148.

18. World Health Organization. Comparison among different methods for the diagnosis of varicocele. Fertil Steril. 1985;43:575–82.
19. Carlsen E, Andersen AG, Buchreitz L, Jørgensen N, Magnus O, Matulevicuus V, Nermoen I, Petersen JH, Punab M, Suominen J, Zilaitiene B, Giwercman A. Inter-observer variation in the results of the clinical andrological examination including estimation of testicular size. Int J Androl. 2000;23(4):248–53. https://doi.org/10.1046/j.1365-2605.2000.00240.x. PMID: 10886429.
20. Stahl P, Schlegel PN. Standardization and documentation of varicocele evaluation. Curr Opin Urol. 2011;21(6):500–5. https://doi.org/10.1097/MOU.0b013e32834b8698. PMID: 21926627.
21. Male Infertility Best Practice Policy Committee of the American Urological Association; Practice Committee of the American Society for Reproductive Medicine. Report on optimal evaluation of the infertile male. Fertil Steril. 2006;86(5 Suppl 1):S202–9. https://doi.org/10.1016/j.fertnstert.2006.08.029. PMID: 17055823.
22. Lee J, Binsaleh S, Lo K, Jarvi K. Varicoceles: the diagnostic dilemma. J Androl. 2008;29:143–6.
23. Atasoy C, Fitoz S. Gray-scale and color Doppler sonographic findings in intratesticular varicocele. J Clin Ultrasound. 2001;29:369–73.
24. Eskew LA, Watson NE, Wolfman N, et al. Ultrasonographic diagnosis of varicoceles. Fertil Steril. 1993;60:693–7.
25. Metin A, Bulut O, Temizkan M. Relationship between the left spermatic vein diameter measured by ultrasound and palpated varicocele and Doppler ultrasound findings. Int Urol Nephrol. 1991;23:65–8.
26. Pierik FH, Vreeburg JT, Stijnen T, et al. Improvement of sperm count and motility after ligation of varicoceles detected with colour Doppler ultrasonography. Int J Androl. 1998;21:256–60.
27. Pilatz A, Altinkilic B, Köhler E, Marconi M, Weidner W. Color Doppler ultrasound imaging in varicoceles: is the venous diameter sufficient for predicting clinical and subclinical varicocele? World J Urol. 2011;29(5):645–50. https://doi.org/10.1007/s00345-011-0701-4. Epub 2011 May 24. PMID: 21607575.
28. Meacham RB, Townsend RR, Rademacher D, Drose JA. The incidence of varicoceles in the general population when evaluated by physical examination, gray scale sonography and color Doppler sonography. J Urol. 1994;151(6):1535–8. https://doi.org/10.1016/s0022-5347(17)35295-3. PMID: 8189565.
29. Cina A, Minnetti M, Pirronti T, Vittoria Spampinato M, Canadè A, Oliva G, Ribatti D, Bonomo L. Sonographic quantitative evaluation of scrotal veins in healthy subjects: normative values and implications for the diagnosis of varicocele. Eur Urol. 2006;50(2):345–50. https://doi.org/10.1016/j.eururo.2006.02.055. Epub 2006 Mar 10. PMID: 16542771.
30. Sarteschi LM, Paoli R, Bianchini M, Menchini Fabris GF. Lo studio del varicocele con eco-color-Doppler. G Ital Ultrasonologia. 1993;4:43–9.
31. Chiou RK, Anderson JC, Wobig RK, Rosinsky DE, Matamoros A Jr, Chen WS, Taylor RJ. Color Doppler ultrasound criteria to diagnose varicoceles: correlation of a new scoring system with physical examination. Urology. 1997;50(6):953–6. https://doi.org/10.1016/S0090-4295(97)00452-4. PMID: 9426729.
32. Bertolotto M, Cantisani V, Drudi FM, Lotti FV. Classification and pitfalls. Andrology. 2021;9(5):1322–30. https://doi.org/10.1111/andr.13053. Epub 2021 Jun 8. PMID: 34038625; PMCID: PMC8596817.
33. Freeman S, Bertolotto M, Richenberg J, Belfield J, Dogra V, Huang DY, Lotti F, Markiet K, Nikolic O, Ramanathan S, Ramchandani P, Rocher L, Secil M, Sidhu PS, Skrobisz K, Studniarek M, Tsili A, Tuncay Turgut A, Pavlica P, Derchi LE, Members of the ESUR-SPIWG WG. Ultrasound evaluation of varicoceles: guidelines and recommendations of the European Society of Urogenital Radiology Scrotal and Penile Imaging Working Group (ESUR-SPIWG) for detection, classification, and grading. Eur Radiol. 2020;30(1):11–25. https://doi.org/10.1007/s00330-019-06280-y. Epub 2019 Jul 22. PMID: 31332561.

34. Bellastella G, Carotenuto R, Caiazzo F, Longo M, Cirillo P, Scappaticcio L, et al. Varicocele: an endocrinological perspective. Front Reprod Health. 2022;4:863695. https://doi.org/10.3389/frph.2022.863695.
35. Chiba K, Ramasamy R, Lamb DJ, Lipshultz LI. The varicocele: diagnostic dilemmas, therapeutic challenges and future perspectives. Asian J Androl. 2016;18(2):276–81. https://doi.org/10.4103/1008-682x.167724.
36. Practice Committee of the American Society for Reproductive Medicine; Society for Male Reproduction and Urology. Report on varicocele and infertility: a committee opinion. Fertil Steril. 2014;102(6):1556–60. https://doi.org/10.1016/j.fertnstert.2014.10.007.
37. Franco A, Proietti F, Palombi V, Savarese G, Guidotti M, Leonardo C, et al. Varicocele: to treat or not to treat? J Clin Med. 2023;12(12) https://doi.org/10.3390/jcm12124062.
38. Cho KS, Seo JT. Effect of varicocelectomy on male infertility. Korean J Urol. 2014;55(11):703–9. https://doi.org/10.4111/kju.2014.55.11.703.
39. Zampieri N, Bosaro L, Costantini C, Zaffagnini S, Zampieri G. Relationship between testicular sperm extraction and varicocelectomy in patients with varicocele and nonobstructive azoospermia. Urology. 2013;82(1):74–7. https://doi.org/10.1016/j.urology.2013.03.037.
40. Takeshima T, Yumura Y, Kuroda S, Kato Y, Noguchi K, Iwasaki A. Effect of varicocele repair in patients with nonobstructive azoospermia. J Reprod Med. 2017;62(5–6):311–6.
41. Esteves SC, Miyaoka R, Roque M, Agarwal A. Outcome of varicocele repair in men with nonobstructive azoospermia: systematic review and meta-analysis. Asian J Androl. 2016;18(2):246–53. https://doi.org/10.4103/1008-682X.169562.
42. Birowo P, Prasetyo DT, Pujianto DA, Atmoko W, Rasyid N, Sini IR. Effect of varicocele repair on sperm retrieval rate and testicular histopathological patterns in men with nonobstructive azoospermia. Asian J Androl. 2022;24(1):85–9. https://doi.org/10.4103/aja.aja_29_21.
43. Kohn JR, Haney NM, Nichols PE, Rodriguez KM, Kohn TP. Varicocele repair prior to assisted reproductive technology: patient selection and special considerations. Res Rep Urol. 2020;12:149–56. https://doi.org/10.2147/rru.S198934.
44. Schlegel PN. Is assisted reproduction the optimal treatment for varicocele-associated male infertility? A cost-effectiveness analysis. Urology. 1997;49(1):83–90. https://doi.org/10.1016/s0090-4295(96)00379-2.
45. Machen GL, Sandlow JI. Extended indications for varicocelectomy. F1000Res. 2019:8. https://doi.org/10.12688/f1000research.19579.1.
46. Guercio C, Patil D, Mehta A. Hypogonadism is independently associated with varicocele repair in a contemporary cohort of men in the USA. Asian J Androl. 2019;21(1):45–9. https://doi.org/10.4103/aja.aja_61_18.
47. Tanrikut C, Goldstein M, Rosoff JS, Lee RK, Nelson CJ, Mulhall JP. Varicocele as a risk factor for androgen deficiency and effect of repair. BJU Int. 2011;108(9):1480–4.
48. Zohdy W, Kamal EE, Ibrahim FA. The effect of varicocelectomy on serum testosterone. Andrology. 2011;31(4):548–52.
49. Zini A, Dohle G. Are varicoceles associated with increased deoxyribonucleic acid fragmentation? Fertil Steril. 2011;96(6):1283–7. https://doi.org/10.1016/j.fertnstert.2011.10.016.
50. Paick S, Choi WS. Varicocele and testicular pain: a review. World J Mens Health. 2019;37(1):4–11. https://doi.org/10.5534/wjmh.170010.
51. Franco I. Laparoscopic varicocelectomy in the adolescent male. Curr Urol Rep. 2004;5(2):132–6.
52. Gorber ED, Chan PT, Zini A, et al. Microsurgical treatment of persistent or recurrent varicocele. Fertil Steril. 2004;82:718–22.
53. Jin L, Yao Q, Wu S, Dai G, Xiang H, Liu X, Xue B. Evaluation of clinical effects of microsurgical subinguinal varicocelectomy with and without testicular delivery. Andrologia. 2020;52(6):e13605. https://doi.org/10.1111/and.13605.
54. Wunsch R, Efinger K. The interventional therapy of varicocele amongst children, adolescents and young men. Eur J Radiol. 2005;53:46–56.

55. Flacke S, Schuster M, Kovacs A, et al. Embolization of varicoceles: pretreatment sperm motility predicts later pregnancy in partners of infertile men. Radiology. 2008;248:540–9.
56. Halpern J, Mittal S, Pereira K, Bhatia S, Ramasamy R. Percutaneous embolization of varicocele: technique, indications, relative contraindications, and complications. Asian J Androl. 2016;18(2):234–8. https://doi.org/10.4103/1008-682X.169985. PMID: 26658060; PMCID: PMC4770492.
57. Sze DY, Kao JS, Frisoli JK, et al. Persistent and recurrent postsurgical varicoceles: venographic anatomy and treatment with N-butyl cyanoacrylate embolization. J Vasc Interv Radiol. 2008;19:539–45.
58. Zuckerman AM, Mitchell SE, Venbrux AC, et al. Percutaneous varicocele occlusion: long-term follow-up. J Vasc Interv Radiol. 1994;5(2):315–9. https://doi.org/10.1016/s1051-0443(94)71492-5. PMID: 8186601.
59. Kawashima K, Kanno T, Tadano K. Robots in laparoscopic surgery: current and future status. BMC Biomed Eng. 2019;1:12. https://doi.org/10.1186/s42490-019-0012-1. PMID: 32903302; PMCID: PMC7422514.
60. Corcione F, Esposito C, Cuccurullo D, Settembre A, Miranda N, Amato F, Pirozzi F, Caiazzo P. Advantages and limits of robot-assisted laparoscopic surgery: preliminary experience. Surg Endosc Other Interv Tech. 2005;19:117–9.
61. Teng J, Jia Z, Ai X, Luo X, Guan Y, Hao X, Fei W. Robotic-assisted laparoscopic artery-sparing varicocelectomy using indocyanine green fluorescence angiography: initial experience. Andrologia. 2020;52(11):e13774.
62. Gudeloglu A, Brahmbhatt JV, Parekattil SJ. Robotic microsurgery in male infertility and urology—taking robotics to the next level. Transl Androl Urol. 2014;3(1):102.
63. McCullough A, Elebyjian L, Ellen J, Mechlin C. A retrospective review of single-institution outcomes with robotic-assisted microsurgical varicocelectomy. Asian J Androl. 2018;20(2):189–94. https://doi.org/10.4103/aja.aja_45_17. PMID: 29086759; PMCID: PMC5858106.
64. Napolitano L, Pandolfo SD, Aveta A, Cirigliano L, Martino R, Mattiello G, Celentano G, Barone B, Rosati C, La Rocca R, Spena G, Spirito L. The management of clinical varicocele: robotic surgery approach. Front Reprod Health. 2022;4:791330. https://doi.org/10.3389/frph.2022.791330. PMID: 36303643; PMCID: PMC9580646.
65. Hassani-Bafrani H, Najaran H, Razi M, Rashtbari H. Berberine ameliorates experimental varicocele-induced damages at testis and sperm levels; evidences for oxidative stress and inflammation. Andrologia. 2019;51(2):e13179. https://doi.org/10.1111/and.13179. Epub 2018 Oct 17. PMID: 30334274.
66. Moshtaghion S-M, Malekinejad H, Razi M, Shafie-Irannejad V. Silymarin protects from varicocele-induced damages in testis and improves sperm quality: evidence for E2f1 involvement. Syst Biol Reprod Med. 2013;59:270–80. https://doi.org/10.3109/19396368.2013.794253.
67. Moslemi MK, Tavanbakhsh S. Selenium-vitamin E supplementation in infertile men: effects on semen parameters and pregnancy rate. Int J Gen Med. 2011;4:99–104. https://doi.org/10.2147/IJGM.S16275. PMID: 21403799; PMCID: PMC3048346.
68. Martin-Hidalgo D, Bragado MJ, Batista AR, Oliveira PF, Alves MG. Antioxidants and male fertility: from molecular studies to clinical evidence. Antioxidants (Basel). 2019;8(4):89. https://doi.org/10.3390/antiox8040089. PMID: 30959797; PMCID: PMC6523199.
69. Tremellen K, Miari G, Froiland D, Thompson J. A randomised control trial examining the effect of an antioxidant (Menevit) on pregnancy outcome during IVF-ICSI treatment. Aust N Z J Obstet Gynaecol. 2007;47:216–21. https://doi.org/10.1111/j.1479-828X.2007.00723.x.
70. Zhou X, Liu F, Zhai S. Effect of L-carnitine and/or L-acetyl-carnitine in nutrition treatment for male infertility: a systematic review. Asia Pac J Clin Nutr. 2007;16(Suppl 1):383–90. PMID: 17392136.

71. Sigman M, Glass S, Campagnone J, Pryor JL. Carnitine for the treatment of idiopathic asthenospermia: a randomized, double-blind, placebo-controlled trial. Fertil Steril. 2006;85(5):1409–14. https://doi.org/10.1016/j.fertnstert.2005.10.055. Epub 2006 Apr 5. PMID: 16600222.
72. Lenzi A, Sgrò P, Salacone P, Paoli D, Gilio B, Lombardo F, Santulli M, Agarwal A, Gandini L. A placebo-controlled double-blind randomized trial of the use of combined l-carnitine and l-acetyl-carnitine treatment in men with asthenozoospermia. Fertil Steril. 2004;81(6):1578–84. https://doi.org/10.1016/j.fertnstert.2003.10.034. PMID: 15193480.
73. Gharagozloo P, Gutierrez-Adan A, Champroux A, Noblanc A, Kocer A, Calle A, Perez-Cerezales S, Pericuesta E, Polhemus A, Moazamian A, et al. A novel antioxidant formulation designed to treat male infertility associated with oxidative stress: promising preclinical evidence from animal models. Hum Reprod (Oxf Engl). 2016;31:252–62. https://doi.org/10.1093/humrep/dev302.
74. Kizilay F, Altay B. Evaluation of the effects of antioxidant treatment on sperm parameters and pregnancy rates in infertile patients after varicocelectomy: a randomized controlled trial. Int J Impot Res. 2019;1 https://doi.org/10.1038/s41443-018-0109-4.
75. Surai PF, Blesbois E, Grasseau I, et al. Fatty acid composition, glutathione peroxidase and superoxide dismutase activity and total antioxidant activity of avian semen. Comp Biochem Physiol B Biochem Mol Biol. 1998;120(3):527–33.
76. Irvine DS. Glutathione as a treatment for male infertility. Rev Reprod. 1996;1(1):6–12. https://doi.org/10.1530/ror.0.0010006. PMID: 9414432.
77. Dahlen CR, Reynolds LP, Caton JS. Selenium supplementation and pregnancy outcomes. Front Nutr. 2022;9:1011850. https://doi.org/10.3389/fnut.2022.1011850. PMID: 36386927; PMCID: PMC9659920.
78. Scott R, MacPherson A, Yates RW, Hussain B, Dixon J. The effect of oral selenium supplementation on human sperm motility. Br J Urol. 1998;82(1):76–80. https://doi.org/10.1046/j.1464-410x.1998.00683.x. PMID: 9698665.
79. Greco E, Iacobelli M, Rienzi L, Ubaldi F, Ferrero S, Tesarik J. Reduction of the incidence of sperm DNA fragmentation by oral antioxidant treatment. J Androl. 2005;26(3):349–53. https://doi.org/10.2164/jandrol.04146. PMID: 15867002.
80. Showell MG, Mackenzie-Proctor R, Brown J, Yazdani A, Stankiewicz MT, Hart RJ. Antioxidants for male subfertility. Cochrane Database Syst Rev. 2014;(12):CD007411. https://doi.org/10.1002/14651858.CD007411.pub3. Epub 2014 Dec 15. Update in: Cochrane Database Syst Rev. 2019 Mar 14;3:CD007411. doi:10.1002/14651858.CD007411.pub4. PMID: 25504418.
81. Agarwal A, Cannarella R, Saleh R, Harraz AM, Kandil H, Salvio G, Boitrelle F, Kuroda S, Farkouh A, Rambhatla A, Zini A, Colpi G, Gül M, Kavoussi P, Hamoda TAA, Ko E, Calik G, Toprak T, Pinggera GM, Park HJ, Ghayda RA, Minhas S, Busetto GM, Bakırcıoğlu ME, Kadioglu A, Chung E, Russo GI, Calogero AE, Ambar RF, Jayasena CN, Shah R. Impact of antioxidant therapy on natural pregnancy outcomes and semen parameters in infertile men: a systematic review and meta-analysis of randomized controlled trials. World J Mens Health. 2023;41(1):14–48. https://doi.org/10.5534/wjmh.220067. Epub 2022 Sep 7. PMID: 36102104; PMCID: PMC9826914.
82. Skoog SJ, Roberts KP, Goldstein M, Pryor JL. The adolescent varicocele: what's new with an old problem in young patients? Pediatrics. 1997;100(1):112–21. https://doi.org/10.1542/peds.100.1.112.
83. Masson P, Brannigan RE. The varicocele. Urol Clin North Am. 2014;41(1):129–44. https://doi.org/10.1016/j.ucl.2013.08.001.
84. Grasso M, Lania C, Castelli M, Galli L, Franzoso F, Rigatti P. Low-grade left varicocele in patients over 30 years old: the effect of spermatic vein ligation on fertility. BJU Int. 2000;85(3):305–7. https://doi.org/10.1046/j.1464-410x.2000.00437.x.

85. Will MA, Swain J, Fode M, Sonksen J, Christman GM, Ohl D. The great debate: varicocele treatment and impact on fertility. Fertil Steril. 2011;95(3):841–52. https://doi.org/10.1016/j.fertnstert.2011.01.002.
86. Damsgaard J, Joensen UN, Carlsen E, Erenpreiss J, Blomberg Jensen M, Matulevicius V, et al. Varicocele is associated with impaired semen quality and reproductive hormone levels: a study of 7035 healthy young men from six European countries. Eur Urol. 2016;70(6):1019–29. https://doi.org/10.1016/j.eururo.2016.06.044.
87. Cannarella R, Calogero AE, Condorelli RA, Giacone F, Aversa A, La Vignera S. Management and treatment of varicocele in children and adolescents: an endocrinologic perspective. J Clin Med. 2019;8(9) https://doi.org/10.3390/jcm8091410.
88. Kozakowski KA, Gjertson CK, Decastro GJ, Poon S, Gasalberti A, Glassberg KI. Peak retrograde flow: a novel predictor of persistent, progressive and new onset asymmetry in adolescent varicocele. J Urol. 2009;181(6):2717–22; discussion 23. https://doi.org/10.1016/j.juro.2009.02.038.
89. Palani A, Cannarella R, Saleh R, Salvio G, Harraz AM, Crafa A, Bahar F, Bocu K, Kumar N, Kothari P, Pinggera GM, Cayan S, Colpi GM, Atmoko W, Shah R, Agarwal A. Impact of varicocele repair on assisted reproductive technique outcomes in infertile men: a systematic review and meta-analysis. World J Mens Health. 2024; https://doi.org/10.5534/wjmh.240132.
90. Mostafa T, Anis T, Imam H, El-Nashar AR, Osman IA. Seminal reactive oxygen species-antioxidant relationship in fertile males with and without varicocele. Andrologia. 2009;41(2):125–9. https://doi.org/10.1111/j.1439-0272.2008.00900.x.
91. Fallara G, Tang S, Pang KH, Pozzi E, Belladelli F, Schifano N, Capogrosso P, Alnajjar HM, Montorsi F, Salonia A, Castiglione F, Muneer A, ESSM Scientific Collaboration and Partnership (ESCAP). Treatment of persistent or recurrent varicoceles: a systematic review. Eur Urol Focus. 2023;9(3):531–40. https://doi.org/10.1016/j.euf.2022.11.008. Epub 2022 Nov 25. PMID: 36443199.
92. Russo GI, Serefoglu EC. Management of recurrent varicocele. In: Esteves S, Cho CL, Majzoub A, Agarwal A, editors. Varicocele and male infertility. Cham: Springer; 2019. https://doi.org/10.1007/978-3-319-79102-9_27.
93. Rotker K, Sigman M. Recurrent varicocele. Asian J Androl. 2016;18(2):229–33. https://doi.org/10.4103/1008-682X.171578. PMID: 26806078; PMCID: PMC4770491.
94. Çayan S, Orhan İ, Akbay E, Kadıoğlu A. Systematic review of treatment methods for recurrent varicoceles to compare post-treatment sperm parameters, pregnancy and complication rates. Andrologia. 2019;51(11):e13419. https://doi.org/10.1111/and.13419. Epub 2019 Oct 1. PMID: 31576594.
95. Chen SS. Predictive factors of successful redo varicocelectomy in infertile patients with recurrent varicocele. Andrologia. 2014;46(7):738–43. https://doi.org/10.1111/and.12142. Epub 2013 Jul 28. PMID: 23889601.

Chapter 9
Fertility Preservation and Oncofertility

Israel Maldonado Rosas, Christina Anagnostopoulou, and Zhongwei Huang

Fertility Analysis Prior to Cancer Treatment

Oncofertility Protocols

Introduction

Oncofertility plays a crucial role in the treatment of patients who are facing a cancer diagnosis or other medical conditions that may impact their long-term fertility. These protocols aim to preserve the reproductive potential of male patients before they undergo potentially fertility-damaging treatments such as chemotherapy, radiation therapy, or surgery. Healthcare providers must be informed about the impact of oncological treatment on male fertility, and they must counsel the patients to undergo fertility preservation or refer them to an assisted reproduction clinic before instituting gonadotoxic treatments. Additionally, oncofertility protocols require close collaboration between oncologists and fertility specialists to ensure the best possible outcomes for patients. Individuals facing a cancer diagnosis should discuss their fertility preservation options with their healthcare team as early as possible to maximize their chances of preserving their male fertility. Sperm cryopreservation is

I. M. Rosas (✉)
Citmer Reproductive Medicine, IVF LAB, Mexico City, Mexico
e-mail: imaldonado@citmer.mx

C. Anagnostopoulou
Future Life Akeso, Athens, Greece

Z. Huang
NUS Bia Echo Asia Centre for Reproductive Longevity and Equality, National University of Singapore, Department of Obstetrics and Gynaecology, National University Health Systems, Singapore, Singapore
e-mail: obgzwh@nus.edu.sg

E. Chung et al. (eds.), *Advances in Andrology*,
https://doi.org/10.1007/978-3-032-29112-7_9

a routine practice for the male fertility preservation of postpubertal men—adolescent and adult patients. Several fertility clinics also offer testicular tissue preservation for prepubertal patients.

Semen Analysis (Health and Viability of Sperm, One-Time or Multiple Collections)

Semen analysis is a test that evaluates the quality and viability of sperm [76]. It is a crucial tool for evaluating male fertility and is especially important for cancer patients who want to preserve their sperm before undergoing treatment. By understanding the quality of their sperm, men can make informed decisions about their fertility preservation options. The evaluation of semen parameters is based on the standards and references listed in the WHO laboratory manual for the examination and processing of human semen. It considers parameters such as volume, viability, motility, concentration, and morphology [76]. Sperm can be damaged in different ways during cancer treatment, and the consequences of freezing and thawing can result in deleterious effects on the functional parameters of their gametes [39]. Therefore, it is relevant that a personalized evaluation of the semen is carried out before the conservation process, considering not only the characteristics of the semen analysis but also the cryopreservation method that can be performed, the types of cancer afflicting the patient and his age [34, 50]. For example, if a man has a low sperm count before treatment, doctors may recommend sperm banking before starting therapy. Additionally, it is recommended to collect semen samples on two or more occasions with at least a week between collections. Sperm parameters can naturally fluctuate between ejaculates [39] and it may be necessary if the cancer patient is considering preserving fertility, to perform multiple semen analyses to obtain a more reliable image of the quality of their sperm [39]. Depending on the urgency to institute life-saving medical treatment to the men, it is reasonable to offer cryopreservation or sperm banking with the first semen sample, whereby only suitable semen samples are frozen for future utility based on the semen analysis. This can potentially reduce the time to cryopreservation of sperm and the commencement of vital medical treatment for the patients.

Prepubertal Male Fertility Preservation

Preservation of Testicular Tissues

The optimal method for fertility preservation in male cancer patients is the cryopreservation of spermatozoa acquired either by semen collection or by testicular biopsy. However, this option is not available to prepubertal patients. Testicular tissue freezing is an alternative experimental approach that provides the chance for fertility restoration. Testicular tissue contains spermatogonial stem cells (SSC) that can be transplanted to restore spermatogenesis. [12] Different options exist to cryopreserve SSC: as testicular cell suspension (TCS), as enriched TCS, or as testicular tissue (TT). After cryopreservation and thawing of testicular tissue, it can be used for either autologous SSC transplantation (SSCT) or TT grafting. In contrast, in case of TCS cryopreservation, the option of a TT graft is not available. [46].

A. Spermatogonial Stem Cells (SSC)

The spermatogonial stem cells, the most primitive spermatogonia, located in the basement membrane of the seminiferous tubules, are the key to spermatogenesis as they have the ability for self-renewal and differentiation to daughter cells [57]. Cryopreserved SSCs potentially restore spermatogenesis after thawing, transplantation, and colonization of the testicular niche. However, the number of SSCs obtained after testicular biopsy of prepubertal patients is limited, while the success of future SSC transplantation or TT grafting depends on the availability and number of viable SSCs [46]. Therefore, maintaining a good number of SSCs is crucial, and the selection and standardization of an efficient cryopreservation method determine the success of fertility restoration. There are options to increase the number of SSCs by the enrichment of testicular cell suspension [19] or by the culture and propagation of SSCs in vitro [40].

B. Testicular Cell Suspension (TCS)

TCS is a valid approach for SSC preservation in prepubertal patients [46]. The dissociation procedure of testicular tissue is an important first step for preparing single-cell suspension. The enzymatic dissociation involving the use of collagenase, hyaluronidase, and DNAase results in high cell numbers; however, the enzymes may adversely affect cell integrity [60]. Alternatively, mechanical tissue disaggregation has been suggested as a faster method for preparing TCS, with reproducible results without causing cell damage [60]. There are several methods to enrich human spermatogonia, such as differential plating, fluorescence, and magnetic-activated cell sorting strategies. [73].

The vitrification of human TCS in open pulled straws has been tried, and promising results have been obtained in terms of cell viability [56]. Testicular cell suspensions have been frozen using the novel cryopiece, lowering DNA Fragmentation Index (DFI) compared to freezing in straws [37].

C. Testicular Tissue Cryopreservation (TTC). Controlled and Uncontrolled Slow Freezing and Vitrification

Controlled slow freezing (CSF) of testicular tissues has been found to be a valid method for fertility preservation in prepubertal patients before gonadotoxic treatment [31]. Tissue pieces are placed in cryovials containing cryoprotectant medium with Dimethylsulfoxide and Human Serum Albumin [9, 31]. The cryovials are equilibrated for 15 min on ice water and then cooled at a rate of -1 °C/min [9]. When the temperature of the cryovials reaches -80 °C, they are stored in liquid nitrogen. The examination of these testicular tissues after thawing by light microscopy (LM) and immunohistochemistry (IHM) has shown that spermatogonia, Sertoli cells, and stromal compartment remained viable and retained the integrity of their cellular structures after slow freezing [31].

The disadvantages of controlled slow freezing include the need for expensive equipment and the time-consuming freezing program. On the contrary, the employment of uncontrolled slow freezing (USF) has simplified the cryopreservation procedure. According to the USF protocol, the samples were equilibrated in a cryoprotective medium containing 1.5 M DMSO and sucrose and then placed in a -80 °C freezer. As a result, the samples were cooled at approximately 1C^0/min [7]. USF with 1.5 M DMSO has efficiently preserved human testicular tissue regarding spermatogonial number and testicular cell ultrastructure.

Vitrification, a simple and inexpensive yet effective testicular tissue cryopreservation method, was studied using a mouse model [6]. The tissue pieces were immersed in cryoprotectant containing DMSO and ethylene glycol before vitrification.

In cases where there is limited testicular tissue, the microinjection of single seminiferous tubules with cryoprotectant followed by vitrification is a valid approach to testicular cryopreservation as it maintains tubule structural integrity, protects germ cells, and prevents apoptosis [22].

A comparison between CSF, USF, and vitrification demonstrated that all three methods were efficient in maintaining the structural integrity and cellular morphology of the testicular tissue and ensuring the survival of SSCs and Sertoli cells [29].

Testicular Tissue for Male Fertility Restoration

Spermatogonial Stem Cell Transplantation (SSCT) (Spermatogonial Stem Cell Culture, Actual Application)

The use of spermatogonial stem cells (SSCs) holds immense promise for fertility preservation in men undergoing gonadotoxic treatments like chemotherapy and radiation, especially in childhood patients who are at risk of cancer treatment-related infertility. SSCs are adult stem cells found in the testes and are the basis for initiating spermatogenesis [15]. Unlike mature sperm, SSCs can be retrieved from testicular tissue biopsies and potentially offer a long-term source for sperm production [12, 59]. This approach, known as Spermatogonial Stem Cell Transplantation (SSCT), involves transplanting SSCs back into the testes of a recipient testis to restore spermatogenesis for sperm production [27]. This technique involves isolating and cultivating SSCs in vitro, which can then be used for various applications such as germ cell transplantation or in vitro spermatogenesis. Current research focuses on optimizing culture conditions to enhance SSC proliferation and maintain their "stemness." While successful in animal models, challenges remain in adapting these techniques for human SSC culture and more research is required to address the limitations in in vitro culture and ensure its safety and efficacy in humans [12, 27]. Ongoing research aims to refine techniques and address challenges to broaden the applicability of SSC transplantation in clinical settings.

Tissue Grafting

Cryopreservation of testicular tissue is still considered an experimental method to preserve the fertility of prepubertal patients before they begin therapies for cancer treatment [16, 30]. Testicular tissue grafting involves transplanting testicular tissue from the testes to another location (like the abdomen), potentially for sperm retrieval in the future [30]. Maintaining the tissues in vivo may be more suitable for complete tissue maturation with germ cell proliferation and differentiation [30]. Fayomi and collaborators [16] demonstrated in a castrated pubertal rhesus macaque model that cryopreserved testicular tissue can be autologously grafted under the skin and matured to produce functional spermatozoa, competent to fertilize rhesus oocytes and produce the birth of a healthy baby [16]. These results suggest that testicular tissue grafting offers potential future applications for young patients who want to preserve their fertility. However, while research on testicular tissue grafting in animals shows some promise, successful sperm retrieval and use for human fertility treatments haven't been consistently achieved. This area of research remains promising for the near future, but there are still ethical and clinical considerations to be finalized before this approach can be offered to all patients.

Human In Vitro Gametogenesis (IVG)

In vitro gametogenesis (IVG) is the procedure employed for the production of spermatids through extracorporeal spermatogenesis in culture [51]. IVG is an alternative approach for male fertility restoration, recommended in patient groups who are facing a high risk of contamination with malignant cells and who, therefore, need to avoid SSCT transplantation. Spermatozoa derived from primitive spermatogonia in vitro may later be used by ICSI to fertilize oocytes. IVG consists of the 2D or 3D culture of testicular cells or organotypic culture of testicular tissue. Functional haploid spermatids have been generated from human SSCs by a three-dimensional system using a matrigel matrix [67]. Additionally, the long-term organotypic culture of testicular tissue from prepubertal boys resulted in the differentiation of germ cells (GC) to a post-meiotic stage [13]. The latest approach is based on creating testicular organoids using a 3D culture system generated from testicular cell suspensions that might allow for more precise replication of the SSC niche [54].

Although promising, the IVG procedure has not yet been completely successful in humans, and until today, human spermatogenesis has progressed only to the spermatid stage. The main challenges that occur are safety issues, as the functionality of key meiotic checkpoints has not yet been investigated [35].

Current Status of In Vitro Gametogenesis (IVG) Research

IVG is a revolutionary advancement in reproductive biology with the potential to transform fertility treatments. Research on the preservation, proliferation, differentiation, and transplantation of spermatogonial stem cells (SSC) or testicular tissue demonstrated that IVG is a promising method to preserve the fertility of children with cancer and men with azoospermia [8]. Currently, research is focused on improving culture systems, providing a 3D structure for cells to grow on, and mimicking the extracellular matrix of the testis, which is crucial for an adequate cell-cell interaction that allows the development of sperm [58]. On the other hand, researchers have achieved significant progress in generating functional sperm and eggs from pluripotent stem cells in mice and are still working to fully understand the complex process of germline development, which is crucial for successful IVG in humans [8, 28]. There are still some years left before this technology can be used in human reproduction, and as IVG research progresses, it is essential to develop clear and ethical guidelines to ensure the appropriate utility of this technology [41].

Postpubertal Male Fertility Preservation

Methods of Sperm Retrieval

Masturbation and Ejaculation

The most simplistic, safe, and low-cost method for sperm retrieval is by masturbation [49]. The patient should be informed that the entire ejaculate should be collected in the sterile cups provided [2]. When the patient prefers to produce the sample at home, the specimen should be brought at the laboratory within an hour while kept at body temperature [2]. However, in urgent indications of gonadotoxic treatment, sperm retrieval is performed regardless of abstinence [74]. In cases of low sperm quality, the patient is advised to repeat the procedure in order to increase the amount of sperm cryopreserved [75].

Oncologic Testicular Sperm Extraction ("Onco-TESE"), Testicular Sperm Extraction (TESE), Testicular Sperm Aspiration (TESA), and Microdissection Testicular Sperm Extraction (MicroTESE)

Epididymal and Testicular Retrieval Techniques
Sperm retrieval by ejaculation is ineffective in cases of non-obstructive azoospermia (NOA), which is common in men with testicular cancer. There are several techniques for obtaining sperm from the epididymis, such as percutaneous epididymal sperm aspiration (PESA) and epididymal sperm aspiration (MESA), while

testicular sperm aspiration (TESA) and testicular sperm extraction (TESE) are used for sperm retrieval from the testis. PESA or TESA is commonly used in men with obstructive azoospermia.

In TESA, a needle is inserted into the testis with negative pressure, and the fluid containing spermatozoa is aspirated [18]. TESE is an open biopsy in which a small portion of the testis containing seminiferous tubules is extracted [14]. If no spermatozoa are found, after dissection of the seminiferous tubules and observation under the inverted microscope in the laboratory, more incisions may be done on other areas of the ipsilateral testis or the contralateral testis.

MicroTESE is a modified technique, in which the biopsy is performed by using a surgical microscope. Spermatogenesis areas may be identified more clearly under magnification 6–8x and more spermatozoa are extracted while extracting smaller testicular tissue fragments [43].

TESE, which can be performed at the same time as orchiectomy (onco-TESE), is a valid option for fertility preservation for some testicular cancer patients. This method, described by Schrader et al., is a useful technique for sperm retrieval before gonadotoxic therapy in azoospermic cancer patients [61].

Sperm Preservation

Sperm Cryopreservation (Determining Factors Include Age, Number of Children, and Semen Quality)

Sperm cryopreservation, or sperm freezing, is a process for preserving sperm cells for later use [20]. This technique offers men the opportunity to father children at a future date despite potential changes in fertility by cancer treatment. Semen should be collected and frozen before the patient begins cancer treatment, especially if the treatment involves chemotherapy or pelvic radiation [32]. Men with normal semen parameters have a higher success rate with cryopreservation. However, even men with lower sperm counts may benefit from sperm banking, especially with advanced techniques like intracytoplasmic sperm injection (ICSI) [20, 32]. Sperm quality tends to decline with age [3], this implies that sperm banking at a younger age offers a better chance of successful cryopreservation and future use. For prepubescent boys who have not yet begun producing sperm, testicular tissue extraction and cryopreservation may be an option. This tissue can potentially be used in the future to produce mature sperm in a lab setting, although this is still an experimental technique [20, 32]. The decision to have children is personal and depends on the patient and his significant others. Some men may choose to cryopreserve sperm if they already have children and want to expand their family in the future; others may choose this procedure if they are not sure whether they want to have children or anticipate future medical conditions that will affect fertility due to cancer treatment [44].

A. Slow Freezing Procedures

Principles and Challenges of Sperm Slow Freezing

The slow freezing technique is a well-established method for cryopreserving human sperm, which is crucial for ART and fertility preservation [25]. This traditional method involves a gradual decrease in temperature using a controlled-rate freezer. Cryoprotectants, chemicals that protect cells during freezing, are added to the sperm sample [53]. Slow, controlled cooling allows for the controlled formation of extracellular ice crystals, minimizing damage to the sperm cells. However, crystal formation during the freezing process remains the biggest obstacle [47]. This process can still cause some sperm to lose motility, viability, and DNA integrity [25, 53] and the recovery rate of functional sperm after cryopreservation remains critical in infertile men [53]. Slow freezing is not ideal for cryopreservation of single or small numbers of spermatozoa [25]. This process requires specialized equipment and trained personnel [63]. While slow freezing remains the gold standard, research continues to explore faster and potentially more efficient freezing methods like vitrification to improve semen preservation in cancer patients.

B. Vitrification. Vitrification Procedure

Principles and Challenges of Sperm Vitrification

Vitrification is a rapid freezing technique replacing traditional slow freezing methods for sperm cryopreservation [4]. Unlike conventional freezing, vitrification uses high concentrations of cryoprotectants to prevent ice crystal formation, a major cause of sperm damage [62, 69]. The sperm suspension is plunged into liquid nitrogen extremely rapidly, transforming it into a glass-like state. Vitrification offers several advantages: faster freezing times, improved sperm motility post-thaw, and potentially better fertilization rates than slow freezing [69]. However, challenges remain. The complex vitrification procedure requires specialized equipment and skilled technicians [69]. Additionally, the long-term effects of vitrification on sperm function and DNA integrity are still under investigation. Sperm vitrification is currently applied in samples with reduced sperm concentration and volume [68, 77]. Studies suggested that vitrification may offer slightly better post-thaw motility and survival rates for sperm compared to slow freezing [4]. However, both methods remain efficacious, and the preferred technique depends on factors such as clinic expertise and equipment availability.

C. Single Sperm Freezing Procedure

Principles and Challenges of Single Sperm Freezing

Single sperm freezing, also known as single spermatozoon cryopreservation, is a technique used to preserve a single sperm cell for future use in assisted reproductive technologies like intracytoplasmic sperm injection (ICSI). Cryopreservation of a few sperm is performed to avoid repeated sperm retrievals in patients with non-obstructive azoospermia and/or severe oligozoospermia. In addition, it is also a way to preserve sperm such that they are free from side effects of any treatment regimen, particularly cancer treatment [39]. This technique involves freezing individual sperm cells instead of a whole semen sample. It's primarily used for men with very low sperm counts and is often used in conjunction with ICSI during ART. To cryopreserve a reduced number of sperm, some strategies have been implemented such as the use of non-biological carriers such as cryoloops, cryotops, and others, which seem promising since they allow good percentages of motile and viable sperm to be recovered [68]. Although single sperm freezing is a highly specialized procedure with lower success rates compared to freezing whole semen samples, this technique requires specialized equipment and highly skilled technicians [38, 68] but proves to be an essential option in patients with extremely low sperm counts.

D. Success Rate of Vitrification and Slow Freezing

Various studies attempt to describe the most appropriate technique to achieve the highest cryosurvival rate of human gametes. Cryopreservation is complex because it requires several protocols, freezing carriers, and cryoprotectant agents [47]. Sperm cryopreservation success rates can vary depending on individual factors like initial sperm quality, freezing technique, and storage duration [68]. Studies suggest that vitrification may offer slightly better post-thaw motility and survival rates for sperm compared to slow freezing with lower levels of DNA damage [45, 68, 77]. Studies haven't specifically focused on the outcomes of cryopreservation of sperm from cancer patients, but overall sperm survival rates exceed 70% with good motility and fertilization potential post-thaw [45, 47, 77]. Slow freezing has success rates of 50–70% for sperm survival [47, 68]. A study examining microRNA (miRNA) changes in sperm after cryopreservation (slow freezing or vitrification) showed that any cryopreservation alters miRNA compared to fresh sperm. This is of utmost importance since sperm-derived miRNAs are delivered to oocytes and can influence fertilization and embryo development. Novel miRNA biomarkers may contribute to effective molecular assessment of sperm quality after thawing [52]. It is still not known which sperm cryopreservation technique provides the best post-thawing results since there is still no standard method that optimizes in all aspects the recovery of sperm parameters affected by freezing and thawing.

Fertilization Methods. Assisted Reproductive Technologies (ART)

In Vitro Fertilization (IVF)

Conventional in vitro fertilization (C-IVF) is a simple, non-invasive method of fertilization mostly applied to non-male infertility cases. C-IVF consists of the co-incubation of sperm with the oocytes overnight. The final concentration of sperm in the fertilization dish is 100, 000–200, and 000 motile spermatozoa/ml; however, it can vary in different IVF lab protocols from 20, 000 to 1, 000, 000/ml. Excess amount of sperm inseminated exposes the oocytes to the risk of abnormal fertilization (polyspermia). At approximately 16–18 post insemination, pronuclear check for fertilization is performed under the microscope. In most clinics c-IVF is performed only in couples with males presenting normal sperm concentration and motility. According to populational studies of fertile men, sperm concentration is considered normal above $15x10^6$/ml and total motility above 42% [76]. However, freezing and subsequent thawing of sperm results to the decrease of sperm motility and fertilizing ability [33, 42]. Furthermore, the amount of sperm cryopreserved before oncological treatment is often limited, and may not be enough for one or multiple treatments with c-IVF. On the contrary, the ICSI procedure requires only a much smaller number of viable spermatozoa for fertilization. These facts should be considered when selecting the fertilization technique that is most adequate for the specific couple.

Intracytoplasmic Sperm Injection (ICSI)

ICSI is the fertilization technique that is routinely used in cases of male infertility and cryopreserved samples of cancer patients. It is suitable for ejaculated sperm and also for PESA, TESA, and TESE samples. In contrast to c-IVF, only a few functional sperm are required in order to achieve fertilization with ICSI. ICSI includes the selection, catching, and immobilization of a single spermatozoon under the inverted microscope. The next step of the procedure is the injection of the spermatozoon into the oocyte. At 16–18 h following insemination, the oocytes are checked for the presence of two pronuclei. During ICSI, the selection of a competent spermatozoon for fertilization may be facilitated by using morphologically selected sperm injection (IMSI) or physiological ICSI (PICSI) [17]. In cases that only immotile spermatozoa are present, there exist several methods for the identification of viable sperm such as the hypo-osmotic swelling test (HOST), the use of pentoxifylline and theophylline, and the laser-assisted immotile sperm selection (LAISS) [65].

ART Success Rates in Cancer Patients

Oncological treatments may have a negative impact on male fertility. Fertility in patients with testicular cancer who have not cryopreserved sperm samples before treatment is significantly decreased after treatments and radiotherapy. These patients experienced the most detrimental effect on IVF outcomes post-therapy [26]. Testicular cancer survivors have a better prognosis in terms of fertility compared to hematological cancer, Hodgkin's disease, or lymphoma [43, 70]. The differences between oncological patients are due to the severity of the chemotherapy treatment which varies according to the type of cancer [43].

In patients who have already banked ejaculated sperm or TESE samples before gonadotoxic treatment, ART success rates with ICSI are similar to those of non-cancer patients. According to a prospective review of the assisted reproduction outcomes with banked semen before oncological treatment, almost 40% of the patients were able to achieve a live birth, regardless of the type of ART used or the type of malignancy they suffered from [1].

A 2021 retrospective study, comparing ART outcomes in male cancer patients, did not find any differences in pregnancy and live birth rate, regardless of the type of sperm sample used, either fresh or frozen and thawed. [48]. However, higher embryo utilization and cryopreservation rates have been noted when using the frozen-thawed sample, and consequently higher cumulative pregnancy rates for patients who had performed fertility preservation [48].

According to a meta-analysis and systematic review of 69 non-randomized studies, with 32,234 patients who attempted to cryopreserve a sperm sample before or during treatment, the utility rate of frozen sperm was 9%, while the pregnancy and delivery rates after ART were 28% and 20%, respectively. The authors concluded that sperm banking before or during oncological treatment is an effective male fertility preservation method [36].

Oncofertility and Ethical Considerations

Oncofertility service offers cancer patients the chance to preserve their fertility before undergoing treatments that may damage reproductive organs or gametes (eggs and sperm) [20]. Many children and young adults diagnosed with cancer may survive treatment due to the advances made in medical oncology treatments. Therefore, fertility preservation can be a safe, affordable, and successful option for these patients. Treatments should be applied as soon as possible after cancer diagnosis and be recommended according to the disease process and individual patient preference [44, 66]. However, ethical considerations do arise, particularly in relation to informed consent and decision-making capacity. A cancer diagnosis can be shocking and potentially impact a patient's ability to fully understand their fertility options [10]. Clinicians must ensure clear communication and address social or religious beliefs that may influence the patients' decisions [10, 23, 24]. Besides, storing gametes or gonads for prolonged periods of time raises ethical and moral questions, many of which remain unanswered to date. The existence of uncertainties in the protocols and strategies, with success rates of using preserved eggs or sperm for future pregnancy vary, which deserves further examination at the ethical and politico-legal level to make concrete plans to ensure the smooth execution of oncofertility services [10, 20]. Another crucial point to consider is the future posthumous use of deceased individuals' preserved tissues and cells [10], which are currently prohibited in many nations and countries [64, 71, 72]. To address all these ethical considerations, there must be open and honest communication between patients, oncologists, and fertility specialists with the inclusion of bioethicists, policymakers, and legislators. Continued research and discussions are needed to ensure equitable access and responsible implementation of oncofertility practices.

Prepubertal Population (Includes Boys and Teenagers Who Have Not Achieved Puberty Yet)

Preservation of fertility in prepubertal pediatric patients remains experimental; however, with the recent scientific advances in the use of spermatogonial stem cells and testicular tissue transplantation, the future of oncofertility for these patients is promising [21]. There are several ethical considerations that oncofertility must consider when treating infantile or prepubertal patients, such as informed consent, the application of fertility preservation techniques that are still in the experimental phase, and long-term storage of the genetic material [55]. In addition to all of these, medical personnel must be able to address, together with the family, complex issues such as the uncertainties of the results of fertility preservation in children and the financial limitations related to procedures and storage [21, 55]. It is recommended that a multidisciplinary team be involved to evaluate each case individually and offer personalized advice to the patients and families with options that exist to preserve fertility. It is vital to maintain open communication with the provision of comprehensive advice for families before the parents can make informed decisions to preserve fertility for their children.

Postpubertal Population (Can Include Teenagers Below 21 Years Old and Adult Men)

For men who can ejaculate, sperm cryopreservation (sperm banking) is the only established method of fertility preservation [20]. Oncologists must ensure patients understand the potential risks and benefits of fertility preservation options, considering their age, diagnosis, and prognosis [44]. Discussions about alternative family-building options like adoption or surrogacy are also crucial [10, 44]. For teenagers approaching adulthood, assessing their decision-making capacity is vital, as well as comprehending the consequences of cancer treatment and fertility preservation [5]. Another essential point to be informed to men is the existence of a potential risk of genetic damage in the sperm collected after the start of therapy, which is why it is recommended to collect sperm before starting treatment and to ensure the quality of the sperm sample and DNA integrity. In addition, ICSI allows the future use of cryopreserved sperm, even when the number of sperm is very limited [44]. Open communication and emotional support are essential to navigate these complex decisions [10]. Although scientific advances continue to improve fertility preservation in cancer patients, challenges still exist to meet the various fertility needs of prepubertal and postpubertal patients. The need to allocate resources to perform research in this area, in conjunction with clinical practice, will allow more robust options to address fertility preservation in patients of all age.

Future Perspectives

Current advances in reproductive technologies have provided fertility preservation options for males with oncofertility needs. The technologies available are suitable for postpubertal males, even for males who are azoospermic or have anejaculation, while immature testicular tissue cryopreservation remains the only alternative for prepubertal boys which is still considered experimental [11]. Concerted efforts should be invested in pushing the science of fertility preservation, especially on gonadal tissue cryopreservation, in vitro maturation, and gamete formation, to ensure that patients of all ages and medical conditions have equal reproductive rights and access to oncofertility services. Importantly, with the advent of advanced fertility cryopreservation techniques, the active involvement of bioethicists, policy-makers, and legislators is essential for the appropriate use of these technologies, funding support, governance, and access for all patients with oncofertility needs. In particular, the topic of posthumous use of the precious gametes from these patients and its implications to the deceased and his family must be explored with definitive guidelines as well as legislation put in place to prevent ambiguity and regret.

Conclusion

Fertility preservation in males is still fraught with challenges, as described previously. The emphasis placed on advancing medical technologies for fertility preservation must be matched by an equal emphasis on ensuring access to oncofertility services for both children and adults. This is a joint effort by a multidisciplinary team that consists of the oncology and fertility specialists, counselors, pediatricians, and advanced andrology laboratory team backed by a supportive healthcare administrative team. Furthermore, global advocacy on this vital issue, such as efforts from the Global Andrology Forum in collaboration with andrology societies around the world, will allow boys and men from any part of the world to access oncofertility services nearest to them at affordable prices with proven efficacy.

References

1. Agarwal A, Ranganathan P, Kattal N, Pasqualotto F, Hallak J, Khayal S, Mascha E. Fertility after cancer: a prospective review of assisted reproductive outcome with banked semen specimens. Fertil Steril. 2004;81(2):342–8. https://doi.org/10.1016/j.fertnstert.2003.07.021. PMID: 14967371. PMID: 14770428
2. Agarwal A, Ong C, Durairajanayagam D. Contemporary and future insights into fertility preservation in male cancer patients. Transl Androl Urol. 2014;3(1):27–40.
3. Ajayi AF, Onaolapo MC, Omole AI, Adeyemi WJ, Oluwole DT. Mechanism associated with changes in male reproductive functions during ageing process. Exp Gerontol. 2023;179:112232.

4. Antonouli S, Di Nisio V, Messini C, Daponte A, Rajender S, Anifandis G. A comprehensive review and update on human fertility cryopreservation methods and tools. Front Vet Sci. 2023;10:1151254. https://doi.org/10.3389/fvets.2023.1151254.
5. Ataman LM, Laronda MM, Gowett M, Trotter K, Anvari H, Fei F, Ingram A, Minette M, Suebthawinkul C, Taghvaei Z, Torres-Vélez M, Velez K, Adiga SK, Anazodo A, Appiah L, Bourlon MT, Daniels N, Dolmans MM, Finlayson C, Gilchrist RB, Gomez-Lobo V, Greenblatt E, Halpern JA, Hutt K, Johnson EK, Kawamura K, Khrouf M, Kimelman D, Kristensen S, Mitchell RT, Moravek MB, Nahata L, Orwig KE, Pavone ME, Pépin D, Pesce R, Quinn GP, Rosen MP, Rowell E, Smith K, Venter C, Whiteside S, Xiao S, Zelinski M, Goldman KN, Woodruff TK, Duncan FE. A synopsis of global frontiers in fertility preservation. J Assist Reprod Genet. 2022;39(8):1693–712. https://doi.org/10.1007/s10815-022-02570-5.
6. Baert Y, Goossens E, van Saen D, Ning L, in't Veld P, Tournaye H. Orthotopic grafting of cryopreserved prepubertal testicular tissue: in search of a simple yet effective cryopreservation protocol. Fertil Steril. 2012;97(5):1152–7.e1–2. https://doi.org/10.1016/j.fertnstert.2012.02.010. Epub 2012 Feb 25. PMID: 22369773
7. Baert Y, Van Saen D, Haentjens P, In't Veld P, Tournaye H, Goossens E. What is the best cryopreservation protocol for human testicular tissue banking? Hum Reprod. 2013;28(7):1816–26. https://doi.org/10.1093/humrep/det100. Epub 2013 Apr 7. PMID: 23569082
8. Botigelli RC, Carly G, Braz AR. Denicol Anna Carolina. In vitro gametogenesis from embryonic stem cells in livestock species: recent advances, opportunities, and challenges to overcome. J Anim Sci. 2023;101:skad137. https://doi.org/10.1093/jas/skad137.
9. Braye A, Tournaye H, Goossens E. Setting up a cryopreservation Programme for immature testicular tissue: lessons learned after more than 15 years of experience. Clin Med Insights Reprod Health. 2019;13:1179558119886342. https://doi.org/10.1177/1179558119886342. PMID: 31798308; PMCID: PMC6868573
10. Carvalho BR, Kliemchen J, Woodruff TK. Ethical, moral and other aspects related to fertility preservation in cancer patients. JBRA Assist Reprod. 2017;21(1):45–8. https://doi.org/10.5935/1518-0557.20170011.
11. Chen L, Dong Z, Chen X. Fertility preservation in pediatric healthcare: a review. Front Endocrinol (Lausanne). 2023;14:1147898.
12. David S, Orwig KE. Spermatogonial stem cell culture in oncofertility. Urol Clin North Am. 2020;47(2):227–44. https://doi.org/10.1016/j.ucl.2020.01.001.
13. De Michele F, Poels J, Vermeulen M, Ambroise J, Gruson D, Guiot Y, Wyns C. Haploid germ cells generated in organotypic culture of testicular tissue from Prepubertal boys. Front Physiol. 2018;9:1413. https://doi.org/10.3389/fphys.2018.01413. PMID: 30356879; PMCID: PMC6190924.
14. Esteves SC, Varghese AC. Laboratory handling of epididymal and testicular spermatozoa: what can be done to improve sperm injections outcome. J Hum Reprod Sci. 2012;5(3):233–43.
15. Fayomi AP, Orwig KE. Spermatogonial stem cells and spermatogenesis in mice, monkeys and men. Stem Cell Res. 2018;29:207–14. https://doi.org/10.1016/j.scr.2018.04.009.
16. Fayomi AP, Peters K, Sukhwani M, Valli-Pulaski H, Shetty G, Meistrich ML, Houser L, Robertson N, Roberts V, Ramsey C, Hanna C, Hennebold JD, Dobrinski I, Orwig KE. Autologous grafting of cryopreserved prepubertal rhesus testis produces sperm and offspring. Science. 2019;363(6433):1314–9. https://doi.org/10.1126/science.aav2914.
17. Garrido N, Gül M, Jindal S, Vogiatzi P, Saleh R, Durairajanayagam D, Parmegiani L, Boitrelle F, Colpi GM, Agarwal A. How to select healthy sperm for intracytoplasmic sperm injection in samples with high sperm DNA fragmentation? Panminerva Med. 2023;65(2):148–58. https://doi.org/10.23736/S0031-0808.23.04870-X. Epub 2023 May 16. PMID: 37194246
18. Gorgy A, Podsiadly BT, Bates S, Craft IL. Testicular sperm aspiration (TESA): the appropriate technique. Hum Reprod. 1998;13(4):1111–3. https://doi.org/10.1093/humrep/13.4.1111. PMID: 9619581
19. Guo J, Cairns BR. Isolation and enrichment of Spermatogonial stem cells from human testis tissues. Curr Protoc Stem Cell Biol. 2019;49(1):e77. https://doi.org/10.1002/cpsc.77. Epub 2019 Jan 4. PMID: 30609304

20. Gupta D, Singh S, Shukla S, Shrivastava S. Oncofertility: treatment options from bench to bedside. Cancer Pathog Ther. 2023;1(4):284–9. https://doi.org/10.1016/j.cpt.2023.05.001.
21. Halpern JA, Das A, Faw CA, Brannigan RE. Oncofertility in adult and pediatric populations: options and barriers. Transl Androl Urol. 2020;9(Suppl 2):S227–38. https://doi.org/10.21037/tau.2019.09.27.
22. Han S, Zhao L, Yang C, Xu J, Yao C, Huang C, Zhang H, Ji Z, Luo J, Guo Y, Hong Y, Liu F, Zhou X, Zhou Z, Huang Y, Li Z. Vitrification with microinjection of single seminiferous tubules: an efficient cryopreservation approach for limited testicular tissue. Reprod Biomed Online. 2021;43(4):687–99. https://doi.org/10.1016/j.rbmo.2021.06.026. Epub 2021 Jul 3. PMID: 34556414
23. Hanselin MR, Roybal DL, Leininger TB. Ethics and oncofertility: a call for religious sensitivity. J Oncol Pract. 2017;13(7):e582–9. https://doi.org/10.1200/JOP.2016.020487.
24. Hashiloni-Dolev Y. Posthumous Reproduction (PHR) in Israel: Policy Rationales Versus Lay People's Concerns, a Preliminary Study, 39 Cult. Med. Psychiatry. 2015;634:636.
25. Huang C, Tang YL, Hu JL, Zhou WJ, Huang ZH, Luo XF, Li Z, Zhu WB. Update on techniques for cryopreservation of human spermatozoa. Asian J Androl. 2022;24(6):563–9. https://doi.org/10.4103/aja20229.
26. Huyghe E, Matsuda T, Daudin M, Chevreau C, Bachaud JM, Plante P, Bujan L, Thonneau P. Fertility after testicular cancer treatments: results of a large multicenter study. Cancer. 2004;100(4):732–7. https://doi.org/10.1002/cncr.11950.
27. Ibtisham F, Honaramooz A. Spermatogonial stem cells for in vitro spermatogenesis and in vivo restoration of fertility. Cells. 2020;9(3):745. https://doi.org/10.3390/cells9030745.
28. Ishikura Y, Ohta H, Sato T, Murase Y, Yabuta Y, Kojima Y, Yamashiro C, Nakamura T, Yamamoto T, Ogawa T, Saitou M. In vitro reconstitution of the whole male germ-cell development from mouse pluripotent stem cells. Cell Stem Cell. 2021;28(12):2167–2179.e9. https://doi.org/10.1016/j.stem.2021.08.005.
29. Kabiri D, Safrai M, Gropp M, Hidas G, Mordechai-Daniel T, Meir K, Revel A, Imbar T, Reubinoff B. Establishment of a controlled slow freezing-based approach for experimental clinical cryopreservation of human prepubertal testicular tissues. F S Rep. 2021;3(1):47–56. https://doi.org/10.1016/j.xfre.2021.11.001. PMID: 35386499; PMCID: PMC8978083
30. Kanbar M, Delwiche G, Wyns C. Fertility preservation for prepubertal boys: are we ready for autologous grafting of cryopreserved immature testicular tissue? Ann Endocrinol (Paris). 2022;83(3):210–7. https://doi.org/10.1016/j.ando.2022.04.006.
31. Keros V, Hultenby K, Borgström B, Fridström M, Jahnukainen K, Hovatta O. Methods of cryopreservation of testicular tissue with viable spermatogonia in pre-pubertal boys undergoing gonadotoxic cancer treatment. Hum Reprod. 2007;22(5):1384–95. https://doi.org/10.1093/humrep/del508. Epub 2007 Jan 26. PMID: 17259225
32. Kobayashi H, Tamura K, Tai T, Nagao K, Nakajima K. Semen cryopreservation as an oncofertility treatment in 122 Japanese men with cancer: a decade-long study. Reprod Med Biol. 2017;16(4):320–4. https://doi.org/10.1002/rmb2.12044.
33. Kopeika J, Thornhill A, Khalaf Y. The effect of cryopreservation on the genome of gametes and embryos: principles of cryobiology and critical appraisal of the evidence. Hum Reprod Update. 2015;21(2):209–27. https://doi.org/10.1093/humupd/dmu063. Epub 2014 Dec 17. PMID: 25519143
34. Ku JY, Park NC, Jeon TG, Park HJ. Semen analysis in cancer patients referred for sperm cryopreservation before chemotherapy over a 15-year period in Korea. World J Mens Health. 2015;33(1):8–13. https://doi.org/10.5534/wjmh.2015.33.1.8.
35. Lei Q, van Pelt AMM, Hamer G. In vitro spermatogenesis: why meiotic checkpoints matter. Curr Top Dev Biol. 2023;151:345–69. https://doi.org/10.1016/bs.ctdb.2022.04.009. Epub 2022 Jun 9. PMID: 36681476
36. Li Q, Lan QY, Zhu WB, Fan LQ, Huang C. Fertility preservation in adult male patients with cancer: a systematic review and meta-analysis. Hum Reprod Open. 2024;2024(1):hoae006. https://doi.org/10.1093/hropen/hoae006. PMID: 38389980; PMCID: PMC10882264

37. Lin F, Zheng B. Cryopreservation of human spermatozoa by freezing testicular seminiferous tubule with novel cryopiece. Andrologia. 2022;54(3):e14356. https://doi.org/10.1111/and.14356. Epub 2021 Dec 26. PMID: 34957581; PMCID: PMC9285044
38. Liu S, Li F. Cryopreservation of single-sperm: where are we today? Reprod Biol Endocrinol. 2020;18(1):41. https://doi.org/10.1186/s12958-020-00607-x.
39. Liu X, Liu B, Liu S, Xian Y, Zhao W, Zhou B, Xiao X, Wang L, Zhu X, Shu B, Jiang M, Li F. Male cancer patient sperm cryopreservation for fertility preservation: 10-year monocentric experience. Basic Clin Androl. 2021;31(1):24. https://doi.org/10.1186/s12610-021-00140-w.
40. Martin LA, Seandel M. Propagation of adult SSCs: from mouse to human. Biomed Res Int. 2013;2013:384734. https://doi.org/10.1155/2013/384734. Epub 2013 Jan 1. PMID: 23484114; PMCID: PMC3581147
41. Matthews Kirstin RW, Daniel M. Can we do that here? An analysis of US federal and state policies guiding human embryo and embryoid research. J Law Biosci. 2022;9(1):lsac014. https://doi.org/10.1093/jlb/lsac014.
42. Nijs M, Ombelet W. Cryopreservation of human sperm. Hum Fertil (Camb). 2001;4(3):158–63. https://doi.org/10.1080/1464727012000199232. PMID: 11591273
43. Ogouma L, Berthaut I, Lévy R, Hamid RH, Prades M, Audouin M, Sermondade N, Dupont C. Testicular sperm extraction (TESE) outcomes in the context of malignant disease: a systematic review. Asian J Androl. 2022;24(6):584–90. https://doi.org/10.4103/aja2021129. PMID: 35259785; PMCID: PMC9809488
44. Oktay K, Harvey BE, Partridge AH, Quinn GP, Reinecke J, Taylor HS, Hamish Wallace W, Wang ET, Loren AW. Fertility preservation in patients with cancer: ASCO clinical practice guideline update. JCO. 2018;36:1994–2001. https://doi.org/10.1200/JCO.2018.78.1914.
45. O'Neill HC, Nikoloska M, Ho H, Doshi A, Maalouf W. Improved cryopreservation of spermatozoa using vitrification: comparison of cryoprotectants and a novel device for long-term storage. J Assist Reprod Genet. 2019;36(8):1713–20. https://doi.org/10.1007/s10815-019-01505-x.
46. Onofre J, Baert Y, Faes K, Goossens E. Cryopreservation of testicular tissue or testicular cell suspensions: a pivotal step in fertility preservation. Hum Reprod Update. 2016;22(6):744–61. https://doi.org/10.1093/humupd/dmw029. Epub 2016 Aug 27. PMID: 27566839; PMCID: PMC5099994
47. Ozimic S, Ban-Frangez H, Stimpfel M. Sperm cryopreservation today: approaches, efficiency, and pitfalls. Curr Issues Mol Biol. 2023;45(6):4716–34. https://doi.org/10.3390/cimb45060300.
48. Papler TB, Vrtacnik-Bokal E, Drobnic S, Stimpfel M. The outcome of IVF/ICSI cycles in male cancer patients: retrospective analysis of procedures from 2004 to 2018. Radiol Oncol. 2021;55(2):221–8. https://doi.org/10.2478/raon-2021-0011. PMID: 33675201; PMCID: PMC8042825
49. Parekh NV, Lundy SD, Vij SC. Fertility considerations in men with testicular cancer. Transl Androl Urol. 2020;9(Suppl 1):S14–23. https://doi.org/10.21037/tau.2019.08.08. PMID: 32055481; PMCID: PMC6995852
50. Peluso G, Tisato V, Singh AV, Gemmati D, Scarpellini F. Semen cryopreservation to expand male fertility in cancer patients: Intracase evaluation of semen quality. J Pers Med. 2023;13(12):1654. https://doi.org/10.3390/jpm13121654.
51. Pelzman DL, Orwig KE, Hwang K. Progress in translational reproductive science: testicular tissue transplantation and in vitro spermatogenesis. Fertil Steril. 2020;113(3):500–9. https://doi.org/10.1016/j.fertnstert.2020.01.038. Epub 2020 Feb 25. PMID: 32111477
52. Podgrajsek R, Bolha L, Pungert T, Pizem J, Jazbec K, Malicev E, Stimpfel M. Effects of slow freezing and vitrification of human semen on post-thaw semen quality and miRNA expression. Int J Mol Sci. 2024;25:4157. https://doi.org/10.3390/ijms25084157.
53. Raad G, Lteif L, Lahoud R, Azoury J, Azoury J, Tanios J, Hazzouri M, Azoury J. Cryopreservation media differentially affect sperm motility, morphology and DNA integrity. Andrology. 2018;6(6):836–45. https://doi.org/10.1111/andr.12531.
54. Richer G, Baert Y, Goossens E. In-vitro spermatogenesis through testis modelling: toward the generation of testicular organoids. Andrology. 2020;8(4):879–91. https://doi.org/10.1111/andr.12741. Epub 2020 Jan 9. PMID: 31823507; PMCID: PMC7496450

55. Rowell EE, Lautz TB, Lai K, Weidler EM, Johnson EK, Finlayson C, van Leeuwen K. The ethics of offering fertility preservation to pediatric patients: a case-based discussion of barriers for clinicians to consider. Semin Pediatr Surg. 2021;30(5):151095. https://doi.org/10.1016/j.sempedsurg.2021.151095.
56. Sá R, Cremades N, Malheiro I, Sousa M. Cryopreservation of human testicular diploid germ cell suspensions. Andrologia. 2012;44(6):366–72. https://doi.org/10.1111/j.1439-0272.2012.01290.x. Epub 2012 Mar 15. PMID: 22420610
57. Saitou M, Hayashi K. Mammalian in vitro gametogenesis. Science. 2021;374(6563):eaaz6830. https://doi.org/10.1126/science.aaz6830. Epub 2021 Oct 1. PMID: 34591639
58. Salem M, Khadivi F, Javanbakht P, Mojaverrostami S, Abbasi M, Feizollahi N, Abbasi Y, Heidarian E, Rezaei YF. Advances of three-dimensional (3D) culture systems for in vitro spermatogenesis. Stem Cell Res Ther. 2023;14(1):262. https://doi.org/10.1186/s13287-023-03466-6.
59. Sanou I, van Maaren J, Eliveld J, Lei Q, Meißner A, de Melker AA, Hamer G, van Pelt AMM, Mulder CL. Spermatogonial stem cell-based therapies: taking preclinical research to the next level. Front Endocrinol (Lausanne). 2022;13:850219. https://doi.org/10.3389/fendo.2022.850219.
60. Schneider F, Redmann K, Wistuba J, Schlatt S, Kliesch S, Neuhaus N. Comparison of enzymatic digestion and mechanical dissociation of human testicular tissues. Fertil Steril. 2015;104(2):302–11.e3. https://doi.org/10.1016/j.fertnstert.2015.05.001. Epub 2015 Jun 13. PMID: 26056924
61. Schrader M, Müller M, Sofikitis N, Straub B, Krause H, Miller K. "Onco-tese": testicular sperm extraction in azoospermic cancer patients before chemotherapy-new guidelines? Urology. 2003;61(2):421–5. https://doi.org/10.1016/s0090-4295(02)02264-1. PMID: 12597960
62. Shah D, Rasappan S, Gunasekaran K. A simple method of human sperm vitrification. MethodsX. 2019;6:2198–204. https://doi.org/10.1016/j.mex.2019.09.022.
63. Sieme H, Oldenhof H, Wolkers WF. Sperm membrane behaviour during cooling and cryopreservation. Reprod Domest Anim. 2015;50(Suppl 3):20–6. https://doi.org/10.1111/rda.12594.
64. Simana S. Creating life after death: should posthumous reproduction be legally permissible without the deceased's prior consent? J Law Biosci. 2018;5(2):329–54.
65. Simopoulou M, Gkoles L, Bakas P, Giannelou P, Kalampokas T, Pantos K, Koutsilieris M. Improving ICSI: a review from the spermatozoon perspective. Syst Biol Reprod Med. 2016;62(6):359–71. https://doi.org/10.1080/19396368.2016.1229365. Epub 2016 Sep 20. PMID: 27646677
66. Skaznik-Wikiel ME, Gilbert SB, Meacham RB, Kondapalli LA. Fertility preservation options for men and women with cancer. Rev Urol. 2015;17(4):211–9.
67. Sun M, Yuan Q, Niu M, Wang H, Wen L, Yao C, Hou J, Chen Z, Fu H, Zhou F, Li C, Gao S, Gao WQ, Li Z, He Z. Efficient generation of functional haploid spermatids from human germline stem cells by three-dimensional-induced system. Cell Death Differ. 2018;25(4):749–66. https://doi.org/10.1038/s41418-017-0015-1. Epub 2018 Jan 5. PMID: 29305586; PMCID: PMC5864226
68. Tamburrino L, Traini G, Marcellini A, Vignozzi L, Baldi E, Marchiani S. Cryopreservation of human spermatozoa: functional, molecular and clinical aspects. Int J Mol Sci. 2023;24(5):4656. https://doi.org/10.3390/ijms24054656.
69. Tao Y, Sanger E, Saewu A, Leveille MC. Human sperm vitrification: the state of the art. Reprod Biol Endocrinol. 2020;18(1):17. https://doi.org/10.1186/s12958-020-00580-5.
70. Tournaye H, Goossens E, Verheyen G, Frederickx V, De Block G, Devroey P, Van Steirteghem A. Preserving the reproductive potential of men and boys with cancer: current concepts and future prospects. Hum Reprod Update. 2004;10(6):525–32. https://doi.org/10.1093/humupd/dmh038. Epub 2004 Aug 19. PMID: 15319377
71. Tremellen K, Savulescu J. A discussion supporting presumed consent for posthumous sperm procurement and conception, Reprod Biomed Online. 2015a;30:6–13.

72. Tremellen K, Savulescu J. A discussion supporting presumed consent for posthumous sperm procurement and conception. Reprod Biomed Online. 2015b;30(1):6–13. https://doi.org/10.1016/j.rbmo.2014.10.001.
73. Valli H, Sukhwani M, Dovey SL, Peters KA, Donohue J, Castro CA, Chu T, Marshall GR, Orwig KE. Fluorescence- and magnetic-activated cell sorting strategies to isolate and enrich human spermatogonial stem cells. Fertil Steril. 2014;102(2):566–580.e7. https://doi.org/10.1016/j.fertnstert.2014.04.036. Epub 2014 Jun 2. PMID: 24890267; PMCID: PMC4128386
74. Vinolas C, Raad J, Sonigo C, Sifer C, Sermondade N, Grynberg M. Medical techniques of fertility preservation in the male and female. J Visc Surg. 2018;155(Suppl 1):S3–9. https://doi.org/10.1016/j.jviscsurg.2018.03.009. Epub 2018 May 19. PMID: 29784583
75. Vomstein K, Reiser E, Pinggera GM, Toerzsoek P, Deininger S, Kriesche T, Biasio W, Lusuardi L, Toth B. Sperm banking before gonadotoxic treatment: is it worth the effort? Asian J Androl. 2021;23(5):490–4. https://doi.org/10.4103/aja.aja_16_21. PMID: 33818523; PMCID: PMC8451482
76. World Health Organization. WHO laboratory manual for the examination and processing of human semen. 6th ed. Geneva: WHO Press; 2021.
77. Zhou D, Wang XM, Li RX, Wang YZ, Chao YC, Liu ZZ, Huang ZH, Nie HC, Zhu WB, Tan YQ, Fan LQ. Improving native human sperm freezing protection by using a modified vitrification method. Asian J Androl. 2021;23(1):91–6. https://doi.org/10.4103/aja.aja_29_20.

Chapter 10
Male Contraception: What Is New?

Pallav Sengupta, Sulagna Dutta, Ramadan Saleh, and Ashok Agarwal

Introduction

Male contraception research has lately gained substantial attention as a critical component of family planning and reproductive health strategies. Historically, male contraceptive options have been limited primarily to condoms and vasectomy, which, while effective, present challenges such as compliance issues and irreversible outcomes [1, 2]. The need for innovative male contraceptive methods is underscored by the fact that approximately 40–45% of pregnancies worldwide remain unplanned, indicating a significant gap in available contraceptive options for men [3].

The historical perspective on male contraceptive methods reveals a long-standing reliance on a narrow range of options. Despite extensive research efforts dating back to the 1970s aimed at developing hormonal methods, progress has been slow, with no approved male contraceptive drugs currently available on the market [4, 5]. The limited focus on male contraceptive research, compared to female methods, has contributed to a lack of awareness and acceptance among men regarding their role

P. Sengupta
Department of Biomedical Sciences, College of Medicine, Gulf Medical University, Ajman, UAE

S. Dutta (✉)
Basic Medical Sciences Department, College of Medicine, Ajman University, Ajman, UAE

R. Saleh
Department of Dermatology, Venereology and Andrology, Faculty of Medicine, Sohag University, Sohag, Egypt

Ajyal IVF Center, Ajyal Hospital, Sohag, Egypt

A. Agarwal
Global Andrology Forum, Moreland Hills, OH, USA

E. Chung et al. (eds.), *Advances in Andrology*,
https://doi.org/10.1007/978-3-032-29112-7_10

in family planning [6]. However, recent studies indicate a growing interest among men in effective, reversible, and safe contraceptive methods, suggesting a shift in societal attitudes toward male involvement in reproductive health [7].

Recent advances in male contraception have sparked renewed optimism within the field. Innovative approaches, including hormonal and non-hormonal methods, are currently under investigation, with promising results emerging from clinical trials [8]. Non-hormonal contraceptives, in particular, represent a significant area of interest, as they offer the potential for targeted action with fewer side effects compared to hormonal alternatives [5]. Furthermore, the development of multipurpose prevention technologies (MPTs) that incorporate male contraceptive methods is gaining traction, highlighting the need for integrated solutions that address both contraception and sexually transmitted infection prevention [9]. Thus, the landscape of male contraception is evolving, driven by historical limitations, recent advancements, and an increasing demand for innovative solutions. As research continues to progress, it is essential to foster awareness and acceptance of male contraceptive options, ensuring that men can actively participate in family planning and reproductive health decisions.

This chapter aims to provide a comprehensive overview of male contraception, tracing its historical development, examining recent advances, and highlighting the urgent need for innovative solutions.

Current Landscape of Male Contraception

Conventional Methods: Condoms, Vasectomy, Withdrawal

Conventional methods of male contraception, including condoms, vasectomy, and withdrawal, play a crucial role in family planning. Each method presents unique advantages and challenges, influencing their acceptance and utilization among men. Condoms are a widely used barrier method that not only prevent pregnancy but also protect against sexually transmitted infections (STIs). Their effectiveness is contingent upon correct and consistent use, with typical use resulting in a failure rate of approximately 18% per year [10]. Despite their accessibility and dual protective benefits, some men report decreased sexual pleasure and spontaneity as significant drawbacks, which can affect consistent usage [11]. Furthermore, cultural perceptions and misconceptions about condoms can hinder their acceptance, particularly in regions where male involvement in contraceptive decisions is limited [12].

Vasectomy, a surgical procedure that involves the occlusion or severance of the vas deferens, is recognized as one of the most effective forms of permanent contraception for men, boasting a success rate exceeding 99% [13]. The procedure is minimally invasive and associated with low complication rates, making it a favorable option for men who are certain about not wanting future children [14]. However, societal stigma and misinformation regarding its impact on sexual function can deter men from considering this option. Studies indicate that many men fear a loss of libido or sexual satisfaction post-vasectomy, despite evidence suggesting that sexual function may remain unchanged or even improve for some couples [15, 16]. The decline in vasectomy rates in recent years, particularly among younger men, highlights the need for improved education and outreach regarding this method [17]. Withdrawal, or coitus interruptus, is another traditional method of contraception. While it is cost-free and requires no medical intervention, its effectiveness is significantly lower than that of condoms or vasectomy, with a typical use failure rate of about 22% per year [18]. The method relies heavily on the ability of the male partner to withdraw before ejaculation, which can be challenging and often leads to unintended pregnancies. Furthermore, withdrawal does not provide protection against STIs, limiting its appeal as a standalone contraceptive method [19]. Therefore, while conventional methods such as condoms, vasectomy, and withdrawal offer various options for male contraception, their effectiveness and acceptance are influenced by cultural attitudes, misconceptions, and personal preferences. Enhanced education and counseling are essential to address these barriers and promote informed decision-making among men regarding their contraceptive choices.

Limitations and Challenges of Current Methods

The development and implementation of male contraceptive methods face several limitations and challenges that hinder their widespread acceptance and use. One significant barrier is the prevailing social and cultural norms surrounding male involvement in family planning. Research indicates that traditional gender roles often position contraceptive responsibility primarily with women, which can lead to reluctance of men to engage in family planning discussions and decisions [20]. This reluctance is compounded by a lack of awareness and understanding of male contraceptive options, as many men express concerns about potential side effects and their impact on sexual function [21–23]. Such fears can deter men from considering hormonal methods, despite evidence suggesting that these methods can be effective and reversible [23]. Moreover, the current male contraceptive landscape is limited, primarily offering only condoms and vasectomy as viable options. While condoms are widely used, they are often associated with issues of compliance and reduced sexual satisfaction, leading to inconsistent use [2]. Vasectomy, on the other hand, presents challenges related to its permanence and the stigma surrounding surgical interventions [1]. The lack of diverse and easily accessible male contraceptive methods contributes to a significant gap in these services, particularly in low- and middle-income countries where the demand for male contraceptive options is high [24].

Another critical challenge is the insufficient research and development of new male contraceptive methods. Although there are promising candidates, such as hormonal gels and non-hormonal agents like lonidamine, many of these options remain in the experimental phase and have not yet reached the market [6, 25, 26]. This slow progress can be attributed to various factors, including funding limitations, regulatory hurdles, and the historical focus on female contraceptive methods [26]. Furthermore, the complexity of male reproductive physiology poses additional scientific challenges in developing effective contraceptive agents that do not compromise sexual health [27].

Global and Cultural Perspectives on Male Contraception

The global landscape of male contraception is characterized by diverse cultural perspectives and varying levels of acceptance, which significantly influence its uptake and development. Historically, male contraceptive options have been limited primarily to condoms and vasectomy, with the latter often viewed as a permanent solution that poses challenges in the context of changing family dynamics and increasing divorce rates [28]. This limitation has led to a growing demand for novel, reversible male contraceptive methods that can empower men to take a more active role in family planning [29].

Cultural attitudes toward male contraception vary widely across regions. In many parts of Sub-Saharan Africa, for instance, traditional gender roles often dictate that family planning responsibilities fall predominantly on women, leading to a lack of male involvement in contraceptive decision-making [30]. However, recent studies indicate a shift in this paradigm, with increasing awareness and acceptance of male contraceptive methods among men, particularly when educational initiatives are implemented [31, 32]. For example, in Uganda, targeted family planning programs have shown that higher education levels correlate with increased modern contraceptive use among men, suggesting that education plays a critical role in shaping attitudes toward male involvement in contraception [31]. Moreover, the perception of male contraceptives is often clouded by myths and misinformation. Concerns about potential side effects, such as impacts on sexual function and fertility, have been significant barriers to acceptance [30]. Research indicates that addressing these fears through comprehensive education and counseling can enhance willingness of men to engage with contraceptive options [33]. For instance, studies in Uganda have highlighted the effectiveness of peer outreach and mass media campaigns in improving attitudes of men toward contraception [33]. Despite the progress in awareness and education, the actual uptake of male contraceptive methods remains low globally, with vasectomy prevalence reported at only 0.9% among men [33]. This underscores the need for continued advocacy and development of male contraceptive options that are culturally sensitive and address the unique needs of different populations [34]. The integration of male contraceptives into broader reproductive health strategies is essential for achieving equitable family planning goals and improving overall reproductive health outcomes [35].

Hormonal Approaches

Testosterone-Based Therapies

Testosterone-based therapies have emerged as a pivotal area of research in male contraception, primarily due to their dual role in managing testosterone levels and influencing spermatogenesis. Exogenous testosterone administration has been shown to suppress the hypothalamic-pituitary-gonadal (HPG) axis, leading to decreased production of gonadotropins and subsequent inhibition of spermatogenesis. This suppression is particularly effective in certain populations, such as East Asian men, where testosterone alone can achieve azoospermia, which is essential for contraceptive efficacy [36, 37]. However, in other demographics, such as Caucasians, additional agents, typically progestins, are required to enhance the contraceptive effect of testosterone [37].

The mechanisms underlying the influence of testosterone on fertility are complex. Testosterone is crucial for normal spermatogenesis, as it regulates Sertoli cell function and the maturation of germ cells [38]. Studies have demonstrated that testosterone levels must be maintained within a specific range to support spermatogenesis effectively; both excessive and insufficient levels can lead to infertility [39]. For instance, high doses of testosterone can lead to increased serum testosterone but may not adequately suppress intratesticular testosterone levels, which are critical for sperm production [40]. Conversely, the cessation of testosterone therapy often results in the resumption of spermatogenesis, indicating that the effects of testosterone on fertility can be reversible [41]. The combination of testosterone with antiandrogens, such as cyproterone acetate, has also shown promise in achieving azoospermia while managing testosterone levels effectively [42].

Mechanism of Action

The mechanism of action of hormonal contraceptives for male contraception primarily involves the suppression of the HPG axis, which is crucial for regulating male reproductive hormones. Hormonal contraceptives typically utilize a combination of androgens, such as testosterone, and progestins to achieve this suppression. The administration of exogenous testosterone, whether through injections or implants, serves to maintain androgen levels necessary for male physiological functions while simultaneously inhibiting endogenous testosterone production and spermatogenesis [26, 43, 44].

When testosterone levels are artificially elevated through hormonal contraceptives, the feedback mechanism to the hypothalamus and pituitary gland is altered. Specifically, high levels of testosterone lead to decreased secretion of gonadotropin-releasing hormone (GnRH) from the hypothalamus, which in turn reduces the release of luteinizing hormone (LH) and follicle-stimulating hormone (FSH) from the anterior pituitary [26]. This reduction in LH and FSH is critical, as these hormones are essential for stimulating the Leydig cells in the testes to produce testosterone and for promoting spermatogenesis, respectively. Consequently, the suppression of these hormones results in a significant decrease in intratesticular testosterone levels, leading to the arrest of spermatogenesis and ultimately resulting in azoospermia or severe oligozoospermia [26, 43]. The addition of progestins to the regimen enhances the contraceptive effect by further suppressing gonadotropin levels. Progestins act synergistically with testosterone to inhibit the secretion of LH and FSH more effectively than testosterone alone, thereby providing a more robust contraceptive effect [43, 45]. This dual-hormone approach not only suppresses sperm production but also maintains the physiological levels of testosterone necessary for male health, thereby minimizing side effects associated with testosterone-only regimens [44]. Moreover, the role of kisspeptin in the regulation of the HPG axis has garnered attention in recent studies. Kisspeptin, a neuropeptide that stimulates GnRH secretion, is sensitive to feedback from sex steroids. Its modulation could provide a novel target for male contraceptive development, potentially allowing for more refined control over spermatogenesis without the complete suppression of testosterone [46]. The ongoing research into the roles of various hormones, including kisspeptin, continues to inform the development of more effective and reversible male contraceptive methods [43, 44].

Current Research and Trials

Current research on hormonal male contraception has gained significant momentum in recent years, reflecting a growing recognition of the need for male contraceptive options that are both effective and reversible. Traditional male contraceptive methods, such as condoms and vasectomy, have limitations, including high failure rates and irreversibility, respectively [47]. Consequently, the exploration of hormonal male contraceptives has become a focal point in reproductive health research.

Recent clinical trials have demonstrated promising results for hormonal male contraceptives, particularly those combining testosterone with progestins. These combinations have been shown to effectively suppress gonadotropin levels, leading to a significant reduction in sperm production [23, 43, 48]. For instance, a study involving a combined nestorone-testosterone gel reported that it successfully suppressed serum gonadotropins to levels associated with effective contraception [48]. Furthermore, efficacy trials enrolling approximately 2000 men have indicated that these hormonal methods may achieve effectiveness comparable to female hormonal contraceptives [49]. By administering exogenous hormones, such as testosterone and progestins, researchers aim to lower intratesticular testosterone levels, thereby inhibiting sperm production [50, 51]. This approach not only provides a reversible contraceptive option but also maintains male physiological functions due to the androgenic support provided by testosterone [23, 43]. Despite the advancements, challenges remain in the development of male hormonal contraceptives. Concerns regarding side effects, such as mood changes and cardiovascular risks, have been noted in various studies [32, 52]. For example, mood alterations were reported in participants of a clinical trial involving a testosterone-progestin gel, highlighting the importance of monitoring psychological well-being during such trials [52]. Additionally, the long-term implications of hormonal administration on male health, particularly concerning cardiovascular and prostate health, are still under investigation [51].

The landscape of male contraception is evolving, with several hormonal methods currently in various stages of clinical trials. Notably, agents such as Dimethandrolone Undecanoate (DMAU) and 11β-methyl-nortestosterone dodecylcarbonate (11β-MNTDC) are being evaluated for their safety and efficacy [44]. As of mid-2023, two hormonal male contraceptive methods are undergoing phase II clinical trials, indicating a promising future for the field [53]. The integration of hormonal methods into family planning could facilitate shared responsibility between partners, ultimately enhancing reproductive health choices for couples [3, 54]. Continued research is essential to address safety concerns and to ensure the successful implementation of these contraceptive methods in clinical practice.

Efficacy and Safety Profiles

Clinical trials have demonstrated that various hormonal regimens can effectively suppress serum gonadotropins to levels associated with effective contraception. For instance, the combination of nestorone and testosterone gel has shown promising results in suppressing serum FSH and LH to levels that inhibit spermatogenesis [48, 55]. Additionally, studies have indicated that oral progestins such as cyproterone acetate (CPA) and levonorgestrel (LNG) can also achieve significant suppression of gonadotropin levels, making them viable candidates for male hormonal contraceptive regimens [4, 56]. The efficacy of these methods is comparable to female hormonal contraceptives, with success rates often exceeding 90% in achieving azoospermia [57]. Safety profiles of hormonal male contraceptives are critical for their acceptance and use. While the majority of studies report mild to moderate adverse effects, such as mood changes and weight gain, serious adverse events (AEs) remain rare. Notably, the risk of thrombotic events, a significant concern with female hormonal contraceptives, has not been prominently reported in male trials [32]. However, caution is warranted, particularly for older men or those with pre-existing cardiovascular conditions, as certain progestins may increase the risk of blood coagulation and inflammation [50]. The careful selection of progestins and monitoring of cardiovascular health are essential components of developing safe hormonal contraceptive options for men.

Moreover, the acceptability of male hormonal contraceptives is influenced by cultural and psychosocial factors. Surveys indicate a strong willingness among men to engage in contraceptive responsibilities, reflecting changing attitudes toward male involvement in family planning [43]. However, the psychological impact of hormonal treatments, including mood disturbances, necessitates thorough evaluation during clinical trials [52]. Addressing these concerns is crucial for the successful integration of male hormonal contraceptives into mainstream contraceptive options.

Non-testosterone Hormonal Methods

Non-testosterone hormonal male contraceptive methods represent a burgeoning area of research aimed at expanding male contraceptive options beyond traditional methods such as condoms and vasectomy. These methods primarily focus on the inhibition of spermatogenesis through the modulation of hormonal pathways without relying solely on testosterone. The underlying principle involves the suppression of gonadotropin release from the pituitary gland, which is crucial for sperm production in the testes. This can be achieved through the use of progestins or other hormonal agents that do not include testosterone, thereby offering an alternative approach to male contraception [43, 45].

Recent advancements in non-testosterone hormonal contraceptive methods have shown promise in clinical trials. For instance, compounds such as selective androgen receptor modulators (SARMs) and other non-steroidal agents have been explored for their potential to suppress spermatogenesis effectively while minimizing androgenic side effects [43, 45]. These methods aim to provide reversible and effective contraception, addressing the unmet need for male-controlled family planning options. The interest in these alternatives is underscored by studies indicating a significant demand among men and women for safe and effective male contraceptive methods [3, 23]. Moreover, the development of non-testosterone hormonal contraceptives could alleviate some of the concerns associated with testosterone-based methods, such as potential cardiovascular risks and hormonal imbalances [50, 51]. By utilizing different hormonal pathways, these methods may offer a more favorable safety profile while maintaining efficacy in preventing pregnancy. The exploration of these alternatives is particularly relevant in light of the increasing recognition of the roles of men in family planning and reproductive health [23, 58]. Despite the progress made, challenges remain in the commercialization and widespread acceptance of non-testosterone hormonal contraceptives. Regulatory hurdles, public awareness, and cultural attitudes toward male contraception play significant roles in the successful introduction of these methods to the market [28, 49, 59]. Continued research and development efforts are essential to refine these contraceptive options, ensuring they meet the needs and preferences of potential users while providing reliable and reversible contraception [26, 36] (Fig. 10.1).

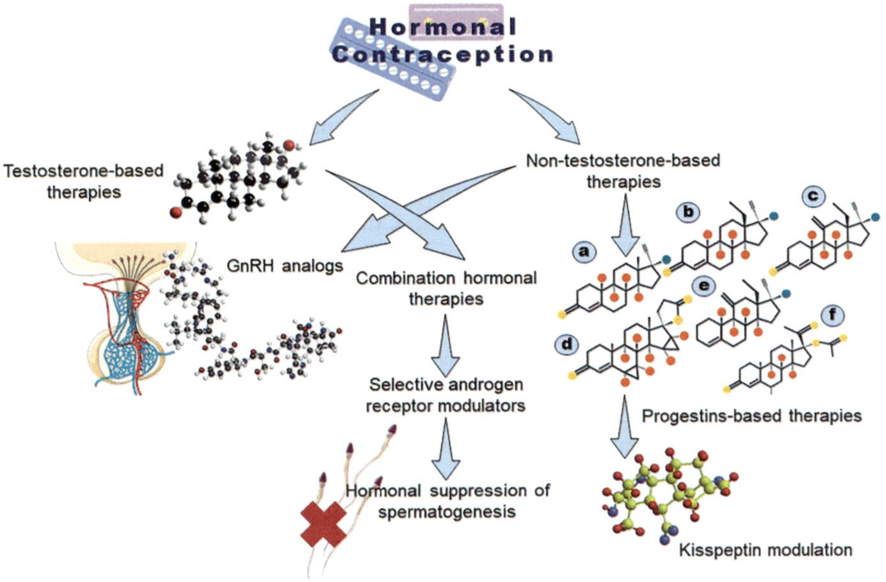

Fig. 10.1 Mechanisms of hormonal male contraception, categorized into testosterone-based and non-testosterone-based therapies. Testosterone-based therapies suppress gonadotropins to inhibit spermatogenesis, while GnRH analogs and combination hormonal therapies (testosterone with progestins) enhance contraceptive efficacy. Selective androgen receptor modulators (SARMs) and hormonal suppression of spermatogenesis further regulate male fertility. Non-testosterone-based therapies include progestin-based treatments, utilizing synthetic progestins such as (**a**) Norethindrone, (**b**) Levonorgestrel, (**c**) Etonogestrel, (**d**) Drospirenone, (**e**) Desogestrel, and (**f**) Medroxyprogesterone acetate, which work by suppressing LH and FSH to inhibit sperm production. Kisspeptin modulation represents an emerging approach targeting GnRH secretion

GnRH Analogs

GnRH analogs have emerged as promising male contraceptive methods due to their ability to modulate the HPG axis, thereby suppressing spermatogenesis and testosterone production. GnRH analogs can be categorized into agonists and antagonists, both of which have demonstrated efficacy in reducing fertility in various animal models and clinical settings. The mechanism of action primarily involves the inhibition of LH and FSH secretion from the pituitary gland, leading to decreased intratesticular testosterone levels and subsequent suppression of sperm production [23].

Research indicates that the administration of GnRH analogs can effectively suppress gonadotropin levels, resulting in a significant reduction in sperm output. For instance, studies have shown that the use of GnRH agonists can lead to reversible infertility by inducing a state of hypogonadism, characterized by low levels of testosterone and sperm count [23, 60]. In a study involving male mice, a recombinant GnRH-based fusion protein achieved 100% contraceptive efficacy, highlighting the potential for immunocontraceptive strategies that target GnRH [61]. Furthermore, the use of GnRH vaccines has been explored, demonstrating the ability to induce long-lasting contraceptive effects by eliciting an immune response against GnRH, thereby preventing its physiological action [62].

The reversibility of GnRH analogs is a significant advantage, as fertility can be restored upon cessation of treatment. This characteristic is particularly appealing for male contraceptive methods, as it allows for family planning without permanent alterations to reproductive function [23, 63]. Clinical trials have shown that GnRH analogs, such as deslorelin, can be administered in a slow-release format, providing sustained contraceptive effects with minimal side effects [64]. Additionally, the potential for GnRH analogs to be used in combination with other hormonal agents may enhance their contraceptive efficacy while maintaining a favorable safety profile [60]. Thus, GnRH analogs represent a viable option for male contraception, with their ability to effectively suppress spermatogenesis and testosterone production. Ongoing research into the optimization of these agents, including the development of long-acting formulations and immunocontraceptive vaccines, holds promise for expanding the contraceptive options available to men, thereby contributing to more equitable family planning strategies [60, 63].

Combination Hormonal Therapies

Combination hormonal therapies represent a promising avenue for male contraception, leveraging the synergistic effects of androgens and progestins to effectively suppress spermatogenesis. The fundamental mechanism underlying these therapies involves the suppression of the HPG axis, which is achieved through the administration of exogenous testosterone in combination with progestins. This combination not only inhibits the secretion of gonadotropins, LH, and FSH, but also provides androgenic support necessary for maintaining male physiological functions [2, 43]. Recent studies have demonstrated that such combinations can lead to sperm concentrations below the threshold for fertility, comparable to the efficacy of female hormonal contraceptives [2, 49].

The efficacy of combination hormonal therapies has been substantiated through various clinical trials. For instance, a randomized controlled trial indicated that the administration of testosterone alongside different progestins, such as Nestorone, resulted in significant suppression of gonadotropin levels and subsequent spermatogenesis [55, 56]. The findings suggest that these therapies can achieve effective contraception while maintaining a favorable safety profile, with minimal adverse effects reported [32, 59]. Moreover, the flexibility in administration routes—ranging from transdermal gels to long-acting injections—enhances the acceptability and adherence to these contraceptive methods [23]. Despite the promising results, the path to market for male hormonal contraceptives remains complex, influenced by regulatory guidelines and societal perceptions [50]. Studies indicate that men often feel less informed about hormonal contraceptives compared to their female counterparts, which can hinder their willingness to engage with these options [65].

The future of combination hormonal therapies in male contraception is bright, as ongoing research continues to refine these methods. Innovations in hormonal agents, such as the development of SARM with dual androgenic and progestational activities, hold promise for enhancing the effectiveness and safety of male contraceptives [66]. As societal norms evolve and awareness increases, combination hormonal therapies may soon become a viable and widely accepted option for male contraception, providing couples with greater control over family planning.

Non-hormonal Approaches

Physical Barrier Methods beyond Condoms

Physical barrier methods of contraception, primarily represented by condoms, have long been recognized for their role in preventing pregnancy and sexually transmitted infections (STIs). However, the exploration of additional physical barrier methods beyond condoms is essential for expanding male contraceptive options. Current research indicates a growing interest in alternative methods that can complement or serve as substitutes for traditional barrier methods. One promising avenue is the development of intraurethral devices, which are designed to block sperm passage through the urethra. These devices could provide a reversible and non-invasive alternative to vasectomy, which remains a popular but permanent solution for male contraception [67]. The intraurethral approach could potentially allow for easier adoption among men who are hesitant to undergo surgical procedures. Moreover, the efficacy of such devices in preventing pregnancy while also offering protection against STIs remains a critical area of investigation [19]. Another innovative concept involves the use of gels or films that can be applied to the penis before intercourse. These products would act as a physical barrier to sperm, similar to condoms, but may offer additional benefits such as enhanced sensation or ease of use. Research has shown that the acceptability of such methods could be high among men, particularly if they are marketed effectively [68]. Furthermore, the integration of these products with existing contraceptive methods could enhance dual protection strategies, where users combine barrier methods with hormonal or long-acting reversible contraceptives (LARCs) to maximize efficacy against unintended pregnancies and STIs [69].

Vas-Occlusive Techniques

Vas-occlusive techniques, particularly vasectomy, have emerged as a pivotal method for male contraception, offering a reliable and effective means of preventing unwanted pregnancies. Vasectomy involves the surgical occlusion of the vas deferens, thereby preventing sperm from being included in the ejaculate. This method is recognized for its high efficacy, with failure rates reported to be less than 1% when performed correctly [70, 71].

The traditional vasectomy procedure has evolved significantly, incorporating techniques such as the no-scalpel vasectomy (NSV), which minimizes tissue trauma and enhances recovery times [72]. Recent advancements have also introduced non-invasive methods, such as laser coagulation, which utilize high-frequency ultrasound imaging to achieve occlusion while reducing complications associated with traditional surgical approaches [73]. These innovations are crucial as they may increase male acceptance of vasectomy by addressing common concerns regarding surgical risks and recovery [73]. Despite its effectiveness, vasectomy has faced challenges regarding its perception and uptake. Cultural attitudes, misinformation, and concerns about long-term health effects have historically limited its acceptance in various populations [33, 74]. However, studies indicate that vasectomy is a cost-effective contraceptive method, particularly when integrated into broader family planning programs [33]. Moreover, the procedure is associated with minimal complications, and recent reviews suggest that it does not significantly increase the risk of prostate cancer, countering prevalent myths surrounding the procedure [70, 71]. In addition to traditional vasectomy, emerging techniques such as the Reversible Inhibition of Sperm Under Guidance (RISUG) and the development of hydrogel-based systems for non-invasive occlusion are being explored [75, 76]. RISUG involves the injection of a polymer into the vas deferens, which can be reversed using a specific chemical treatment, thus offering a potentially reversible alternative to traditional vasectomy [75]. Similarly, ultrasound-induced hydrogels represent a novel approach that allows for real-time monitoring and the possibility of recanalization, thereby enhancing the flexibility of male contraceptive options [76].

The future of male contraception may also include the integration of nanotechnology, which promises to enhance the safety and efficacy of vas-occlusive methods. Nanomaterials can facilitate targeted drug delivery and controlled release, potentially improving the reversibility and effectiveness of male contraceptive methods [77]. As research continues to advance, these innovative techniques may provide men with more choices, addressing the long-standing need for effective male contraceptive options beyond condoms and surgical sterilization.

Reversible Inhibition of Sperm Under Guidance

RISUG represents a significant advancement in male contraceptive methods, providing a non-hormonal, long-term solution that is both effective and reversible. Developed as an alternative to traditional vasectomy, RISUG utilizes a polymeric gel composed of styrene maleic anhydride (SMA) dissolved in dimethyl sulfoxide (DMSO) [75, 78]. This innovative approach allows for a non-scalpel injection into the vas deferens, creating a physical barrier that obstructs sperm transport while simultaneously inducing biochemical changes that impair sperm function [79]. The mechanism of action for RISUG is multifaceted. Upon injection, the polymeric gel alters the local pH environment within the vas deferens, leading to acrosomal damage in spermatozoa, which is crucial for fertilization [78, 80]. Studies have demonstrated that this alteration results in a significant reduction in sperm motility and viability, effectively inducing a state of azoospermia [75, 80]. Furthermore, the interaction between the sperm membrane and the polyelectrolytic nature of the SMA leads to the destabilization of essential enzymes required for fertilization, further enhancing its contraceptive efficacy [76].

Clinical trials have reported a contraceptive efficacy rate exceeding 97%, positioning RISUG as a promising candidate for male contraception [80]. One of the most compelling features of RISUG is its reversibility. The reversal process can be achieved through the administration of sodium bicarbonate ($NaHCO_3$) or DMSO, which flushes the RISUG gel from the vas deferens [81]. Research indicates that $NaHCO_3$ may facilitate a quicker restoration of fertility compared to DMSO, although the precise mechanisms remain to be fully elucidated [81]. This aspect of RISUG addresses a significant concern regarding male contraceptive methods: the ability to restore fertility after cessation of use, which is often a barrier to acceptance among potential users [79]. The safety profile of RISUG has been rigorously evaluated through multiple phases of clinical trials, confirming its biocompatibility and minimal side effects [82]. Unlike hormonal contraceptives, which can lead to systemic side effects, the localized action of RISUG minimizes the risk of adverse reactions, making it an attractive option for men seeking to take an active role in family planning [83]. Moreover, the non-invasive nature of the procedure, combined with its long-lasting effects, positions RISUG as a viable alternative to existing male contraceptive methods, which are predominantly limited to condoms and vasectomy [84].

Vasalgel

Vasalgel, a novel male contraceptive method, represents a significant advancement in the field of reproductive health, particularly in providing men with a long-acting reversible contraceptive (LARC) option. Developed as a high-molecular-weight polymer of styrene-alt-maleic acid (SMA), Vasalgel is administered via intravasal injection into the vas deferens, effectively blocking sperm transport while allowing for potential reversibility [85]. This method contrasts sharply with traditional vasectomy, which is considered permanent and lacks a straightforward reversal process [81]. The mechanism of action of Vasalgel involves the formation of a gel-like barrier within the vas deferens, which obstructs the passage of sperm from the testes to the ejaculate. Studies in animal models, including rabbits and rhesus monkeys, have demonstrated that Vasalgel can induce azoospermia, thereby achieving effective contraception [85, 86]. Notably, the reversibility of Vasalgel has been a focal point of research, with evidence suggesting that fertility can be restored through a secondary injection of $NaHCO_3$, which dissolves the polymer at a high pH [87]. This feature is particularly appealing for men who wish to retain the option of fatherhood in the future.

Clinical trials and studies have shown promising results regarding the efficacy and safety of Vasalgel. In a study involving adult male rhesus monkeys, no conceptions occurred post-injection, indicating a high contraceptive efficacy [86]. Furthermore, research has indicated that the effectiveness of Vasalgel can last for extended periods, with some estimates suggesting a duration of efficacy comparable to existing long-acting contraceptive methods [88]. The biocompatibility of the polymer and the absence of systemic hormonal effects further enhance its appeal as a non-hormonal contraceptive alternative [89]. Despite its potential, Vasalgel is still in the developmental phase, with ongoing studies required to fully assess its long-term effects and safety in humans [81]. The lack of extensive human trials raises questions about its market readiness, as well as concerns regarding the long-term stability of the polymer within the human body [81]. Moreover, the social implications of introducing a male contraceptive method like Vasalgel are profound, as it could shift the dynamics of contraceptive responsibility and family planning [6].

Novel Approaches and Research

Thermal Methods

Thermal methods as male contraceptive strategies have garnered increasing attention in recent years, particularly due to their potential to exploit the temperature sensitivity of male fertility. The underlying principle is that elevated temperatures can adversely affect spermatogenesis and sperm quality, leading to temporary or permanent infertility. This phenomenon is well-documented across various species, including insects and mammals, where thermal stress has been shown to compromise male reproductive capabilities significantly [25, 90].

Research indicates that male fertility is particularly vulnerable to thermal stress, with studies demonstrating that exposure to elevated temperatures can disrupt spermatid elongation and impair sperm motility [91]. For instance, in the model organism Drosophila melanogaster, heat stress has been linked to a reduction in sperm viability and overall fertility, with males experiencing a decline in reproductive success following exposure to high temperatures [91, 92]. Similarly, in mammals, it has been observed that spermatocytes are susceptible to damage during spermatogenesis when exposed to elevated temperatures, leading to decreased sperm quality and quantity [25, 90]. The concept of using thermal methods for male contraception is not merely theoretical; experimental approaches have demonstrated the feasibility of inducing temporary infertility through controlled heat exposure. For example, studies have shown that heat waves can lead to significant reductions in sperm production and viability in various insect models, suggesting that similar principles could be applied to mammalian systems [91]. The potential for recovery of fertility after a return to normal temperatures has also been documented, indicating that thermal methods could be designed for reversible contraception [92]. Moreover, the specificity of thermal effects on male fertility presents an opportunity for targeted contraceptive strategies. For instance, heat-induced infertility can be selectively applied to males without affecting female fertility, thus allowing for controlled breeding practices in agricultural settings or wildlife management [93]. This specificity is crucial, as it minimizes the risk of unintended consequences on female reproductive health and population dynamics. In addition to the direct effects of temperature on sperm quality, there is evidence that thermal stress can have transgenerational effects on fertility, potentially influencing offspring viability and reproductive success [91]. This aspect underscores the complexity of thermal methods as contraceptive strategies, as they may not only impact the immediate generation but also future generations through altered reproductive dynamics.

Ultrasound Techniques

Ultrasound techniques have emerged as a promising avenue for male contraception, leveraging advancements in imaging technology to assess and potentially modulate male reproductive health. The application of ultrasound in this context primarily revolves around its ability to visualize and evaluate the male reproductive organs, particularly the testes and associated structures, which are critical for sperm production and overall fertility. One of the key ultrasound modalities employed is shear wave elastography (SWE), which assesses the elasticity of testicular tissue. This technique has been shown to provide insights into parenchymal damage that can adversely affect sperm production [94]. By evaluating the mechanical properties of testicular tissue, SWE can identify abnormalities that may lead to infertility, thus serving as a diagnostic tool that could inform contraceptive strategies. Furthermore, the integration of Doppler ultrasound allows for the assessment of blood flow to the testes, which is vital for spermatogenesis [95]. This dynamic analysis can help in understanding how alterations in blood supply may influence reproductive function and could be targeted in contraceptive approaches. Moreover, ultrasound has been utilized to monitor assisted reproductive techniques, such as the induction of spermiation and ovulation through hormonal manipulation [96]. This monitoring capability could be adapted for contraceptive purposes, where ultrasound could guide interventions aimed at temporarily suppressing spermatogenesis. The non-invasive nature of ultrasound makes it an attractive option for developing male contraceptive methods, as it minimizes the risks associated with surgical or pharmacological interventions. The relationship between ultrasound findings and hormonal profiles further underscores the potential of this technology in male contraception. For instance, ultrasound can be used to correlate testicular volume and sperm parameters, providing a comprehensive view of male reproductive health [97]. This correlation is crucial, as hormonal regulation plays a significant role in spermatogenesis, and understanding these dynamics could lead to the development of ultrasound-guided hormonal contraceptive methods. In addition to its diagnostic capabilities, ultrasound may also facilitate the exploration of novel contraceptive techniques. For example, targeted ultrasound applications could potentially disrupt sperm motility or viability, thereby preventing fertilization without the systemic effects associated with hormonal contraceptives [98]. This approach aligns with the growing interest in non-hormonal contraceptive methods, which are often preferred by men due to concerns about side effects and long-term health implications. Despite the promising applications of ultrasound in male contraception, challenges remain. The lack of standardization in ultrasound techniques and the subjective nature of some diagnostic interpretations can hinder the widespread adoption of these methods [98]. Ongoing research and multicenter studies are essential to establish standardized protocols and validate the efficacy of ultrasound-based contraceptive strategies.

Chemosterilization

Chemosterilization as a male contraceptive method represents a novel approach in the field of reproductive health, aiming to provide men with effective and reversible options for fertility control [99]. This method involves the use of chemical agents to induce sterility in males, effectively preventing sperm production without the need for surgical intervention. The underlying principle of chemosterilization is to disrupt the normal physiological processes of spermatogenesis, thereby reducing sperm count to levels that are insufficient for fertilization. Research into chemosterilization has drawn parallels with existing hormonal contraceptive methods, which also target the HPG axis to suppress spermatogenesis [100]. While hormonal methods have shown promise in clinical trials, the development of chemosterilization offers an alternative that may circumvent some of the side effects associated with hormonal treatments, such as mood disorders and libido changes [23, 32].

One of the key advantages of chemosterilization is its potential for reversibility. Unlike vasectomy, which is often considered a permanent solution, chemosterilization could allow for the restoration of fertility following cessation of chemical treatment. This aspect is particularly appealing to men who may wish to retain the option of fatherhood in the future [67, 101]. Moreover, the acceptability of chemosterilization could be enhanced by its non-invasive nature, which may appeal to men who are hesitant about surgical procedures [7, 68].

The efficacy of chemosterilization has been demonstrated in various studies, with agents such as lufenuron showing effectiveness in sterilizing target populations in agricultural settings [102]. Although the application of such agents in human male contraception is still under investigation, the principles of chemosterilization could be adapted from these findings. Despite the potential benefits, the implementation of chemosterilization as a male contraceptive method faces several challenges. Public perception and acceptance of chemical methods may be influenced by concerns regarding safety and long-term health effects, which have historically hindered the development of male contraceptives [23, 102]. Additionally, regulatory hurdles and the need for extensive clinical trials to establish safety and efficacy will be critical in advancing chemosterilization from experimental stages to practical application [4, 5].

Immunological Approaches

Immunological approaches to male contraception represent a burgeoning field of research that seeks to provide effective, reversible, and safe contraceptive options for men. Traditional methods, primarily hormonal, have faced significant challenges, including concerns over side effects and the efficacy of drug delivery systems [3]. In contrast, immunological strategies focus on targeting specific proteins involved in sperm function and development, thereby offering a non-hormonal alternative. One promising avenue in immunological male contraceptive development involves the use of epididymal sperm proteins as vaccine targets. Research has indicated that proteins such as Sperm Factor Protein 2 can be utilized to elicit an immune response that inhibits sperm motility and function [103]. This approach is particularly appealing because it can potentially lead to a multivalent vaccine that targets multiple sperm antigens, thereby enhancing contraceptive efficacy [103]. The immunogenicity of these proteins is crucial, as a successful vaccine must provoke a robust immune response without causing adverse effects [103].

Another innovative immunological strategy involves inhibiting retinoic acid biosynthesis, which is essential for spermatogenesis. Studies have shown that compounds like bisdichloroacetyldiamines can effectively suppress spermatogenesis by interfering with retinoic acid synthesis in the testes [104]. This method not only reduces sperm production but also maintains testosterone levels, which is vital for preserving secondary sexual characteristics and overall male health [104]. The dual benefit of maintaining hormonal balance while achieving contraceptive effects makes this approach particularly attractive. Moreover, the development of non-hormonal contraceptives has gained momentum due to the increasing demand for male contraceptive options that do not disrupt hormonal homeostasis.

Emerging Technologies and Innovations

Gene Editing and Male Contraception

Gene editing technologies, particularly CRISPR/Cas9, have emerged as transformative tools in the field of reproductive biology, offering novel avenues for the development of male contraceptives. Recent studies have identified several testis-enriched genes that are critical for male fertility, presenting potential targets for non-hormonal contraceptive strategies. For instance, the knockout of specific genes such as bromodomain testis-specific protein (BRDT) and protein phosphatase 3 catalytic subunit gamma (PPP3CC) has demonstrated their dispensability for male reproduction, suggesting their viability as targets for contraceptive development [105]. Furthermore, the Rhox gene family, predominantly expressed in Sertoli cells and germ cells, has been implicated in spermatogenesis, with targeted ablation resulting in impaired fertility [106]. This highlights the potential of gene editing to disrupt critical pathways in sperm development without the hormonal side effects associated with traditional contraceptives. The identification of genes such as PRSS55, which is essential for sperm motility, further underscores the promise of gene editing in male contraception. Disruption of PRSS55 has been shown to lead to male infertility in murine models, making it a compelling candidate for targeted gene editing approaches aimed at developing reversible contraceptive methods [107]. Similarly, the MEIG1-PACRG complex, crucial for spermiogenesis, has been identified as a potential target for non-hormonal contraceptive development, with studies indicating that its disruption can significantly impair sperm maturation [108]. The ability to precisely edit these genes using CRISPR/Cas9 technology allows for the exploration of their roles in male fertility and the potential to develop targeted contraceptive interventions. Moreover, the advancement of gene editing techniques, including base editing and prime editing, enhances the precision of genetic modifications, reducing the risk of off-target effects that could compromise male reproductive health [109, 110]. These innovations enable researchers to make specific alterations to the genome, thereby facilitating the development of contraceptive methods that are both effective and safe. The ongoing exploration of genetic loci influencing reproductive behavior and fertility further supports the notion that genetic factors play a significant role in male reproductive health, with implications for contraceptive development [110]. Despite the promising landscape of gene editing for male contraception, challenges remain in translating these findings into clinical applications. The identification of reproductive tract-specific genes and their functional characterization is essential for advancing drug development [110]. Moreover, while significant progress has been made, no male contraceptive agents have yet received regulatory approval, highlighting the need for continued research and development in this area [111]. The integration of genetic insights with innovative gene editing technologies holds the potential to revolutionize male contraception, providing men with greater reproductive autonomy and contributing to family planning efforts globally.

Targeting Sperm Motility and Function

Targeting sperm motility and function represents a promising avenue for the development of male contraceptive methods. Sperm motility is a critical determinant of male fertility, as it directly influences the ability of sperm to navigate through the female reproductive tract and successfully fertilize the ovum. Recent research has identified several molecular and physiological pathways that regulate sperm motility, which can be exploited for contraceptive purposes. One of the key players in sperm motility is the CatSper calcium channel, which is essential for the hyperactivated motility required for effective sperm navigation. Studies have shown that disruption of CatSper function leads to impaired sperm motility and reduced fertility in various animal models [112, 113]. Specifically, CatSper-null sperm exhibit atypical beating patterns and are less capable of migrating through the female reproductive tract, underscoring the importance of this channel in male fertility [112]. Furthermore, the regulation of calcium homeostasis through CatSper channels is crucial for sperm hyperactivation, a process that enhances motility and is necessary for penetrating the zona pellucida during fertilization [113]. In addition to calcium signaling, mitochondrial function plays a pivotal role in sperm motility. The mitochondrial membrane potential (MMP) is a critical factor that influences sperm motility and viability. Research indicates that spermatozoa with low MMP are less capable of undergoing the acrosome reaction, which is vital for fertilization [114]. Consequently, targeting mitochondrial function could provide a novel approach to male contraception by impairing sperm motility without affecting spermatogenesis [115] (Fig. 10.2).

Recent advancements in pharmacological interventions have also highlighted the potential of using soluble adenylyl cyclase (sAC) inhibitors as a means to control sperm motility. sAC inhibitors can effectively block both progressive and hyperactivated motility, thereby preventing sperm from reaching the ovum [116]. This method allows for a rapid onset of action, making it suitable for on-demand

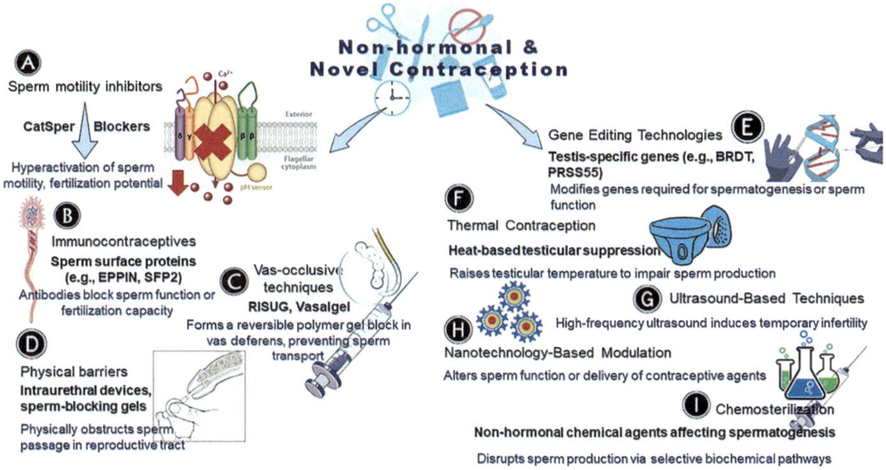

Fig. 10.2 Various non-hormonal and novel male contraceptive approaches categorized by their mechanisms of action. (**a**) Sperm motility inhibitors target calcium ion channels (e.g., CatSper blockers) to prevent hyperactivation and fertilization. (**b**) Immunocontraceptives block sperm surface proteins (e.g., EPPIN, SFP2) to impair sperm function. (**c**) Vas-occlusive techniques such as RISUG and Vasalgel create reversible polymer gel blocks in the vas deferens to obstruct sperm transport. (**d**) Physical barriers include intraurethral devices and sperm-blocking gels that physically prevent sperm passage. (**e**) Gene editing technologies modify testis-specific genes (e.g., BRDT, PRSS55) essential for spermatogenesis or sperm function. (**f**) Thermal contraception raises testicular temperature to impair sperm production. (**g**) Ultrasound-based techniques use high-frequency ultrasound to induce temporary infertility. (**h**) Nanotechnology-based modulation alters sperm function or delivers targeted contraceptive agents. (**i**) Chemosterilization disrupts spermatogenesis using non-hormonal chemical agents that interfere with biochemical pathways. These emerging contraceptive technologies aim to expand male contraceptive options while ensuring effectiveness and reversibility

contraception. The ability to administer such inhibitors immediately before intercourse could provide a practical and reversible contraceptive option for men. Moreover, natural compounds have been explored for their contraceptive potential by reducing sperm motility. For instance, the root powder of Ruellia tuberosa has been shown to significantly decrease sperm count and motility in animal models, suggesting its efficacy as an anti-fertility agent [117]. This highlights the potential for developing herbal or plant-based contraceptives that target sperm function. Thus, targeting sperm motility and function offers a multifaceted approach to male contraception. By focusing on key regulatory mechanisms such as calcium signaling through CatSper channels, mitochondrial function, and pharmacological interventions, researchers are paving the way for innovative contraceptive methods. These strategies not only aim to reduce sperm motility but also preserve overall spermatogenesis, thereby ensuring that hormonal balance and fertility can be maintained when desired.

Smart Contraceptives: Wearables and Digital Health Tools

The integration of wearables and digital health tools into contraceptive methods can facilitate real-time monitoring and management of reproductive health. For instance, devices that track physiological parameters could potentially be used to inform users about their fertility status, thereby enhancing the effectiveness of contraceptive methods [77]. The application of nanotechnology in contraceptive development is also noteworthy; it allows for the creation of microneedle systems for hormone delivery, which could be integrated into wearable devices [9]. Such advancements not only promise improved efficacy but also address issues of user compliance and convenience, which are often barriers to effective contraception [118].

Digital health tools are increasingly recognized for their role in improving contraceptive use among reproductive-age individuals. These tools can provide personalized information and reminders, thereby enhancing user engagement and adherence to contraceptive methods [118]. For men, the potential for digital platforms to facilitate education about new contraceptive options is particularly relevant. Research indicates that many men are unaware of the full range of contraceptive options available to them, which underscores the need for targeted educational interventions [67, 118]. Furthermore, the acceptance of wearable technologies is growing, as evidenced by the increasing market presence of such devices [119]. This trend suggests a readiness among consumers to embrace innovative contraceptive solutions that leverage digital health advancements. Moreover, the concept of multipurpose prevention technologies (MPTs) is gaining traction in the development of male contraceptives. MPTs aim to provide dual protection against unintended pregnancies and STIs, a critical consideration in male contraceptive development [9]. The male condom remains the most widely recognized MPT, yet there is a pressing need for additional options that can be seamlessly integrated into the daily lives of men [120]. The development of wearables that can deliver hormonal contraception or provide real-time fertility tracking could significantly enhance male involvement in family planning, thereby promoting shared responsibility in reproductive health decisions [121].

Sociocultural and Ethical Considerations

Men's Attitudes toward Contraception

Attitudes of men toward contraception are shaped by a complex interplay of cultural, social, and individual factors. A significant body of research indicates a growing willingness among men to engage in contraceptive practices, particularly with the advent of new male contraceptive methods. For instance, a survey involving over 9000 men across nine countries revealed that between 28.5% and 71.4% expressed a readiness to use hormonal male contraceptives, highlighting a considerable demand for male contraceptive options [122]. This willingness is further supported by studies indicating that men desire a variety of contraceptive choices, reflecting a shift toward shared responsibility in family planning [48]. However, the acceptance of men of contraception is often influenced by prevailing gender norms and societal expectations. Research has shown that perceptions of men of masculinity can significantly impact their attitudes toward contraceptive use. For example, men may feel societal pressure to conform to traditional masculine norms that discourage them from taking an active role in family planning [123]. This is compounded by the fear of negative social repercussions, such as disapproval from peers, which can deter men from initiating contraceptive use [123]. Furthermore, misconceptions about the effects of contraceptive methods on sexual performance and satisfaction can also hinder acceptance [21, 124].

In various cultural contexts, the dynamics of male involvement in family planning reveal both opportunities and barriers. Studies in Sub-Saharan Africa, for instance, have identified that while men may express a willingness to use contraceptives, concerns about side effects and impacts on sexual function often prevail [21, 125]. In contrast, qualitative studies in Western contexts suggest that men are increasingly open to sharing contraceptive responsibilities with their partners, indicating a shift toward more egalitarian attitudes [126]. This is particularly evident in settings where couples engage in discussions about family planning, which significantly enhances involvement of men and acceptance of contraceptive methods [127, 128]. Moreover, the role of education and socio-economic status cannot be overlooked. Higher levels of education among men correlate with increased acceptance and use of contraceptive methods, as educated men are more likely to engage in discussions about family planning with their partners [129, 130]. This suggests that educational interventions could play a crucial role in transforming attitudes toward male contraception and enhancing overall family planning practices.

Societal Impact of Male Contraceptive Methods

The societal impact of male contraceptive methods is multifaceted, influencing not only individual reproductive choices but also broader social dynamics and gender roles. As male contraceptive options expand, they hold the potential to shift traditional paradigms surrounding family planning and reproductive health. This shift is particularly significant in contexts where women have historically borne the brunt of contraceptive responsibilities and associated health risks. Research indicates that the introduction of male contraceptive methods could lead to a more equitable distribution of contraceptive responsibilities between genders. For instance, studies have shown that men are increasingly willing to share the contraceptive burden, particularly when motivated by the adverse effects their partners experience from female contraceptives [101, 131]. This willingness is echoed in qualitative analyses that highlight the desire of men to alleviate the contraceptive load from women, suggesting a potential for improved relationship dynamics and shared decision-making in reproductive health [132]. Moreover, the involvement of men in contraceptive decision-making has been linked to higher satisfaction in relationships, as joint decisions foster egalitarian interactions [132]. The societal acceptance of male contraceptive methods may also challenge existing stigmas associated with male participation in family planning. In many cultures, traditional gender norms discourage men from engaging in contraceptive discussions or using methods perceived as feminine [133]. However, as awareness and education about male contraceptives grow, there is potential for destigmatization, which could lead to increased utilization of these methods [134]. The role of social networks in shaping attitudes toward contraception is significant, as peer influence and familial discussions can enhance acceptance and uptake of male contraceptive methods [135]. Furthermore, the potential for male contraceptives to reduce unintended pregnancies is substantial, particularly in regions with low contraceptive prevalence. Modeling studies suggest that the introduction of novel male contraceptive methods could significantly decrease unintended pregnancies, thereby positively impacting public health outcomes [136]. This is particularly relevant in settings where current contraceptive use is limited, as new methods may attract individuals who have previously been disengaged from family planning initiatives [136].

Educational initiatives aimed at increasing knowledge about male contraceptive options are crucial for enhancing their societal acceptance and use. Evidence suggests that higher education levels among men correlate with more positive attitudes toward contraceptive use [30]. Thus, targeted educational programs that address misconceptions and provide comprehensive information about male contraceptives could facilitate greater male involvement in reproductive health decisions.

Ethical Considerations in Male Contraceptive Methods

The development and distribution of male contraceptive methods present a complex landscape of ethical considerations that intertwine medical, social, and cultural dimensions. As male contraceptives advance from research to market, it is imperative to address the ethical implications surrounding their efficacy, safety, and societal acceptance. First, the ethical principle of informed consent is paramount in the clinical trials and eventual distribution of male contraceptive methods. Participants in clinical trials must be fully informed about potential side effects and the long-term implications of using these contraceptives. Research has shown that fear of side effects significantly influences the willingness of men to adopt modern contraceptive methods, often leading them to rely on traditional methods instead [137]. This highlights the necessity for transparent communication regarding the risks and benefits associated with new male contraceptive options, paralleling the established practices in female contraceptive methods [32]. Moreover, ethical considerations must extend to the design of clinical trials, ensuring that they are inclusive and representative of diverse populations to avoid biases that could affect the generalizability of the findings [138].

Secondly, the societal implications of male contraceptive methods must be carefully considered. The historical context of contraceptive responsibility has predominantly placed the burden on women, which has fostered a culture of gender inequity in reproductive health [139]. The introduction of male contraceptives could challenge these norms, promoting shared responsibility in family planning. However, this shift may also provoke resistance from traditional societal structures that view male involvement in contraception as non-conformist [54]. Therefore, ethical frameworks must address these societal dynamics, advocating for educational initiatives that enhance the understanding of men of contraceptive options and their role in reproductive health [140]. Furthermore, the potential for coercion in contraceptive use raises significant ethical concerns. As male contraceptive methods become available, there is a risk that some men may feel pressured to use these methods to satisfy their partners' reproductive desires, undermining the autonomy of both partners [59]. It is crucial to establish guidelines that protect individual choice and promote mutual decision-making in contraceptive practices, ensuring that both partners are equally informed and consenting [141]. Additionally, the intersection of legal, ethical, and religious considerations cannot be overlooked. In many cultures, contraceptive use is influenced by religious beliefs that may oppose artificial methods of birth control. Therefore, the development of male contraceptives must navigate these complexities, ensuring that products are not only scientifically sound but also culturally sensitive [142]. Engaging with community leaders and stakeholders in discussions about male contraceptive options can facilitate a more ethical approach to their introduction and acceptance [58].

Future Directions and Conclusion

The future directions in male contraceptive research are promising yet complex, reflecting a growing recognition of the need for effective male contraceptive options. Despite the historical emphasis on female contraceptives, there is a burgeoning interest among both men and women for safe, reversible male contraceptive methods. Recent studies indicate that while hormonal and non-hormonal male contraceptives are under development, progress has been slow, and commercialization remains distant [3, 84]. Notably, efficacy trials have shown that male hormonal contraceptives can be as effective as female counterparts, suggesting that these methods may soon be viable options in the market [49]. Furthermore, the exploration of MPTs that combine male contraceptive methods with other health benefits is gaining traction, which could enhance their appeal and uptake [9].

Integrating male contraception into public health policy is essential for addressing the unmet need for contraceptive options. Current public health frameworks often overlook male involvement in family planning, which can lead to ineffective communication and service delivery [143]. For male contraceptives to be effectively integrated, public health campaigns must educate both men and women about the benefits and responsibilities associated with male contraceptive use. This requires a shift in societal norms, where men are encouraged to participate actively in contraceptive decision-making [21]. Additionally, healthcare providers play a crucial role in facilitating access to male contraceptives, and training programs should be implemented to equip them with the necessary knowledge and skills [144]. Thus, the landscape of male contraception is evolving, driven by scientific advancements and changing societal attitudes. The development of new male contraceptive methods, alongside a growing recognition of the roles of men in family planning, presents an opportunity to reshape reproductive health paradigms. However, for these advancements to translate into real-world impact, it is imperative to integrate male contraceptive options into public health policies and practices effectively. This integration will not only enhance contraceptive choice but also promote shared responsibility in family planning, ultimately contributing to better reproductive health outcomes globally [145]. As research continues to progress, the anticipation for novel male contraceptive methods remains high, with the potential to significantly alter the dynamics of reproductive health.

References

1. Manetti G, Honig S. Update on male hormonal contraception: is the vasectomy in jeopardy? Int J Impot Res. 2010;22(3):159–70.
2. Roth MY, Shih G, Ilani N, Wang C, Page ST, Bremner WJ, et al. Acceptability of a transdermal gel-based male hormonal contraceptive in a randomized controlled trial. Contraception. 2014;90(4):407–12.

3. Gava G, Meriggiola MC. Update on male hormonal contraception. Ther Adv Endocrinol Metab. 2019;10:2042018819834846.
4. Wang C, Festin MP, Swerdloff RS. Male hormonal contraception: where are we now? Curr Obstet Gynecol Rep. 2016;5:38–47.
5. Nickels L, Yan W, Dantzer R. Nonhormonal male contraceptive development—strategies for progress. Pharmacol Rev. 2024;76(1):37–48.
6. Plana O. Male contraception: research, new methods, and implications for marginalized populations. Am J Mens Health. 2017;11(4):1182–9.
7. Le Guen M, Ventola C, Bohet A, Moreau C, Bajos N. Men's contraceptive practices in France: evidence of male involvement in family planning. Contraception. 2015;92(1):46–54.
8. Johnston DS. Pre-clinical and early clinical considerations for the development of non-hormonal contraceptives for men. Andrology. 2024;12(7):1558–67.
9. Vahdat HL, Nickels LM. Common ground: the opportunity of male contraceptives as MPTs. Front Reprod Health. 2023;5:1278709.
10. Mohamad Al-Ali B, Shamloul R, Ramsauer J, Bella AJ, Scrinzi U, Treu T, et al. The effect of vasectomy on the sexual life of couples. J Sex Med. 2014;11(9):2239–42.
11. Zhang X, Eisenberg ML. Vasectomy utilization in men aged 18–45 declined between 2002 and 2017: results from the United States National Survey for Family Growth data. Andrology. 2022;10(1):137–42.
12. Yahyazadeh SR, Sadighi Gilani MA, Karimi A. Vasectomy reversal: unilateral versus bilateral vasovasostomy. Andrologia. 2021;53(9):e14178.
13. White AL, Davis RE, Billings DL, Mann ES. Men's vasectomy knowledge, attitudes, and information-seeking behaviors in the Southern United States: results from an exploratory survey. Am J Mens Health. 2020;14(4):1557988320949368.
14. Thummalachetty N, Mathur S, Mullinax M, DeCosta K, Nakyanjo N, Lutalo T, et al. Contraceptive knowledge, perceptions, and concerns among men in Uganda. BMC Public Health. 2017;17:1–9.
15. Shattuck D, Perry B, Packer C, Quee DC. A review of 10 years of vasectomy programming and research in low-resource settings. Glob Health Sci Pract. 2016;4(4):647–60.
16. Amory JK, Jessen JW, Muller C, Berger RE. Vasectomy by epithelial curettage without suture or cautery: a pilot study in humans. Asian J Androl. 2010;12(3):315.
17. Patel HR, Solanki H, Dharaviya P. A comparative study of scalpel versus no scalpel vasectomy. Int Surg J. 2018;5(5):1708–12.
18. Guo DP, Lamberts RW, Eisenberg ML. Relationship between vasectomy and sexual frequency. J Sex Med. 2015;12(9):1905–10.
19. Cheng LG, White K, Jarlenski M, Hwang K. Patient-reported influence of sociopolitical issues on post-dobbs vasectomy decisions. JAMA Netw Open. 2025;8(1):e2454430-e.
20. Kabagenyi A, Jennings L, Reid A, Nalwadda G, Ntozi J, Atuyambe L. Barriers to male involvement in contraceptive uptake and reproductive health services: a qualitative study of men and women's perceptions in two rural districts in Uganda. Reprod Health. 2014;11:1–9.
21. Cartwright AF, Lawton A, Brunie A, Callahan RL. What about methods for men? A qualitative analysis of attitudes toward male contraception in Burkina Faso and Uganda. Int Perspect Sex Reprod Health. 2020;46:153.
22. Najafi FS, Rahman HA, Juni MH. Barriers to modern contraceptive practices among selected married women in a public university in Malaysia. Global J Health Sci. 2011;3(2):50.
23. Wang C, Swerdloff RS. Hormonal approaches to male contraception. Curr Opin Urol. 2010;20(6):520–4.
24. Moreira LR, Ewerling F, Barros AJ, Silveira MF. Reasons for nonuse of contraceptive methods by women with demand for contraception not satisfied: an assessment of low and middle-income countries using demographic and health surveys. Reprod Health. 2019;16:1–15.

25. Gong S, Zhu S, Zhou P, Cheng CY, Li W, Yao W, et al. Discovering a reversible male contraceptive agent derived from Lonidamine. ACS Omega. 2023;8(20):18245–54.
26. Yuen F, Nguyen BT, Swerdloff RS, Wang C. Continuing the search for a hormonal male contraceptive. Best Pract Res Clin Obstet Gynaecol. 2020;66:83–94.
27. Cheng CY, Mruk DD. A local autocrine axis in the testes that regulates spermatogenesis. Nat Rev Endocrinol. 2010;6(7):380–95.
28. Frankiewicz M, Połom W, Matuszewski M. Can the evolution of male contraception lead to a revolution? Review of the current state of knowledge. Cent Eur J Urol. 2017;71(1):108.
29. Drevet JR. Epididymal approaches to male contraception. Basic Clin Androl. 2018;28(1):12.
30. Namasivayam A, Lovell S, Namutamba S, Schluter PJ. Predictors of modern contraceptive use among women and men in Uganda: a population-level analysis. BMJ Open. 2020;10(2):e034675.
31. Tumwesigye R, Kigongo E, Nakiganga S, Mbyariyehe G, Nabeshya J, Kabunga A, et al. Uptake and associated factors of male contraceptive method use: a community-based cross-sectional study in Northern Uganda. Open Access J Contracept. 2023:129–37.
32. Abbe C, Roxby AC. Assessing safety in hormonal male contraception: a critical appraisal of adverse events reported in a male contraceptive trial. BMJ Sex Reprod Health. 2020;46(2):139–46.
33. Jacobstein R, Radloff S, Khan F, Mimno K, Pal M, Snell J, et al. Down but not out: vasectomy is faring poorly almost everywhere—we can do better to make it a true method option. Glob Health Sci Pract. 2023;11(1)
34. Nieschlag E, Nieschlag S. Why we need more methods for male contraception. Andrology. 2023;11(3):421–4.
35. Wang C, Blithe D, Page S, Serfaty D, Ware RS, editors. Progress in male contraception: a brief summary of the third international congress on male contraception, May 2022. International Congress on Male Contraception. p. 2022.
36. Nieschlag E. Clinical trials in male hormonal contraception. Contraception. 2010;82(5):457–70.
37. Thirumalai A, Page ST. Male hormonal contraception. Annu Rev Med. 2020;71(1):17–31.
38. O'Hara L, Smith LB. Androgen receptor roles in spermatogenesis and infertility. Best Pract Res Clin Endocrinol Metab. 2015;29(4):595–605.
39. Patel AS, Leong JY, Ramos L, Ramasamy R. Testosterone is a contraceptive and should not be used in men who desire fertility. World J Men Health. 2019;37(1):45–54.
40. Zhang X-W, Zhang C, Zhang W, Yang D, Meng S, Wang P, et al. Suppression of spermatogenesis by testosterone undecanoate-loaded injectable in situ-forming implants in adult male rats. Asian J Androl. 2016;18(5):791–7.
41. Crosnoe-Shipley LE, Elkelany OO, Rahnema CD, Kim ED. Treatment of hypogonadotropic male hypogonadism: case-based scenarios. World J Nephrol. 2015;4(2):245.
42. El Meliegy A, Motawi A, Abd El Salam MA. Systematic review of hormone replacement therapy in the infertile man. Arab J Urol. 2018;16(1):140–7.
43. Page ST, Blithe D, Wang C. Hormonal male contraception: getting to market. Front Endocrinol. 2022;13:891589.
44. Long JE, Lee MS, Blithe DL. Update on novel hormonal and nonhormonal male contraceptive development. J Clin Endocrinol Metabol. 2021;106(6):e2381–e92.
45. Ilani N, Liu PY, Swerdloff RS, Wang C. Does ethnicity matter in male hormonal contraceptive efficacy? Asian J Androl. 2011;13(4):579.
46. Yu H, Liu J, Han Y, Chen C, Meng F. Correlation between serum Kisspeptin and spermatogenic function in men. BioRxiv. 2019:810572.
47. Kroopnick JM, Lee MS, Blithe DL. Development of new hormonal male contraception for the couple. Andrology. 2024;
48. Anawalt BD, Roth MY, Ceponis J, Surampudi V, Amory JK, Swerdloff RS, et al. Combined nestorone–testosterone gel suppresses serum gonadotropins to concentrations associated with effective hormonal contraception in men. Andrology. 2019;7(6):878–87.

49. Meriggiola MC, Goulis DG. Contraceptive counseling: shared decision on contraceptive choices. Andrology. 2024;12(7):1525–8.
50. Zitzmann M. Would male hormonal contraceptives affect cardiovascular risk? Asian J Androl. 2018;20(2):145–8.
51. Ahmed H, Memon A, Hoda F, Alvares J. The male birth control pill–A new approach to family planning and population control. Int J Health Plann Manag. 2024;39(5):1652–7.
52. Yuen F, Wu S, Thirumalai A, Swerdloff RS, Page ST, Liu PY, et al. Preventing secondary exposure to women from men applying a novel nestorone/testosterone contraceptive gel. Andrology. 2019;7(2):235–43.
53. Louwagie EJ, Quinn GF, Pond KL, Hansen KA. Male contraception: narrative review of ongoing research. Basic Clin Androl. 2023;33(1):30.
54. Sidhom K, Bal DS, Ramjiawan R, Patel P. The landscape of male contraception: a narrative review. Can Urol Assoc J. 2024;18(10)
55. Roth MY, Ilani N, Wang C, Page ST, Bremner WJ, Swerdloff RS, et al. Characteristics associated with suppression of spermatogenesis in a male hormonal contraceptive trial using testosterone and Nestorone® gels. Andrology. 2013;1(6):899–905.
56. Zitzmann M, Rohayem J, Raidt J, Kliesch S, Kumar N, Sitruk-Ware R, et al. Impact of various progestins with or without transdermal testosterone on gonadotropin levels for non-invasive hormonal male contraception: a randomized clinical trial. Andrology. 2017;5(3):516–26.
57. Roth M, Amory J. Pharmacologic development of male hormonal contraceptive agents. Clin Pharmacol Ther. 2011;89(1):133–6.
58. Khourdaji I, Zillioux J, Eisenfrats K, Foley D, Smith R. The future of male contraception: a fertile ground. Transl Androl Urol. 2018;7(Suppl 2):S220.
59. Roth MY, Amory JK, editors. Beyond the condom: frontiers in male contraception, Seminars in reproductive medicine. Thieme Medical Publishers; 2016.
60. Amory JK. Development of novel male contraceptives. Clin Transl Sci. 2020;13(2):228–37.
61. Minhas V, Shrestha A, Wadhwa N, Singh R, Gupta SK. Novel sperm and gonadotropin-releasing hormone-based recombinant fusion protein: achievement of 100% contraceptive efficacy by co-immunization of male and female mice. Mol Reprod Dev. 2016;83(12):1048–59.
62. Pinkham R, Eckery D, Mauldin R, Gomm M, Hill F, Vial F, et al. Longevity of an immunocontraceptive vaccine effect on fecundity in rats. Vaccine: X. 2022;10:100138.
63. Matsumoto N, Tomiyasu J, Hagino K, Matsui M, Yanagawa Y. Contraceptive effect of a gonadotropin-releasing hormone vaccine on captive male brown bears (Ursus arctos). Reprod Domest Anim. 2024;59(9):e14707.
64. Lucas X. Clinical use of deslorelin (GnRH agonist) in companion animals: a review. Reprod Domest Anim. 2014;49:64–71.
65. Borrero S, Farkas A, Dehlendorf C, Rocca CH. Racial and ethnic differences in men's knowledge and attitudes about contraception. Contraception. 2013;88(4):532–8.
66. Mahmoud A, T'Sjoen G. Male hormonal contraception: where do we stand? Eur J Contracept Reprod Health Care. 2012;17(3):179–86.
67. Amory JK. Male contraception. Fertil Steril. 2016;106(6):1303–9.
68. Dorman E, Bishai D. Demand for male contraception. Expert Rev Pharmacoecon Outcomes Res. 2012;12(5):605–13.
69. Pazol K, Kramer MR, Hogue CJ. Condoms for dual protection: patterns of use with highly effective contraceptive methods. Public Health Rep. 2010;125(2):208–17.
70. Yang F, Li J, Dong L, Tan K, Huang X, Zhang P, et al. Review of vasectomy complications and safety concerns. World J Men Health. 2020;39(3):406.
71. Lu W-H, Liang X-W, Gu Y-Q, Wu W-X, Bo L-W, Zheng T-G, et al. A randomized, controlled, multicenter contraceptive efficacy clinical trial of the intravas device, a nonocclusive surgical male sterilization. Asian J Androl. 2014;16(3):432–6.

72. Labrecque M. Are evidence-based vasectomy surgical techniques performed in low-resource countries? Gates Open Res. 2019:3.
73. Cilip CM, Pierorazio PM, Ross AE, Allaf ME, Fried NM. High-frequency ultrasound imaging of noninvasive laser coagulation of the canine vas deferens. Lasers Surg Med. 2011;43(8):838–42.
74. Bintoro T, Murti B, Sutisna E. Relationship of knowledge and attitudes with male participation in vasectomy in Indonesia. Medico-Legal Update. 2021;21(1)
75. Ansari AS, Badar A, Balasubramanian K, Lohiya NK. Contraception with RISUG® and functional reversal through DMSO and NaHCO3 in male rabbits. Asian J Androl. 2017;19(4):389–95.
76. Wang Z-Q, Liu Z-Q, Zhao C-H, Zhang K, Kang Z-J, Qu T-R, et al. An ultrasound-induced self-clearance hydrogel for male reversible contraception. ACS Nano. 2022;16(4):5515–28.
77. Su Z, Diao T, McGuire H, Yao C, Yang L, Bao G, et al. Nanomaterials solutions for contraception: concerns, advances, and prospects. ACS Nano. 2023;17(21):20753–75.
78. Subramanian B, Agarwal T, Ghorai SK, Mandal P, Chattopadhyay S, Basak P, et al. Biocompatible polyvinyl alcohol and RISUG® blend polymeric films with spermicidal potential. Biomed Mater. 2019;14(3):035017.
79. Khilwani B, Badar A, Ansari AS, Lohiya NK. RISUG® as a male contraceptive: journey from bench to bedside. Basic Clin Androl. 2020;30:1–12.
80. Kumar S, Roy S, Chaudhury K, Sen P, Guha SK. Study of the micro-structural properties of RISUG®—A newly developed male contraceptive. J Biomed Mater Res Part B Appl Biomater. 2008;86(1):154–61.
81. Lohiya NK, Ansari AS, Sadasukhi TC, Pachera S, Khilwani B, Dhaked RK. RISUG® offers early contraception: an experience during phase III clinical trials. J Reprod Healthc Med. 2022;3:11.
82. Sharma RS, Mathur AK, Singh R, Das HC, Singh GJ, Toor DPS, et al. Safety & efficacy of an intravasal, one-time injectable & non-hormonal male contraceptive (RISUG): a clinical experience. Indian J Med Res. 2019;150(1):81–6.
83. Mathew V, Bantwal G. Male contraception. Indian J Endocrinol Metab. 2012;16(6):910–7.
84. Kim J, So B, Heo Y, So H, Jo JK. Advances in male contraception: when will the novel male contraception be available? World J Men Health. 2024:42.
85. Waller D, Bolick D, Lissner E, Premanandan C, Gamerman G. Reversibility of Vasalgel™ male contraceptive in a rabbit model. Basic Clin Androl. 2017;27:1–9.
86. Colagross-Schouten A, Lemoy M-J, Keesler RI, Lissner E, VandeVoort CA. The contraceptive efficacy of intravas injection of Vasalgel™ for adult male rhesus monkeys. Basic Clin Androl. 2017;27:1–7.
87. Tropp J. Biomaterial platforms offer capability of efficacious male contraceptives. Springer; 2022.
88. Buck KA, Stadick JL, Frazier ML. Preparing for sperm-targeted contraception: college students' perceptions and intentions related to non-hormonal intravas injectable gel. Public Health Nurs. 2020;37(5):639–46.
89. Howard SA, Benhabbour SR. Non-hormonal contraception. J Clin Med. 2023;12(14):4791.
90. Hurley LL, McDiarmid CS, Friesen CR, Griffith SC, Rowe M. Experimental heatwaves negatively impact sperm quality in the zebra finch. Proc R Soc B Biol Sci. 1871;2018(285):20172547.
91. Sales K, Vasudeva R, Dickinson ME, Godwin JL, Lumley AJ, Michalczyk Ł, et al. Experimental heatwaves compromise sperm function and cause transgenerational damage in a model insect. Nat Commun. 2018;9(1):4771.
92. Meena A, De Nardo AN, Maggu K, Sbilordo SH, Roy J, Snook RR, et al. Fertility loss and recovery dynamics after repeated heat stress across life stages in male Drosophila melanogaster: patterns and processes. R Soc Open Sci. 2024;11(10):241082.

93. Costa SG, Magalhães S, Santos I, Zélé F, Rodrigues LR. A sex-specific trade-off between pesticide resistance and tolerance to heat-induced sterility in Tetranychus urticae. Evol Appl. 2024;17(9):e70014.
94. Varma D, Ullah IK, Thakur MK. Role of testicular elastography in the evaluation of male infertility: a comparative cross-sectional study. Int J Res Med Sci. 2023;11(5):1754.
95. de Carvalho CF, Magalhães JR, Magalhães AM, Guimarães KCDS, de Moraes RS, de Sousa DB, et al. Pulsed-wave Doppler Ultrasound in canine reproductive system–Part 2: use in the routine. Res Soc Dev. 2021;10(5):e52610515352-e
96. Holtze S, Lukač M, Cizelj I, Mutschmann F, Szentiks CA, Jelić D, et al. Monitoring health and reproductive status of olms (Proteus anguinus) by ultrasound. PLoS One. 2017;12(8):e0182209.
97. Condorelli R, Calogero AE, La Vignera S. Relationship between testicular volume and conventional or nonconventional sperm parameters. Int J Endocrinol. 2013;2013(1):145792.
98. Lotti F, Maggi M. Ultrasound of the male genital tract in relation to male reproductive health. Hum Reprod Update. 2015;21(1):56–83.
99. Sengupta P. Chemosterilization: spermatogenesis, steroidogenesis, reproductive functions, and behavior; from historical perspective to contemporary practice. J Basic Clin Reprod Sci. 2013;2(1):1–2.
100. Sengupta P, Dutta S. Chemosterilization in male: 'past and present' in reproductive biology. Biomed Pharmacol J. 2022;15(1):1–4.
101. Laurent C, Mieusset R, Soufir JC, Perrin J. Real-life users of hormonal or thermal male contraception: an analysis of female partners' motivation, experience, and satisfaction: Andrology. 2024.
102. Moya P, Flores S, Ayala I, Sanchis J, Montoya P, Primo J. Evaluation of lufenuron as a chemosterilant against fruit flies of the genus Anastrepha (Diptera: Tephritidae). Pest Manag Sci Formerly Pesticide Science. 2010;66(6):657–63.
103. Khan SA, Jadhav SV, Suryawanshi AR, Bhonde GS, Gajbhiye RK, Khole VV. Evaluation of contraceptive potential of a novel epididymal sperm protein SFP2 in a mouse model. Am J Reprod Immunol. 2011;66(3):185–98.
104. Amory JK, Muller CH, Shimshoni JA, Isoherranen N, Paik J, Moreb JS, et al. Suppression of spermatogenesis by bisdichloroacetyldiamines is mediated by inhibition of testicular retinoic acid biosynthesis. J Androl. 2011;32(1):111–9.
105. Sun J, Lu Y, Nozawa K, Xu Z, Morohoshi A, Castaneda JM, et al. CRISPR/Cas9-based genome editing in mice uncovers 13 testis-or epididymis-enriched genes individually dispensable for male reproduction. Biol Reprod. 2020;103(2):183–94.
106. Welborn JP, Davis MG, Ebers SD, Stodden GR, Hayashi K, Cheatwood JL, et al. Rhox8 ablation in the Sertoli cells using a tissue-specific RNAi approach results in impaired male fertility in mice. Biol Reprod. 2015;93(1):8, 1–14.
107. Kobayashi K, Endo T, Matsumura T, Lu Y, Yu Z, Matzuk MM, et al. Prss55 but not Prss51 is required for male fertility in mice. Biol Reprod. 2020;103(2):223–34.
108. Hasse TA, Zhang Z, Huang Y-M. In silico discovery of potential inhibitors targeting the MEIG1-PACRG complex for male contraceptive development. bioRxiv 2024:2024.12.16.628759.
109. Choubisa V, Sharma S. Unveiling neural network potential in forecasting CRISPR effects and off-target prophecies for gene editing. Int J Sci Res Arch. 2023;10(1):252–9.
110. Robertson MJ, Kent K, Tharp N, Nozawa K, Dean L, Mathew M, et al. Large-scale discovery of male reproductive tract-specific genes through analysis of RNA-seq datasets. BMC Biol. 2020;18:1–28.
111. Service CA, Puri D, Hsieh T-C, Patel DP. Emerging concepts in male contraception: a narrative review of novel, hormonal and non-hormonal options. Ther Adv Reprod Health. 2023;17:26334941221138323.

112. Chung J-J, Miki K, Kim D, Shim S-H, Shi HF, Hwang JY, et al. CatSperζ regulates the structural continuity of sperm Ca2+ signaling domains and is required for normal fertility. elife. 2017;6:e23082.
113. Lee K-H, Hwang JY. Ca2+ homeostasis and male fertility: a target for a new male contraceptive system. Anim Cells Syst. 2024;28(1):171–83.
114. Agnihotri SK, Agrawal AK, Hakim BA, Vishwakarma A, Narender T, Sachan R, et al. Mitochondrial membrane potential (MMP) regulates sperm motility. In Vitro Cell Dev Biol Anim. 2016;52:953–60.
115. Kaur K, Allahbadia G, Singh M. Efforts to generate a male contraception just by prevention of sperm motility acquirement in epididymis without influencing the physiology of spermatogenesis: yet still a little far goal. J Obst Gynecol Surg. 2021;2(1):1–3.
116. Balbach M, Rossetti T, Ferreira J, Ghanem L, Ritagliati C, Myers RW, et al. On-demand male contraception via acute inhibition of soluble adenylyl cyclase. Nat Commun. 2023;14(1):637.
117. Pardeshi MH, Deshmukh AA, Gajare KA. Ruellia tuberosa Linn. acts as anti-fertility agent that reduces sperm count, motility and viability in male Swiss albino mice (Mus-musculus). Int J Curr Pharm Res. 2017;9(1):105–9.
118. Opatunji FO, Sowunmi CO. The role of digital health tools in improving contraceptive use among reproductive age women. Int J Health Psychol Res. 2024;12(1):18–33.
119. Stănescu DF, Romaşcanu MC, editors. An explorative study on users' motivation and adoption of wearables technologies using the technology acceptance model (TAM). International Psychological Applications Conference and Trends (InPACT); 2022.
120. Weerasinghe M, Agawane S, Karandikar N, Fisher J, Sastry J. Examining the place of the female condom in India's family planning program: A qualitative investigation of the attitudes and opinions of key stakeholders in Pune, India. BMC Public Health. 2022;22(1):1675.
121. Campelia GD, Adashi EY, Amory JK. Shared risk and shared responsibility: the ethics of male contraceptives. Andrology. 2024;
122. Hardee K, Croce-Galis M, Gay J. Are men well served by family planning programs? Reprod Health. 2017;14(1):14.
123. Newmann SJ, Zakaras JM, Dworkin SL, Withers M, Ndunyu L, Gitome S, et al. Measuring men's gender norm beliefs related to contraception: development of the masculine norms and family planning acceptance scale. Arch Sex Behav. 2021;50:2691–702.
124. Tekakwo A, Nabirye RC, Nantale R, Oguttu F, Nambozo B, Wani S, et al. Enablers and barriers of male involvement in the use of modern family planning methods in Eastern Uganda: a qualitative study. Contracep Repro Med. 2023;8(1):49.
125. Nguyen BT. Male contraceptive acceptability versus male acceptance of contraceptive responsibility. Andrology. 2024;12(7):1585–9.
126. Amouroux M, Mieusset R, Desbriere R, Opinel P, Karsenty G, Paci M, et al. Are men ready to use thermal male contraception? Acceptability in two French populations: New fathers and new providers. PLoS One. 2018;13(5):e0195824.
127. Adera A, Belete T, Gebru A, Hagos A, Gebregziabher W. Assessment of the role of men in family planning utilization at Edaga-Hamuse town, Tigray, North Ethiopia. Am J Nurs Sci. 2015;4(4):174.
128. Wondim G, Degu G, Teka Y, Diress G. Male involvement in family planning utilization and associated factors in Womberma District, Northern Ethiopia: community-based cross-sectional study. Open Access J Contracept. 2020:197–207.
129. Shruthee S, Deepanchakravarthi V. Family planning from a male perspective: observations from a community-based cross-sectional study in Chennai, Tamil Nadu. Indian J Community Med. 2023;48(6):930–3.
130. Kassa M, Abajobir AA, Gedefaw M. Level of male involvement and associated factors in family planning services utilization among married men in Debremarkos town, Northwest Ethiopia. BMC Int Health Hum Rights. 2014;14:1–8.

131. Reynolds-Wright JJ, Cameron NJ, Anderson RA. Will men use novel male contraceptive methods and will women trust them? A systematic review. J Sex Res. 2021;58(7):838–49.
132. Meyer D, Heiden-Rootes K, Sledge R, Salas J. The role of couple dynamics in contraception decision-making. Couple Family Psychol Res Pract. 2024;13(1):15.
133. Blackstone SR, Iwelunmor J. Determinants of contraceptive use among Nigerian couples: evidence from the 2013 Demographic and Health Survey. Contracep Reprod Med. 2017;2:1–8.
134. Kabunga A, Kigongo E, Acanga A, Tumwesigye R, Auma AG, Musinguzi M, et al. Qualitative study on stigma as a barrier to emergency contraceptive pill use among university students in the Lango subregion, Uganda. BMJ Open. 2024;14(2):e079478.
135. Dombola GM, Manda WC, Chipeta E. Factors influencing contraceptive decision making and use among young adolescents in urban Lilongwe, Malawi: a qualitative study. Reprod Health. 2021;18:1–11.
136. Dorman E, Perry B, Polis CB, Campo-Engelstein L, Shattuck D, Hamlin A, et al. Modeling the impact of novel male contraceptive methods on reductions in unintended pregnancies in Nigeria, South Africa, and the United States. Contraception. 2018;97(1):62–9.
137. Islam MS. Determinants of contraceptive method choice in Bangladesh: male perspectives. South East Asia J Public Health. 2013;3(1):50–6.
138. Long JE, Lee MS, Blithe DL. Male contraceptive development: update on novel hormonal and nonhormonal methods. Clin Chem. 2019;65(1):153–60.
139. Hoga LA, Rodolpho JR, Sato PM, Nunes MC, Borges AL. Adult men's beliefs, values, attitudes and experiences regarding contraceptives: a systematic review of qualitative studies. J Clin Nurs. 2014;23(7–8):927–39.
140. Osuafor GN, Akokuwebe ME, Idemudia ES. Male involvement in Family Planning decisions in Malawi and Tanzania: what are the determinants? Int J Environ Res Public Health. 2023;20(6):5053.
141. Wang C, Meriggiola MC, Amory JK, Barratt CL, Behre HM, Bremner WJ, et al. Practice and development of male contraception: European Academy of Andrology and American Society of Andrology guidelines. Andrology. 2024;12(7):1470–500.
142. Hapsari A, Aftabuddin SK, editors. The estimation of male contraceptive methods' development considering legal, ethical, and religious aspects. 2nd International Conference on Sports Sciences and Health 2018 (2nd ICSSH 2018). Atlantis Press; 2019.
143. Böttcher B, Abu-El-Noor M, Abu-El-Noor N. Choices and services related to contraception in the Gaza strip, Palestine: perceptions of service users and providers. BMC Womens Health. 2019;19:1–8.
144. Lince-Deroche N, Hendrickson C, Moolla A, Kgowedi S, Mulongo M. Provider perspectives on contraceptive service delivery: findings from a qualitative study in Johannesburg, South Africa. BMC Health Serv Res. 2020;20:1–10.
145. Prol B, Klein S, Rennie C, Andelija S. Respondent Demographics and Contraceptive Use Patterns in the United States: a national survey of family growth analysis. Cureus. 2024;16:e53121.

Chapter 11
Advances in Surgery for Male Infertility

Luca Boeri, Mirko Preto, and Marco Falcone

Introduction

Couple's infertility is a rinsing issue worldwide, affecting nearly 15% of couples of reproductive age [46]. Male factor infertility (MFI) accounts for approximately 20% of cases, while a combination of male and female factors contributes to 30% of infertility cases [12, 46]. Several causes of MFI have been identified thus including hormonal diseases, genetic conditions, gonadotoxic treatment, metabolic disorders, and urogenital infections [10, 13, 26]. However, infertility remains idiopathic in its nature in about 30% of cases [76]. Varicocele, for instance, is one of the most common causes of MFI. Its treatment has been debated for years in the last decades, but recent systematic reviews and meta-analysis have confirmed that varicocele repair may improve pregnancy rates and sperm concentration in adult infertile men [27]. Nonetheless, due to the lack of randomized controlled studies, it has not yet been determined which type of surgical approach is associated with better outcomes.

Semen quality impairment is usually associated with subfertility [11], but azoospermia represents the most severe form of MFI. Azoospermia, meaning the absence of sperm in the ejaculate after centrifugation, is categorized in clinical practice into obstructive azoospermia (OA) and non-obstructive azoospermia (NOA).

NOA is a common clinical condition, accounting for approximately 1% of all men and 10% of all infertile men [46]. NOA has multiple etiologies including primary testicular dysfunction, impairment of the hypothalamus-pituitary-gonadal (HPG) axis, acquired causes such as cryptorchidism, and exposure to gonadotoxic

L. Boeri (✉)
IRCCS Fondazione Ca' Granda Ospedale Maggiore Policlinico, Milan, Italy

M. Preto · M. Falcone
A.O.U. Città della Salute e della Scienza di Torino—Presidio Molinette—Clinica Urologica, Turin, Italy
e-mail: marco.falcone@unito.it

E. Chung et al. (eds.), *Advances in Andrology*,
https://doi.org/10.1007/978-3-032-29112-7_11

chemotherapy and/or pelvic radiation and genetic causes such as Klinefelter's syndrome and Y chromosome microdeletions [18]. Men with NOA usually have small testicular volume, high FSH values, and normal semen volume [14]. NOA men usually have small and isolated foci of residual spermatogenesis within the testes; therefore, surgical sperm retrieval and intracytoplasmic sperm injection (ICSI) are valuable treatment options to father a child.

OA is the absence of spermatozoa in the sediment of a centrifuged sample of ejaculate due to obstruction. It is less common than NOA and occurs in 20%–40% of men with azoospermia [46]. The location of the obstruction can be at any site between the testis and the ejaculatory ducts, but the most common is at epididymis. Moreover, obstruction can be due to several causes thus including infections, trauma, post-surgery, congenital (usually associated with CFTR gene mutations), or idiopathic. Additionally, other causes like ejaculatory duct obstruction resulting from surgery, trauma, or congenital Mullerian duct cysts can also cause OA [46]. Men with OA usually have normal FSH, testes of normal size, and epididymal enlargement. Moreover, OA men generally have normal sperm production, and thus, sperm retrieval from the testis, epididymis, or even vas deferens is a potential viable option. For retrieval from the epididymis, either microsurgical epididymal sperm aspiration or percutaneous epididymal sperm aspiration may be performed [12]. Moreover, in cases where the precise location of obstruction is identified, surgery (reconstructive or to relieve obstruction) can be a definitive treatment for the infertility case.

Since spermatogenesis is not impaired in OA men, sperm retrieval can be achieved in approximately 90%–100% of cases [46]. Conversely, in NOA men, with a wide variability among cohorts and techniques, positive sperm retrieval has been reported in up to 50% of patients [21]. Of note, one of the most important challenges in infertility research is to identify reliable predictors of positive sperm retrieval in NOA cases. In fact, numerous predictive factors have been investigated, including clinical parameters, serum hormones, surgical approach, and testicular histology, but no definitive predictors have been associated with successful retrieval [9, 21, 46]. In addition, new surgical advancements have been proposed in men with azoospermia and in those with varicocele to improve sperm retrieval and sperm recovery. In this chapter, we will revise the new advances in surgery for male infertility and their impact on semen quality and pregnancy outcomes.

TESE Old but Gold

- *Classic TESE: Limitations*

As previously mentioned, in patients with NOA, sperm retrieval can be performed due to the existence of isolated islands of active spermatogenesis within the testicles. Different SR techniques have been described in the literature for this purpose, such as: Testicular Fine Needle Aspiration (TFNA), Conventional Testicular

Sperm Extraction (c-TESE), testicular sperm aspiration (TESA), and Microdissection TESE (micro-TESE) [46]. c-TESE is an option for sperm retrieval in NOA patients for ICSI. c-TESE can be performed under either local anesthesia with or without intravenous sedation or epidural anesthesia. Usually, a transverse 2 cm incision is made through the anterior scrotal skin, dartos, and tunica vaginalis. The albuginea is incised for ~1 cm. Gentle pressure is made onto the testis to extrude testicular parenchyma. A small fragment (~5 × 5 mm) is excised with sharp scissors and placed in sperm culture media. A single or multiple specimens can be extracted from the same incision [77]. This procedure can be performed with a single or multiple incisions of the tunica albuginea. Through multiple c-TESE, the tunica albuginea is incised transversely in several regions of the testicular poles, followed by a light compression and excision of the protruding tissue which is sent for processing and analysis using microscopy. The appropriate number of biopsies during c-TESE is still a matter of debate. A previous study showed that the sperm retrieval rate (SRR) was 37.5% and 49% among patients undergoing single and multiple biopsy [74]. In a recent study, Falcone et al. analyzed NOA men with poor chance of retrieval (testicular volume <10 cc and FSH >12.4 UI/L) undergoing c-TESE vs. combined trifocal and m-TESE procedures. They found that SRR was higher in the combination group than c-TESE (29.4% vs. 26.9%, $p < 0.03$) [25]. Potential complications after c-TESE are persistent pain, edema, infection, hydrocele, hematoma, androgen deficiency to atrophy, and testicular failure. Intratesticular hematomas are frequent after c-TESE but most cases resolve spontaneously, without significantly compromising testicular function. Some authors have reported that excision of a large volume of testicular parenchyma by c-TESE might be associated with a high risk of transient or permanent reduction in testosterone levels due to testicular devascularization. However, testosterone decline after surgery is usually small, and recovery to baseline levels is expected up to 18 months after TESE [24]. Recent studies assessing patients with NOA have found an overall success rate in SR ranging from 30% to 50%, with testicular sperm obtaining in all etiologic categories, encompassing cryptorchidism, orchitis, genetics, radiotherapy or chemotherapy, and idiopathic [21]. Nonetheless, c-TESE is still considered as a "random" procedure as testicular biopsy is performed without the opportunity to select seminiferous tubules that are more likely to contain spermatozoa. In addition, the gross testicular biopsy does not preserve intratesticular blood vessel, with potential consequences in terms of testicular health. For these reasons, several advances in surgical technique have been introduced in the last decades.

- *Micro-TESE: Update on SR Data*

The micro-TESE was initially described by Schlegel in 1999. This technique emerged with the proposal to be the gold standard for SR, because it is minimally invasive, safe, and limits the impairment of testicular function, with a high sperm retrieval rate. This procedure is performed under general anesthesia. A transverse equatorial incision is made, and each side of the tunica albuginea is gently pulled apart with the aid of two surgical hemostats. The seminiferous tubules are then examined carefully and systematically prior to manipulation under at least 25x magnification using a surgical microscope. Optimal tubules (i.e., those likely to contain sperm), which are generally larger and more opaque, are taken entirely whenever possible. Bipolar cautery should be used to limit postoperative bleeding as well as tissue damage. Once an adequate number of tubules are selected, processing should occur as previously described [65]. M-TESE is now considered the gold standard for SR in NOA men [12, 46]. In terms of complications, studies reported a lower rate of testicular hematoma and fibrosis, a lower reduction in testicular volume (>2 ml) and a lower drop in serum testosterone levels compared to c-TESE [22]. Conversely, the superiority of m-TESE compared to classic procedure in terms of SRR is still debated.

A previous review that summarized seven studies between 1999 and 2013 reported a SRR of 16.7%–45.0% for c-TESE and 42.9%–63.0% for m-TESE group [22]. Subsequently, a meta-analysis of 15 studies with almost 2000 patients demonstrated that m-TESE had a 1.5× greater likelihood of successful sperm retrieval compared to c-TESE [4]. This meta-analysis, that included only comparative studies, also showed that c-TESE yield a twofold improvement in sperm retrieval compared to TESA. More recently, Corona et al. [21] assessed 21,404 patients in a total of 117 studies and showed that c-TESE/micro-TESE resulted in an SR rate of up to 50% in NOA men with no differences between the surgical techniques. Retrieved sperm resulted in a live birth rate of up to 28%. The authors also recognized the low quality of the included studies and claimed a sufficiently powerful and well-designed randomized controlled trial to compare micro-TESE with c-TESE in men with NOA.

The main factors limiting the widespread adoption of micro-TESE (m-TESE) are its higher cost and the need for specialized microsurgical training. Success in male infertility microsurgery is heavily dependent on the surgeon's microsurgical skills. Laboratory-based practice is known to enhance microsurgical skills improving the surgeon's confidence and reduces stress and operating time, benefiting both the patient and the surgeon [44]. Therefore, more dedicated microsurgical training is needed to promote the diffusion of m-TESE.

Since SRR after TESE is relatively low (up to 50%), it is of paramount importance to select the best candidate for this procedure. Several studies have investigated potential predictors of positive sperm retrieval in NOA men.

- Testis volume has been classically correlated to spermatogenesis. However, its predictive role in NOA men is uncertain. A meta-analysis revealed that testis volume significantly predicted SRR, specifically a mean volume higher than 12.5 mL predicted a SRR >60% with an accuracy of 86.2% ($p < 0.0001$) and a specificity and sensitivity of 73% and 74%, respectively [21]. Conversely, a study including only m-TESE procedures found that testis volume had limited value in predicting positive sperm retrieval in patients with NOA (AUC 0.63), mostly due to low specificity [42].
- Male age has been correlated with deterioration in ejaculated semen parameters and increased serum FSH concentrations. Age has been inconsistently associated with SRR after TESE, particularly in Klinefelter's patients. Overall, male age is

not considered a reliable predictor of TESE success in both the general population and in men with chromosomal abnormalities [9].

- Hormonal Parameters: Follicle-stimulating hormone (FSH) and testosterone (T) are both required to promote full spermatogenesis; in addition, their serum levels reflect both the pituitary and testicular function in physiological and pathological conditions. However, their role as predictors of spermatogenesis in patients with NOA is, however, questionable. Serum FSH concentrations have been suggested, in some isolated reports, to predict sperm retrieval in conventional TESE. Other studies have reported FSH levels to inversely correlate with the number of germ cells present and stages of spermatogenesis [58]. However, while high serum FSH levels may provide a more global representation of the level of spermatogenic dysfunction within a testis, there still may be small foci of spermatogenesis that can be identified and retrieved during m-TESE. Similarly, inconclusive data exist regarding the association between testosterone levels and SRR [17]. More recently, Pozzi et al. investigated the role of AMH as predictor of SRR. They found that men with iNOA with lower levels of AMH had a significantly higher percentage of successful SR at surgery. A threshold of <4 ng/ml for circulating AMH ensured satisfactory sensitivity, specificity, and positive predictive values in the context of positive SR at m-TESE [57].
- Testis Histology: There is great consensus about the close relationship between different histopathological categories and m-TESE outcome. Patients with Sertoli cells only syndrome (SCO) have the lowest probability of SSR (22.5%–41%), while patients with hypospermatogenesis (HS) have the best chances of sperm retrieval (73%–100%), and patients with late maturation arrest (MA) have better prognosis (SRR 27%–86%) compared to those with early MA (SRR 27%–40%) [28]. The role of histology has been also conformed in men undergoing salvage m-TESE [14]. Unfortunately, since preoperative testicular biopsy is not recommended by current Guidelines, histology is only obtained after the initial TESE but it can guide the decision to undergo a salvage procedure [46].
- Others: Men with cryptorchidism might have sperm impairment but also azoospermia. Sperm retrieval is reported to be 52%–75% in clinical series [17]. Klinefelter syndrome is the most common karyotype abnormality in infertile men. These men have typically small, atrophic testes, and hypergonadotropic hypogonadism, with tubular hyalinization as the prevalent histopathological pattern [56]. Most Klinefelter men are azoospermic, but residual foci of spermatogenesis can be found with TESE. Reported rates of sperm retrieval in this group are wide (ranging 12%–75%), but real-life series have shown an overall reduced chance of SR compared to men without genetic abnormalities [9, 20]. Lastly, various gene products, long noncoding RNAs, or transcripts in the ejaculate have been investigated as predictors of positive SR, but results are still experimental.

As a whole, there are still several open questions and gray areas around TESE both in terms of procedural effectiveness and predictors of success to select the best candidate for this procedure.

In terms of surgical efficacy, several optimizations have been introduced in the last decades.

- *Advanced TESE*

Several new and promising technologies have recently emerged to aid urologists in sperm retrieval for male infertility. Techniques such as multiphoton microscopy (MPM), Raman spectroscopy (RS), and full-field optical coherence tomography (FFOCT) can assist in distinguishing tubules with and without spermatogenesis during micro-TESE procedures, a role that can potentially also be fulfilled by Doppler ultrasound (US). Additionally, ORBEYE technology presents itself as a viable alternative to traditional microscopy techniques.

Multiphoton Microscopy

MPM provides high-resolution images in real time without the need for physical extraction. It uses a pulsed femtosecond near-infrared laser with two/three low-energy photons to generate excitation of intrinsic fluorophores, resulting in auto-fluorescence. Among the advantages of this technique are the depth of penetration (up to 400 μm below the surface) and the unnecessity of additional coloring (which can damage spermatozoa).

Furthermore, this technique helps pinpoint sperm-containing tubules while preserving Leydig cells and enables the visualization of peritubular fibrosis, a common feature in testes with defective spermatogenesis.

In a pilot study conducted by Najari et al., MPM exhibited a 92% concordance rate in diagnosis compared to Hematoxylin and eosin (H&E) staining in men with non-obstructive azoospermia (NOA). Still, there are some concerns regarding laser intensity and ethical issues in assisted reproduction. Especially, safety concerns include the risk of DNA damage, potentially leading to genetic abnormalities in IVF (in vitro fertilization) gametes, though rodent models show minimal phototoxicity, human validation is essential [39, 50, 59].

Raman Spectroscopy

Raman spectroscopy (RS) is a laser-based technique used in reproductive medicine to assess sperm DNA integrity and identify spermatozoa capable of zona pellucida binding. It operates on the principle of inelastic scattering from molecular vibrations and the generation of the so-called Raman spectra. In rat models, RS showed high sensitivity and specificity in detecting spermatogenesis in Sertoli cell-only histology, suggesting potential for improving sperm retrieval rates with RS-guided micro-TESE. This technique, although non-invasive and non-destructive, needs further evaluation of safety in human use. Additionally, the RS offers real-time analysis, but each assessment consumes approximately 2 min, with results potentially affected by light contamination [52].

Full-Field Optical Coherence Tomography

FFOCT, a technique based on white-light interference microscopy using a 150-W halogen lamp, offers high-resolution imaging of unprocessed tissue. Its advantages include speed (1 frame/s) and safe light from a 150-W halogen lamp, suitable for IVF with ICSI. In an animal study, FFOCT was able to distinguish between tubules with and without spermatogenesis in specimens from a busulfan-treated rodent model, specifically FFOCT identified spermatogenesis by detecting a bright signal emanating from the unique microtubular structure in sperm tails [60]. Yet, limitations of this technique include the absence of cellular details, the limited imaging depth, and the inability to image live specimens. Its efficacy in human testicular tissue remains unexplored, leaving uncertainty about its ability to identify spermatogenesis due to the complex cellular structures.

ORBEYE

The ORBEYE 4 K 3D microscope is a surgical exoscope, or "camera," designed to enhance urological microsurgical procedures such as microepididymal sperm aspiration (MESA) or micro-TESE. It features two Sony 4 K (4096 × 2160 pixels) Exmor R CMOS image sensors, which enable high sensitivity, low noise, and a wide color range image. Positioned over the surgical field, the exoscope projects the image onto two 140-cm (55-inch) monitors, allowing for active 3D viewing with lightweight passive light 3D glasses.

In urology, ORBEYE was compared to traditional operating microscopes for vasectomy reversal in a prospective randomized controlled animal trial, finding no significant differences in terms of patency, operating time, or granuloma formation [6].

Another study examined operating times and surgeon fatigue for urological microsurgery, showing potentially shorter varicocelectomy times with ORBEYE. To summarize, ORBEYE offers logistical advantages such as maneuverability and an ergonomic design, but comes with a higher cost. It may also pose challenges for surgical assistants due to the rotated view projected onto the monitor [45].

Ultrasonography

Testicular imaging is of great interest for men with NOA due to the invasiveness of biopsies and the limited predictive ability of clinical characteristics. Ultrasound (US) is being investigated as a non-invasive and widely accessible method for evaluating patients undergoing testicular sperm retrieval.

In NOA men, testicular structure and blood flow are significantly altered, often showing decreased or absent intratesticular arterial flow compared to normal testes. Conversely, men with obstructive azoospermia (OA) typically have uniform flow patterns similar to controls [29]. Previous studies have suggested a correlation between testicular blood flow and volume in young boys, indicating a potential relationship between blood flow and testicular function during spermatogenesis.

Studies on patients with NOA have shown that sperm quality is highest in testicular areas with high sperm perfusion. High levels of perfusion correlate with a greater success rate of sperm retrieval from TESE [35]. Additionally, researchers developed a non-invasive method using Doppler ultrasound (US) for testicular screening, which has low sensitivity but high specificity: This method is particularly useful for predicting the absence of spermatozoa and avoiding areas of absent spermatogenesis.

In a study conducted in 2001 by Belenky et al., it was found that ultrasound-guided testicular sperm aspiration (TESA) was a safe and accurate method for sperm retrieval in patients with NOA when compared to "blind" TESA. However, no significant differences were observed between the two groups in terms of pregnancy rates in the female partners of the patients [2].

In a 2019 study, contrast-enhanced ultrasound (CEUS) was used 10 days prior to testicular sperm aspiration (TESA) in 70 men, 46 with non-obstructive azoospermia (NOA), and others with obstructive azoospermia (OA). The study found that CEUS-guided TESA with cognitive fusion did not improve sperm retrieval outcomes in NOA patients. This could be due to the imprecise correlation between biopsy sites and the main perfusion areas analyzed by CEUS [80].

Finally, research conducted by Herwig et al. on patients with azoospermia undergoing testicular sperm extraction (TESE) biopsy revealed that areas of high tissue perfusion exhibited high sperm quality. Additionally, their findings demonstrated a correlation between the number of motile sperm isolated from tissue samples and the intensity of tissue perfusion as determined by color Doppler ultrasound (US) [36].

Although US shows considerable promise as a prognostic tool for sperm retrieval, its true strength can only be confirmed through external validation. However, there are some limitations to its use in this context. The effectiveness of US outcomes heavily relies on the skills of the operator.

Moreover, previous studies examining testicular perfusion with Doppler US were limited to locating main arteries in the testes and were unable to resolve microvasculature. However, dense microvasculature significantly contributes to high blood testicular perfusion, which correlates with focal spermatogenesis [51]. Despite the mentioned limitations, Doppler ultrasound (US) holds significant potential as an effective tool to aid in sperm retrieval procedures.

Artificial Intelligence

AI has been largely used to better predict SRR after TESE by integrating various predictors and machine learning methods [82]. However, a few reports have also proposed AI to guide surgical approaches. Ichioka et al. used AI to develop a systematic procedure for micro-TESE to maximize surface area and achieve a high sperm retrieval rate. Using a three-dimensional (3D) simulation model, they found that longitudinal incision on the tunica albuginea and following transverse slicing incisions in the testicular parenchyma maximized the surface area and improved the SRR of micro-TESE [37].

Idiopathic Obstructive Azoospermia

Obstructive azoospermia (OA) is the absence of spermatozoa in two centrifuged samples of ejaculate due to obstruction. It occurs in 40% of azoospermia, and it is less common than non-obstructive azoospermia [46].

In case of OA, obstruction may occur at various levels along the male reproductive tract, including the testes, epididymis, rete testis, efferent ducts, and ejaculatory ducts.

When diagnosing OA, a typical patient will have a normal FSH level indicative of normal spermatogenesis, normal-sized testes, and enlarged epididymis observed on ultrasound (US) imaging. This is because the main site of obstruction is often at the epididymal level [46].

It can be challenging to differentiate OA from late maturation arrest, as both conditions can present with normal gonadotropins level and normal testicular size. In such cases, surgical exploration is usually required to determine the underlying cause.

The treatment of OA aims to retrieve sperm, and it involves either microsurgical reconstruction or sperm aspiration/retrieval without reconstruction.

The choice between reconstruction and sperm retrieval is influenced by factors such as the desired number of children, previous surgical history, past fertility as a couple, the female partner's age, female infertility factors, religious beliefs, the potential for natural conception, and financial consideration [46].

It is not so uncommon to resolve an OA especially if we consider that of the 600.000 men undergoing vasectomy annually in the USA, up to 6% eventually seek vasectomy reversal.

- Intratesticular Obstruction

In case of intratesticular obstruction, TESE is the only recommended method for retrieving sperm.

- Epididymal Obstruction

For bilateral absence of vas deferens, microsurgical procedures such as MESA or PESA are indicated. TESE and percutaneous techniques like testicular sperm aspiration (TESA) can also be performed. Typically, one MESA procedure provides sufficient material for several Assisted Reproductive Technology (ART) cycles with a high fertilization rate.

For OA secondary to acquired epididymal obstruction, and with a female partner having good ovarian reserve, microsurgical vasoepididymostomy (VE) is recommended. Various techniques, such as end-to-side and intussusception, have been proposed.

Before microsurgery, and in cases where recanalization is impossible, epididymal spermatozoa should be retrieved intra-operatively by MESA and cryopreserved for subsequent ART procedures.

- Vas Deferens Obstruction

Vas Deferens Obstruction After Vasectomy

In case of vas deferens obstruction after vasectomy, microsurgical vasectomy reversal is necessary.

It can be performed for the desire to have more children, post-vasectomy pain management, or as treatment for iatrogenic (herniorrhaphy, orchidopexy, hydrocelectomy), traumatic, or infectious causes of obstruction.

The reported patency and pregnancy rates are 90%–97% and 52%–73%, respectively. The average time to patency is 1.7–4.3 months, and late failure is rare (0%–12%).

Robot-assisted vasovasostomy has similar success, but larger studies are needed to define its benefits over standard microsurgical procedures. The absence of spermatozoa in vas deferens fluid during surgery suggests secondary epididymal obstruction; in this case, microsurgical VE may be indicated.

Vas deferens Obstruction at the Inguinal Level

In case of vas deferens obstruction secondary to iatrogenic damage (hernial surgery or orchidopexy), correction surgery is not possible. In these cases, TESE, MESA, or PESA or proximal vas deferens sperm aspiration should be done, and sperm retrieval is used for ART.

- Ejaculatory Duct Obstruction

The treatment of ejaculatory duct obstruction depends on its etiology.

Transurethral resection of the ejaculatory ducts (TURED) can be used in post-inflammatory obstruction and cystic obstruction. In cases of obstruction caused by an intraprostatic cyst, treatment typically requires incision, unroofing, or aspiration of the cyst. Intraoperative TRUS makes this procedure safer.

Pregnancy rates after TURED are 20%–25%, with complications including epididymitis, UTI, gross hematuria, hematospermia, urinary reflux into the ejaculatory ducts and seminal vesicles.

Alternative therapeutic strategies include seminal vesiculoscopy, balloon dilatation or laser incision, MESA, PESA, TESE, proximal vas deferens sperm aspiration, and seminal vesicle-ultrasonically guided aspiration.

Microsurgical VE

Between 1978 and 2005, most VE surgeries utilized end-to-end or end-to-side technique. After 2005, the majority of studies employed the intussusception technique (LIVE—longitudinal intussusception vasoepididymostomy), resulting in a larger diameter for flow from the epididymal tubule to the vas, leading to improved outcomes compared to perpendicular placement of two sutures in the epididymal tubule or 3-suture triangulation technique. The LIVE technique permits accurate approximation of the 300- to 400-micron vasal lumen to the 150- to 250-micron epididymal tubule lumen [81]. However, studies suggested that there is no significant difference in operative time between the 2 suture transverse and LIVE techniques [3].

The European Association of Urology (EAU) guidelines suggest that the patency rate after VE is between 65% and 85%, and cumulative pregnancy rates range between 21% and 44% [46]. However, these values vary widely in the literature due to differences in surgical techniques, surgeon experience, and absence of a standardized definition.

The end-to-end or end-to-side techniques developed between 1978 and 2005 have a patency rate of 61.1% and 70%, respectively, whereas the intussusception technique/LIVE technique results in 90% of patency rate and 40% of pregnancy rates. In contrast, pregnancy rates for end-to-end or end-to-side are 26.9%. In Yoon et al. meta-analysis, the patency is reported as 64.1% (95% CI: 58.5%–69.3%), and the pregnancy rate is 31.1% (95% CI: 26.9%–35.7%) [81]. The mean time to reach patency ranges from 2.8 to 9.6 months. Notably, the variability in reported patency percentages is attributed to the lack of standardized definition. Yoon et al. found that among 42 studies, 15 studies did not specifically define patency, while others used different criteria such as the presence of spermatozoa or motile spermatozoa, with varying concentration threshold. Surgeon skills also influence patency rates.

The mean time to achieve pregnancy is reported between 6.9 and 9.9 months. Comparing pregnancy rates is challenging due to the lack of a specific definition for pregnancy, which can be defined biochemically or clinically detected by ultrasound.

Anastomosis sites are also a significant predictor of patency and pregnancy rates (*p*-value = 0.035). The patency rate was 22.2% for head anastomosis, 63.3% for body anastomosis, and 87.0% for tail anastomosis. In their meta-analysis, Yoon et al. compared the patency rate of different sites of anastomosis; particularly in the caudal or corpus area, anastomosis was found to be favorable for patency rate in microsurgical VE (RR = 1.17%; 95% CI: 1.01%–1.35%; *P* value = 0.04).

Predictors of pregnancy are various and include male and female age, sperm concentration, and forward motility. According to Peng et al., overall patency and live birth rate after VE are 76.3% and 34.8%, respectively [54].

Vasectomy Reversal

Vasectomy stands as safe and effective male contraceptive method chosen by 42–60 million men globally, constituting the preference for 6%–8% of married couples.

Vasectomy encompasses a spectrum of surgical techniques, typically executed in two distinct steps: vas deferens isolation and subsequent vas occlusion.

The first step of vasectomy includes two main different way of vas isolation

- Conventional Vasectomy (CV).
- Minimally Invasive Vasectomy (MIV)—including no-scalpel vasectomy (NSV).
- Conventional Vasectomy (CV) does not require specific instruments and it is performed by making either one midline incision or bilateral scrotal incisions (among 1.5–3 cm) using a scalpel, then the vas is grasped with a towel clip or an Allis forceps.
- No-scalpel vasectomy (NSV) was developed in 1974 in China by Dr. Li Shunqiang, and it was the first minimally invasive technique for vasectomy. To be defined NSV is necessary for the approach to the vas deferens the use of vas ring clamp and vas dissector (both of which have been specially designed for no-scalpel vasectomy. The vas ring clamp is placed around the vas, perivasal tissue, and overlying skin before making the skin opening and creates a skin opening of ≤10 mm by piercing the skin with the vas dissector followed by spreading the tissue overlying the vas with the vas dissector or similar. This technique allows to leave the skin opening unsutured either as a single midline opening or as bilateral openings [49].
- Minimally Invasive Vasectomy (MIV) should be performed either as an open access approach or a closed access approach, in fact it is possible to isolate the vas deferens—with vas ring clamp or other similar instruments—before or after skin incision, depending on the characteristics of the patient's tissues.

It can be performed one midline (just below the penoscrotal junction) or bilateral scrotal (at the level of the penoscrotal junction or higher) skin incision, but to date there is no evidence in favor of one or other approach, so it depends on the surgeon's preference.

Vas Occlusion

Various techniques of vas occlusion have been described, and it is good to point out that, virtually, all techniques of vasectomy use complete division of the vas with or without excision of a segment; in fact, according to AUA guide lines, there is no consistent evidence supporting the superiority, in terms of effectiveness, of section, and excision of a portion of the vas deferens over the section alone.

- Fascial interposition (FI) involves the placement of a layer of the internal spermatic fascia between the two divided vas ends, and it is usually combined with ligation and excision or mucosal cautery
- Ligation technique with the occlusion of the vas with ligatures (from 1 to 3 on each ends) with division and excision of vas segment of 1 cm approximately.
- Clips technique with the occlusion of the vas with clips with division and excision between the clips.
- Folding back technique which provides the fold and suture of each divided vas end on itself.
- Mucosal cautery (MC) applying thermal or electrical cautery to vasal mucosa, creating a scar tissue plug, minimizing the damage to the nearby tissue, occluding the vas lumen.

Vasectomy reversal encompasses surgical techniques aimed at reconstructing the interrupted spermatic pathway, specifically through vasovasostomy (VV) and vasoepididymostomy (VE).

Vasovasostomy can be performed with various anastomotic techniques:

- One-Layer Technique: It is a full-thickness suture through all layers of the vas, and there is also a modified one-layer technique, in which an additional layer of interrupted seromuscolar suture is placed. This technique is relatively simple and fast and it does not require specific microsurgical instrumentation, but does not account for discrepant lumen size.
- Two-Layer Technique: An inner layer of suture is placed to bring the mucosa together; then an outer layer closing the seromuscolar layers is placed.

These two techniques have been compared demonstrating similar patency outcomes.

Vasoepididymostomy has been previously described.

Robotic Vasectomy Reversal

In 2003, Schoor et al. conducted the first study using an ex vivo rat model to assess the feasibility of robotic-assisted VR [67].

Following this, in 2010 Parekattil et al. published the first series of robotic VR compared with microsurgical VR performing a three-layer [53].

The robot-assisted VR begins in the same way as microsurgical VR: A paramedian incision is made and the testis is delivered from the scrotum, the site of vasectomy is identified, and the proximal and distal ends of the vas deferens are isolated using towel clips and fine hemostats taking care not to injure the blood supply further than it was during the vasectomy. The ends of the vas deferens are transected, the ends are approximated using a vasovasostomy clamp, and then, the robot is brought into the operating field. The robotic anastomosis starts with loading two microforceps into the robot. The surgeon uses 9–0 nylon sutures to perform the anastomosis according to the various techniques discussed, depending on his or her preference; at the end, the third arm of the robot can be loaded with scissors to cut the sutures. After performing the microsurgical part of the anastomosis, the robot is pulled away from the operating table and the anastomosis is covered with perivasal tissue and the scrotal wounds are closed.

The robotic technique, compared with the microsurgical technique, allows better preservation of vascular support, and the use of robotic arms in anastomosis increases its accuracy by reducing hand tremor and imprecision.

Literature available on VR highlights several advantages of robotic surgery over microscopic surgery. These include a decrease in operative time (97 min in the VR vs 120 min in the microscopic technique), an increase in patency rate (96% in VR cases vs 80% in microsurgical cases), and a reduction in the learning curve (11 h of robot course and VR practice vs 40 h go microsurgey course.

Disadvantages of robotic VR include high costs, the necessity of a specialized team, and specialized microsurgical robotic instruments. Additionally, there's the challenge of inferior magnification (×10–15) compared to a microscope (×20–30), particularly evident during VE. Consequently, current literature primarily focuses on vasovasostomy (VV) due to this magnification limitation.

Onco-TESE

Definition and Indications

Sperm cryopreservation is widely recognized as an effective method of preserving male fertility in patients affected by testicular cancer (TC). In cases of azoospermia, cryptozoospermia or failure to retrieve sperm (due to medical, cultural, or religious factors), a TESE specifically called onco-TESE, either performed with microscope or using conventional methods, can be indicated to preserve fertility; however, data regarding onco-TESE are currently limited in the literature [48].

Given the youthfulness of patients and the high rates of cancer-specific survival, preserving fertility is a crucial consideration in the treatment of TC, as it may result in a temporary or permanent decrease in fertility. This concern is particularly relevant due to the growing prevalence of infertility among couples, notably in developed countries, and the fact that TC itself poses a risk factor for infertility. A significant proportion of TC patients (approximately 50%) exhibit abnormalities in seminal fluid parameters even before treatment initiation. These changes can range from mild to severe, with azoospermia observed in around 10%–15% of cases.

The initial instance of onco-TESE, involving testicular biopsy and cryopreservation of viable sperm prior to orchiectomy for TC, was documented by Res et al. in 1997 [61]. Subsequently, the term "onco-TESE" was coined by Schrader et al. in 2003 [68], when they presented the first retrospective series on onco-TESE, encompassing 31 azoospermic TC patients. This series also involved non-germ cell tumors, including Hodgkin Disease ($n = 7$) and Non-Hodgkin lesions ($n = 10$).

In the most recent literature analysis of 2023 [19], a total of 23 articles were retrieved investigating onco-TESE conducted before the onset of gonadotoxic treatment (Table 11.1). Among these articles, the majority (15) were either case reports or case series, while 8 were retrospective studies. Collectively, 139 onco-TESE procedures were executed, with 108 performed on individuals diagnosed with azoospermia. The retrospective investigations documented positive sperm retrieval rates ranging from 33% to 83%. Case reports primarily detailed TESE procedures resulting in the retrieval and cryopreservation of spermatozoa. The utilization of retrieved sperm was assessed in 6 retrospective studies and 8 case reports, encompassing a total of 22 ICSI cycles, leading to 17 pregnancies or live births. TESE was the most frequently performed technique (94 cases), followed by micro-TESE described in 45 cases. Importantly, the Onco-TESE procedure did not delay the initiation of adjuvant therapy in any case, supporting its oncological safety.

Table 11.1 List of papers investigating onco-TESE outcomes

Study	Study type	Sample size	AZO[1]. *n*	OAT[2] or Crypt[3] *n*	Others[4] *n*	Cancer type	Surgery	SRR[5] *n* (%)	ART[6]
Res et al. [61]	Case report	1	1	–	–	SGCT[7]	TESE[12]	1 (100)	1 LB[14]
Schrader et al. [68]	Retrospective study	31	31	–	–	8 SGCT, 6 NSGCT[8], 7 HD[9], 10 NHL[10]	TESE	14 (45.2)	1 miscarriage and 1 LB
Binsaleh et al. [7]	Case report	2	2	–	–	2 NGCT	m-TESE[13]	1 (50)	1 pregnancy
Carmignani et al. [16]	Case report	4	4	–	–	2 SGCT; 2 NSGCT	m-TESE	3 (75)	1 ICSI[15]
Descombe et al. [23]	Case report	2	1	1	–	1 SGCT; 2NSGCT	TESE	2 (100%)	1 LB
Hallak et al. [33]	Retrospective study	5	5	–	–	1 SGCT, 5 NGTT[11]	m-TESE	4 (80.0)	1 LB
Safsaf et al. [64]	Case report	1	1	–	–	1 SGCT	TESE	1 (100)	None
Furuhashi et al. [30]	Retrospective study	6	4	2	–	3 SGCT, 2 NSGCT, 1 NGTT	TESE	4 (66,7)	1 pregnancy
Berookhim and Mulhall [5]	Retrospective study	21	11	2	8	N/A	TESE	8 (38.1)	None
Haddad et al. [32]	Case report	1	–	1	–	1 SGCT	TESE	1 (100)	None
Roque et al. [63]	Case report	1	1	–	–	1 SGCT	TESE	1 (100)	1 LB
Luján et al. [43]	Case report	1	1	–	–	1 SGCT	TESE	1 (100)	1 LB
Pindoria et al. [55]	Case report	1	1	–	–	1 epididymal papillary cystadenocarcinoma	TESE and m-TESE	1 (100)	1 LB
Tsutsumi et al. [75]	Case report	2	2	–	–	2 SGCT	TESE	1 (50)	None
Kuroda et al. [41]	Case report	1	1	–	–	1 SGCT	m-TESE	1 (100)	None

Sener et al. [70]	Case report	1	–	1	–	1 SGCT	TESE	1 (100)	None
Takeshima et al. [73]	Case report	1	1	–	–	1 epidermal cyst	TESE	1 (100)	None
Hayashi et al. [34]	Case report	1	1	–	–	1 SGCT	TESE	1 (100)	1 LB
Blecher et al. [8])	Retrospective study	13	12	1	–	3 SGCT; 4 NSGCT; 4 NGTT; 2 benign lesions	m-TESE	10 (83)	1 miscarriage; 6 LB
Giwerc et al. [31]	Retrospective study	24	9	5	10	13 SGCT; 11 NSGCT	TESE	14 (58,3)	1 ICSI
Scott et al. [69]	Retrospective study	9	9	–	–	N/A	m-TESE	7 (78%)	None
Symeonidis et al. [72]	Case report	1	1	–	–	NSGCT	m-TESE	1 (100)	None
Cirigliano et al. [19]	Retrospective study	9	9	–	–	4 SGCT; 5 NSGCT	m-TESE	3 (33,3)	1 miscarriage 1 LB

Varicocele

Effect of Varicocele on Male Fertility

Varicocele is a common risk factor for male infertility. Although varicocele is present in nearly 15% of the general male population, it is important to note that not all men with varicocele experience infertility and the degree of impact can vary. Varicocele is found in approximately 35%–40% of men presenting with infertility. Specifically, the incidence of varicocele among men with primary infertility is around 35%–44%, while among men with secondary infertility, it ranges from 45% to 81% [38]. The impact on male fertility is evident through observed alterations in semen analysis in 25% of men with varicocele. Agarwal et al. identified reduced sperm count, impaired mobility, and abnormal morphology in men with varicocele compared to those without the condition [1].

Several factors have been suggested as contributing to a multifactorial decline in fertility:

- Scrotal Hyperthermia: The retrograde venous reflux from major veins, more frequently the left renal vein or the inferior vena cava, toward the veins of the pampiniform plexus can elevate testicular temperature with inhibition of spermatogenesis. In addition to this, in hyperthermic environments, germ cells undergo apoptosis as a consequence of increased oxidative stress.
- Increase in Hydrostatic Pressure and Hypoxia: Venous reflux within the pampiniform plexus induces increased venous pressure, vessel dilation, and venous stasis. The compromised venous drainage induces high hydrostatic pressures within the venules of the microcirculation in the testis. When the venous pressure exceeds the arteriolar pressure, it leads to hypoxia and ischemic damage to the testicular tissues through inflammatory reactions and the hypoxia induction factor (HIF) pathway, ultimately resulting in impaired sperm quality and a decrease in quantity (10). Moreover, elevated endovascular pressure on the venous vessel walls may result in an increased release of reactive oxygen species (ROS).
- Oxidative Stress: In the presence of varicocele, the heightened ROS levels cause ROS-mediated peroxidative damage to the sperm plasma membranes, rich in polyunsaturated fatty acids, and DNA mutations and fragmentation at both nuclear and mitochondrial levels, resulting in cellular apoptosis and a change in the fertilizing capacity of the spermatozoa.
- Backflow of Renal and/or Adrenal Metabolites Within the Venous Plexus of the Testis: These might contribute to vasodilatory effect and worsening of venous stasis.
- Hormonal Alterations. Varicoceles are believed to have a negative impact on the functioning of Sertoli and Leydig cells, leading to an alteration in the hypothalamic–pituitary–gonadal axis. Specifically, a time-dependent dysfunction of Leydig cells may be observed in men aged over 30 with varicoceles, resulting in diminished testosterone production and consequent changes in the spermatogenesis process which is controlled by testosterone signaling.

- Testicular Immune Microenvironment Disorder: In infertile men, an increasing number of studies highlight the detrimental impact of varicocele on the testicular immune system. The dysregulation of the testicular immune system is primarily influenced by alterations in inflammatory pathways and changes in the permeability and structure of the BTB, leading to the development of anti-sperm antibodies (ASAs). When ASAs are present, they bind to sperm, resulting in sperm agglutination, apoptosis of sperm cells, and a reduction in sperm motility. It has been observed that in men with varicocele, the autoimmune anti-sperm reaction is accompanied by a more significant decrease in semen quality (concentration, motility, and morphology), along with acrosome reaction disorders and increased DNA fragmentation. These disorders are linked to the extent of oxidative stress, with ASA-positive varicocele men exhibiting ROS production 2.8 and 3.5 times greater than that observed in ASA-negative varicocele patients and fertile men, respectively.

Nevertheless, none of these mechanisms can independently provide an exact explanation for the deleterious effects of varicoceles on testicular function.

Updated Data Regarding the Impact of Treatment of Male Infertility

The current guidelines provided by the European Association of Urology (EAU) and the American Urologic Association (AUA), as well as the American Society of Reproductive Medicine (ASRM), recommend varicocele repair for men with a clinical varicocele, one or more semen abnormalities, and otherwise unexplained infertility in a couple where the female partner has a good ovarian reserve [46, 66]. EAU guidelines also indicate that varicocele repair may lead to the presence of sperm in the ejaculate for males with non-obstructive azoospermia.

One of the markers used to measure the impact of varicocele repair on male infertility is the evaluation of semen parameters, as they may reflect men's health and testicular function. There is increasing evidence that varicocele repair led to improvement of DNA fragmentation and outcomes of assisted reproductive techniques (ART) [40].

Another emerging tool for evaluating male infertility and predicting outcomes of pregnancy, either natural or with the use of ART, after varicocele repair is the evaluation of sperm DNA fragmentation along with oxidative stress. Recent studies describe the benefits of varicocelectomy in improving DNA integrity, oxidative stress, and semen parameters, resulting in an improvement in male fertility. Notably, varicocele repair in randomized clinical trials has shown a 75% increase in sperm concentration, an 8% improvement in morphology, and a 5.2% enhancement in motility [15]. More recently, a systematic review and meta-analysis including only prospective randomized and nonrandomized studies showed that varicocele treatment improved pregnancy rates (odds ratio 1.29; 95% confidence interval [CI]

1.00–1.65; $p = 0.048$) and sperm concentration (mean difference 12.34 million/ml, 95% CI 3.49–21.18; $p = 0.006$) compared with observation [27].

Various surgical approaches are available for varicocele repair, with the open approach being one of the most commonly used techniques. Updated data regarding the impact of treatment on male infertility have recently become available. Recent evidence suggests that the use of microscope or surgical loupes during the procedure may result in lower rates of recurrence and complications compared to procedures performed without them [79].

Over the years, there has been a growing interest in assessing the advantages of incorporating microsurgery into the surgical treatment of varicocele, due to its resolution that enables excellent identification of anatomical structures. Recent evidence highlights the efficacy of microsurgical varicocelectomy compared to various varicocelectomy techniques. This approach not only diminishes postoperative complications and the risk of varicocele recurrence compared to other surgical techniques but also slightly improves pregnancy rates. However, as a drawback, microsurgical treatment is characterized by longer operative times. Comparing traditional open, laparoscopic, and microsurgical varicocelectomy, hydrocele rates were 13%, 20%, and 0.7%, respectively. Moreover, the microsurgical approach showed a 2.1% recurrence rate, contrasting with 4.3% and 14.9% for laparoscopic and traditional open methods, while improvements in semen parameters and birth rates were similar across all techniques. Despite the higher cost of maintaining an operating microscope, along with the investment in microsurgical training, studies have questioned whether traditional loupe magnification is sufficient. Despite better visualization with loupes, surgical outcomes were comparable to the standard approach, highlighting the clear superiority of the surgical microscope in terms of complications and recurrence rates. This evidence emphasizes the essential role of the operating microscope in achieving high-quality varicocelectomy.

In conclusion, considering all the above data, subinguinal microsurgical varicocelectomy is considered the current gold standard for repair.

Endovascular Varicocele Treatment: Lights and Shadows

Endovascular treatment of varicoceles involves the use of imaging guidance and catheter-based interventions to occlude or redirect blood flow within the affected veins. This can be achieved through various techniques, such as coil embolization, sclerotherapy, or balloon occlusion.

Despite the diversity of embolic materials used in varicocele embolization, no studies have shown the superiority of any particular agent. Nevertheless, technical success rates ranging from 95% to 100% have been reported in series published over the past decade.

Major advantages of endovascular treatment of varicocele are the minimally invasive nature: day surgery procedure under local anesthesia, fast recovery, and return to work. However, recurrent rates are reported to be higher compared to microsurgical approach. Complications associated with this procedures are rare mostly related to chemical orchitis and transient testicular pain [46].

Robotic Varicocelectomy, the Use of 3D Videomicroscope

In the 1970s, the operative microscope made its debut in male infertility procedures. Technological innovations in infertility procedures have progressed notably with the incorporation of the da Vinci robotic platform (Intuitive Surgical, Inc., Sunnyvale, CA, USA) into microsurgical procedures.

Varicocele ligation can be performed through various approaches: retroperitoneal (high ligation via open incision or laparoscopic), inguinal, or subinguinal. Evidence suggests that the microsurgical subinguinal approach carries lower risks of recurrence and postoperative complications such as hydrocele and testicular atrophy compared to other methods. Therefore, instead of merely adapting the laparoscopic approach to robotic assistance, initial reports of robotic-assisted varicocelectomy opted for adapting the gold standard subinguinal approach. This decision was influenced by the advantages offered by the robotic in terms of visualization, maneuverability, and precision.

Comparative studies between standard microsurgery and robot-assisted microsurgery showed similar outcomes, with operative times gradually decreasing as surgeons gained experience. The Da Vinci platform allowed for real-time Doppler ultrasonography to assess the location of arteries and veins, contributing to the safety and efficacy of the procedure.

Varicocele Repair for Elevated Sperm DNA Fragmentation

Research indicates that men with varicocele show significantly higher levels of sperm DNA fragmentation (SDF) compared to controls, irrespective of their fertility status [47]. A meta-analysis by Wang et al., encompassing 12 studies (7 assessing SDF in varicocele patients and 6 evaluating surgical outcomes), demonstrated that varicocele was linked to significantly higher SDF levels compared to controls, with a mean difference (MD) of 9.84% (95% CI = 9.19–10.49; $p < 0.00001$). Varicocele treatment led to a significant reduction in SDF levels compared to the control group (MD of −3.37%; 95% CI −4.09 to −2.65; $p < 0.00001$) [78].

A recent review by Roque and Esteves, analyzing 21 studies with over 1200 subjects, explored the impact of varicocele ligation on SDF. The authors noted a consistent decrease in SDF across all studies during a follow-up period ranging from 3 to 12 months [62]. Some studies reported lower SDF values in couples who conceived compared to those who did not. Smit et al. utilized the Sperm Chromatin

Structure Assay (SCSA) in 49 patients before and after varicocelectomy, reporting a significant reduction in SDF values post-surgery (MD = 5%; $p = 0.019$). Among these subjects, 37% conceived spontaneously, and 22% conceived with Assisted Reproductive Technology (ART). SDF levels were significantly lower in patients who conceived, either spontaneously or with ART (26.6% ± 13.7%), compared to those who did not conceive (37.3% ± 13.9%) ($p = 0.013$) [71].

Controversies and Limitations

Major limitation is the low quality evidence of the included studies. Most are retrospective case series, single center thus opening the possibility of selection bias. In terms of technical developments, costs associated with robotics and advanced imaging technology cannot be affordable by all countries.

Future Directions

One of the most debated topics in male infertility is the identification of accurate predictors of successful sperm retrieval (SR) following TESE. Despite recent advances in artificial intelligence and advanced imaging technologies, further improvements are still needed. The ideal marker should be a cost-affordable, easily tested serum predictor of SRR. In this way, epigenetic or genetic factors, integrated with artificial intelligence predictive models, would be ideal to overcome the lack of understanding for sperm recovery.

Conclusion

Multiple new promising technologies have emerged recently to assist urologists during sperm retrieval for a male with infertility or to improve sperm recovery in men with varicocele. The use of MPM, RS, and FFOCT during a micro-TESE procedure can help distinguish tubules with and without spermatogenesis, a role that can also be potentially played by Doppler US. ORBEYE technology can be used as a valid alternative to the traditional microscopy technique. Robotic approach has been introduced in vasectomy reversal and in men with varicocele, but results are still not superior to microscopic approach. All these advantages are associated with higher costs, which cannot be sustained by all countries. Health economics should always be considered when introducing new developments in clinical practice.

References

1. Agarwal A, Sharma R, Harlev A, Esteves SC. Effect of varicocele on semen characteristics according to the new 2010 World Health Organization criteria: a systematic review and meta-analysis. Asian J Androl. 2016;18:163–70.
2. Belenky A, Avrech OM, Bachar GN, Zuckerman Z, Ben Rafael Z, Fisch B, Cohen M. Ultrasound-guided testicular sperm aspiration in azoospermic patients: a new sperm retrieval method for intracytoplasmic sperm injection. J Clin Ultrasound. 2001;29:339–43.
3. Belker AM, Thomas AJ, Fuchs EF, Konnak JW, Sharlip ID. Results of 1,469 microsurgical vasectomy reversals by the Vasovasostomy Study Group. J Urol. 1991;145:505–11.
4. Bernie AM, Mata DA, Ramasamy R, Schlegel PN. Comparison of microdissection testicular sperm extraction, conventional testicular sperm extraction, and testicular sperm aspiration for nonobstructive azoospermia: a systematic review and meta-analysis. Fertil Steril. 2015;104:1099–1103.e13.
5. Berookhim BM, Mulhall JP. Outcomes of operative sperm retrieval strategies for fertility preservation among males scheduled to undergo cancer treatment. Fertil Steril. 2014;101:805–11. https://doi.org/10.1016/j.fertnstert.2013.11.122.
6. Best JC, Gonzalez D, Alawamlh OAH, Li PS, Ramasamy R. Use of 4K3D video microscope in male infertility microsurgery. Urol Video J. 2020;7:100046.
7. Binsaleh S, Sircar K, Chan PTK. Feasibility of simultaneous testicular microdissection for sperm retrieval and ipsilateral testicular tumor resection in azoospermic men. J Androl. 2004;25:867–71. https://doi.org/10.1002/j.1939-4640.2004.tb03155.x.
8. Blecher GA, Chung E, Katz D, Kim SHK, Bailie J. Onco-testicular sperm extraction (onco-TESE): a contemporary concept review and report of Australian sperm retrieval rates and fertility outcomes. Urology. 2022;160:109–16.
9. Boeri L, Palmisano F, Preto M, Sibona M, Capogrosso P, Franceschelli A, Ruiz-Castañé E, Sarquella-Geli J, Bassas-Arnau L, Scroppo FI, et al. Sperm retrieval rates in non-mosaic Klinefelter patients undergoing testicular sperm extraction: what expectations do we have in the real-life setting? Andrology. 2020;8:680–7.
10. Boeri L, Pederzoli F, Capogrosso P, Abbate C, Alfano M, Mancini N, Clementi M, Montanari E, Montorsi F, Salonia A. Semen infections in men with primary infertility in the real-life setting. Fertil Steril. 2020;113:1174–82.
11. Boeri L, Belladelli F, Capogrosso P, Cazzaniga W, Candela L, Pozzi E, Valsecchi L, Papaleo E, Viganò P, Abbate C, et al. Normal sperm parameters per se do not reliably account for fertility: a case-control study in the real-life setting. Andrologia. 2021;53:e13861.
12. Boeri L, Capogrosso P, Ortensi I, Miacola C, Cai T, Verze P, Salonia A, Giammusso B, Palmieri A. Diagnostic and therapeutic workup of male infertility: results from a Delphi consensus panel. Int J Impot Res. 2021;35:1.
13. Boeri L, Capogrosso P, Ventimiglia E, Cazzaniga W, Pozzi E, Belladelli F, Pederzoli F, Alfano M, Abbate C, Montanari E, et al. Testicular volume in infertile versus fertile white-European men: a case-control investigation in the real-life setting. Asian J Androl. 2021;23:501.
14. Boeri L, Bebi C, Dente D, Greco E, Turetti M, Capece M, Cocci A, Cito G, Preto M, Pescatori E, et al. Outcomes and predictive factors of successful salvage microdissection testicular sperm extraction (mTESE) after failed classic TESE: results from a multicenter cross-sectional study. Int J Impot Res. 2022;34:795–9.
15. Cannarella R, Shah R, Hamoda TA-AA-M, Boitrelle F, Saleh R, Gul M, Rambhatla A, Kavoussi P, Toprak T, Harraz AM, et al. Does varicocele repair improve conventional semen parameters? A meta-analytic study of before-after data. World J Mens Health. 2024;42:92–132.
16. Carmignani L, Gadda F, Gazzano G, Ragni G, Paffoni A, Rocco F, Colpi GM. Testicular sperm extraction in cancerous testicle in patients with azoospermia: a case report. Hum Reprod. 2007;22:1068–72. https://doi.org/10.1093/humrep/del468.

17. Caroppo E, Colpi GM. Prediction models for successful sperm retrieval in patients with non-obstructive azoospermia undergoing microdissection testicular sperm extraction: is there any room for further studies? J Clin Med. 2021;10:5538.
18. Cioppi F, Rosta V, Krausz C. Genetics of azoospermia. Int J Mol Sci. 2021;22:3264.
19. Cirigliano L, Falcone M, Gül M, Preto M, Ceruti C, Plamadeala N, Peretti F, Ferro I, Scavone M, Gontero P. Onco-TESE (Testicular Sperm Extraction): insights from a tertiary center and comprehensive literature analysis. Med Kaunas Lith. 2023;59:1226.
20. Corona G, Pizzocaro A, Lanfranco F, Garolla A, Pelliccione F, Vignozzi L, Ferlin A, Foresta C, Jannini EA, Maggi M, et al. Sperm recovery and ICSI outcomes in Klinefelter syndrome: a systematic review and meta-analysis. Hum Reprod Update. 2017;23:265–75.
21. Corona G, Minhas S, Giwercman A, Bettocchi C, Dinkelman-Smit M, Dohle G, Fusco F, Kadioglou A, Kliesch S, Kopa Z, et al. Sperm recovery and ICSI outcomes in men with non-obstructive azoospermia: a systematic review and meta-analysis. Hum Reprod Update. 2019;25:733–57.
22. Deruyver Y, Vanderschueren D, Van der Aa F. Outcome of microdissection TESE compared with conventional TESE in non-obstructive azoospermia: a systematic review. Andrology. 2014;2:20–4.
23. Descombe L, Chauleur C, Gentil-Perret A, Aknin-Seifer I, Tostain J, Lévy R. Testicular sperm extraction in a single cancerous testicle in patients with azoospermia: a case report. Fertil Steril. 2008;90:443.e1–4. https://doi.org/10.1016/j.fertnstert.2007.07.1308.
24. Eliveld J, van Wely M, Meißner A, Repping S, van der Veen F, van Pelt AM. The risk of TESE-induced hypogonadism: a systematic review and meta-analysis. Hum Reprod Update. 2018;24:442–54.
25. Falcone M, Boeri L, Timpano M, Cirigliano L, Preto M, Russo GI, Peretti F, Ferro I, Plamadeala N, Gontero P. Combined trifocal and microsurgical testicular sperm extraction enhances sperm retrieval rate in low-chance retrieval non-obstructive azoospermia. J Clin Med. 2022;11:4058.
26. Fallara G, Cazzaniga W, Boeri L, Capogrosso P, Candela L, Pozzi E, Belladelli F, Schifano N, Ventimiglia E, Abbate C, et al. Male factor infertility trends throughout the last 10 years: report from a tertiary-referral academic andrology centre. Andrology. 2021;9:610–7.
27. Fallara G, Capogrosso P, Pozzi E, Belladelli F, Corsini C, Boeri L, Candela L, Schifano N, Dehò F, Castiglione F, et al. The effect of varicocele treatment on fertility in adults: a systematic review and meta-analysis of published prospective trials. Eur Urol Focus. 2023;9:154–61.
28. Flannigan R, Bach PV, Schlegel PN. Microdissection testicular sperm extraction. Transl Androl Urol. 2017;6:745–52.
29. Foresta C, Garolla A, Bettella A, Ferlin A, Rossato M, Candiani F. Doppler ultrasound of the testis in azoospermic subjects as a parameter of testicular function. Hum Reprod Oxf Engl. 1998;13:3090–3.
30. Furuhashi K, Ishikawa T, Hashimoto H, Yamada S, Ogata S, Mizusawa Y, Matsumoto Y, Okamoto E, Kokeguchi S, Shiotani M. Onco-testicular sperm extraction: testicular sperm extraction in azoospermic and very severely oligozoospermic cancer patients. Andrologia. 2013;45:107–10. https://doi.org/10.1111/j.1439-0272.2012.01319.x.
31. Giwerc A, Chebbi A, Dupuis H, Chiavelli H, Cornu J-N, Pfister C, Safsaf A, Rives N, Sibert L. Onco-TESE and testicular cancer. Prog Urol. 2021;31:293–302. https://doi.org/10.1016/j.purol.2020.09.019.
32. Haddad N, Al-Rabeeah K, Onerheim R, Zini A. Is ex vivo microdissection testicular sperm extraction indicated for infertile men undergoing radical orchiectomy for testicular cancer? Case report and literature review. Fertil Steril. 2014;101:956–9. https://doi.org/10.1016/j.fertnstert.2013.12.052.
33. Hallak J, Cocuzza M, Sarkis AS, Athayde KS, Cerri GG, Srougi M. Organ-sparing microsurgical resection of incidental testicular tumors plus microdissection for sperm extraction and cryopreservation in Azoospermic patients: surgical aspects and technical refinements. Urology. 2009;73:887–91.; discussion 891–892. https://doi.org/10.1016/j.urology.2008.08.510.

34. Hayashi K, Inamoto T, Azuma H, Masuda H, Oku H. A case of congenital single testis with testicular cancer patient and azoospermia who was able to collect spermatozoa with ipsilateral Onco-TESE. Clin Case Rep. 2021;9:535–9. https://doi.org/10.1002/ccr3.3576.
35. Herwig R, Tosun K, Pinggera GM, Soelder E, Moeller KT, Pallwein L, Frauscher E, Bartsch G, Wildt L, Illmensee K. Tissue perfusion essential for spermatogenesis and outcome of testicular sperm extraction (TESE) for assisted reproduction. J Assist Reprod Genet. 2004;21:175–80.
36. Herwig R, Tosun K, Schuster A, Rehder P, Glodny B, Wildt L, Illmensee K, Pinggera G-M. Tissue perfusion-controlled guided biopsies are essential for the outcome of testicular sperm extraction. Fertil Steril. 2007;87:1071–6.
37. Ichioka K, Matsui Y, Terada N, Negoro H, Goto T, Ogawa O. Three-dimensional simulation analysis of microdissection testicular sperm extraction for patients with non-obstructive azoospermia. Andrology. 2020;8:1214–21.
38. Jarow JP, Coburn M, Sigman M. Incidence of varicoceles in men with primary and secondary infertility. Urology. 1996;47:73–6.
39. Katz MJ, Huland DM, Ramasamy R. Multiphoton microscopy: applications in urology and andrology. Transl Androl Urol. 2014;3:77–83.
40. Kirby EW, Wiener LE, Rajanahally S, Crowell K, Coward RM. Undergoing varicocele repair before assisted reproduction improves pregnancy rate and live birth rate in azoospermic and oligospermic men with a varicocele: a systematic review and meta-analysis. Fertil Steril. 2016;106:1338–43.
41. Kuroda S, Kondo T, Mori K, Yasuda K, Asai T, Sanjo H, Yakanaka H, Takeshima T, Kawahara T, Kato Y, et al. Successful onco-testicular sperm extraction from a testicular cancer patient with a single testis and azoospermia. Clin Exp Reprod Med. 2018;45:44–7. https://doi.org/10.5653/cerm.2018.45.1.44.
42. Li H, Chen L-P, Yang J, Li M-C, Chen R-B, Lan R-Z, Wang S-G, Liu J-H, Wang T. Predictive value of FSH, testicular volume, and histopathological findings for the sperm retrieval rate of microdissection TESE in nonobstructive azoospermia: a meta-analysis. Asian J Androl. 2018;20:30–6.
43. Luján S, Guzman-Ordaz D, Rogel R, Broseta E, Pellicer A, Boronat F. ONCO-TESE: obtaining spermatozoa after radical orchiectomy for testicular tumour and azoospermia. Actas Urol Esp. 2016;40:64–7. https://doi.org/10.1016/j.acuro.2015.06.009.
44. Mehta A, Li PS. Male infertility microsurgical training. Asian J Androl. 2013;15:61–6.
45. Meltzer AJ, Hallbeck MS, Morrow MM, Lowndes BR, Davila VJ, Stone WM, Money SR. Measuring ergonomic risk in operating surgeons by using wearable technology. JAMA Surg. 2020;155:444–6.
46. Minhas S, Bettocchi C, Boeri L, Capogrosso P, Carvalho J, Cilesiz NC, Cocci A, Corona G, Dimitropoulos K, Gül M, et al. European association of urology guidelines on male sexual and reproductive health: 2021 update on male infertility. Eur Urol. 2021;S0302–2838(21):01982–5.
47. Moazzam A, Sharma R, Agarwal A. Relationship of spermatozoal DNA fragmentation with semen quality in varicocele-positive men. Andrologia. 2015;47:935–44.
48. Moody JA, Ahmed K, Horsfield C, Pedersen MRV, Yap T, Shabbir M. Fertility preservation in testicular cancer - predictors of spermatogenesis. BJU Int. 2018;122:236–42.
49. Moon HJ. Minimally invasive vas surgery using a newly designed double-ringed clamp. World J Urol. 2010;28:205–8.
50. Najari BB, Ramasamy R, Sterling J, Aggarwal A, Sheth S, Li PS, Dubin JM, Goldenberg S, Jain M, Robinson BD, et al. Pilot study of the correlation of multiphoton tomography of ex vivo human testis with histology. J Urol. 2012;188:538–43.
51. Nariyoshi S, Nakano K, Sukegawa G, Sho T, Tsuji Y. Ultrasonographically determined size of seminiferous tubules predicts sperm retrieval by microdissection testicular sperm extraction in men with nonobstructive azoospermia. Fertil Steril. 2020;113:97–104.e2.
52. Osterberg EC, Laudano MA, Ramasamy R, Sterling J, Robinson BD, Goldstein M, Li PS, Haka AS, Schlegel PN. Identification of spermatogenesis in a rat sertoli-cell only model using Raman spectroscopy: a feasibility study. J Urol. 2014;192:607–12.

53. Parekattil SJ, Gudeloglu A, Brahmbhatt J, Wharton J, Priola KB. Robotic assisted versus pure microsurgical vasectomy reversal: technique and prospective database control trial. J Reconstr Microsurg. 2012;28:435–44.
54. Peng J, Zhang Z, Yuan Y, Cui W, Song W. Pregnancy and live birth rates after microsurgical vasoepididymostomy for azoospermic patients with epididymal obstruction. Hum Reprod Oxf Engl. 2017;32:284–9.
55. Pindoria N, Miki Y, Tay A, Chandra A, Anderson C, Zacharakis E, Shabbir M. Epididymal papillary cystadenocarcinoma metastasising to the testis in a patient with infertility managed with Onco-microTeSE. J Surg Case Rep. 2016;2016:rjw191. https://doi.org/10.1093/jscr/rjw191.
56. Pozzi E, Boeri L, Capogrosso P, Palmisano F, Preto M, Sibona M, Franceschelli A, Ruiz-Castañé E, Sarquella-Geli J, Bassas-Arnau L, et al. Rates of hypogonadism forms in Klinefelter patients undergoing testicular sperm extraction: a multicenter cross-sectional study. Andrology. 2020;8:1705–11.
57. Pozzi E, Raffo M, Negri F, Boeri L, Saccà A, Belladelli F, Cilio S, Ventimiglia E, Arma A, d' Pagliardini L, et al. Anti-Müllerian hormone predicts positive sperm retrieval in men with idiopathic non-obstructive azoospermia-findings from a multi-centric cross-sectional study. Hum Reprod Oxf Engl. 2023;38:1464–72.
58. Punjani N, Kang C, Schlegel PN. Two decades from the introduction of microdissection testicular sperm extraction: how this surgical technique has improved the management of NOA. J Clin Med. 2021;10:1374.
59. Ramasamy R, Sterling J, Fisher ES, Li PS, Jain M, Robinson BD, Shevchuck M, Huland D, Xu C, Mukherjee S, et al. Identification of spermatogenesis with multiphoton microscopy: an evaluation in a rodent model. J Urol. 2011;186:2487–92.
60. Ramasamy R, Sterling J, Manzoor M, Salamoon B, Jain M, Fisher E, Li PS, Schlegel PN, Mukherjee S. Full field optical coherence tomography can identify spermatogenesis in a rodent sertoli-cell only model. J Pathol Inform. 2012;3:4.
61. Res U, Res P, Kastelic D, Stanovnik M, Kmetec A, Merlo A. Birth after treatment of a male with seminoma and azoospermia with cryopreserved-thawed testicular tissue. Hum Reprod Oxf Engl. 2000;15:861–4.
62. Roque M, Esteves SC. Effect of varicocele repair on sperm DNA fragmentation: a review. Int Urol Nephrol. 2018;50:583–603.
63. Roque M, Sampaio M, Salles PGDO, Geber S. Onco-testicular sperm extraction: birth of a healthy baby after fertility preservation in synchronous bilateral testicular cancer and azoospermia. Andrologia. 2015;47:482–5. https://doi.org/10.1111/and.12292.
64. Safsaf A, Sibert L, Cleret J-M, Perdrix A, Milazzo J-P, Gobet F, Mace B, Rives N. Concomitant unilateral and synchronous bilateral testis cancer in azoospermic dizygotic twins: differential management of fertility preservation. Fertil Steril. 2011;95:2434.e11–3. https://doi.org/10.1016/j.fertnstert.2011.01.153.
65. Schlegel PN. Testicular sperm extraction: microdissection improves sperm yield with minimal tissue excision. Hum Reprod Oxf Engl. 1999;14:131–5.
66. Schlegel PN, Sigman M, Collura B, De Jonge CJ, Eisenberg ML, Lamb DJ, Mulhall JP, Niederberger C, Sandlow JI, Sokol RZ, et al. Diagnosis and treatment of infertility in men: AUA/ASRM guideline part II. Fertil Steril. 2021;115:62–9.
67. Schoor RA, Ross L, Niederberger C. Robotic assisted microsurgical vasal reconstruction in a model system. World J Urol. 2003;21:48–9.
68. Schrader M, Müller M, Sofikitis N, Straub B, Krause H, Miller K. "Onco-tese": testicular sperm extraction in azoospermic cancer patients before chemotherapy-new guidelines? Urology. 2003;61:421–5.
69. Scott C, Omar K, Alnajjar HM, Alifrangis C, Ahmed K, Muneer A. A patient-centric pathway for testicular cancer —A multicentre study investigating the uptake of semen cryopreservation and impact on treatment. Andrology. 2021;9:823–8. https://doi.org/10.1111/andr.12984.

70. Sener TE, Ozveren B, Tinay I, Cam K, Turkeri L. Clinical case discussion: bilateral synchronous testicular cancer and organ-sparing surgery. Eur Urol Focus. 2018;4:737–9. https://doi.org/10.1016/j.euf.2016.08.003.
71. Smit M, Romijn JC, Wildhagen MF, Veldhoven JLM, Weber RFA, Dohle GR. Decreased sperm DNA fragmentation after surgical varicocelectomy is associated with increased pregnancy rate. J Urol. 2013;189:S146–50.
72. Symeonidis EN, Tsifountoudis I, Anastasiadis A, Mutomba WF, Kotakidou R, Hatzichristou D, Dimitriadis F. Synchronous bilateral testicular cancer with discordant histopathology occurring in a 20-year-old patient: a case report and review of the literature. Urol J. 2021;90:434–41. https://doi.org/10.1177/03915603211028556.
73. Takeshima T, Yamamoto M, Takamoto D, Mochizuki T, Kuroda S, Kawahara T, Izumi K, Teranishi J-I, Miyoshi Y, Otani M, et al. High orchiectomy and ipsilateral testicular sperm extraction in a man with a testicular tumor and Klinefelter syndrome: a case report. IJU Case Rep. 2018;2:65–8. https://doi.org/10.1002/iju5.12037.
74. Tournaye H, Liu J, Nagy PZ, Camus M, Goossens A, Silber S, Van Steirteghem AC, Devroey P. Correlation between testicular histology and outcome after intracytoplasmic sperm injection using testicular spermatozoa. Hum Reprod Oxf Engl. 1996;11:127–32.
75. Tsutsumi S, Kawahara T, Takeshima T, Chiba S, Uemura K, Otani M, Shimokihara K, Hayashi Y, Mochizuki T, Takamoto D, et al. Onco-testicular sperm extraction (onco-TESE) for bilateral testicular tumors: two case reports. J Med Case Rep. 2017;11:139. https://doi.org/10.1186/s13256-017-1303-6.
76. Ventimiglia E, Pozzi E, Capogrosso P, Boeri L, Alfano M, Cazzaniga W, Matloob R, Abbate C, Viganò P, Montorsi F, et al. Extensive assessment of underlying etiological factors in primary infertile men reduces the proportion of men with idiopathic infertility. Front Endocrinol. 2021;12:801125.
77. Vieira M, Bispo de Andrade MA, Santana-Santos E. Is testicular microdissection the only way to retrieve sperm for non-obstructive azoospermic men? Front Reprod Health. 2022;4:980824.
78. Wang Y-J, Zhang R-Q, Lin Y-J, Zhang R-G, Zhang W-L. Relationship between varicocele and sperm DNA damage and the effect of varicocele repair: a meta-analysis. Reprod Biomed Online. 2012;25:307–14.
79. Wang J, Xia S-J, Liu Z-H, Tao L, Ge J-F, Xu C-M, Qiu J-X. Inguinal and subinguinal micro-varicocelectomy, the optimal surgical management of varicocele: a meta-analysis. Asian J Androl. 2015;17:74–80.
80. Xue H, Wang S-Y, Cui L-G, Hong K. Can contrast-enhanced ultrasound increase or predict the success rate of testicular sperm aspiration in patients with azoospermia? AJR Am J Roentgenol. 2019;212:1054–9.
81. Yoon YE, Lee HH, Park SY, Moon HS, Kim DS, Song S-H, Kim DK. The role of vasoepididymostomy for treatment of obstructive azoospermia in the era of in vitro fertilization: a systematic review and meta-analysis. Asian J Androl. 2018;21:67–73.
82. You JB, McCallum C, Wang Y, Riordon J, Nosrati R, Sinton D. Machine learning for sperm selection. Nat Rev Urol. 2021;18:387–403.

Chapter 12
Innovation in Management of Ejaculatory Duct Obstruction

Raghavender Kosgi, Balagobi Balasingam, and Vineet Malhotra

Introduction

Ejaculatory duct obstruction (EDO) is an uncommon cause of obstructive azoospermia which leads to male subfertility. It may cause severe oligo-astheno teratozoospermia in case of partial EDO and azoospermia in case of complete EDO. Among various causes for male subfertility, EDO is one of the conditions, which will be curable with the hope of natural conception provided female evaluation is normal.

Incidence of EDO in male sub-fertile patients is about 1–5% [1, 2]. Majority of the patients with EDO are diagnosed only during evaluation of male subfertility. Some patients may also present to urologist or andrologist with the complaints of painful ejaculation, perineal pain, genital pain and hematospermia [1].

High index of clinical suspicion is needed to identify EDO due to its rare occurrence. Patients with low volume, acidic ejaculate (<1.5 ml, pH <7) with absent fructose showing azoospermia on semen analysis may have complete bilateral EDO. Patients with partial EDO may present with low volume, acidic ejaculate with reduced fructose and severe oligozoospermia (<5 mil/ml). Patients with unilateral, either complete or partial EDO, may often go unnoticed due to patent contralateral ejaculatory duct.

To distinguish ejaculatory duct obstruction (EDO) from non-obstructive azoospermia (NOA), key diagnostic tools include semen analysis, hormonal testing

R. Kosgi (✉)
Department of Andrology and Men's Health, Apollo Hospitals, Jubilee Hills, Hyderabad, Telangana, India

B. Balasingam
Department of Surgery, Faculty of Medicine, University of Jaffna, Jaffna, Sri Lanka

V. Malhotra
VNA Hospital, New Delhi, India

E. Chung et al. (eds.), *Advances in Andrology*,
https://doi.org/10.1007/978-3-032-29112-7_12

and imaging. EDO typically presents with low semen volume, acidic pH, absent fructose and azoospermia. Hormone levels (FSH, LH, testosterone) are normal. Transrectal ultrasound (TRUS) may reveal dilated seminal vesicles or cysts. In contrast, NOA shows normal semen volume and pH, with elevated FSH and often small testes, reflecting testicular failure. Testicular biopsy confirms spermatogenesis in EDO but shows impaired spermatogenesis in NOA. Thus, hormonal profiles and TRUS are critical for differentiation, supported by testicular biopsy if needed [2].

Management of EDO depends upon the aetiology. TURED is a gold standard procedure for congenital cystic obstruction of minimally invasive new endoscopic interventions with image guidance will enhance the accuracy of diagnosis and surgical outcomes. This chapter highlights the conventional therapies and newer innovations for the management of ejaculatory duct obstruction.

Anatomy of Ejaculatory Duct

Spermatozoa are generated within the seminiferous tubules of the testes under the influence of hormonal factors, including FSH and testosterone. The epididymis connects seamlessly with the vas deferens, which then merges with the emerging ducts from the seminal vesicles (SV), forming the ejaculatory ducts (EDs). These EDs typically penetrate the central zone of the prostate and open into the prostatic urethra on each side of the seminal colliculus (verumontanum) as slit like opening [3]. Despite variations in anatomy [4, 5], the ED typically courses obliquely for 1–2 cm within the prostate at a 75-degree angle [4]. The typical dimensions of the seminal vesicles are 4.5–5.5 cm in length and 1.5 cm in width.

The ejaculatory duct is divided into three sections: a proximal extra prostatic portion, a middle intraprostatic portion, and a brief distal segment within the verumontanum close to the prostatic urethra [6]. These ducts, measuring 1–2 cm in length, are lined with cuboidal or pseudostratified epithelium, resembling the lining of the seminal vesicles in the proximal and distal portions.

The ED originates from the Wolffian duct during the 8–12 weeks of gestation, coinciding with testosterone production [7], similar to the development of the epididymis body and tail, vas deferens, and seminal vesicles. Conversely, the prostate gland originates from the endoderm, which invaginates into the surrounding mesenchyme [8].

The prostatic utricle, a remnant of the Müllerian duct, is located between the openings of the EDs at the verumontanum and is non-communicating [9]. While the existence of a valve or sphincter-like mechanism (known as 'sphincter spermaticus') has been postulated at the junction of the ejaculatory ducts and the urethra, it is now widely believed that the acute angle of duct insertion serves to maintain ejaculatory continence and prevent urinary reflux.

Regarding fluid composition, prostatic fluid contributes approximately 0.5 mL to the ejaculate and is acidic in pH, while the seminal vesicles produce an alkaline fluid containing prostaglandins and fructose, comprising 1.5–2.0 mL (~50–80% of total semen volume) of the seminal fluid.

Patho-physiology of Ejaculatory Duct Obstruction and Male Infertility

Infertility, characterized by the inability to conceive after a year of regular unprotected sexual intercourse, affects around 15–20% of couples worldwide [10], with approximately half of these cases attributed to male factors either alone or in conjunction with female factors [11]. Among the various male infertility issues, ejaculatory duct obstruction (EDO) is relatively rare but can be effectively treated, potentially enabling affected men to naturally impregnate their partners.

The reported incidence of EDO among men seeking fertility assistance ranges from 1% to 5%. Azoospermia or severe oligozoospermia [1], coupled with low ejaculate volume, may indicate EDO.

EDO can arise from congenital or acquired conditions. Acquired EDO often stems from factors such as seminal vesicle calculi, scar formation due to inflammation at the prostate level due to prior urethral catheterization, urethral trauma, previous transurethral procedures like bladder-neck incision, transurethral resection of the prostate (TURP) [12], prostate cryotherapy and high-intensity focused ultrasound (HIFU).

Congenital causes include atresia or stenosis of the ejaculatory ducts, Müllerian duct (utricular) or Wolffian duct (diverticular) cysts. Prostatic cysts, more prevalent in infertile men than the general population, can compress ejaculatory ducts, leading to EDO and subsequent infertility [13].

Midline cysts, classified as sperm-containing or non-sperm-containing, pose challenges in differentiation. Non-sperm-containing cysts, known as utricle cysts and Müllerian duct cysts [14]. Utricle cysts are endodermal in origin and typically located midline near the verumontanum contrast to Müllerian duct cysts are mesodermal in origin and are located near the base of the prostate [15]. Sperm-containing cysts, such as Wolffian or ejaculatory duct cysts, are less common and paramedian in location within the prostate gland behind the prostatic urethra [16].

EDO patients often lack relevant antecedent history. Patients with congenital or non-infectious causes may have better outcomes than those with infectious causes. A significant proportion of idiopathic EDO cases exhibits cystic fibrosis gene (CFTR) mutations, particularly the 5 T polymorphism, warranting genetic evaluation [17].

Diagnosis of EDO

In cases of suspected ejaculatory duct obstruction (EDO), a thorough medical history should include inquiries about infertility, painful ejaculation, urinary symptoms, past surgeries, medications, family history and lifestyle factors.

Patients typically present with reduced ejaculatory volume or infertility, sometimes with painful ejaculation, hematospermia. Additional symptoms may include decreased ejaculation force, perineal or lower back discomfort, chronic scrotal pain and dysuria [18]. These symptoms of ejaculatory duct obstruction (EDO) can mimic those of prostatitis or epididymitis, emphasizing the importance of excluding common differential diagnosis [17].

Physical examination involves assessing the genitalia, conducting a digital rectal examination (DRE) to evaluate the prostate and performing a neurological and systemic examination. The finding of palpable vasa deferential and seminal vesicle can help differentiate EDO from the congenital bilateral absence of vas deferens (CBAVD).

Laboratory investigations such as semen analysis, hormonal assays and genetic testing, along with imaging studies like transrectal ultrasound or MRI, may be conducted based on clinical findings. A comprehensive approach enables clinicians to accurately diagnose and manage EDO, guiding further testing, treatment decisions and patient counselling to optimize reproductive health.

Semen Analysis and Hormone Profile

Semen analysis plays a crucial role in the diagnosis of EDO. In cases of bilateral complete EDO, semen analysis manifests with acidic semen (pH <7.2), azoospermia, low ejaculate volume (<1.5 mL) and low (<13 μmol per ejaculate) or absent fructose levels [12]. Partial obstructions may present with oligo- or oligo-asthenoteratozoospermia, where ejaculate volume and fructose levels may be normal. Additionally, semen analysis may show signs of hematospermia.

It is suggested that a small volume of acidic azoospermia semen and absence of fructose in a patient with palpable vasa deferentia is pathognomonic for EDO. However, the absence of one or more of these features cannot exclude EDO.

Hormonal assessments, including testosterone, FSH, LH, prolactin and oestradiol levels, are conducted in male infertility evaluations to assess testicular function and rule out endocrine disorders. While not diagnostic of EDO, they provide valuable insights when interpreted alongside clinical and diagnostic findings.

Transrectal Ultrasonography (TRUS)

Transrectal ultrasound (TRUS) utilizing a 5–7 MHz probe has become the standard imaging method in ejaculatory duct obstruction (EDO) due to its non-invasive nature compared to the previously employed vasography [20].

TRUS reveals midline cysts, enlarged seminal vesicles (cross section width >1.5 cm) or ejaculatory ducts (diameter >2.3 mm), hyperechoic areas indicating calculi and absence of the vas deferens [21]. However, TRUS only provides static anatomical details, lacking functional information regarding seminal vesicle emptying. Furthermore, some patients with EDO may have normal TRUS findings and abnormal TRUS findings don't confirm the diagnosis of EDO, as even fertile men may exhibit dilated seminal vesicles, depending on sexual abstinence duration.

Consequently, dilated seminal vesicles are sensitive but not specific indicators of EDO. TRUS alone may yield false-positive EDO diagnoses in up to 50% of cases, emphasizing its sensitivity but limited specificity [21].

Seminal Vesicle Aspiration

Under transrectal ultrasound (TRUS) guidance, a 22-gauge, 7-inch spinal needle is used to aspirate seminal vesicle (SV) fluid for analysis, aiming to detect sperm presence [22]. Typically, in healthy men, SVs don't contain motile sperm. Diagnosis of ejaculatory duct obstruction (EDO) is often based on finding more than three sperm per high-power microscopic field (400×).

Engin et al. found that only half of TRUS-obstructive cases showed sperm in SV aspiration [23], suggesting combining SV aspiration with TRUS for better diagnostic accuracy. Harvested sperm from SVs can be utilized in assisted reproductive technology (ART) procedures, enhancing fertility options [24].

Seminal Vesicle Chromotubation

Following transrectal ultrasound (TRUS)-guided seminal vesicle (SV) aspiration, a 5 mL diluted dye solution like indigo carmine or methylene blue is injected into the SV. Subsequently, the outflow of dye from the prostatic urethra is observed through cystourethroscopy [21].

This technique serves to confirm obstruction and can also be utilized post-endoscopic transurethral resection of the ejaculatory duct (TURED) to verify resolution of obstruction [21].

Seminal Vesiculography

Combining transrectal ultrasound (TRUS)-guided injection of a non-ionic contrast agent into the seminal vesicles with fluoroscopy allows for comprehensive evaluation of anatomical and functional aspects of the ejaculatory duct (ED) [25].

The absence of contrast within the urethra and bladder, coupled with enlarged seminal vesicles, indicates obstruction. This imaging examination also assesses vas patency through retrograde vasography in about two-thirds of patients [26].

Seminal Tract Washout

Seminal tract washout is a diagnostic and therapeutic procedure in EDO. It involves flushing out the seminal tract with a solution to remove any obstructive material or debris, aiming to restore fertility. This procedure can be conducted in conjunction with other investigations/treatments such as seminal vesicle aspiration or endoscopic procedures like transurethral resection of the ejaculatory duct (TURED) [27].

Seminal tract washout aims to clear obstructions and facilitate the passage of sperm, potentially improving fertility outcomes in individuals with EDO. However, its efficacy can vary depending on the underlying cause and severity of obstruction. Close monitoring and follow-up assessments are necessary to evaluate the success of seminal tract washout in treating EDO.

Vasography

Vasography involves making an incision or puncture in the vas deferens, followed by injecting a contrast agent. The blockage is confirmed through radiologic or fluoroscopic observation, showing normal vasa deferentia, enlarged seminal vesicles and the absence of contrast in the bladder and urethra [1].

Despite being historically regarded as the preferred method for diagnosing ejaculatory duct obstruction (EDO) and allowing for sperm collection for cryopreservation, scrotal vasography has been supplanted by transrectal ultrasound (TRUS). TRUS, which offers high accuracy without invasiveness, has become the standard imaging diagnostic tool due to the invasive nature and associated risks, such as vasal stenosis or stricture, of vasography [28].

Endorectal MRI

Identification of ejaculatory duct obstruction (EDO) via T2-weighted MRI entails observing an ED diameter over 2 mm, along with factors like SV wall thickness or enhanced wall signal [29].

Relying solely on MRI may over diagnose EDO, leading to unnecessary surgeries. Engin et al. compared MRI and transrectal ultrasound (TRUS) in 218 infertile men, suggesting TRUS as the primary assessment method, with MRI reserved for inconclusive TRUS results. MRI, pricier than TRUS, might miss calcifications [30].

Manometry

Seen as an enhancement of seminal vesicle (SV) chromotubation, ejaculatory duct (ED) manometry assesses SV pressure using a spinal needle linked to a 3-way stopcock. Eisenberg et al. examined ED open pressure using this technique and verified obstruction relief post-transurethral resection of the ejaculatory ducts (TURED). Their study observed a decrease in pressure from an average of 116 cm H_2O (range 80–150) to 54 cm H_2O (range 10–82) following ED resection [31].

Diagnostic Seminal Vesiculoscopy

Diagnostic seminal vesiculoscopy is a small endoscope to directly visualize and evaluate ED and SV seminal vesicles. This procedure can provide valuable diagnostic information on EDO, seminal vesicle cysts/calcifications or other anomalies that may contribute to male infertility [32].

(a) *Management of Ejaculatory Duct Obstruction*

After the diagnosis of obstructive azoospermia due to ejaculatory duct obstruction, based on zero sperm count, acidic pH and absent /low fructose, which is confirmed by imaging (TRUS/MRI of reproductive organs), we offer the couple various options like endoscopic interventions (TURED +_ image guided, TSV) and assisted reproductive techniques. After shared decision making with the couple, we proceed with the treatment accordingly. Management of ejaculatory duct obstruction depends upon the aetiology. Endoscopic interventions are cost effective therapy for EDO. In our practice, most of the male sub-fertile patients opt for endoscopic procedures.

Reversible or treatable ejaculatory duct obstruction (EDO), such as midline cysts or distal duct obstruction, can often be managed with transurethral resection of the ejaculatory ducts (TURED), especially when TRUS shows dilated seminal vesicles and cysts. These cases typically restore sperm to the ejaculate and may enable natural conception. In contrast, non-treatable EDO involves extensive fibrosis, congenital bilateral absence of the vas deferens (CBAVD) or proximal obstruction with absent seminal vesicle dilation. Reconstruction is not possible in such cases, and sperm retrieval with assisted reproductive techniques (e.g., IVF/ICSI) is required. Imaging and endoscopic findings help guide treatment feasibility [32].

(b) *Trans Urethral Resection of Ejaculatory Duct (TURED)*

TURED is indicated for relieving ejaculatory duct obstruction. It may be because of post inflammatory obstruction or cystic obstruction [1, 33]. Relief of EDO achieves symptomatic improvement in patients with painful ejaculation and/or hematospermia [34]. In case of subfertility by improving semen parameters, it improves the fertility outcomes.

TURED was first described by Farley and Barnes in 1973, which involves the use of a 24F resectoscope and an electrocautery loop for the resection of ejaculatory ducts at the level of verumontanum. It may remove the part of verumontanum [35].

Success of TURED is noted by visualization of milky/cloudy fluid flowing from resection site. Avoiding coagulation cautery usage and using only pure cutting current minimize scarring and prevent restenosis of ED [1, 35].

Minor modifications to above standard technique have been introduced to reduce the complications of TURED. Using a bipolar cautery, balloon dilatation, using holmium laser energy and smaller monopolar resection loop are such technical modifications [36–38]. Intra operative TRUS usage is more useful in making TURED a safe procedure.

Outcomes of TURED: Semen quality improvement and patency of ejaculatory ductal system are noted in up to 59% and 94% of cases after TURED, respectively [21, 39, 40]. In men with complete EDO, 60% of them will have sperms in the ejaculate after TURED, out of which about 38% will show normal semen parameters [38, 41]. Natural pregnancy rates of 12–31% were reported after TURED [21, 39–43].

Complications of TURED: The incidence of TURED complications ranges from 4% to 26% [21, 38, 39, 42, 44]. Epididymo-orchitis, urinary tract infection, haematuria, hematospermia, reflux of urine into ejaculatory ducts and seminal vesical vesicles are known complications. In cases of partial EDO, it may cause azoospermia due to complete stenosis (1).

Damage to bladder neck and external urinary sphincter, obstructive scar at the ED orifice may also result in acute urinary retention, retrograde ejaculation, incontinence of urine and/or a secondary obstruction with persistent azoospermia. Erectile dysfunction and perforation of rectum were also reported [45].

Prognostic Factors for Surgical Success in TURED

Surgical outcomes of TURED are directly related to aetiology of ejaculatory duct obstruction. Patients with congenital cystic ED obstruction had more significant postoperative improvement in semen parameters than those with traumatic or post inflammatory ED obstructions [44].

Natural pregnancy rates were higher in congenital group than those with acquired EDO group. Patients with partial ED obstruction have shown better improvement in semen parameters than those with complete obstruction [39, 42].

(c) *Therapeutic Trans Utricular Seminal Vesiculoscopy (TSV)*

Trans utricular seminal vesiculoscopy (TSV) technique was first described by Yang et al. in 2002 [43]. It is useful in identification and resolving obstructions caused by stones, debris and clots. TSV technique involves insertion of a 6 or 9F vesiculoscope in a retrograde fashion through the ejaculatory duct natural lumen or by presumptive ED orifice puncture and incision with holmium laser at the wall of the prostatic utricle [46].

In a study done by, Wang et al. 21 patients with partial or complete EDO who underwent TSV were followed for 1 year [46]. Improvement of semen parameters was noted in 90% (19) of patients, and four couples (19%) achieved pregnancy naturally.

In another study involving 22 men with EDO, Xu et al. noted that 7 patients with stones (31.8%) had shown significant semen parameter improvements, and 6 couples (27%) achieved natural conception [47].

Complex anatomy of ejaculatory duct makes TSV, a challenging procedure. Chen et al. were in 2018 described four types of ED orifices using vesiculoscopy. They found type C in majority of the patients, followed by type D [48].

Types of ED Orifices

Type A—ED orifice clearly observed from the urethra.
Type B—ED orifice covered by a thin white membrane.
Type C—ED not visualized but punctured successfully in the presumptive location.
Type D—ED orifice not visualized and puncture not successful.

In difficult cases where ED orifice is not visible, TURED will be the treatment of choice. TSV also useful in patients with painful ejaculation and hematospermia to relieve symptoms. It is both diagnostic and therapeutic for seminal vesicle stones, clots and stricture of ED. Strictures can be incised with Holmium laser [46–48].

Complications of TSV include the possibility of seminal vesicle perforation, erectile dysfunction, reflux of urine into the ejaculatory duct, epididymitis, stenosis or rectourethral fistula [48]. Dilatation of the ED with a 9F seminal vesiculoscope reduces the complications [47].

(d) *Image Guided Interventions*

(i) *TRUS/Fluoroscopy Guided Balloon Dilation*
TRUS guided balloon dilatation of ED was first described by Jarow et al. [49]. In their case report, SV puncture was done under TRUS guidance. A 0.035-inch heavy-duty straight guidewire was used for catheter advancement through the occluded ED. Under urethroscopic visualization, 4 mm diameter balloon will be correctly positioned inside the ED. Fluoroscopy can also be used for this purpose with the use of contrast. For adequate dilatation, balloon was inflated twice after positioning correctly. Later on, balloon dilation under CT guidance was proposed [50]. Data is available only for relief of chronic pelvic pain [49, 51].

(ii) *TRUS Guided Prostatic Cyst Aspiration*
Midline prostatic cysts (MPC) are found in about 5.8% of fertile men and 10–17% of infertile men [48, 53]. Under TRUS guidance and under local anaesthesia, an 18-gauge 20 cm-long needle is inserted into the MPC. A 20 mL syringe is used to aspirate the fluid and examined at 400× magnification to verify the presence of sperms [52].

In a retrospective cohort study done by Lotti et al., 11 patients with cysts >0.25 mL underwent TRUS guided cyst aspiration [52]. Sperm counts improved in all patients 1 month later but this improvement was temporary. Three months after the procedure, due to increased volume of cyst, the sperm count declined,

After 1-year follow-up, 4 patients achieved natural pregnancy and one by intracytoplasmic sperm injection (ICSI). Cysts larger than 0.117 ml might affect fertility and treatment of which may enhance outcomes. Self-limiting, mild haematuria is noted after TRUCA (TRUS guided cyst aspiration) [52].

(e) *Assisted Reproductive Techniques (ART)—Sperm Retrieval with ICSI*

Though endoscopic interventions are cost effective and curative options for sub-fertile male with EDO, these are not feasible in all patients. Restenosis of ED orifice, sub-optimal semen parameter improvements after surgery have been reported. Few couples may choose ART directly. In these situation ART, particularly ICSI is a viable alternative [39, 40, 47, 53]. Even though female partner is not at fault, unfortunately she is subjected to ICSI in many cases. In patients with partial EDO and sub optimal postoperative semen parameter improvement, ejaculate sperms can be used for ICSI. In patients with complete EDO not amenable for surgery, amenable but not willing for surgery and in patients with failed surgical intervention, surgical sperm retrieval is an alternative method. In patients with EDO, mechanism of spermatogenesis is intact and shows normal spermatogenesis.

Sperm retrieval is successful in almost all these patients. Sperm harvesting can be done from epididymis, testis and seminal vesicles. Sperm retrieval can be done percutaneously with PESA/MESA/TESA and by open surgery with TESE [54]. Ultrasound guided seminal vesicle aspiration and proximal vas deference sperm aspiration can also be tried in these patients. Micro-TESE is usually not required in these patients. Aetiology of obstructive azoospermia and surgical technique have little influence on surgical sperm retrieval rates and outcomes of ICSI. In men with obstructive azoospermia including EDO, live birth rates with ICSI have been reported in the range of 32–36% [55].

(f) *Management of Functional EDO*

Functional EDO is an uncommon cause of ED obstruction, commonly noted in patients with neurological issues. It is associated with spinal cord lesions, multiple sclerosis, diabetic neuropathy, iatrogenic neural damage after retroperitoneal lymph nodes dissection (RPLND), pelvic surgery or medications like alpha-blockers, anti-psychotics, thiazide diuretics and tricyclic antidepressants. After TURED some patients with persistent dilatation of seminal vesicle, may have functional EDO [56]. Functional EDO may impair the sperm transport. There is no effective medication for dealing with functional EDO. Off label phosphodiesterase inhibitors (PDE5I) were tried in diabetic patients with minimal benefit [56, 57]. Sperm retrieval with ICSI is the only effective way for these patients to deal with male subfertility.

Summary

Ejaculatory duct obstruction (EDO) is a reversible cause of male infertility, typically presenting with low ejaculate volume, acidic pH, absent fructose and azoospermia or severe oligospermia. Initial evaluation includes semen analysis, hormonal profiling (usually normal in EDO) and physical examination. Key imaging includes transrectal ultrasound (TRUS), identifying dilated seminal vesicles, cysts or calcifications; MRI may be adjunctive. Diagnosis is confirmed with testicular biopsy or seminal vesiculography when needed. Management depends on obstruction type: treatable cases undergo transurethral resection of the ejaculatory ducts (TURED), while non-treatable cases require assisted reproductive techniques like sperm retrieval with IVF/ICSI (Fig. 12.1).

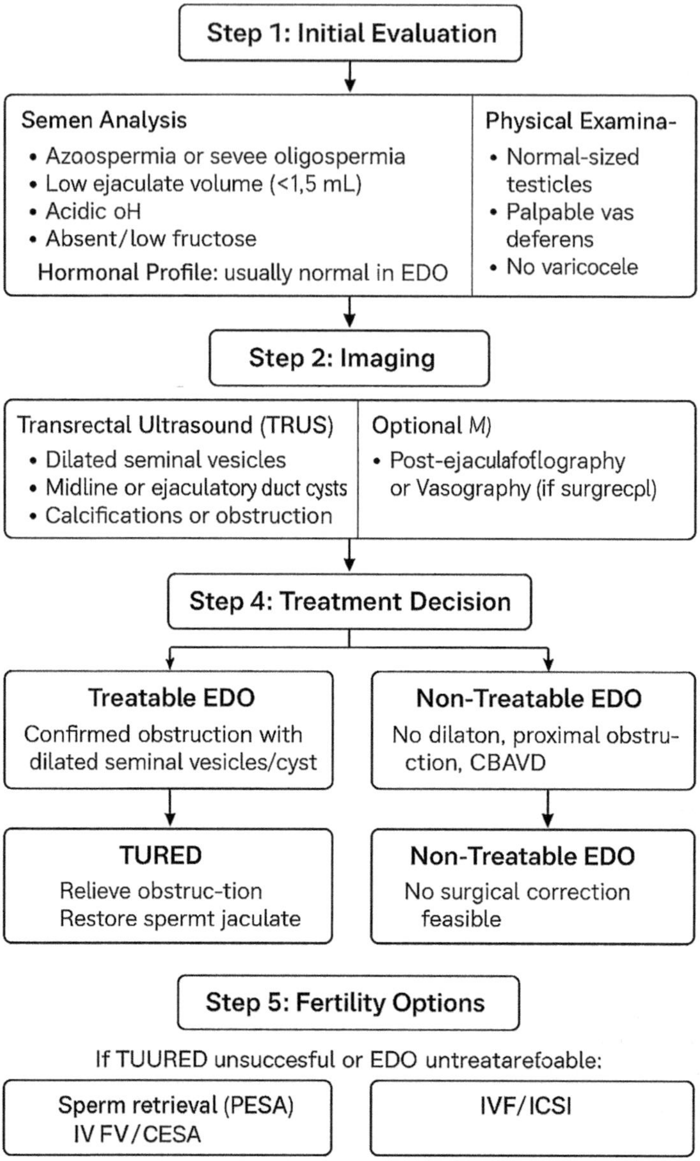

Fig. 12.1 Algorithm to approach ejaculatory duct obstruction

References

1. Avellino GJ, Lipshultz LI, Sigman M, Hwang K. Transurethral resection of the ejaculatory ducts: etiology of obstruction and surgical treatment options. Fertil Steril. 2019;111:427–43.
2. Modgil V, Rai S, Ralph DJ, Muneer A. An update on the diagnosis and management of ejaculatory duct obstruction. Nat Rev Urol. 2016;13:13–20.
3. Mathangasinghe Y, Samaranayake UMJE, Dolapihilla BN, Anthony DJ, Malalasekera AP. Morphology of ejaculatory ducts: a systematic review. Clin Anat. 2020;33:1164–75.
4. Li ZY, Xu Y, Liu C, Xiao ZM, Luo BH, Xu GW, et al. Anatomical study of the seminal vesicle system for transurethral seminal vesiculoscopy. Clin Anat. 2019;32:244–52.
5. Banner MP, Hassler R. The normal seminal vesiculogram. Radiology. 1978;128:339–44.
6. Nguyen HT, Etzell J, Turek PJ. Normal human ejaculatory duct anatomy: a study of cadaveric and surgical specimens. J Urol. 1996;155:1639–42.
7. Schoenwolf GC, et al. Larsen's human embryology. 4th ed. Churchill Livingstone Elsevier; 2009. p. 511.
8. Jurewicz M, Gilbert BR. Imaging and angiography in male factor infertility. Fertil Steril. 2016;105:1432–42.
9. McIntyre M. The incidence of proximal ejaculatory duct in transrectal ultrasound guided biopsy specimens. Presented at the South Eastern Section American Urological Association Annual Meeting. Miami, 11–14 March, 2010.
10. Cox CM, Thoma ME, Tchangalova N, Mburu G, Bornstein MJ, Johnson CL, Kiarie J. Infertility prevalence and the methods of estimation from 1990 to 2021: a systematic review and meta-analysis. Hum Reprod Open. 2022;2022(4):hoac051. https://doi.org/10.1093/hropen/hoac051. PMID: 36483694; PMCID: PMC9725182.
11. Choy JT, Eisenberg ML. Male infertility as a window to health. Fertil Steril. 2018;110:810–4.
12. Pryor JP, Hendry WF. Ejaculatory duct obstruction in sub fertile males: analysis of 87 patients. Fertil Steril. 1991;56:725–30.
13. Kim ED, et al. The prevalence of cystic abnormalities of the prostate involving the ejaculatory ducts as detected by transrectal ultrasound. Int Urol Nephrol. 1997;29:647–52.
14. Kirkali Z, et al. Cysts of the prostate, seminal vesicles and diverticulum of the ejaculatory ducts. Eur Urol. 1991;20:77–80.
15. Elder JS, Mostwin JL. Cyst of the ejaculatory duct/urogenital sinus. J Urol. 1984;132:768–71.
16. Shebel HM, Farg HM, Kolokythas O, El-Diasty T. Cysts of the lower male genitourinary tract: embryologic and anatomic considerations and differential diagnosis. Radiographics. 2013;33:1125–43.
17. Jarvi K, et al. Cystic fibrosis transmembrane conductance regulator and obstructive azoospermia. Lancet. 1995;345:1578.
18. Fisch H. Transurethral resection of the ejaculatory ducts. Curr Surg Techn Urol. 1992;5:2–7.
19. Johnson CW, Bingham JB, Goluboff ET, Fisch H. Transurethral resection of the ejaculatory ducts for treating ejaculatory symptoms. BJU Int. 2005;95:117–9.
20. Jarow JP. Transrectal ultrasonography of infertile men. Fertil Steril. 1993;60:1035–9.
21. Purohit RS, Wu DS, Shinohara K, Turek PJ. A prospective comparison of 3 diagnostic methods to evaluate ejaculatory duct obstruction. J Urol. 2004;171:232–5. discussion 235–6.
22. Healy MW, Yauger BJ, James AN, Jezior JR, Parker P, Dean RC. Seminal vesicle sperm aspiration from wounded warriors. Fertil Steril. 2016;106:579–83.
23. Engin G, Celtik M, Sanli O, Aytac O, Muradov Z, Kadioglu A. Comparison of transrectal ultrasonography and transrectal ultrasonography-guided seminal vesicle aspiration in the diagnosis of the ejaculatory duct obstruction. Fertil Steril. 2009;92:964–70.
24. Orhan I, Onur R, Cayan S, Koksal IT, Kadioglu A. Seminal vesicle sperm aspiration in the diagnosis of ejaculatory duct obstruction. BJU Int. 1999;84:1050–3.

25. Jones TR, Zagoria RJ, Jarow JP. Transrectal US-guided seminal vesiculography. Radiology. 1997;205:276–8.
26. Katz D, Mieza M, Nagler HM. Ultrasound guided transrectal seminal vesiculography: a new approach to the diagnosis of male reproductive tract abnormalities (abstract 330). J Urol. 1994;151:310A.
27. Colpi GM, Negri L, Scroppo FI, Grugnetti C, Patrizio P. Seminal tract washout: a new diagnostic tool in complicated cases of male infertility. J Androl. 1994;15(Suppl):17S–22S. PMID: 7721670.
28. Schroeder-Printzen I, Ludwig M, Kohn F, Weidner W. Surgical therapy in infertile men with ejaculatory ductobstruction: technique and outcome of a standardized surgical approach. Hum Reprod. 2000;15:1364–8.
29. Guo Y, Liu G, Yang D, Sun X, Wang H, Deng C, et al. Role of MRI in assessment of ejaculatory duct obstruction. J Xray Sci Technol. 2013;21:141–6.
30. Engin G, Kadioğlu A, Orhan I, Akdol S, Rozanes I. Transrectal US and endorectal MR imaging in partial and complete obstruction of the seminal duct system. A comparative study. Acta Radiol. 2000;41:288–95.
31. Eisenberg ML, Walsh TJ, Garcia MM, Shinohara K, Turek PJ. Ejaculatory duct manometry in normal men and in patients with ejaculatory duct obstruction. J Urol. 2008;180:255–60.
32. Song T, Zhang X, Zhang L, Zhang F, Fu WJ. Transurethral seminal vesiculoscopy in the diagnosis and treatment of seminal vesicle stones. Chin Med J. 2012;125(8):1475–8. PMID: 22613656.
33. Elder JS, et al. Cyst of the ejaculatory duct/urogenital sinus. J Urol. 1984;132:768.
34. Manohar T, Ganpule A, Desai M. Transrectal ultrasound- and fluoroscopic-assisted transurethral incision of ejaculatory ducts: a problem-solving approach to non-malignant hematospermia due to ejaculatory duct obstruction. J Endourol. 2008;22:1531–5.
35. Farley S, Barnes R. Stenosis of ejaculatory ducts treated by endoscopic resection. J Urol. 1973;109:664–6.
36. Jiang HT, Yuan Q, Liu Y, Liu ZQ, Zhou ZY, Xiao KF, et al. Multiple advanced surgical techniques to treat acquired seminal duct obstruction. Asian J Androl. 2014;16:912–6.
37. Sabanegh E Jr, Thomas A Jr. Modified resectoscope loop for transurethral resection of the ejaculatory duct. Urology. 1994;44:909–10.
38. Tu XA, Zhuang JT, Zhao L, Zhao LY, Zhao JQ, Lu KL, et al. Transurethral bipolar plasma kinetic resection of ejaculatory duct for treatment of ejaculatory duct obstruction. J Xray Sci Technol. 2013;21:293–302.
39. Kadioglu A, Cayan S, Tefekli A, Orhan I, Engin G, Turek PJ. Does response to treatment of ejaculatory duct obstruction in infertile men vary with pathology? Fertil Steril. 2001;76:138–42.
40. Turek PJ, Magana JO, Lipshultz LI. Semen parameters before and after transurethral surgery for ejaculatory duct obstruction. J Urol. 1996;155:1291–3.
41. Schroeder-Printzen I, Ludwig M, Kohn F, Weidner W. Surgical therapy in infertile men with ejaculatory duct obstruction: technique and outcome of a standardized surgical approach. Hum Reprod. 2000;15:1364–8.
42. El-Assmy A, El-Tholoth H, Abouelkheir RT, Abou-El-Ghar ME. Transurethral resection of ejaculatory duct in infertile men: outcome and predictors of success. Int Urol Nephrol. 2012;44:1623–30.
43. Yang SC, Rha KH, Byon SK, Kim JH. Trans utricular seminal vesiculoscopy. J Endourol. 2002;16:343–5.
44. Netto NR Jr, Esteves SC, Neves PA. Transurethral resection of partially obstructed ejaculatory ducts: seminal parameters and pregnancy outcomes according to the etiology of obstruction. J Urol. 1998;159:2048–53.
45. Vazquez-Levin MH, Dressler KP, Nagler HM. Urine contamination of seminal fluid after transurethral resection of the ejaculatory ducts. J Urol. 1994;152(6 Pt 1):2049–52.

46. Wang H, Ye H, Xu C, Liu Z, Gao X, Hou J, et al. Transurethral seminal vesiculoscopy using a 6F vesiculoscope for ejaculatory duct obstruction: initial experience. J Androl. 2012;33:637–43.
47. Xu B, Niu X, Wang Z, Li P, Qin C, Li J, et al. Novel methods for the diagnosis and treatment of ejaculatory duct obstruction. BJU Int. 2011;108:263–6.
48. Chen R, Wang L, Sheng X, Piao SG, Nian XW, Cheng X, et al. Transurethral seminal vesiculoscopy for recurrent hemospermia: experience from 419 cases. Asian J Androl. 2018;20:438–41.
49. Jarow JP, Zagoria RJ. Antegrade ejaculatory duct recanalization and dilation. Urology. 1995;46:743–6.
50. Kayser O, Osmonov D, Harde J, Girolami G, Wedel T, Schafer P. Less invasive causal treatment of ejaculatory duct obstruction by balloon dilation: a case report, literature review and suggestion of a CT- or MRI-guided intervention. Ger Med Sci. 2012;10:Doc06.
51. Lawler LP, Cosin O, Jarow JP, Kim HS. Transrectal US-guided seminal vesiculography and ejaculatory duct recanalization and balloon dilation for treatment of chronic pelvic pain. J Vasc Interv Radiol. 2006;17:169–73.
52. Lotti F, Corona G, Cocci A, Cipriani S, Baldi E, Degl'Innocenti S, et al. The prevalence of midline prostatic cysts and the relationship between cyst size and semen parameters among infertile and fertile men. Hum Reprod. 2018;33:2023–34.
53. Esteves SC, Roque M, Bedoschi G, Haahr T, Humaidan P. Intracytoplasmic sperm injection for male infertility and consequences for offspring. Nat Rev Urol. 2018;15:535–62.
54. Miyaoka R, Orosz JE, Achermann AP, Esteves SC. Methods of surgical sperm extraction and implications for assisted reproductive technology success. Panminerva Med. 2019;61:164–77.
55. Esteves SC, Lee W, Benjamin DJ, Seol B, Verza S Jr, Agarwal A. Reproductive potential of men with obstructive azoospermia undergoing percutaneous sperm retrieval and intracytoplasmic sperm injection according to the cause of obstruction. J Urol. 2013;189:232–7.
56. Font MD, Pastuszak AW, Case JR, Lipshultz LI. An infertile male with dilated seminal vesicles due to functional obstruction. Asian J Androl. 2017;19:256–7.
57. La Vignera S, Condorelli RA, Vicari E, Lotti F, Favilla V, Morgia G, et al. Seminal vesicles and diabetic neuropathy: ultrasound evaluation after prolonged treatment with a selective phosphodiesterase-5 inhibitor. Andrology. 2013;1:245–50.

Chapter 13
Male Fertility Regeneration: Is It Possible?

Adriano Fregonesi, Mehmet Yilmaz, and Selçuk Sarikaya

Introduction

In the rapidly evolving landscape of reproductive medicine, the quest to decipher and remediate male infertility is a pinnacle of scientific endeavor and human hope. This chapter delves into the frontier of male fertility regeneration, an area burgeoning with the promise of innovative technologies and groundbreaking research that challenges the boundaries of current medical practices [1]. As we stand on the cusp of potential revolutions in health and science, this discussion extends beyond mere academic interest, touching on the profound aspects of human experience, the desire for parenthood, and the continuation of genetic legacy [1].

Through the sophisticated realms of stem cells and regenerative medicine, the capacity to mend once irrevocable damage leads to male infertility. By harnessing the latest advancements in spermatogonial stem cell and hormonal therapies, this review aims to illuminate the sophisticated interplay between biology, technology, and hope. Furthermore, it addresses the pressing ethical and legal implications of such profound interventions in human life and fertility issues [2].

A. Fregonesi (✉)
Department of Surgery, Discipline/Area of Urology, Faculty of Medical Sciences, University of Campinas (UNICAMP), Campinas, São Paulo, Brazil

Faculty of Medicine of Jundiaí, Jundiaí, São Paulo, Brazil

M. Yilmaz
Mediclin Kraichgau-Klinik, Urology, Bad Rappenau, Germany

S. Sarikaya
University of Health Sciences, Gulhane Research and Training Hospital, Department of Urology, Ankara, Turkey

E. Chung et al. (eds.), *Advances in Andrology*,
https://doi.org/10.1007/978-3-032-29112-7_13

It is not merely a prelude to academic discourse but a clarion call to the scientific community to pursue solutions to one of humanity's most sensitive challenges. Through this exploration, we seek to expand our scientific horizons and offer tangible hope to countless individuals dreaming of realizing their fullest potential in family life. Let us proceed with caution and optimism, guided by science and tempered by the ethical considerations that such profound work necessitates [3] (Fig. 13.1).

1. *Stem Cells and Regenerative Male Fertility*

What Are Stem Cells?

Stem cells are versatile cells that are crucial for regenerative medicine and research. They possess a unique ability to self-renew and differentiate into various cell types, making them building blocks of tissues and organs. Stem cells can be classified based on their differentiation capacity into totipotent, pluripotent, multipotent, oligopotent, and unipotent cells. Additionally, they can be categorized by their origin, including the bone marrow, amniotic cells, adipose tissue, umbilical cord, and placental tissue. Stem cells play a vital role in replenishing mature cell compartments and have been utilized in treating genetic blood diseases, pain states, and neurodegenerative conditions such as Parkinson's and Alzheimer's diseases. Stem cells offer promise in replacing damaged neurons, advancing drug development, and regenerating fertility [4].

Totipotent: Stem cells are produced by the fusion of an egg and sperm cell. The cells produced by the first few divisions of the fertilized egg are also totipotent. These cells can differentiate into embryonic and extra-embryonic cell types [5].

Pluripotent: Stem cells are descendants of totipotent cells and can differentiate into cells derived from any of the three germ layers [5].

Multipotent: Stem cells can produce only cells of a closely related family of cells (e.g., HSCs differentiate into red blood cells, white blood cells, platelets, etc.) [5].

Unipotent: Cells can produce only one cell type but have the property of self-renewal, which distinguishes them from non-stem cells (e.g., muscle stem cells) [6].

Stem cells are physiological reservoirs for normal cell turnover and tissue regeneration after injury. These cells represent the natural proliferative compartment of the mature cells. Stem cells are present in all body organs and tissues and are located in a special anatomical setup called the niche [6].

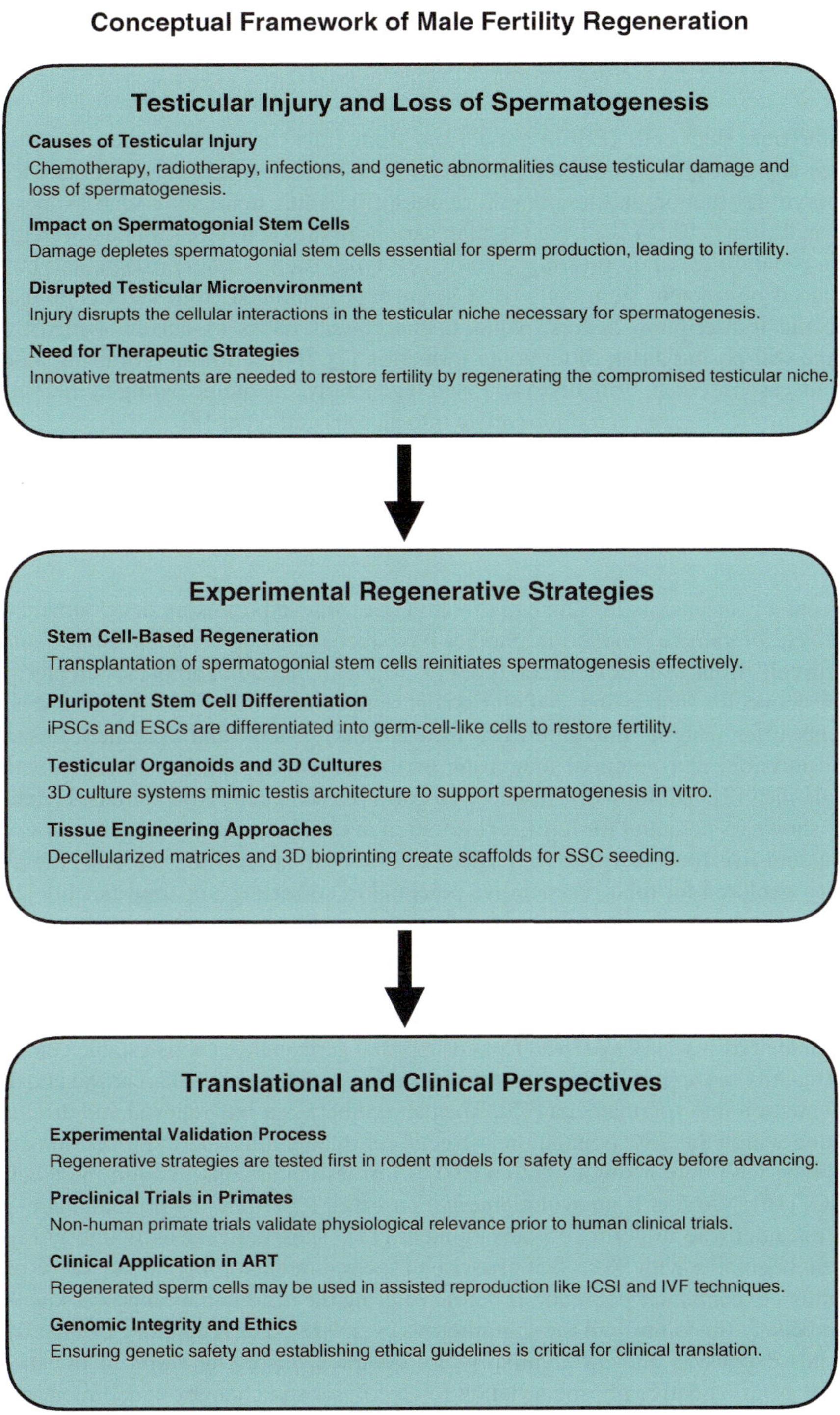

Fig. 13.1 Conceptual framework of male fertility regeneration

What Are the Differences Between Embryonic, Adult, and Induced Pluripotent Stem Cells?

Embryonic stem cells (ESCs) are derived from embryos and have the potential to form any cell type in the body; however, their use raises ethical concerns due to embryo destruction and teratoma formation [7]. Adult stem cells, such as mesenchymal stem cells (MSCs), are found in various tissues and have limited differentiation capabilities, often forming specific cell types such as fat, cartilage, and bone. Induced pluripotent stem cells (iPSCs) are reprogrammed from adult cells using specific transcription factors, avoiding the ethical issues associated with ESCs, while still posing a risk of teratoma formation [7]. iPSCs offer a promising model for disease research, drug discovery, and regenerative medicine owing to their ability to mimic diseases and differentiate into various cell types [8].

Stem Cells in Male Reproduction

Recent advancements in stem cell research have shown promising developments in the field of gamete production. Studies have focused on deriving male and female germ cells from various stem cell types [9, 10], with particular emphasis on pluripotent stem cells, such as induced pluripotent stem cells (iPSCs) [11]. These advancements offer insights into infertility mechanisms, genetic and epigenetic disease transmission, and potential diagnostic and treatment approaches in reproductive medicine [12]. Additionally, research on germline stem cell (GSCs) transplantation has shown its potential for fertility restoration in clinical settings, wildlife conservation, and livestock breeding [13]. Stem cell-derived extracellular vesicles are also being explored for their regenerative potential in correcting impaired fertility [14]. These advancements hold promise for revolutionizing regenerative approaches in the field of reproductive medicine.

Spermatogonial stem cells (SSCs) are pivotal in initiating and maintaining spermatogenesis in mice and serve as the foundation for continuous sperm production and male fertility. SSCs derived from primordial germ cells establish stable colonies postnatally to support lifelong spermatogenesis by undergoing self-renewal and differentiation into spermatozoa [15]. The balance between self-renewal and differentiation within the SSC population is crucial for maintaining sperm production after puberty, with only a small fraction (0.03%) of testicular cells in adult mice being SSCs [16]. NANOS is an evolutionarily conserved RNA-binding protein that plays an essential role in germ cell development [17]. Spermatogenesis is tightly regulated, beginning with SSCs that give rise to spermatogonial progenitors. These progenitors expand their populations before entering the differentiation process, which is precisely timed through the seminiferous cycle [18]. The regulatory mechanisms of this expansion and differentiation are complex, involving shifts in metabolic states from oxidative phosphorylation to glycolysis and changes in cell membrane composition, which affect cell-cell contact and responses to extracellular cytokines [19]. Techniques such as spermatogonial transplantation have been developed to quantify SSCs based on their regenerative capacity, highlighting the functional definition of stem cells [20]. Moreover, the isolation of spermatogonia from mouse testes has been refined to obtain nearly pure populations of undifferentiated spermatogonia, facilitating further research on SSC biology and its application in addressing male infertility [21]. Recent studies have explored the effects of various factors on SSC proliferation and spermatogenesis, including the role of epididymosomes and bone marrow-derived mesenchymal stem cells (BM-MSCs), which have shown promise in enhancing SSC proliferation and differentiation in vitro [22]. Additionally, the blood-testis barrier (BTB) is a critical component of spermatogenesis, with specific claudins necessary for SSC transmigration and colonization [23]. Understanding the molecular mechanisms regulating SSC function, including the gene expression patterns associated with spermatogenesis, is essential for developing novel stem cell-based therapies for assisted reproduction and fertility restoration in humans. This comprehensive approach to studying SSCs and their contribution to spermatogenesis in mice underscore their potential for advancing male fertility treatments and understanding reproductive biology [9].

How Do Stem Cells Contribute to Testicular Regeneration?

Stem cells have emerged as a promising avenue for promoting testicular regeneration and addressing male infertility issues stemming from various causes, such as chemotherapy, radiation, and genetic factors. The ability of mesenchymal stem cells (MSCs) to differentiate into specialized cells and their self-renewal capacity make them effective in treating testicular degeneration, as highlighted by research indicating their efficacy in regenerating damaged testicular elements [24]. Specifically, bone marrow-derived mononuclear cells have been shown to recover testicular cells in cyclophosphamide-treated rats, thereby improving hormonal regulation and spermatogenesis [25]. Furthermore, human umbilical cord perivascular cells (HUCPVCs), a type of MSC, have demonstrated potential in supporting the expansion of spermatogonial stem cells (SSCs) and promoting germ cell regeneration in vivo, suggesting their role in repairing the human testicular niche [26]. The regenerative capacity of SSCs, particularly after chemotherapy-induced damage, is supported by molecular changes that enhance their mitotic activity and responsiveness to growth factor signaling, which are crucial for germline recovery [27]. Additionally, certain populations of spermatogonia identified through the expression of specific markers have been found to be essential for efficient testicular regeneration post-injury, expanding the stem cell activity pool for rapid tissue repair [28]. Human umbilical cord mesenchymal stem cells (HUC-MSCs) have also been investigated for their ability to promote spermatogenic regeneration and have shown promising results in enhancing germ cell-specific gene expression [29]. Bone marrow-derived mesenchymal stem cells (BMSCs) have the potential to transdifferentiate into spermatogenic-like cells, further supporting the possibility of endogenous fertility recovery [30]. The intricate balance between SSC self-renewal and differentiation is regulated by growth factors and intrinsic signaling pathways, underscoring the importance of understanding SSC biology for therapeutic applications [31]. Research on testis stem cells, including the generation of cells with embryonic-like potential from adult testis germ cells, has opened new avenues for patient-specific stem cell therapies [32]. Finally, the fundamental biology of testicular stem cells (TSCs) and their role in spermatogenesis provide a foundation for developing techniques such as TSC transplantation and grafting, offering hope for fertility restoration in cancer patients [33].

What Is the Role of Stem Cells in Sperm Production and Gametogenesis?

Spermatogonial stem cells (SSCs) play a pivotal role in spermatozoa production and the broader process of gametogenesis, ensuring the continuity of male fertility across generations. SSCs, the most primitive spermatogonia in the testis, have a dual capacity for self-renewal and differentiation. This unique ability allows them to maintain a stable pool of stem cells while generating daughter cells that undergo differentiation to become mature spermatozoa, thus transmitting genetic information to subsequent generations [22]. Spermatogenesis, which begins with SSCs, is crucial for producing a sufficient number of specialized gametes to maintain normal fertility [34]. SSC maintenance involves a complex interplay between niche and intrinsic factors. Growth factors, such as GDNF, FGF, and EGF, play significant roles in regulating SSC self-renewal and proliferation through various signaling pathways, including Ras-ERK1/2, PI3K/Akt, and MEK/ERK-mTOR [31, 35]. Additionally, transcription factors such as OCT4, PLZF, and FOXO1 directly influence SSC self-renewal and proliferation [36]. This intricate regulatory network ensures the continuous generation of functional spermatozoa [31]. Recent advancements have highlighted the potential of SSCs in regenerative medicine. Techniques such as spermatogonial transplantation and in vitro spermatogenesis (IVS) have been developed, offering hope for fertility restoration in cases of male infertility [37]. These applications underscore the importance of SSCs not only in the natural process of gametogenesis but also in medical interventions aimed at overcoming challenges associated with male fertility [38]. Furthermore, the dynamic behavior of SSCs, including their ability to balance self-renewal and differentiation at the population level, exemplifies the concept of "population asymmetry" [39]. This balance is critical for lifelong sperm production and maintenance of fertility. Understanding the role of SSCs in spermatozoa production and gametogenesis is fundamental to both basic biological research and the development of therapeutic strategies for male infertility.

Regenerative Medicine Approaches Using Stem Cells

Mesenchymal Stem Cells (MSCs) in Male Reproductive Regeneration

MSCs are multipotent stem cells that can differentiate into various cell types and exert strong paracrine effects, making them a promising tool for regenerative medicine. Their ability to secrete growth factors and cytokines can modulate the testicular microenvironment, promoting tissue repair and regeneration in the testis.

- *Mechanisms of MSCs in Spermatogenesis*
  - *Differentiation into Germ Cells*: MSCs derived from the bone marrow, adipose tissue, and umbilical cord have been shown to differentiate into germ cell-like cells in vitro [30]. This differentiation is often induced by specific culture conditions or growth factors that mimic the testicular niche [30].
  - *Paracrine Effects*: MSCs secrete extracellular vesicles and soluble factors that can enhance spermatogenesis by promoting the proliferation and survival of spermatogonial stem cells (SSCs). These factors include fibroblast growth factor (FGF2), which supports SSC self-renewal.
  - *Immunomodulatory Properties*: MSCs can modulate the immune system, reducing inflammation and oxidative stress in the testicular microenvironment, which is often associated with infertility.
- *Applications of MSCs in Male Infertility:* MSCs have been tested in animal models of male infertility, including non-obstructive azoospermia (NOA) and chemotherapy-induced infertility. Studies have shown that MSC transplantation can lead to the recovery of spermatogenesis and improved fertility outcomes [30]. For example, bone marrow-derived MSCs (BMSCs) have been shown to integrate into seminiferous tubules and express spermatogonial stem cell markers [30].

Despite these promising results, several challenges remain to be addressed. The exact mechanisms by which MSCs contribute to spermatogenesis are not fully understood, and the long-term safety and efficacy of MSC transplantation in humans require further investigation.

Tissue Engineering and Biomaterials in Male Reproductive Regeneration

Tissue engineering combines cells, biomaterials, and growth factors to create functional tissue substitutes. In the context of male infertility, this approach aims to reconstruct the testicular microenvironment to support spermatogenesis.

- *Key Strategies in Tissue Engineering*

1. *Scaffolds and Biomaterials*: Scaffolds made from natural or synthetic materials, such as decellularized testicular matrix (DTM) or polylactic-co-glycolic acid (PLGA), provide structural support for cell attachment and growth [36]. These scaffolds can be seeded with SSCs or MSCs to create a bioartificial testis [36].
2. *3D Culture Systems*: Three-dimensional (3D) culture systems, including bioreactors and microfluidic devices, have been developed to mimic the complex testicular microenvironment of the seminiferous tubules. These systems allow spatial and temporal regulation of growth factors and hormones, which are critical for spermatogenesis [36].
3. *In Vitro Spermatogenesis (IVS)* involves the generation of functional spermatozoa from SSCs in vitro. This approach has been successful in animal models; however, achieving complete spermatogenesis in humans remains challenging because of the complexity of the process [36].

- *Applications of Tissue Engineering*
  Tissue engineering has the potential to address several clinical scenarios, including:
  - *Fertility Preservation for Prepubertal Boys*: Tissue engineering can be used to preserve immature testicular tissue in prepubertal boys undergoing gonadotoxic treatment. This approach involves cryopreserving testicular tissue and using bioengineering techniques to optimize grafting outcomes.
  - *Treatment of Non-obstructive Azoospermia*: Tissue engineering strategies, such as the use of scaffolds seeded with SSCs, may provide a novel treatment for NOA by restoring the testicular niche and promoting spermatogenesis [36].
  - *Development of Artificial Testes*: Advances in tissue engineering could lead to the creation of artificial testes that can support spermatogenesis and hormone production, offering a potential solution for severe testicular damage.

Spermatogonial Stem Cells (SSCs) in Male Reproductive Regeneration

SSCs are the foundation of spermatogenesis, as they are responsible for the continuous production of spermatozoa throughout a male's life. SSC dysfunction or depletion is a common cause of male infertility [40].

- *Role of SSCs in Spermatogenesis:* SSCs have two key functions: self-renewal to maintain the stem cell pool and differentiation to produce mature spermatozoa [22, 36]. The regulation of SSCs is tightly controlled by the testicular niche, which includes somatic cells such as Sertoli cells and peritubular myoid cells, as well as a complex interplay of hormones and growth factors [41].

- *Therapeutic Applications of SSCs*
  - SSC transplantation has been successfully used in animal models to restore fertility in cases of SSC depletion [36]. This approach involves isolating SSCs from a fertile donor or the patient's own tissue, expanding them in vitro and transplanting them back into the recipient's testes [36].
  - *In Vitro Spermatogenesis*: SSCs can be cultured in vitro to produce spermatozoa, which can then be used in Assisted Reproductive Technologies (ARTs), such as in vitro fertilization (IVF) or intracytoplasmic sperm injection (ICSI), for research purposes and potential future applications.
  - *Gene Editing and Correction*: SSCs can be used as a platform for gene editing to correct genetic mutations that cause male infertility. This approach has the potential to prevent the transmission of genetic disorders to future generations.

In Vitro Spermatogenesis (IVS) and Its Challenges

IVS is a groundbreaking technology that generates functional spermatozoa from SSCs or induced pluripotent stem cells (iPSCs) in vitro. This approach has the potential to treat various forms of male infertility, including NOA, and preserve fertility in individuals undergoing gonadotoxic treatments [42].

- *Recent Advances in IVS*
  - *Mouse Models*: IVS has been successfully achieved in mouse models with the generation of functional spermatozoa that can produce viable offspring.
  - *Human Applications*: Although IVS in humans is still in its infancy, recent studies have made progress in culturing human SSCs and inducing their differentiation into haploid male germ cells.
  - *Technological Innovations*: Advances in tissue engineering, such as the development of bioreactors and microfluidic systems, have improved the efficiency of IVS by providing a more physiological environment for spermatogenesis.
- *Challenges in IVS*
  - *Complexity of Spermatogenesis*: Spermatogenesis is a highly regulated process involving multiple stages of cell proliferation, differentiation, and maturation. Replicating this process in vitro is a significant technical challenge.
  - *Epigenetic and Genetic Stability*: Ensuring the epigenetic and genetic stability of spermatozoa generated through IVS is critical for their functionality and safety in clinical applications.
  - *Ethical Considerations*: The use of IVS raises ethical concerns, particularly regarding the potential for misuse in reproductive technologies.

Challenges and Ethical Considerations in Stem Cell-Based Fertility Regeneration

The use of stem cells in fertility treatment presents a complex array of ethical concerns and challenges, reflecting the broader societal, regulatory, and clinical implications of this rapidly evolving field [12]. One of the primary ethical concerns revolves around the sources of stem cells, particularly the use of human embryonic stem cells (hESCs), which raises significant ethical dilemmas owing to the destruction of human embryos [12]. This issue has historically limited the development of hESC-based clinical therapies, although the advent of induced pluripotent stem cells (iPSCs) has somewhat mitigated these concerns by providing an alternative that does not require the destruction of embryos [12, 43]. However, iPSCs introduce their own ethical challenges, including the potential for abnormal reprogramming and tumor generation during stem cell therapy, as well as the prohibition of their use in human cloning, germ cell production, or embryo creation [12, 44]. Informed consent is another critical ethical challenge, necessitating clear communication with patients about the risks, benefits, and unproven nature of stem cell-based fertility treatments [12, 45]. The need for balanced and complete scientific reporting and public communication is paramount to ensure that patients and the public are well informed about the potential and limitations of these treatments [12, 46]. Regulatory frameworks and ethical guidelines are essential for navigating the ethical landscape of stem cell use in fertility treatment, addressing issues such as beneficence, justice, and equitable access to treatment [12, 47]. Moreover, the clinical application of stem cells in fertility treatments must be normalized and standardized to effectively address ethical issues [12, 48]. The societal consequences of stem cell-based fertility treatments, including the potential to alter traditional concepts of parenthood and family, warrant careful consideration. Researchers, clinicians, and bioethics committees must engage in responsible clinical implementation processes that consider the broad societal impact of innovative treatments [12, 49]. Collectively, these ethical concerns and challenges underscore the need for a multidisciplinary approach involving regulators, scientists, clinicians, professional societies, and patient advocacy groups to collaboratively articulate expectations and develop ethical frameworks for the proper development and delivery of stem cell-based fertility treatments [12, 50].

Hormonal Therapies

Hormonal Imbalances and Fertility

Hormonal Imbalances Can Have a Significant Impact on Male Fertility

Hormonal imbalances significantly affect sperm production and quality, thereby affecting fertility. Follicle-stimulating hormone (FSH) and luteinizing hormone (LH) are pivotal in initiating and maintaining spermatogenesis, and imbalances in these hormones are correlated with altered sperm parameters [51]. Testosterone, which is produced under LH stimulation, is essential for spermatogenesis, and lower serum testosterone levels are associated with reduced semen quality [52]. Conversely, higher testosterone levels have been shown to be positively correlated with sperm count and motility, suggesting a protective role in maintaining sperm quality [53]. Prolactin and estradiol, although less directly involved in spermatogenesis, have been observed to negatively affect sperm quality when their levels are abnormal. Elevated prolactin levels are associated with decreased sperm motility, morphology, and viability [54]. In summary, specific hormonal imbalances, particularly those involving FSH, LH, testosterone, prolactin, and estradiol, significantly affect sperm production and quality, underscoring the need for comprehensive hormonal evaluation in the assessment of male infertility [13, 54].

Advancements in Hormonal Treatments

Current Testosterone and Gonadotropin-Based Therapies

1. *Gonadotropin Therapy*
   Gonadotropins, including human chorionic gonadotropin (hCG) and follicle-stimulating hormone (FSH), are the cornerstone treatments for male infertility, particularly in cases of hypogonadotropic hypogonadism. These therapies mimic the natural hypothalamic-pituitary-gonadal (HPG) axis to stimulate testosterone production and spermatogenesis [14, 55, 56].

   - *Indications and Prognostic Factors*: Gonadotropin therapy is primarily indicated for *hypogonadotropic hypogonadism* [14], including *congenital hypogonadotropic hypogonadism (CHH)* [15]. It has also shown utility in *non-obstructive azoospermia (NOA)*, where recombinant gonadotropins may retrieve viable sperm [15, 57]. The efficacy can vary, underscoring the need for *personalized approaches and research into predictive biomarkers*, with efforts to identify predictors of response to gonadotropin therapy to optimize outcomes [21, 22].

- *Mechanism of Action*: hCG acts like luteinizing hormone (LH), stimulating Leydig cells to produce testosterone, whereas FSH directly supports Sertoli cells in the testes, promoting spermatogenesis [14, 58, 59].
- *Efficacy*: Studies have shown that combined hCG and FSH therapy can *restore spermatogenesis in 75%–80% of men with CHH* [15, 55]. In patients with NOA, recombinant gonadotropins have been shown to retrieve viable sperm [15, 57]. Novel protocols involving "reboot" therapy with high-dose hCG and FSH injections have shown promising results in restoring spermatogenesis in men with severe oligospermia or azoospermia, with 74% of treated patients demonstrating improved semen parameters [18].
- *Side Effects*: The provided sources did not explicitly detail the side effects of gonadotropin therapy.

2. *Selective Estrogen Receptor Modulators (SERMs)*
   SERMs, such as *clomiphene citrate*, are widely used to modulate the HPG axis. They inhibit negative feedback on the hypothalamus, increasing endogenous gonadotropin release and, subsequently, testosterone production [15, 60].

   - *Indications and Prognostic Factors*: SERMs are particularly effective in men with *idiopathic infertility or hypergonadotropic hypogonadism* [16, 60]. They are often used empirically to enhance sperm parameters in men with normal gonadotropin levels [16, 61]. However, their use is often empirical because of the *limited availability of high-quality Randomized Controlled Trials (RCTs)*, highlighting the need for more robust studies to establish standardized protocols [21, 62, 63].
   - *Mechanism of Action*: SERMs inhibit the negative feedback of estradiol on the hypothalamus, leading to an increased pulsatile release of GnRH. This, in turn, stimulates the pituitary gland to release more LH and FSH, thereby increasing endogenous testosterone production and promoting spermatogenesis [16, 60].
   - *Efficacy*: SERMs have been shown to be effective in improving sperm parameters in select patients, particularly those with idiopathic infertility or hypergonadotropic hypogonadism [16, 60].

Aromatase Inhibitors (AIs)

Aromatase inhibitors block the conversion of testosterone to estradiol, thereby maintaining higher testosterone levels and improving spermatogenesis. They are particularly beneficial for men with a low testosterone-to-estradiol ratio [16, 59, 60].

- *Indications and Prognostic Factors*: AIs are particularly beneficial for *men with a low testosterone-to-estradiol ratio* [16, 60]. Their efficacy has been observed in select patients, although their use remains controversial due to limited evidence from randomized controlled trials [17, 40, 60]. Further research is required to establish standardized treatment protocols [21, 62, 63].

- *Mechanism of Action*: AIs prevent the enzyme aromatase from converting androgens (such as testosterone) into estrogens (such as estradiol), thereby increasing systemic and intratesticular testosterone levels, which are crucial for spermatogenesis [16, 59].
- *Efficacy*: AIs have been shown to *improve sperm count and motility in selected patients* [17, 60]. Optimizing intratesticular testosterone (ITT) levels through such therapies can improve sperm retrieval outcomes in patients with NOA [20, 40].

1. *Testosterone Therapy*
   While exogenous testosterone is contraindicated in men seeking fertility because of its suppressive effects on spermatogenesis, certain formulations and adjunct therapies are being explored to mitigate these effects [17, 41].

   - *Indications and Prognostic Factors*: Exogenous testosterone replacement therapy (TRT) is *contraindicated in men seeking fertility* because it reduces endogenous testosterone production and impairs spermatogenesis [17, 41]. However, strategies such as combining TRT with hCG or FSH may be employed to *preserve spermatogenesis* in hypogonadal men who require testosterone replacement while desiring fertility [17, 22, 64].
   - *Mechanism of Action*: Exogenous testosterone suppresses the hypothalamic-pituitary-gonadal (HPG) axis, leading to a decrease in endogenous LH and FSH, which are essential for natural testosterone production and spermatogenesis [17, 41].
   - *Efficacy*: Testosterone therapy is *not effective for restoring male fertility*; rather, it *impairs* spermatogenesis [17, 41].
   - The primary side effect relevant to fertility is the *suppression of spermatogenesis*, which reduces sperm production [17, 41].

Emerging Therapies and Innovations

1. *Combination Gonadotropin Therapy*

Recent studies suggest that combining hCG with purified FSH (rather than clomiphene-mediated FSH release) may improve spermatogenesis recovery in men with a history of testosterone use [18, 64]. This approach has shown promising results, with 74% of treated patients demonstrating improved semen parameters [18, 64]. *Novel Protocols*: Emerging data support the use of “reboot” therapy, which involves high-dose hCG and FSH injections, to restore spermatogenesis in men with severe oligospermia or azoospermia [18, 42].

2. *Recombinant Gonadotropins*

Recombinant human gonadotropins (rhFSH and rhLH) offer a more purified and standardized alternative to traditional gonadotropin therapy. These agents have been successfully used to stimulate spermatogenesis in men with NOA, with viable sperm retrieved in up to 50% of cases [19, 57]. A study demonstrated that recombinant gonadotropin therapy enabled successful pregnancies via intracytoplasmic sperm injection (ICSI), highlighting its potential as an alternative to sperm [19, 57].

3. *Optimization of Intratesticular Testosterone (ITT) Levels*

Intratesticular testosterone levels are critical for spermatogenesis, particularly during spermiogenesis. Therapies aimed at optimizing ITT levels, such as hCG-based hormonal therapy, have shown promise in improving sperm retrieval outcomes in patients with NOA [20, 40, 59]. *Future Directions*: Research is ongoing to develop protocols that enhance ITT levels while maintaining HPG axis function, potentially offering new hope for men with severe spermatogenic impairment [20, 40, 42].

Challenges and Considerations

1. *Variability in Response*
   The efficacy of hormonal therapies varies widely among individuals, with some men showing minimal improvement despite receiving treatment. This variability underscores the need for personalized approaches and further research on predictive biomarkers [21, 60, 62].
2. *Lack of Randomized Controlled Trials (RCTs)*
   Many therapies, such as SERMs and AIs, are used empirically because of the limited availability of high-quality RCTs. Larger, well-designed studies are needed to establish standardized treatment protocols [21, 62, 63].
3. *Balancing Fertility and Testosterone Replacement Men* requiring testosterone therapy for hypogonadism often face challenges in preserving fertility. Emerging strategies, such as combining TRT with hCG or FSH, aim to address this dilemma [22, 41].

Future Directions

1. *Personalized Medicine*
   Advances in understanding the genetic and molecular underpinnings of spermatogenesis offer opportunities for developing tailored therapies. For example, identifying predictors of response to gonadotropin therapy could help optimize treatment outcomes [22, 42, 55].

2. *Novel Therapeutic Targets*
   Research on the role of growth factors, such as epidermal growth factor-like growth factors, and their interaction with gonadotropins may uncover new therapeutic targets for spermatogenic disorders [23, 59].
3. *Fertility Preservation During Testosterone Therapy*
   Innovative approaches, such as intermittent TRT or adjunctive therapies, are being explored to maintain fertility in hypogonadal men requiring testosterone replacement therapy [23, 41].

Genetic and Epigenetic Factors

Genetic Determinants of Male Infertility

Genetic abnormalities associated with infertility affect approximately 15% of men [65]. The main known genetic causes of male infertility are congenital bilateral absence of the vas deferens associated with cystic fibrosis gene mutations, deletions in the long arm of the Y chromosome, and autosomal and sex chromosomal gene disorders [66]. Considering that more than 2000 genes are responsible for spermatogenesis and spermiogenesis, mutations in these genes can cause male infertility [67].

Chromosomal abnormalities may be numerical or structural (e.g., inversions or translocations) [68]. The most common numerical chromosomal disorder in infertile men is Klinefelter syndrome (KS) [69]. KS is a disorder caused by the presence of an additional X chromosome, and hypogonadism is caused by primary testicular disease [70]. The most common findings in patients with KS are azoospermia and oligospermia [71], with a prevalence of 5% in men with severe oligozoospermia and 10% in men [72]. The most common autosomal structural chromosomal disorders in infertile men are reciprocal Robertsonian translocations and inversions, which are more common in patients with oligozoospermia [66, 68].

The Y chromosome contains the majority of genes that are particularly important for spermatogenesis and the development of male gonads. The last three segments form the male-specific region of the Y chromosome (MSY), and deletions, duplications, and inversions that occur can lead to azoospermia, Sertoli cell-only syndrome, severe oligozoospermia, and spermatogenic arrest [73]. Y chromosome microdeletions are the second most common genetic cause of male infertility, following Klinefelter syndrome. The AZF region on the long arm of the Y chromosome (Yq) contains genes that allow sperm to grow and develop; microdeletions in this region are called AZFa, AZFb, and AZFc deletions [68, 73]. Complete deletions involving the AZFa and AZFb regions have poor prognostic significance for sperm retrieval using TESE. Therefore, TESE is not recommended for these patients, although testicular sperm can be found in 50%–75% of men with AZFc microdeletions [68].

Many X-linked genes are expressed in the testis. It has been reported that X-linked testis expressed 11 (TEX11) and human reproductive homeobox (RHOX) genes are associated with male infertility; a protein encoded by TEX11 plays a role in the pathogenesis of azoospermia, and mutations in the human reproductive homeobox (RHOX) gene (RHOXF1 and RHOXF2/2B) expressed in germ cells have been identified in men with severe oligozoospermia [66]. Kallmann syndrome, which has both X-linked and autosomal genetic components, is defined as idiopathic hypogonadotropic hypogonadism with anosmia or hyposmia and is another problem that can cause infertility in men [73]. This disease is caused by a defect in the migration of GnRH neurons and has specific deletions in the KAL1 (KS 1 sequence) and FGFR1 (fibroblast growth factor receptor 1) genes [74, 75].

The cystic fibrosis transmembrane conductance regulator (CFTR) gene affects the formation of the ejaculatory duct, seminal vesicle, vas deferens, and the distal 2/3 of the epididymis; therefore, men with CFTR abnormalities may experience infertility that prevents sperm transport, including oligospermia, epididymal obstruction, ejaculatory duct obstruction, seminal vesicle abnormalities, congenital unilateral absence of the vas deferens, and congenital bilateral absence of the vas deferens [68, 76].

Epigenetic Modifications and Fertility

Epigenetics involves molecular modifications that affect gene expression without altering DNA sequences [77]. Proper functioning of epigenetic mechanisms during gonadal development and spermatogenesis is essential for normal sperm function and semen production [66]. DNA methylation, post-translational modifications of histones, chromatin remodeling, and gene expression regulation by miRNAs are among the most frequent manifestations of epigenetic modifications that regulate all phases of spermatogenesis and fertilization processes [78]. They are crucial for the differentiation and maturation of cells, particularly spermatozoa [78].

DNA methylation is the process by which a methyl group is transferred by DNA methyltransferases from S-adenosylmethionine to the fifth carbon of the cytosine ring at different methylation sites [79]. Oxidative stress and urinary phthalates can impair DNA methylation [80]. Appropriate and correct DNA methylation leads to proper chromatin condensation in the sperm head, sperm maturation, and fertilization [81]. When methylation is abnormal, there is incomplete or abnormal condensation of sperm chromatin, causing DNA damage, impairing fertilization, and affecting the pregnancy rate [82]. Clinical manifestations include oligozoospermia, teratozoospermia, asthenozoospermia, oligoasthenozoospermia, oligoteratozoospermia, asthenoteratozoospermia, and oligoasthenoteratozoospermia [82].

Histone post-translational protein modifications (PTMs) are vital for the biological regulation of mitosis, spermatogenesis, and sperm functions, such as transcription, DNA repair, DNA replication, and chromosome condensation [78, 83]. For example, acetylation and methylation of H3 and H4 and ubiquitination of H3K4 and

H2B lead to increased gene expression in testicular tissues [66]. At the end of the germ cell differentiation process, which involves DNA repair, recombination, and gene expression of histone PTMs, spermatozoa develop [84]. Failure in histone alteration and/or modification can lead to azoospermia, oligozoospermia, and teratozoospermia [84].

Chromatin remodeling is regulated by ATP-dependent complexes and can function to both activate and repress gene expression [79, 85]. During sperm chromatin remodeling, a large amount of DNA in spermatozoa is packed into a tiny nucleus. Appropriate DNA packaging is essential for normal spermatogenesis and fertility. DNA in mature spermatozoa is densely packed with protamines, and during fertilization, the highly condensed nucleoprotamine must be extracted from this package and rearranged into a nucleosomal complex. Incorrect modifications at any step in these processes can lead to male infertility [78].

Non-coding RNAs (siRNAs, miRNAs, and piRNAs) play essential roles in the epigenetic regulation of gene expression in many cellular processes in eukaryotes. They are expressed in male germ cells, spermatocytes, and round spermatids during spermatogenesis and are involved in the regulation of cell proliferation, apoptosis regulation and inhibition, and cell cycle regulation [79, 86]. Disorders in these processes can lead to non-obstructive azoospermia, asthenozoospermia, and oligoasthenozoospermia [87, 88].

Genetic Screening and Counseling

Karyotyping, a type of chromosomal analysis, is a genetic testing method that identifies numerical chromosomal abnormalities and structural defects. Karyotype abnormalities are the most common type of genetic defect and are observed in patients with azoospermia and oligozoospermia [46, 89]. The most common karyotypic abnormality is Klinefelter syndrome (47, XXY). The EAU Sexual and Reproductive Health Guidelines recommend that all men with azoospermia and oligozoospermia (spermatozoa <five million/mL) should be offered diagnostic standard karyotype analysis and genetic counseling [68].

Men with unilateral absence of the vas deferens and normal kidneys should be screened for cystic fibrosis transmembrane conductance regulator gene mutations [68]. In addition, for men with structural anomalies of the vas deferens, both partners should be screened for CFTR mutations, comprising a minimal panel of common point mutations and the 5 T allele [89].

Y chromosome microdeletions affect AZFa, AZFb, and AZFc on the long arm of the Y chromosome. Y chromosome microdeletion testing is recommended if the sperm concentration is lower than 5×10 U/mL. However, this test is mandatory if the sperm concentration is $<1 \times 10$ units/mL [68].

The latest EAU Sexual and Reproductive Health Guidelines recommend sperm DNA fragmentation (SDF) testing for the evaluation of couples with recurrent pregnancy loss from natural conception and ART failure or men with unexplained infertility [68]. It is also strongly recommended that genetic counseling be provided to all couples in whom genetic abnormalities are detected on genetic testing and to patients with an inherited disease [48].

Lifestyle and Environmental Impact

The Impact of Lifestyle Factors on Male Fertility

Infertility is a common health problem that affects nearly 15% of couples of reproductive age [90]. Many factors directly affect fertility potential and cause infertility. A significant association exists between lifestyle habits and fertility potential [90]. Male infertility is increasingly seen as a consequence of lifestyle and environmental factors such as dietary habits, smoking, adiposity, and use of steroids, alcohol, drugs, and chemicals [91]. These factors can affect semen volume, sperm concentration, motility, and viability [91]. Cigarette smoking causes exposure to chemical and hazardous substances that decrease fertility potential [92]. Alcohol affects the hypothalamus-pituitary-gonadal axis, which in turn affects hormonal levels and Leydig and Sertoli cell functions [92]. Chronic alcohol consumption directly affects sperm maturation, morphology, quality, and hormone levels [92]. Obesity, psychological stress, advanced paternal age, sleep disturbances, mobile phone exposure, and caffeine intake are other factors closely linked to fertility potential [92].

Environmental Exposures and Fertility

High-temperature exposure may also negatively affect sperm quality [93]. Long-duration sitting, radiant heat exposure, varicocele, and cryptorchidism are factors that can cause scrotal hyperthermia [92]. The chemicals present in pesticides, cosmetic products, air, and water can affect hormonal regulation and are called endocrine-disrupting chemicals [94]. These chemicals affect the secretion of luteinizing hormone and follicle-stimulating hormone, which directly affect spermatogenesis and androgen secretion [94]. Pesticides, per- and polyfluorinated alkyl substances, formaldehyde, benzene, bisphenol, and phthalate are the main occupational exposures, and pesticides, dietary factors, alcohol, smoking, bisphenols, phthalates, parabens, and electromagnetic fields are the main environmental exposures related to male infertility [94]. Dibromochloropropane was found to have negative impacts on sperm counts [95]. Certain occupations pose additional risks with different types of exposure [95]. Bakers, welders, metal, glass, and ceramic industry workers, and sedentary job workers who sit for hours are at risk of scrotal heat exposure; pesticide applicators, pesticide producers, and fruit and vegetable harvesters are at risk of pesticide exposure; chemical manufacturing workers, drivers, traffic wardens, and roadway cleaners are at risk of chemical exposure; workers in contraceptive pills or other hormonal agent manufacturing are at risk of hormonal exposure; professional and amateur sportsmen are at risk of recreational/performance-enhancing drugs; and cancer survivors are at risk of exposure to therapeutic treatment [95]. Studies have also investigated the association between environmental and occupational exposure and seminal vesicle lead and cadmium levels, and it was found that exposure was associated with reduced sperm motility, viability, and normal sperm forms [96].

Mitigation Strategies

Reduced stress, changes in dietary habits, healthy eating, increased physical activity, and increased social support positively affect sperm quality in men [90]. Scrotal cooling, which provides an optimal temperature, improves spermatogenesis [93]. Studies have shown the positive effects of antioxidant therapies, including aescin, coenzyme Q10, glutathione, Korean red ginseng, L-carnitine, Nigella sativa, omega-3, selenium, zinc, folate, and menevit, on male infertility [97]. Considering the outcomes of the literature and the factors that affect fertility potential, it is very important to avoid negative lifestyle and environmental factors to increase fertility potential and receive accurate pharmacological, psychological, and dietary support to protect this potential [51].

Innovation in Male Fertility Diagnostics and Supportive Technologies

Emerging Technologies in Male Fertility

Emerging technologies are expected to reshape the evaluation, diagnosis, and treatment of male infertility. Computer-assisted semen analysis techniques and advanced imaging technologies (e.g., ultrasound for microdissection) are becoming increasingly popular for diagnostic precision.

Advanced Diagnostic and Predictive Tools

Innovative technological approaches for *sperm DNA double-strand break diagnosis* are also used to prevent reproductive failure, offering useful insights for preventive healthcare implications and potentially cost-effective solutions. Such diagnostic advancements can guide the selection of appropriate regenerative therapies and predict their success likelihood.

- *Note Regarding Artificial Intelligence (AI)*: The provided sources primarily discuss the application of Artificial Intelligence (AI) in the context of Assisted Reproductive Technologies (ART), such as assessing the quality of oocytes, sperm, and embryos, and automating ART procedures [89, 98]. Since this chapter is strictly focused on male fertility *regeneration* and excludes ART, information on AI's direct role of AI in *regenerative* processes (e.g., optimizing stem cell cultures for spermatogenesis or discovering new regenerative factors) is not available within the given sources. Therefore, a detailed section on AI for regeneration cannot be included at this time based on the available material.

Ethical and Legal Considerations

The ethical concerns mentioned in this section pertain specifically to profound interventions in human life and fertility through regenerative medicine [2].

The use of stem cells in fertility treatment presents a complex array of ethical concerns and challenges, reflecting the broader societal, regulatory, and clinical implications of this rapidly evolving field [12]. One of the primary ethical concerns revolves around the sources of stem cells, particularly the use of human embryonic stem cells (hESCs), which raises significant ethical dilemmas owing to the destruction of human embryos [12]. This issue has historically limited the development of hESC-based clinical therapies, although the advent of induced pluripotent stem cells (iPSCs) has somewhat mitigated these concerns by providing an alternative that does not require the destruction of embryos [12, 43]. However, iPSCs introduce their own ethical challenges, including the potential for abnormal reprogramming and tumor generation during stem cell therapy, as well as the prohibition of their use in human cloning, germ cell production, or embryo creation [12, 44].

Informed consent is another critical ethical challenge, necessitating clear communication with patients about the risks, benefits, and unproven nature of stem cell-based fertility treatments [12, 45]. The need for *balanced and complete scientific reporting and public communication* is paramount to ensure that patients and the public are well informed about the potential and limitations of these treatments [12, 46]. *Regulatory frameworks and ethical guidelines* are essential for navigating the ethical landscape of stem cell use in fertility treatment, addressing issues such as beneficence, justice, and equitable access to treatment [12, 47]. Moreover, the clinical application of stem cells in fertility treatments must be normalized and standardized to effectively address ethical issues [12, 48]. The *societal consequences* of stem cell-based fertility treatments, including the potential to alter traditional concepts of parenthood and family, warrant careful consideration. Researchers, clinicians, and bioethics committees must engage in responsible clinical implementation processes that consider the broad societal impact of innovative treatments [12, 49]. Collectively, these ethical concerns and challenges underscore the need for a multidisciplinary approach involving regulators, scientists, clinicians, professional societies, and patient advocacy groups to collaboratively articulate expectations and develop ethical frameworks for the proper development and delivery of stem cell-based fertility treatments [12, 50].

- *Note on Legal Frameworks and Regulations*: While legal and regulatory frameworks are crucial for reproductive medicine, the provided sources discuss these almost exclusively in the context of Assisted Reproductive Technologies (ART) (e.g., age limits for IVF, donor identity, surrogacy laws across countries) [94, 96, 99]. As this chapter is now strictly focused on male fertility *regeneration* and excludes ART, a detailed discussion of ART-specific legal frameworks is outside the scope of the revised chapter. The general principles of robust regulatory oversight for novel regenerative therapies remain essential, as highlighted in the conclusion [100].

Conclusion

The exploration of male fertility regeneration through stem cell research offers promising avenues for addressing male infertility [101]. The potential of stem cells, particularly spermatogonial and mesenchymal stem cells, to regenerate damaged testicular tissue and restore fertility, highlights a significant breakthrough in medical science [101]. However, the application of these technologies is challenging. Ethical considerations, particularly regarding the use of embryonic stem cells and genetic manipulation of induced pluripotent stem cells, require careful deliberation and robust ethical guidelines [101]. Additionally, the variability in treatment outcomes necessitates a more personalized approach to hormonal therapy tailored to individual profiles and infertility diagnoses [101].

The integration of advanced diagnostic technologies in the evaluation of male infertility could standardize procedures and potentially increase the efficacy of regenerative approaches. However, these technologies require further validation and ethical scrutiny to ensure their safety, effectiveness, and accessibility [102]. Legal and regulatory frameworks also play a crucial role in the adoption and practice of these technologies, varying significantly across jurisdictions and impacting treatment accessibility [102].

As we advance, it is imperative that ongoing research continues to refine these techniques, ensuring that they are both effective and ethically sound. Collaboration among scientists, clinicians, ethicists, and legislators is essential to navigate the complex landscape of male fertility regeneration, ultimately leading to innovative solutions that are both scientifically feasible and ethically sound [103].

Further research is needed to explore the following:

Optimization of MSC Therapy: Investigating the optimal sources of MSCs, their mechanisms of action, and the long-term safety and efficacy of MSC transplantation in humans [104–106].

Advancements in Tissue Engineering: Development of more sophisticated biomaterials and scaffolds that better mimic the testicular niche and support spermatogenesis [104, 107, 108].

Scaling Up IVS: Improving the efficiency and scalability of IVS to make it a viable option for clinical applications [104, 109].

Addressing Ethical and Regulatory Issues: Ensuring that the development and application of these technologies are guided by robust ethical frameworks and regulatory oversight [100].

In conclusion, the combination of stem cell therapy and tissue engineering represents a powerful approach for male reproductive regeneration. Although significant progress has been made, continued research and collaboration among scientists, clinicians, and policymakers are essential to realize the full potential of these technologies [100, 105–110].

References

1. Kumar R, Sharma A, Pattnaik AK, Varadwaj PK. Stem cells: an overview with respect to cardiovascular and renal diseases. J Nat Sci Biol Med. 2010;1(1):43–52.
2. Poliwoda S, Noor N, Downs E, Schaaf A, Cantwell A, Ganti L, et al. Stem cells: a comprehensive review of origins and emerging clinical roles in medical practice. Orthop Rev. 2022;14(3):37498.
3. Mitalipov S, Wolf D. Totipotency, pluripotency and nuclear reprogramming. Adv Biochem Eng Biotechnol. 2009;114:185–99.
4. Jiang Y, Jahagirdar BN, Reinhardt RL, Schwartz RE, Keene CD, Ortiz-Gonzalez XR, et al. Pluripotency of mesenchymal stem cells derived from adult bone marrow. Nature. 2002;418(6893):41–9.
5. Dulak J, Szade K, Szade A, Nowak W, Józkowicz A. Adult stem cells: hopes and hypes of regenerative medicine. Acta Biochim Pol. 2015;62(3):329–37.
6. Young RA. Control of the embryonic stem cell state. Cell. 2011;144(6):940–54.
7. Cable J, Fuchs E, Weissman I, Jasper H, Glass D, Rando TA, et al. Adult stem cells and regenerative medicine: a symposium report. Ann N Y Acad Sci. 2020;1462(1):27–36.
8. Aboul-Soud MAM, Alzahrani AJ, Mahmoud A. Induced pluripotent stem cells (iPSCs)-roles in regenerative therapies, disease modelling and drug screening. Cells. 2021;10(9):2319.
9. Botigelli RC, Guiltinan C, Arcanjo RB, Denicol AC. In vitro gametogenesis from embryonic stem cells in livestock species: recent advances, opportunities, and challenges to overcome. J Anim Sci. 2023;101:skad137.
10. Özdemi̇r AZ, Taştan AŞ. Stem cell applications in female infertility – a rewiev. J Exp Clin Med. 2023;40(1):122–6.
11. Cui YH, Chen W, Wu S, Wan CL, He Z. Generation of male germ cells in vitro from the stem cells. Asian J Androl. 2023;25(1):13.
12. Zhang W, Nie R, Cai Y, Xie W, Zou K. Progress in germline stem cell transplantation in mammals and the potential usage. Reprod Biol Endocrinol. 2022;20(1):59.
13. Saha S, Roy P, Corbitt C, Kakar SS. Application of stem cell therapy for infertility. Cells. 2021;10(7):1613.
14. Qamar AY, Hussain T, Rafique MK, Bang S, Tanga BM, Seong G, et al. The role of stem cells and their derived extracellular vesicles in restoring female and male fertility. Cells. 2021;10(9):2460.

15. Fayomi AP, Orwig KE. Spermatogonial stem cells and spermatogenesis in mice, monkeys and men. Stem Cell Res. 2018;29:207–14.
16. Inoue H, Sakurai T, Hasegawa K, Suzuki A, Saga Y. NANOS3 suppresses premature spermatogonial differentiation to expand progenitors and fine-tunes spermatogenesis in mice. Biol Open. 2022;11(4):bio059146.
17. Suzuki H, Sada A, Yoshida S, Saga Y. The heterogeneity of spermatogonia is revealed by their topology and expression of marker proteins including the germ cell-specific proteins Nanos2 and Nanos3. Dev Biol. 2009;336(2):222–31.
18. Rahbar M, Asadpour R, Azami M, Mazaheri Z, Hamali H. Improving the process of spermatogenesis in azoospermic mice using spermatogonial stem cells co-cultured with epididymosomes in three-dimensional culture system. Life Sci. 2022;310:121057.
19. Önen S, Köse S, Yersal N, Korkusuz P. Mesenchymal stem cells promote spermatogonial stem/progenitor cell pool and spermatogenesis in neonatal mice in vitro. Sci Rep. 2022;12(1):11494.
20. Gul M, Hildorf S, Dong L, Thorup J, Hoffmann ER, Jensen CFS, et al. Review of injection techniques for spermatogonial stem cell transplantation. Hum Reprod Update. 2020;26(3):368–91.
21. van Melis V, Roa-de la Cruz L, Hermann BP. Isolation of undifferentiated spermatogonia from adult and developing mouse testes. Methods Mol Biol Clifton NJ. 2023;2656:179–93.
22. Diao L, Turek PJ, John CM, Fang F, Reijo Pera RA. Roles of spermatogonial stem cells in spermatogenesis and fertility restoration. Front Endocrinol. 2022;13:895528.
23. Kanatsu-Shinohara M, Ogonuki N, Matoba S, Ogura A, Shinohara T. Autologous transplantation of spermatogonial stem cells restores fertility in congenitally infertile mice. Proc Natl Acad Sci. 2020;117(14):7837–44.
24. Ismail HY, Hussein S, Shaker NA, Rizk H, Wally YR. Stem cell treatment trials for regeneration of testicular tissue in laboratory animals. Reprod Sci. 2023;30(6):1770–81.
25. Mousbah AM, El-Samie A, Mohammed E, Elbehery AM, El-Nady AI. Immunohistochemistry and hormonal investigation for spermatogenesis restoration in degenerated testes of rats after bone marrow stem cells transplantation. J Appl Vet Sci. 2020;5(4):47–54.
26. Maghen L, Shlush E, Gat I, Filice M, Barretto TA, Jarvi K, et al. Human umbilical perivascular cells (HUCPVCs): a novel source of mesenchymal stromal-like (MSC) cells to support the regeneration of the testicular niche. Reproduction. 2017;153(1):85–95.
27. La HM, Liao J, Legrand JMD, Rossello FJ, Chan AL, Vaghjiani V, et al. Distinctive molecular features of regenerative stem cells in the damaged male germline. Nat Commun. 2022;13(1):2500.
28. Carrieri C, Comazzetto S, Grover A, Morgan M, Buness A, Nerlov C, et al. A transit-amplifying population underpins the efficient regenerative capacity of the testis. J Exp Med. 2017;214(6):1631–41.
29. Yang RF, Liu TH, Zhao K, Xiong CL. Enhancement of mouse germ cell-associated genes expression by injection of human umbilical cord mesenchymal stem cells into the testis of chemical-induced azoospermic mice. Asian J Androl. 2014;16(5):698.
30. Zhang D, Liu X, Peng J, He D, Lin T, Zhu J, et al. Potential spermatogenesis recovery with bone marrow mesenchymal stem cells in an azoospermic rat model. Int J Mol Sci. 2014;15(8):13151–65.
31. Wei B-H, Hao S-L, Yang W-X. Regulation of spermatogonial stem cell self-renewal and proliferation in mammals. Histol Histopathol. 2022;37(09):825–38.
32. Kee K, Reijo Pera RA, Turek PJ. Testicular germline stem cells. Nat Rev Urol. 2010;7(2):94–100.
33. Goossens E, Jahnukainen K, Mitchell R, van Pelt A, Pennings G, Rives N, et al. Fertility preservation in boys: recent developments and new insights †. Hum Reprod Open. 2020;2020(3):hoaa016.

34. Kubota H, Brinster RL. Spermatogonial stem cells†. Biol Reprod. 2018;99(1):52–74.
35. de Rooij DG. The nature and dynamics of spermatogonial stem cells. Development. 2017;144(17):3022–30.
36. Ibtisham F, Honaramooz A. Spermatogonial stem cells for in vitro spermatogenesis and in vivo restoration of fertility. Cells. 2020;9(3):745.
37. Abdelaal NE, Tanga BM, Abdelgawad M, Allam S, Fathi M, Saadeldin IM, et al. Cellular therapy via spermatogonial stem cells for treating impaired spermatogenesis, non-obstructive azoospermia. Cells. 2021;10(7):1779.
38. Aponte PM, Gutierrez-Reinoso MA, Garcia-Herreros M. Bridging the gap: animal models in next-generation reproductive technologies for male fertility preservation. Life. 2024;14(1):17.
39. Caires K, Broady J, McLean D. Maintaining the male germline: regulation of spermatogonial stem cells. J Endocrinol. 2010;205(2):133–45.
40. Piuzzi NS, Emara A, Chahla J, Mandelbaum BR. Ethical and practical considerations for integrating cellular ("stem cell") therapy into clinical practice. Curr Rev Musculoskelet Med. 2020;13(4):525–9.
41. Alahmad G, Aljohani S, Najjar MF. Ethical challenges regarding the use of stem cells: interviews with researchers from Saudi Arabia. BMC Med Ethics. 2020;21(1):35.
42. Lovell-Badge R, Anthony E, Barker RA, Bubela T, Brivanlou AH, Carpenter M, et al. ISSCR guidelines for stem cell research and clinical translation: the 2021 update. Stem Cell Rep. 2021;16(6):1398–408.
43. Sugarman J, Barker RA, Kerridge I, Lysaght T, Pellegrini G, Sipp D, et al. Tackling ethical challenges of premature delivery of stem cell-based therapies: ISSCR 2018 annual meeting focus session report. Stem Cell Rep. 2018;11(5):1021–5.
44. Volarevic V, Markovic BS, Gazdic M, Volarevic A, Jovicic N, Arsenijevic N, et al. Ethical and safety issues of stem cell-based therapy. Int J Med Sci. 2018;15(1):36–45.
45. Huang FG, Hu J, Liu JF, Gong JP, Liu Y. The ethical issues in the clinical application of stem cells. Int Surg J. 2017;4(3):852–5.
46. Hendriks S, Vliegenthart R, Repping S, Dancet EAF. Broad support for regulating the clinical implementation of future reproductive techniques. Hum Reprod. 2018;33(1):39–46.
47. Lo B, Parham L. Ethical issues in stem cell research. Endocr Rev. 2009;30(3):204–13.
48. Oduwole OO, Huhtaniemi IT, Misrahi M. The roles of luteinizing hormone, follicle-stimulating hormone and testosterone in spermatogenesis and folliculogenesis revisited. Int J Mol Sci. 2021;22(23):12735.
49. Andreassen M, Juul A, Feldt-Rasmussen U, Jørgensen N. Semen quality in patients with pituitary disease and adult-onset hypogonadotropic hypogonadism. Endocr Connect. 2018;7(4):523–33.
50. Zhao W, Jing J, Shao Y, Zeng R, Wang C, Yao B, et al. Circulating sex hormone levels in relation to male sperm quality. BMC Urol. 2020;20(1):101.
51. Wei TC, Huang WJ, Lin ATL, Chen KK. The role of hormones in semen parameters in patients with idiopathic or varicocele-related oligoasthenoteratozoospermia (OAT) syndrome. J Chin Med Assoc. 2013;76(11):624.
52. Dwyer AA, McDonald IR, Quinton R. Current landscape of fertility induction in males with congenital hypogonadotropic hypogonadism. Ann N Y Acad Sci. 2024;1540(1):133–46.
53. Ho CCK, Tan HM. Treatment of hypogonadal infertile males: a review. Sex Med Rev. 2013;1(1):42–9.
54. Fink J, Schoenfeld BJ, Hackney AC, Maekawa T, Horie S. Human chorionic gonadotropin treatment: a viable option for management of secondary hypogonadism and male infertility. Expert Rev Endocrinol Metab. 2021;16(1):1–8.
55. Shiraishi K, Matsuyama H. Gonadotropin actions on spermatogenesis and hormonal therapies for spermatogenic disorders [Review]. Endocr J. 2017;64(2):123–31.
56. Laursen RJ, Elbaek HO, Povlsen BB, Lykkegaard J, Jensen KBS, Esteves SC, et al. Hormonal stimulation of spermatogenesis: a new way to treat the infertile male with non-obstructive azoospermia? Int Urol Nephrol. 2019;51(3):453–6.

57. Çayan S, Altay AB, Rambhatla A, Colpi GM, Agarwal A. Is there a role for hormonal therapy in men with oligoasthenoteratozoospermia (OAT)? J Clin Med. 2024;14(1):185.
58. Madhukar D, Rajender S. Hormonal treatment of male infertility: promises and pitfalls. J Androl. 2009;30(2):95–112.
59. Shiraishi K. Hormonal therapy for non-obstructive azoospermia: basic and clinical perspectives. Reprod Med Biol. 2015;14(2):65–72.
60. Khodamoradi K, Khosravizadeh Z, Parmar M, Kuchakulla M, Ramasamy R, Arora H. Exogenous testosterone replacement therapy versus raising endogenous testosterone levels: current and future prospects. FS Rev. 2021;2(1):32–42.
61. Stocks BT, Oppenheimer AG, Campbell KJ, Lindsey JP, Kohn TP, Alexander JM, et al. Optimal restoration of spermatogenesis after testosterone therapy using human chorionic gonadotropin and follicle-stimulating hormone. Fertil Steril. 2024;S0015–0282(24):02313–6.
62. Herati AS, Kohn TP, Kassiri B. New frontiers in fertility preservation: a hypothesis on fertility optimization in men with hypergonadotrophic hypogonadism. Transl Androl Urol. 2020;9(Suppl 2):S171–7.
63. Pozzi E, Corsini C, Salonia A. Medical therapy for male infertility. Curr Opin Urol. 2025;35(2):157–64.
64. Rambhatla A, Shah R, Pinggera GM, Mostafa T, Atmoko W, Saleh R, et al. Pharmacological therapies for male infertility. Pharmacol Rev. 2025;77(2):100017. PHARMREV-AR-2023-001085.
65. Salonia A, Bettocchi C, Boeri L, Capogrosso P, Carvalho J, Cilesiz NC, et al. European Association of Urology guidelines on sexual and reproductive health-2021 update: male sexual dysfunction. Eur Urol. 2021;80(3):333–57.
66. O'Flynn N. Assessment and treatment for people with fertility problems: NICE guideline. Br J Gen Pract. 2014;64(618):50–1.
67. Agarwal A, Baskaran S, Parekh N, Cho CL, Henkel R, Vij S, et al. Male infertility. Lancet. 2021;397(10271):319–33.
68. Krausz C, Riera-Escamilla A. Genetics of male infertility. Nat Rev Urol. 2018;15(6):369–84.
69. Gunes S, Esteves SC. Role of genetics and epigenetics in male infertility. Andrologia. 2021;53(1):e13586.
70. Hochstenbach R, Hackstein JH. The comparative genetics of human spermatogenesis: clues from flies and other model organisms. Results Probl Cell Differ. 2000;28:271–98.
71. Lanfranco F, Kamischke A, Zitzmann M, Nieschlag E. Klinefelter's syndrome. Lancet. 2004;364(9430):273–83.
72. Sá R, Ferraz L, Barros A, Sousa M. The Klinefelter syndrome and testicular sperm retrieval outcomes. Genes. 2023;14(3):647.
73. Stormont GD, Deibert CM. Genetic causes and management of male infertility. Transl Androl Urol. 2021;10(3):1365372–1372.
74. Foresta C, Garolla A, Bartoloni L, Bettella A, Ferlin A. Genetic abnormalities among severely oligospermic men who are candidates for intracytoplasmic sperm injection. J Clin Endocrinol Metab. 2005;90(1):152–6.
75. Bhagavath B, Layman LC. The genetics of hypogonadotropic hypogonadism. Semin Reprod Med. 2007;25(4):272–86.
76. Boehm U, Bouloux PM, Dattani MT, de Roux N, Dodé C, Dunkel L, et al. Expert consensus document: European Consensus Statement on congenital hypogonadotropic hypogonadism–pathogenesis, diagnosis and treatment. Nat Rev Endocrinol. 2015;11(9):547–64.
77. Bieniek JM, Lapin CD, Jarvi KA. Genetics of CFTR and male infertility. Transl Androl Urol. 2021;10(3):1391–400.
78. Das L, Parbin S, Pradhan N, Kausar C, Patra SK. Epigenetics of reproductive infertility. Front Biosci-Sch. 2017;9(4):509–35.
79. Tahmasbpour Marzouni E, Ilkhani H, Beigi Harchegani A, Shafaghatian H, Layali I, Shahriary A. Epigenetic modifications, a new approach to male infertility etiology: a review. Int J Fertil Steril. 2022;16(1):1–9.

80. Neto FTL, Bach PV, Najari BB, Li PS, Goldstein M. Genetics of male infertility. Curr Urol Rep. 2016;17(10):70.
81. Menezo Y, Dale B, Elder K. The negative impact of the environment on methylation/epigenetic marking in gametes and embryos: a plea for action to protect the fertility of future generations. Mol Reprod Dev. 2019;86(10):1273–82.
82. Carrell DT. The sperm epigenome: implications for assisted reproductive technologies. In: Baldi E, Muratori M, editors. Genetic damage in human spermatozoa [Internet]. Cham: Springer International Publishing; 2019. [cited 2024 May 7]. p. 47–56. Available from: https://doi.org/10.1007/978-3-030-21664-1_3.
83. Rotondo JC, Lanzillotti C, Mazziotta C, Tognon M, Martini F. Epigenetics of male infertility: the role of DNA methylation. Front Cell Dev Biol [Internet]. 2021 [cited 2024 May 7];9. Available from: https://www.frontiersin.org/articles/10.3389/fcell.2021.689624.
84. Schon SB, Luense LJ, Wang X, Bartolomei MS, Coutifaris C, Garcia BA, et al. Histone modification signatures in human sperm distinguish clinical abnormalities. J Assist Reprod Genet. 2019;36(2):267–75.
85. Chioccarelli T, Pierantoni R, Manfrevola F, Porreca V, Fasano S, Chianese R, et al. Histone post-translational modifications and CircRNAs in mouse and human spermatozoa: potential epigenetic marks to assess human sperm quality. J Clin Med. 2020;9(3):640.
86. Rajender S, Avery K, Agarwal A. Epigenetics, spermatogenesis and male infertility. Mutat Res. 2011;727(3):62–71.
87. Song R, Hennig GW, Wu Q, Jose C, Zheng H, Yan W. Male germ cells express abundant endogenous siRNAs. Proc Natl Acad Sci. 2011;108(32):13159–64.
88. Lian J, Zhang X, Tian H, Liang N, Wang Y, Liang C, et al. Altered microRNA expression in patients with non-obstructive azoospermia. Reprod Biol Endocrinol. 2009;7(1):13.
89. Khazaie Y, Nasr Esfahani MH. MicroRNA and male infertility: a potential for diagnosis. Int J Fertil Steril. 2014;8(2):113–8.
90. Kim EJ, Nho JH. Lifestyle interventions for adults with infertility. J Lifestyle Med. 2022;12(2):69–71.
91. Biggs SN, Kennedy J, Lewis SL, Hearps S, O'Bryan MK, McLachlan R, et al. Lifestyle and environmental risk factors for unexplained male infertility: study protocol for Australian Male Infertility Exposure (AMIE), a case–control study. Reprod Health. 2023;20:32.
92. Durairajanayagam D. Lifestyle causes of male infertility. Arab J Urol. 2018;16(1):10–20.
93. Clavijo RI. Lifestyle habits and idiopathic male infertility: are men willing to change? FS Rep. 2021;2(3):266.
94. Marić T, Fučić A, Aghayanian A. Environmental and occupational exposures associated with male infertility. Arh Hig Rada Toksikol. 2021;72(3):101–13.
95. Sharpe RM. Lifestyle and environmental contribution to male infertility. Br Med Bull. 2000;56(3):630–42.
96. Wijesekara GUS, Fernando DMS, Wijerathna S, Bandara N. Environmental and occupational exposures as a cause of male infertility: a caveat. Ceylon Med J. 2015;60(2):52.
97. Yao DF, Mills JN. Male infertility: lifestyle factors and holistic, complementary, and alternative therapies. Asian J Androl. 2016;18(3):410–8.
98. Diaz P, Dullea A, Chu KY, Zizzo J, Loloi J, Reddy R, et al. Future of male infertility evaluation and treatment: brief review of emerging technology. Urology. 2022;169:9–16.
99. Wang TE, Lee CI, Huang CC, Tsao HM, Chang HC, Chang LS, et al. Innovative technology for evaluation of sperm DNA double-strand breaks diagnoses male factor infertility and prevents reproductive failures. Sci Rep. 2023;13:18996.
100. Irani D, Mehrabani D, Karimi-Busheri F. Mesenchymal stem cells in regenerative medicine, possible applications in the restoration of spermatogenesis: a review. Cell J. 2024;26(3):169–84.
101. Margiana R. Enhancing spermatogenesis in non-obstructive azoospermia through mesenchymal stem cell therapy. Curr Stem Cell Res Ther. 2024;19(11):1429–41.
102. El-Naggar L, Khalifa T, Elfeky BA. Use of mesenchymal stem cells in repairing male infertility suffering from oligospermia. J Product Dev. 2022;27(1):141–55.

103. Zhankina R, Baghban N, Askarov M, Saipiyeva D, Ibragimov A, Kadirova B, et al. Mesenchymal stromal/stem cells and their exosomes for restoration of spermatogenesis in non-obstructive azoospermia: a systemic review. Stem Cell Res Ther. 2021;12(1):229.
104. Ün BÇ, Ferah MA, Ün B. Can mesenchymal stem cells ameliorate testicular damage? Current researches. J Surg Med. 2020;4(7):603–7.
105. Modanlou M, Mahdipour M, Mobarak H. Effectiveness of stem cells therapy for male infertility restoration: a systematic review. J Investig Med. 2025;73(2):229–52.
106. Sagaradze G, Monakova A, Basalova N, Popov V, Balabanyan VU, Efimenko A. Regenerative medicine for male infertility: a focus on stem cell niche injury models. Biomed J. 2022;45(4):607–14.
107. Bhaskar R, Gupta MK. Testicular tissue engineering: an emerging solution for in vitro spermatogenesis. In: Biopolymer-based formulations. Elsevier; 2020. p. 835–58.
108. Del Vento F, Vermeulen M, de Michele F, de Michele F, Giudice MG, Giudice MG, et al. Tissue engineering to improve immature testicular tissue and cell transplantation outcomes: one step closer to fertility restoration for prepubertal boys exposed to gonadotoxic treatments. Int J Mol Sci. 2018;19(1):286.
109. Cho IK, Easley CA. Recent developments in in vitro spermatogenesis and future directions. Reprod Med. 2023;4(3):215–32.
110. Diao L, Turek PJ, John CM, Fang F, Reijo Pera RA. Roles of spermatogonial stem cells in spermatogenesis and fertility restoration. Front Endocrinol [Internet]. 2022 [cited 2024 May 7];13. Available from: https://www.frontiersin.org/journals/endocrinology/articles/10.3389/fendo.2022.895528/full.

Chapter 14
Role of AI in Male Infertility

Kadir Bocu, Sunil Jindal, and Hyun Jun Park

Introduction

The quest for parenthood is a profound human endeavor, yet infertility poses a significant challenge for millions of couples globally [1]. While often perceived through a lens focused on female factors, male infertility plays a crucial role, contributing to a substantial number of cases. Male infertility is defined as the inability of a male to cause pregnancy in a fertile female and impacts a significant segment of the global population. Understanding and innovatively addressing male infertility is, therefore, critical to advancing reproductive health [2].

Traditional diagnostic pathways for male infertility mainly rely on semen analysis, which assesses sperm count, motility, and morphology. Additional investigations may encompass hormonal assays, genetic screening, and imaging techniques to determine the underlying etiology [3]. While semen analysis remains a cornerstone, it is hindered by limitations such as inherent subjectivity in interpretation, significant inter-laboratory variability, and an inability to capture the dynamic functional aspects of sperm fully. These conventional methods often fail to detect subtle sperm defects or molecular anomalies that can critically impair fertilization potential, highlighting a pressing need for more objective, accurate, and comprehensive diagnostic tools [4].

K. Bocu (✉)
Department of Urology, Niğde Ömer Halisdemir University Faculty of Medicine, Niğde, Turkey

S. Jindal
Jindal Hospital, Meerut, Uttar Pradesh, India

H. J. Park
Department of Urology, Pusan National University School of Medicine/ Pusan National University Hospital, Pusan, South Korea

E. Chung et al. (eds.), *Advances in Andrology*,
https://doi.org/10.1007/978-3-032-29112-7_14

The field of artificial intelligence (AI) is currently undergoing rapid development and expansion, with significant implications for various aspects of modern life, including communication, industry, and scientific research. The core premise of this field involves creating computer systems that possess the ability to perform tasks typically associated with human intelligence. These tasks include acquiring knowledge from data, solving complex problems, and making informed decisions [5]. AI algorithms excel at processing and analyzing vast datasets, discerning intricate patterns, and generating predictions with remarkable speed and precision. Their applications are pervasive, impacting sectors such as finance, transportation, manufacturing, and, increasingly, healthcare. In medicine, AI plays a crucial role in drug discovery, enhancing diagnostic accuracy, personalizing treatment regimens, and streamlining patient care pathways [6].

This chapter aims to provide a comprehensive review of the current state and prospects of AI applications in the diagnosis, treatment, stratification, and management of male infertility. This paper will explore specific AI methods, including machine learning, deep learning, and computer vision, as well as their applications in areas such as advanced sperm analysis, predicting ART outcomes, and identifying new therapeutic targets. This section will examine the potential of AI to usher in a new era of personalized, effective, and accessible care for male infertility, thereby assisting more couples in achieving their aspiration of parenthood.

Current Diagnostic Methods for Male Infertility

The diagnostic evaluation of male infertility is a multifactorial process designed to identify underlying causes, guide treatment decisions, and provide a prognosis for future fertility. The clinical pathway typically begins with a thorough medical history and physical examination, followed by a series of laboratory and, in some cases, genetic investigations [7]. While these methods form the foundation of current andrology practice, they are accompanied by significant limitations that underscore the need for technological advancement [8].

Traditional Approaches and Their Limitations

Semen Analysis

The cornerstone of male fertility assessment is the semen analysis, also known as a spermogram. This foundational test provides both quantitative and qualitative evaluations of a semen sample, assessing parameters according to guidelines from the World Health Organization (WHO). Key metrics include semen volume, sperm concentration (count), motility (the percentage of moving sperm and their manner of movement), and morphology (the size and shape of sperm). The results are used to classify conditions such as oligozoospermia (low sperm count), asthenozoospermia (poor motility), and teratozoospermia (abnormal morphology) [9].

Limitations Despite its widespread use, conventional semen analysis has significant drawbacks. The assessment, particularly for morphology, is highly subjective and experiences considerable inter- and intra-laboratory variability. An experienced andrologist and a less-experienced technician may arrive at vastly different conclusions from the same sample [10]. Furthermore, semen parameters can vary greatly within the same individual due to factors such as abstinence period, illness, and stress. Most importantly, traditional semen analysis has limited predictive power for functional outcomes, including fertilization success and live birth rates. It provides a snapshot of sperm characteristics but overlooks essential functional aspects such as sperm DNA integrity and acrosomal function, both critical for successful fertilization [11].

Hormonal Assays

In cases where semen analysis results are considered abnormal or where clinical suspicion is warranted, a hormonal evaluation is conducted. This procedure involves blood tests to measure levels of key hormones that regulate sperm production (spermatogenesis) through the hypothalamic-pituitary-gonadal (HPG) axis. The primary hormones assessed included follicle-stimulating hormone (FSH), luteinizing hormone (LH), and testosterone. Abnormal levels can indicate testicular failure (high FSH), hypothalamic or pituitary issues (low FSH/LH), or other endocrine dysfunctions that may be addressed with specific therapies [12].

Limitations While hormonal profiles are useful for identifying specific endocrine disorders, they do not provide a comprehensive view of the patient's condition. A substantial number of infertile males show normal hormone levels, making the test uninformative in these instances. Circadian rhythms, lifestyle factors, and comorbidities also affect hormone levels. This requires careful interpretation and often necessitates repeat testing for confirmation [13].

Genetic Testing

For men with severe male factor infertility, such as non-obstructive azoospermia (absence of sperm in the ejaculate) or severe oligozoospermia, genetic testing is recommended. This includes karyotyping to identify chromosomal abnormalities, such as Klinefelter syndrome (XXY) and testing for microdeletions on the Y-chromosome (AZF deletions), which are known to result in impaired sperm production. Additionally, testing for mutations in the cystic fibrosis transmembrane conductance regulator (CFTR) gene is standard for men with congenital bilateral absence of the vas deferens (CBAVD) [14].

Limitations Current genetic testing is targeted and identifies only a small fraction of the potential genetic causes of male infertility. The vast majority of infertile men with a suspected genetic etiology remain undiagnosed. These tests are often reserved for the most severe cases due to cost and the limited number of identifiable, actionable mutations, leaving a large diagnostic gap for men with moderate, or unexplained infertility [15].

Challenges in Accurate Diagnosis

The limitations inherent in these traditional methods culminate in broader challenges that can impede accurate diagnosis and effective treatment planning.

Subjectivity and Variability in Manual Assessments

The most significant challenge in current andrology diagnostics is the dependence on manual, subjective microscopic assessment. The manual evaluation of sperm morphology exemplifies this issue. Without standardized, objective criteria that can be reliably reproduced, diagnoses can vary dramatically between clinics and even among technicians within the same lab. This lack of standardization complicates clinical decision-making, makes it difficult to compare results from different studies, and can lead to inconsistent patient management strategies [8].

The Need for Enhanced Diagnostic Solutions

The diagnostic gaps left by traditional methods underscore an urgent clinical need for advanced, objective, and comprehensive tools. The ideal diagnostic solution would not only standardize the assessment of conventional parameters but also offer more profound insights into sperm function, molecular integrity, and actual fertilization potential [16]. Such tools must be reproducible, highly accurate, and capable of generating predictive data to guide clinicians toward the most effective and personalized treatment pathways, including decisions on whether to use IUI, IVF, or ICSI. This need for objective, data-driven, and predictive capabilities positions artificial intelligence as a transformative force in the future of male infertility diagnostics [17].

The Potential of Artificial Intelligence in Male Infertility

The advent of artificial intelligence (AI) has emerged as a potent paradigm, poised to address this diagnostic void. By leveraging complex algorithms to analyze data with a level of speed, objectivity, and depth unattainable by humans, AI promises to usher in a new era of precision and personalization in andrology [18].

Overview of AI Technologies

At its core, AI includes a set of computational tools designed to learn from data and perform tasks that usually require human intelligence. In the context of male infertility, two important subfields of AI are especially relevant: machine learning and deep learning [19].

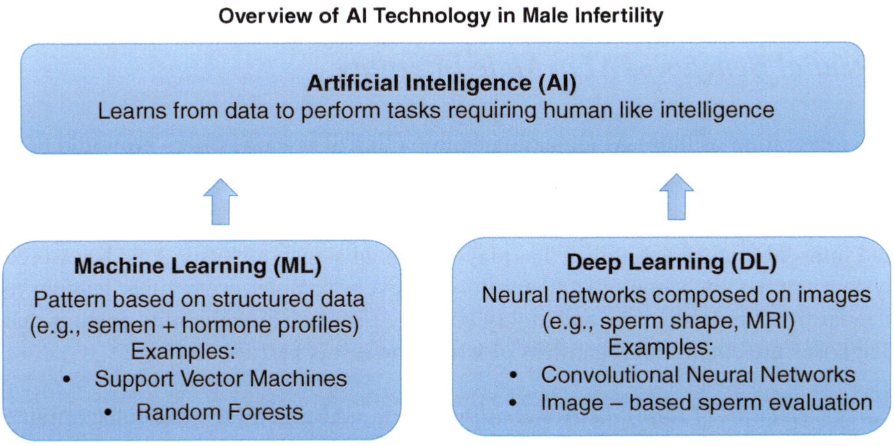

Machine Learning Algorithms

Machine learning (ML) is a subset of AI where algorithms are "trained" on large datasets to recognize patterns and make predictions without being explicitly programmed for that specific task. For example, an ML model can be fed thousands of patient profiles—including semen parameters, hormonal levels, and treatment outcomes—and learn to identify the key factors that predict successful conception [20]. Classic ML techniques, such as support vector machines, random forests, and logistic regression, are adept at classification (e.g., fertile vs. infertile) and prediction tasks based on structured data [21].

Deep Learning Models

Deep learning (DL), a sophisticated subset of machine learning (ML), leverages artificial neural networks composed of multiple processing layers—hence the term "deep." Modeled loosely after the architecture of the human brain, these networks are especially adept at analyzing complex and unstructured data types, such as medical images and genomic sequences [22]. This makes DL particularly promising in the field of male infertility diagnostics. For instance, convolutional neural networks (CNNs), a class of DL models optimized for image recognition, can be trained on large datasets containing tens of thousands of sperm cell images. These networks can discern minute morphological differences between viable and non-viable sperm—variations that are often subtle and subjective when assessed manually under a microscope. By automating and standardizing this evaluation, DL-based systems offer a significant advancement in accuracy, objectivity, and efficiency [23].

Potential Benefits of AI in Male Infertility

The integration of these AI technologies into clinical practice offers profound benefits that directly address the shortcomings of current methods.

Improved Accuracy and Reliability of Diagnosis AI eliminates the subjectivity and inter-laboratory variability that plague manual semen analysis. An AI-powered system applies the same objective criteria to every sample, every time, leading to standardized, reproducible, and highly accurate results. This reliability ensures that diagnoses are consistent regardless of where the test is performed [24].

Early Detection of Reproductive Health Issues AI algorithms can detect minute patterns in semen, hormonal, or genetic data that are invisible to the human eye or undetectable through conventional statistical analysis. By identifying these subtle red flags, AI can potentially signal underlying reproductive health issues much earlier, allowing for proactive intervention and counseling before more significant problems arise [25].

AI Applications in Male Fertility Assessment

The theoretical promise of AI is rapidly translating into practical applications across the entire spectrum of male fertility assessment, from the foundational semen analysis to complex genetic interpretation.

AI in Semen Analysis

AI has recently revolutionized andrology by developing tools that enhance sperm evaluation and selection during ICSI, reducing subjectivity and variability. AI applications now extend to diagnosing and treating male infertility, using ML and artificial neural networks (ANNs) to analyze semen parameters, predict treatment outcomes, and customize therapies. This integration of AI is especially promising for overcoming the complexity and subjectivity of current male infertility diagnostics and treatments [26].

Sperm Morphology

Recent studies have demonstrated that artificial intelligence significantly outperforms human experts in the assessment of sperm morphology. For instance, Mahali et al. integrated Swin Transformer and MobileNetV3 architectures, achieving an impressive 97.6% accuracy, compared to 85% by experienced embryologists, and reduced analysis time by 60% [27]. Similarly, Shahzad et al. (2023) applied deep neural networks (DNNs) and sequential DNNs to 1540 semen samples, identifying 30% more morphological defects than conventional manual evaluation, improving diagnostic precision and treatment planning in assisted reproductive technology (ART) [28]. Furthermore, another study shows that utilizing a convolutional neural network (CNN) model that reached 98.2% accuracy in sperm classification, facilitating more effective sperm selection for ART procedures [29].

Sperm Motility

Advancements in artificial intelligence are significantly transforming the evaluation of sperm motility, presenting promising new avenues for analysis. Utilizing sophisticated algorithms, AI can thoroughly analyze video footage and holographic images of sperm samples. When integrated with Computer-Assisted Sperm Analysis (CASA), this technology facilitates high-throughput assessments and delivers exact evaluations of motility at both the sample level and for individual sperm [30].

For instance, Tsai et al. developed a notable AI-driven image recognition system capable of efficiently and reliably categorizing sperm motility patterns from video data, achieving an accuracy rate of 90%. This innovative system processes information considerably faster than traditional manual methods, significantly reducing the time required for comprehensive motility assessments [31].

In another noteworthy contribution, Kanakasabapathy et al. introduced a smartphone-based diagnostic tool that accurately evaluates motility, alongside critical parameters such as sperm concentration and the total counts of motile and non-motile sperm [32]. Cheon et al. further validated the effectiveness of such smartphone tools, reaching an accuracy of 95% in measuring motility and other semen characteristics, all within 5 min. This is particularly advantageous for remote or underserved regions, as it provides access to advanced reproductive diagnostics for those most in need [33].

Moreover, holographic imaging and microfluidics breakthroughs have enabled more detailed motility analyses. These technologies facilitate the generation of extensive datasets that empower AI algorithms to investigate various parameters of sperm movement, including tail-beating frequency and amplitude. A notable instance is CASAnova, a support vector machine created by Goodson et al., which classified sperm motility with an accuracy rate of 89%, analyzing over 1200 sperm samples [34]. These innovations hold great potential for enhancing diagnostic accuracy in andrology, offering detailed and quantifiable assessments of sperm motility. The outlook appears promising as we leverage these technologies to improve reproductive health.

AI in Sperm DNA Fragmentation

Artificial intelligence provides reliable, non-invasive ways to assess DNA integrity. By analyzing high-resolution images of sperm, machine learning (ML) models can predict DNA fragmentation, connecting physical traits to DNA health. One notable study developed an ML algorithm that used sperm images to predict DNA fragmentation with a 96.71% accuracy rate. This algorithm analyzed more than 2000 sperm images, identifying subtle details in shape and structure linked to DNA fragmentation index (DFI) levels, thus reducing the need for invasive testing [35].

Another study introduced a deep learning model capable of calculating DFI for individual sperm, showing a strong correlation with actual DFI measurements. This model was trained on 24,415 sperm images and validated with a separate set of 15,528 images, achieving a prediction accuracy of 80.15%. This deep learning model's ability to provide accurate DFI assessments from sperm images marks significant progress in non-invasive sperm analysis [36].

Together, these studies demonstrate that AI algorithms can reliably predict DFI from sperm images, offering a valuable tool for selecting sperm with high-quality DNA for ICSI and other assisted reproductive techniques (Fig. 14.1).

The AI vs Human Diagnostic Performance is *based on aggregated findings from multiple peer-reviewed studies cited in the manuscript*, reflecting AI's comparative performance in key areas of male infertility diagnostics. Here's the breakdown for each category and the evidence it draws from:

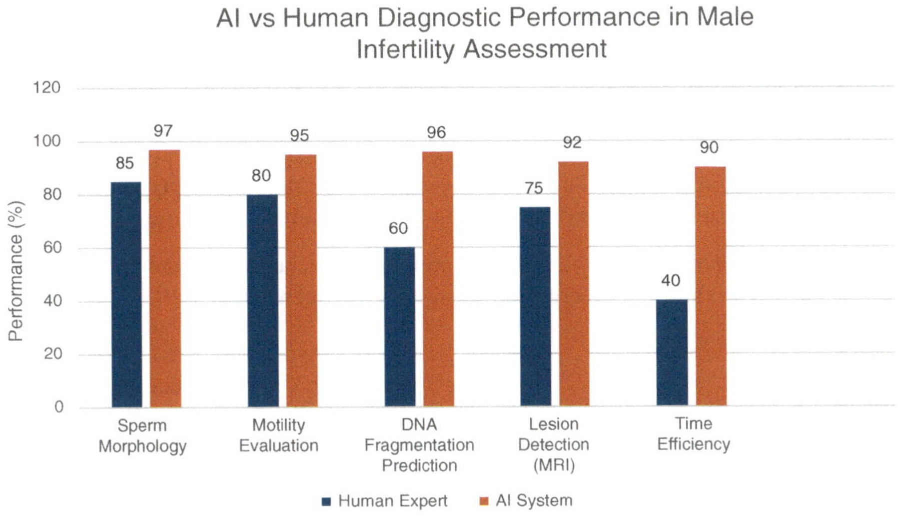

Fig. 14.1 AI vs Human Diagnostic Performance in male infertility assessment

1. *Sperm Morphology*

   Source:

   - Mahali et al. [27] used Swin Transformer + MobileNetV3 with 97.6% accuracy.
   - Shahzad et al. [28] showed AI identified 30% more morphological defects than manual microscopy.
   - Spencer et al. [29] achieved 98.2% classification accuracy using CNNs.

   Human Benchmark: Experienced embryologists are typically around 80%–85% accurate, with variability due to subjectivity [10].

2. *Motility Evaluation*

   Source:

   - Tsai et al. [31] built an AI-based system achieving 90% accuracy.
   - Kanakasabapathy et al. [32] and Cheon et al. [33] reported up to 95% accuracy in smartphone-based AI motility assessment.

   Human Benchmark: Manual motility scoring is subject to bias and observer fatigue, often with 75%–85% consistency.

3. *DNA Fragmentation Prediction*

   Source:

   - Serrano Berenguer et al. [35] developed ML models that reached 96.7% accuracy.
   - Kumar et al. [36] built a deep learning model with 80.15% accuracy in non-invasive DFI prediction.

Human Benchmark: Human prediction without molecular tests is poor—clinicians rely on lab-based tests like SCSA or Comet, not visual judgment.

4. *Lesion Detection (MRI)*

   Source:

   - Feng et al. [37] and Sun et al. [38] showed ML models outperform radiologists in testicular lesion classification and volume estimation.

   Human Benchmark: Radiologist interpretation is accurate but subject to inter-reader variability, with reported sensitivity between 70–80%.

5. *Time Efficiency*

   Source:

   - AI systems complete analyses in seconds to minutes (e.g., sperm classification, DNA analysis, embryo scoring), cutting time by 60–80% [27, 28].

   Human Benchmark: Manual microscopy, DFI tests, or MRI interpretation typically take 15–60 min depending on complexity.

Predictive Models for Fertility Based on Sperm Characteristics

AI moves beyond simple classification to provide accurate predictive insights. ML models can analyze a combination of sperm kinetic patterns (how a sperm swims) and subtle morphological features to predict its likelihood of successfully fertilizing an oocyte. This allows for more informed sperm selection for procedures like Intracytoplasmic Sperm Injection (ICSI), potentially improving ART success rates [39].

AI and Hormonal Profiling

Hormonal profiling enhanced by artificial intelligence (AI) significantly advances endocrine evaluation and fertility management. AI-driven analysis moves beyond traditional isolated hormone measurements—such as follicle-stimulating hormone (FSH), luteinizing hormone (LH), and testosterone—by examining complex interactions and ratios among these hormones to identify specific hormonal signatures linked to various conditions. For example, machine learning (ML) algorithms can differentiate subtypes of testicular failure or predict obstructions affecting fertility [40].

AI in the Treatment of Male Infertility

Artificial intelligence (AI) increasingly transforms male infertility treatment through predictive analytics, personalized care, and integration with assisted reproductive technologies (ARTs). This part explores the multifaceted role of AI in enhancing treatment outcomes, optimizing success rates, and customizing patient management.

AI in Predictive Analytics for Treatment Outcomes

AI uses large datasets such as electronic health records, imaging, genetic profiles, and clinical parameters to forecast disease progression and treatment response in male infertility [17]. ML and DL techniques analyze complex patterns often unseen by clinicians, allowing early detection of factors affecting infertility and predicting treatment success. Predictive analytics helps clinicians make data-driven decisions, improving recovery rates, and patient outcomes by customizing interventions based on individual profiles [41].

AI Models That Predict Success Rates of Different Treatments

Dynamic mathematical and AI models have been developed to estimate the success rates of various infertility treatments such as Intrauterine Insemination (IUI), In Vitro Fertilization–Embryo Transfer (IVF-ET), and Intracytoplasmic Sperm Injection (ICSI) [42]. To simulate treatment outcomes, these models incorporate patient-specific data, including etiology, clinical findings, and laboratory test results. For instance, recent dynamical models demonstrated the ability to predict ART success with stability and sensitivity analyses, highlighting that increased use of IUI and ICSI correlates with better disease control and favorable outcomes. Such models provide a systematic framework for clinicians to assess treatment effectiveness and personalize therapy accordingly [43].

Personalized Treatment Plans with AI Assistance

AI facilitates the creation of personalized treatment plans by integrating diverse patient data—clinical, genetic, hormonal, and imaging—to identify the most effective therapeutic approach. For example, in related reproductive disorders like endometriosis, AI algorithms such as random forest and boosting methods have shown high accuracy in predicting optimal treatments, resulting in improved symptom resolution and reduced treatment switching. These approaches can be adapted for male infertility to enhance the compatibility of initial therapies and reduce trial-and-error in treatment selection [44].

The Role of AI in Radiological Assessment of Male Infertility

AI-enhanced radiological tools improve the diagnostic accuracy of imaging studies used in male infertility evaluation, such as scrotal ultrasound and MRI. AI algorithms rapidly and precisely analyze imaging data to detect abnormalities like varicoceles, testicular lesions, or obstructive pathologies. This advancement facilitates earlier and more accurate diagnoses, guiding targeted therapeutic interventions [37, 38] (Fig. 14.2).

The *workflow of AI in radiologic imaging for male infertility*, specifically in diagnosing conditions like *varicocele, testicular lesions, or obstructive pathologies* using AI-enhanced ultrasound or MRI.

Flowchart Summary

1. *Imaging Data Input* (Ultrasound/MRI of testis, scrotum, or vas deferens)
2. *AI Preprocessing* (Noise reduction, region segmentation, tissue isolation).
3. *Feature Extraction using Deep Learning* (*CNN/Transformer*) (Texture, lesion detection, volume metrics).
4. *Diagnostic Prediction* (AI detects abnormalities—e.g., varicocele, testicular mass, obstruction).
5. *Radiologist-AI Collaboration* (AI results reviewed by experts, improving accuracy & speed).
6. *Clinical Decision Support* (Treatment planning: surgery, hormonal therapy, ART).

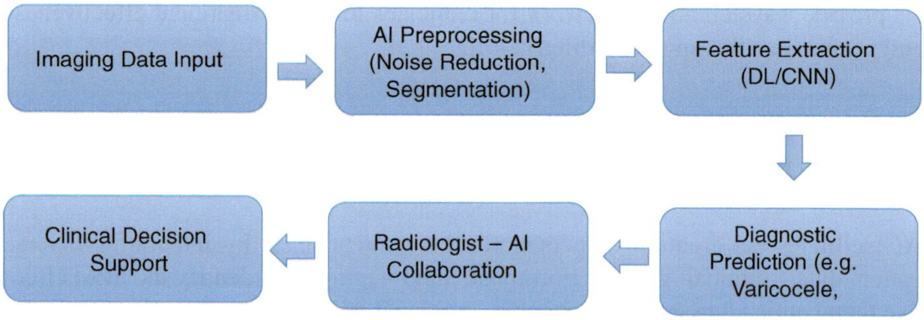

Fig. 14.2 Illustrative overview: AI in radiologic imaging for male infertility

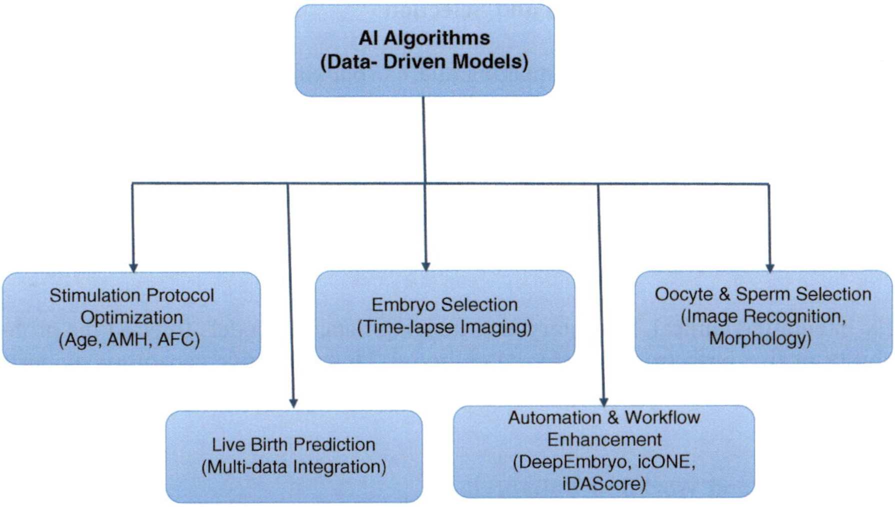

Fig. 14.3 AI integration in assisted reproductive technologies (ARTs)

Integration of AI Techniques in Assisted Reproductive Technologies

Assisted reproductive technologies (ARTs) have transformed the landscape of fertility treatment, but their success relies heavily on optimizing protocols, accurate gamete and embryo selection, and minimizing subjectivity in clinical decisions. Artificial intelligence (AI) has rapidly emerged as a crucial partner in addressing these challenges, applying advanced algorithms to clinical, laboratory, and imaging data. By integrating AI, clinics can increase the precision, personalization, and efficiency of ART procedures [45] (Fig. 14.3).

Stimulation Protocol Optimization

Personalizing ovarian stimulation is a key step in ART. Traditionally, clinicians choose stimulation protocols based on broad clinical criteria, which can result in variable outcomes. By using data such as age, anti-Müllerian hormone (AMH) levels, antral follicle count, and previous cycle responses, AI algorithms can suggest personalized stimulation protocols to optimize oocyte yield and reduce risks like ovarian hyperstimulation syndrome (OHSS) [46].

Oocyte and Sperm Selection

AI-powered image recognition and machine learning models assess morphological and functional characteristics of oocytes and sperm. This automated evaluation improves selection accuracy beyond traditional manual methods, enhancing fertilization potential [47].

Embryo Formation Prediction and Selection

AI systems analyze time-lapse imaging and morphokinetic data to predict embryo viability and developmental potential. These models assist embryologists in selecting embryos with the highest likelihood of implantation and live birth, reducing subjectivity and improving success rates [48].

Live Birth Prediction

By integrating clinical, laboratory, and imaging data, AI models forecast the probability of live birth from transferred embryos. This predictive capability supports clinical decision-making and personalized patient counseling [49].

Automation and Workflow Enhancement

AI streamlines laboratory workflows by automating routine tasks such as image analysis and data interpretation, increasing efficiency, and reducing human error. A systematic review of AI applications in ART reported that AI tools like DeepEmbryo, icONE, and iDAScore improved clinical pregnancy rates by up to 77.3%, implantation accuracy by 92%, and laboratory efficiency by 35% compared to traditional methods. These tools outperformed manual assessments by reducing subjectivity and standardizing workflows, although broader multicenter validation is needed to confirm generalizability [50]. Furthermore, international reviews emphasize that as ART laboratories adopt automation, staffing models must evolve to balance human expertise with AI-driven processes, ensuring quality control and optimal patient outcomes [51].

Ethical and Societal Considerations

Artificial intelligence (AI) in healthcare, including male infertility treatment, raises important ethical and societal issues that must be carefully addressed. Ethical concerns revolve around responsible AI use to protect patient autonomy, fairness, and transparency, while preventing biases that could harm patients. Privacy is essential, given the sensitive nature of health data involved; strong safeguards are necessary to safeguard patient confidentiality and prevent data breaches [52].

Equity is a key aspect, ensuring AI-driven care is accessible to everyone, regardless of socioeconomic or demographic background, and that AI systems do not reinforce existing disparities. Public perception significantly influences AI adoption in healthcare; therefore, educating patients and practitioners about AI's capabilities and limitations is vital to promote informed acceptance. Trust in patients depends on transparency, reliability, and the involvement of human clinicians in AI-assisted diagnoses and treatments [53].

Finally, acceptance and regulation of AI differ across societies, each shaped by unique cultural values and legal frameworks. These regulatory considerations must align with ethical standards and privacy protections to support the responsible global deployment of AI in male infertility care. Addressing these interconnected issues is essential to fully realize AI's potential while minimizing risks and respecting societal values [54].

Future Directions and Trends

Recent innovations in AI have opened new possibilities for understanding and tackling the complexities of male infertility, highlighting promising future directions and trends.

One of the most notable advancements is the use of AI in advanced sperm analysis. AI-powered systems can now detect subtle biomarkers and patterns in sperm samples that are difficult to identify with traditional methods. This improves diagnostic accuracy and allows for earlier intervention, which could lead to better treatment outcomes [55].

Another emerging trend is applying AI to personalize treatment plans. By analyzing large datasets, including genetic, lifestyle, and environmental factors, AI can help customize therapies to individual needs, boosting effectiveness and minimizing side effects. This personalized approach is expected to become a core part of modern reproductive medicine [56].

On a global level, AI can potentially reduce disparities in access to fertility care. In underserved regions, AI-based diagnostic tools can offer affordable and scalable solutions, making high-quality fertility assessments more accessible. Moreover, AI's ability to analyze large datasets can reveal insights into infertility patterns, supporting public health strategies to lower infertility rates worldwide [57].

Conclusion

Traditional diagnostic and therapeutic strategies in male infertility lack the objectivity, depth, and predictive capacity needed for truly personalized care. AI-driven tools address these shortcomings by standardizing semen evaluation, revealing subtle phenotypic and molecular markers, and integrating diverse clinical data to forecast treatment outcomes accurately. Early clinical adoption has already enhanced diagnostic reliability, improved ART success rates, and reduced barriers to care through point-of-care and smartphone-based systems. However, to fully realize these benefits, future research must focus on: (1) large, multicenter validation cohorts to ensure external generalizability; (2) transparent model reporting and ongoing monitoring to reduce bias; (3) robust data governance frameworks to protect patient privacy; and (4) interdisciplinary collaboration among clinicians, computer scientists, ethicists, and regulators. By addressing these challenges, AI can evolve from an adjunct innovation into a core component of evidence-based andrology, ultimately helping more couples achieve their reproductive goals.

References

1. Inhorn MC, Patrizio P. Infertility around the globe: new thinking on gender, reproductive technologies and global movements in the 21st century. Hum Reprod Update. 2015;21(4):411–26. https://doi.org/10.1093/humupd/dmv016.
2. Vander Borght M, Wyns C. Fertility and infertility: definition and epidemiology. Clin Biochem. 2018;62:2–10. https://doi.org/10.1016/j.clinbiochem.2018.03.012.
3. Gül M, Russo GI, Kandil H, Boitrelle F, Saleh R, Chung E, et al. Male infertility: new developments, current challenges, and future directions. World J Mens Health. 2024;42(3):502–17. https://doi.org/10.5534/wjmh.230232.
4. Finelli R, Leisegang K, Tumallapalli S, Henkel R, Agarwal A. The validity and reliability of computer-aided semen analyzers in performing semen analysis: a systematic review. Transl Androl Urol. 2021;10(7):3069–79. https://doi.org/10.21037/tau-21-276.
5. Lungarella M, Iida F, Bongard J, Pfeifer R. 50 years of artificial intelligence: essays dedicated to the 50th anniversary of artificial intelligence. Springer; 2007.
6. Mintz Y, Brodie R. Introduction to artificial intelligence in medicine. Minim Invasive Ther Allied Technol. 2019;28(2):73–81. https://doi.org/10.1080/13645706.2019.1575882.
7. Minhas S, Bettocchi C, Boeri L, Capogrosso P, Carvalho J, Cilesiz NC, et al. European Association of Urology Guidelines on male sexual and reproductive health: 2021 update on male infertility. Eur Urol. 2021;80(5):603–20. https://doi.org/10.1016/j.eururo.2021.08.014.
8. Oehninger S, Ombelet W. Limits of current male fertility testing. Fertil Steril. 2019;111(5):835–41. https://doi.org/10.1016/j.fertnstert.2019.03.005.
9. Boitrelle F, Shah R, Saleh R, Henkel R, Kandil H, Chung E, et al. The sixth edition of the WHO manual for human semen analysis: a critical review and SWOT analysis. Life (Basel). 2021;11(12):1368. https://doi.org/10.3390/life11121368.
10. Eustache F, Auger J. Inter-individual variability in the morphological assessment of human sperm: effect of the level of experience and the use of standard methods. Hum Reprod. 2003;18(5):1018–22. https://doi.org/10.1093/humrep/deg197.
11. Vashisht A, Gahlay GK. Understanding seminal plasma in male infertility: emerging markers and their implications. Andrology. 2024;12(5):1058–77. https://doi.org/10.1111/andr.13563.
12. Concepción-Zavaleta M, Paz Ibarra JL, Ramos-Yataco A, Coronado-Arroyo J, Concepción-Urteaga L, Roseboom PJ, et al. Assessment of hormonal status in male infertility. An update. Diabetes Metab Syndr. 2022;16(3):102447. https://doi.org/10.1016/j.dsx.2022.102447.
13. Trost LW, Mulhall JP. Challenges in testosterone measurement, data interpretation, and methodological appraisal of interventional trials. J Sex Med. 2016;13(7):1029–46. https://doi.org/10.1016/j.jsxm.2016.04.068.
14. Sudhakar DVS, Shah R, Gajbhiye RK. Genetics of male infertility—present and future: a narrative review. J Human Reprod Sci. 2021;14(3):217–27.
15. Xavier M, Salas-Huetos A, Oud M, Aston K, Veltman J. Disease gene discovery in male infertility: past, present and future. Hum Genet. 2021;140(1):7–19.
16. Pandruvada S, Royfman R, Shah TA, Sindhwani P, Dupree JM, Schon S, et al. Lack of trusted diagnostic tools for undetermined male infertility. J Assist Reprod Genet. 2021;38(2):265–76. https://doi.org/10.1007/s10815-020-02037-5.

17. Qaderi K, Sharifipour F, Dabir M, Shams R, Behmanesh A. Artificial intelligence (AI) approaches to male infertility in IVF: a mapping review. Eur J Med Res. 2025;30(1):246. https://doi.org/10.1186/s40001-025-02479-6.
18. Wang R, Pan W, Jin L, Li Y, Geng Y, Gao C, et al. Artificial intelligence in reproductive medicine. Reproduction. 2019;158(4):R139–R54. https://doi.org/10.1530/rep-18-0523.
19. Choi RY, Coyner AS, Kalpathy-Cramer J, Chiang MF, Campbell JP. Introduction to machine learning, neural networks, and deep learning. Transl Vis Sci Technol. 2020;9(2):14. https://doi.org/10.1167/tvst.9.2.14.
20. Venishetty N, Alkassis M, Raheem O. The role of artificial intelligence in male infertility: evaluation and treatment: a narrative review. Uro. 2024;4(2):23–35.
21. Rajula HSR, Verlato G, Manchia M, Antonucci N, Fanos V. Comparison of conventional statistical methods with machine learning in medicine: diagnosis, drug development, and treatment. Medicina (Kaunas). 2020;56(9):455. https://doi.org/10.3390/medicina56090455.
22. Shariaty F, Pavlov V, Baranov M. AI-driven precision oncology: integrating deep learning, radiomics, and genomic analysis for enhanced lung cancer diagnosis and treatment. SIViP. 2025;19(9):693. https://doi.org/10.1007/s11760-025-04244-y.
23. Aktas A, Cap T, Serbes G, Ilhan HO, Uzun H. Advanced multi-level ensemble learning approaches for comprehensive sperm morphology assessment. Diagnostics. 2025;15(12):1564.
24. Chang A, Yang YC, Henthorn D, Cheng YS. P-034 revolutionizing sperm morphology assessment: a novel artificial intelligence optic microscope (AIOM)-powered platform for consistent and reliable analysis in male infertility diagnosis. Hum Reprod. 2024;39(Supplement_1):deae108.411.
25. Agarwal A, Panner Selvam MK, Sharma R, Master K, Sharma A, Gupta S, et al. Home sperm testing device versus laboratory sperm quality analyzer: comparison of motile sperm concentration. Fertil Steril. 2018;110(7):1277–84. https://doi.org/10.1016/j.fertnstert.2018.08.049.
26. Ghayda RA, Cannarella R, Calogero AE, Shah R, Rambhatla A, Zohdy W, et al. Artificial intelligence in andrology: from semen analysis to image diagnostics. World J Mens Health. 2024;42(1):39–61. https://doi.org/10.5534/wjmh.230050.
27. Mahali MI, Leu JS, Darmawan JT, Avian C, Bachroin N, Prakosa SW, et al. A dual architecture fusion and AutoEncoder for automatic morphological classification of human sperm. Sensors (Basel). 2023;23(14):6613. https://doi.org/10.3390/s23146613.
28. Shahzad S, Ilyas M, Lali MIU, Rauf HT, Kadry S, Nasr EA. Sperm abnormality detection using sequential deep neural network. Mathematics. 2023;11(3):515.
29. Spencer L, Fernando J, Akbaridoust F, Ackermann K, Nosrati R. Ensembled deep learning for the classification of human sperm head morphology. Adv Intell Syst. 2022;4(10):2200111.
30. Panner Selvam MK, Moharana AK, Baskaran S, Finelli R, Hudnall MC, Sikka SC. Current updates on involvement of artificial intelligence and machine learning in semen analysis. Medicina (Kaunas). 2024;60(2):279. https://doi.org/10.3390/medicina60020279.
31. Tsai VF, Zhuang B, Pong YH, Hsieh JT, Chang HC. Web- and artificial intelligence-based image recognition for sperm motility analysis: verification study. JMIR Med Inform. 2020;8(11):e20031. https://doi.org/10.2196/20031.
32. Kanakasabapathy MK, Sadasivam M, Singh A, Preston C, Thirumalaraju P, Venkataraman M, et al. An automated smartphone-based diagnostic assay for point-of-care semen analysis. Sci Transl Med. 2017;9(382):eaai7863. https://doi.org/10.1126/scitranslmed.aai7863.
33. Cheon WH, Park HJ, Park MJ, Lim MY, Park JH, Kang BJ, et al. Validation of a smartphone-based, computer-assisted sperm analysis system compared with laboratory-based manual microscopic semen analysis and computer-assisted semen analysis. Investig Clin Urol. 2019;60(5):380–7. https://doi.org/10.4111/icu.2019.60.5.380.
34. Goodson SG, White S, Stevans AM, Bhat S, Kao CY, Jaworski S, et al. CASAnova: a multiclass support vector machine model for the classification of human sperm motility patterns. Biol Reprod. 2017;97(5):698–708. https://doi.org/10.1093/biolre/iox120.
35. Serrano Berenguer L, Hincapié Monsalve S, Lara Cerrillo S, Rosado Iglesias C, Vegas Lozano E, Reverter Comes F, et al. P-101 machine and deep learning models to classify comet assay

tests for sperm DNA fragmentation evaluation. Hum Reprod. 2022;37(Supplement_1):deac107.097.
36. Kumar RS, Sharma S, Halder A, Gupta V. Deep learning-based robust automated system for predicting human sperm DNA fragmentation index. J Human Reprod Sci. 2023;16(1):16–21.
37. Feng Y, Feng Z, Wang L, Lv W, Liu Z, Min X, et al. Comparison and analysis of multiple machine learning models for discriminating benign and malignant testicular lesions based on magnetic resonance imaging radiomics. Front Med. 2023;10:1279622.
38. Sun K, Fan C, Feng Z, Min X, Wang Y, Sun Z, et al. Magnetic resonance imaging based deep-learning model: a rapid, high-performance, automated tool for testicular volume measurements. Front Med. 2023;10:1277535.
39. Badura A, Marzec-Wroblewska U, Kaminski P, Lakota P, Ludwikowski G, Szymanski M, et al. Prediction of semen quality using artificial neural network. J Appl Biomed. 2019;17(3):167–74. https://doi.org/10.32725/jab.2019.015.
40. Kobayashi H, Uetani M, Yamabe F, Mitsui Y, Nakajima K, Nagao K. A new model for determining risk of male infertility from serum hormone levels, without semen analysis. Sci Rep. 2024;14(1):17079. https://doi.org/10.1038/s41598-024-67910-0.
41. Dixon D, Sattar H, Moros N, Kesireddy SR, Ahsan H, Lakkimsetti M, et al. Unveiling the influence of AI predictive analytics on patient outcomes: a comprehensive narrative review. Cureus. 2024;16(5):e59954. https://doi.org/10.7759/cureus.59954.
42. Hafezi SG, Ranjbar M, Ghasemabadi A, Effati S, Naserghandi A, Namakin K, et al. Two dynamical models for male infertility and their stability and sensitivity analysis. Sci Rep. 2025;15(1):18873. https://doi.org/10.1038/s41598-025-03993-7.
43. Mehrjerd A, Rezaei H, Eslami S, Ratna MB, Khadem GN. Internal validation and comparison of predictive models to determine success rate of infertility treatments: a retrospective study of 2485 cycles. Sci Rep. 2022;12(1):7216. https://doi.org/10.1038/s41598-022-10902-9.
44. Latif N, Babe R, Raz K, Zama U, Sherbano S, Zaman F. AI in personalized treatment plans for endometriosis a data-driven approach to therapy selection. Front Health Inform. 2025;13:895–901. https://doi.org/10.63682/fhi2621.
45. Mapari SA, Shrivastava D, Bedi GN, Pradeep U, Gupta A, Kasat PR, et al. Revolutionizing reproduction: the impact of robotics and artificial intelligence (AI) in assisted reproductive technology: a comprehensive review. Cureus. 2024;16(6):e63072. https://doi.org/10.7759/cureus.63072.
46. Ortiz JA, Lledó B, Luque L, Morales R, Myles S, Pérez M, et al. Pharmacogenetic analysis using artificial intelligence (AI) to identify polymorphisms associated with sub-optimal ovarian response and hyper-response. J Assist Reprod Genet. 2025;42:1863–73. https://doi.org/10.1007/s10815-025-03471-z.
47. Amini Mahabadi J, Enderami SE, Nikzad H, Hassani Bafrani H. The use of machine learning for human sperm and oocyte selection and success rate in IVF methods. Andrologia. 2024;2024(1):8165541.
48. Roky MAB, Ray AS, Saad AM. Advancing embryo selection in artificial intelligence-assisted reproductive technologies: a systematic review. Artif Intell Health. 2025;2:1–23. https://doi.org/10.36922/aih.7170.
49. Liu H, Zhang Z, Gu Y, Dai C, Shan G, Song H, et al. Development and evaluation of a live birth prediction model for evaluating human blastocysts from a retrospective study. elife. 2023;12:e83662.
50. Shoham Z. Artificial intelligence in reproductive medicine: transforming assisted reproductive technologies. J IVF-Worldwide. 2025;3(2):1–8.
51. Shirasawa H, Terada Y. Embryologist staffing in assisted reproductive technology laboratories: an international comparative review. Reprod Med Biol. 2025;24(1):e12628.
52. Li F, Ruijs N, Lu Y. Ethics & AI: a systematic review on ethical concerns and related strategies for designing with AI in healthcare. AI. 2023;4(1):28–53.

53. Beltramin D, Lamas E, Bousquet C. Ethical issues in the utilization of black boxes for artificial intelligence in medicine. Stud Health Technol Inform. 2022;295:249–52. https://doi.org/10.3233/shti220709.
54. Bouderhem R. Shaping the future of AI in healthcare through ethics and governance. Human Soc Sci Commun. 2024;11(1):416. https://doi.org/10.1057/s41599-024-02894-w.
55. Marinaro J, Goldstein M. Current and future applications of artificial intelligence to diagnose and treat male infertility. Adv Exp Med Biol. 2025;1469:1–23. https://doi.org/10.1007/978-3-031-82990-1_1.
56. Alowais SA, Alghamdi SS, Alsuhebany N, Alqahtani T, Alshaya AI, Almohareb SN, et al. Revolutionizing healthcare: the role of artificial intelligence in clinical practice. BMC Med Educ. 2023;23(1):689. https://doi.org/10.1186/s12909-023-04698-z.
57. Gbagbo FY, Ameyaw EK, Yaya S. Artificial intelligence and sexual reproductive health and rights: a technological leap towards achieving sustainable development goal target 3.7. Reprod Health. 2024;21(1):196. https://doi.org/10.1186/s12978-024-01924-9.

Chapter 15
Advancements in Sperm and Embryo Selection for ART

Christina Anagnostopoulou, Israel Maldonado, and Paraskevi Vogiatzi

Introduction

Sperm preparation and selection have been established as a main part of assisted reproduction techniques since the first intrauterine insemination (IUI) attempts [1]. Initially, sperm preparation was mainly used as a means to isolate healthy and motile spermatozoa, remove apoptotic spermatozoa, cells, and debris, and improve sperm parameters, thus increasing the efficiency of IUI and in vitro fertilization (IVF).

The spermatozoon not only induces fertilization but also provides half the genetic material to the preimplantation embryo. Increased levels of sperm DNA fragmentation, may adversely affect embryo development and implantation [2]. Even in cases where successful embryo transfers result in pregnancy, genetic alterations to the sperm DNA by oxidative stress, may be inherited by the offspring and lead to epigenetic diseases [3].

As importantly, following fertilization, the sperm basal body converts to a centrosome essential for the early stages of embryogenesis and compaction [4] and, as a result, the presence of an optimally structured spermatozoon is a prerequisite for the following steps of human preimplantation development.

C. Anagnostopoulou (✉)
Future Life Akeso, Athens, Greece

I. Maldonado
Citmer Reproductive Medicine, IVF LAB, Mexico City, Mexico
e-mail: imaldonado@citmer.mx

P. Vogiatzi
Andromed Health and Reproduction, Fertility Diagnostics Laboratory, Maroussi, Greece

E. Chung et al. (eds.), *Advances in Andrology*,
https://doi.org/10.1007/978-3-032-29112-7_15

Similarly, optimal embryo selection has been explored since the early days of assisted reproductive technology (ART). The use of gonadotropins increased the number of oocytes retrieved per IVF cycle, resulting to a larger pool of available embryos for transfer, and higher implantation rates [5]. Furthermore, the turn to single embryo transfer in order to avoid the risks accompanying multiple gestations has made the need for the development of efficient embryo selection tools even more demanding [6].

Nowadays, several embryo selection strategies are available, such as morphology assessment, morphokinetics, metabolomics, and oxidative stress measurement. Additionally, patient groups facing repeated implantation failure (RIM) or unexplained recurrent miscarriage (RM) may benefit from embryo biopsy for preimplantation genetic testing for aneuploidies (PGT-A), a method for the deselection of aneuploid preimplantation embryos. Although it is not always feasible to accurately predict which embryo will implant, the effective selection of the most competent embryo benefits the patients as it decreases the time to pregnancy and in some cases, it even prevents the transfer of aneuploid embryos that would lead to a miscarriage.

This chapter aims to describe and review the most recent and advanced techniques for sperm and embryo selection. More essentially, it aims to unveil the challenges, limitations, and prospects for each one of the currently available selection techniques.

Sperm Preparation and Selection

Conventional Techniques for Sperm Preparation: Swim-Up, Density Gradient, Centrifugation

The techniques used to process sperm samples for use in ART should ensure the selection of the best quality sperm. That is why these techniques focus on the removal of low-quality sperm (including immotile and apoptotic sperm), as well as other cells, such as leukocytes, bacteria, debris, and the rest of the seminal plasma and other harmful substances that may interfere with fertility procedures [7, 8]. Both swim-up and density gradients (DGC) procedures are the conventional and most used techniques for sperm preparation and recovery [7]. Swim-up methods aim at the recovery of motile sperm that migrate from the seminal plasma to a cell-free culture medium [9, 10]. DGC involves the ability of motile sperm to swim through a density gradient made up of colloidal particles during a centrifugation process [7]. The combination of both techniques is used routinely in IVF laboratories and focuses on the recovery of motile sperm. On the other hand, in sperm samples with poor-quality concentration, such as in oligozoospermia or oligoteratozoospermia, it is recommended to only perform a simple wash with culture medium, combined with swim-up, to recover more sperm. Another strategy for optimizing sperm retrieval in asthenozoospermia, oligospermia, or low ejaculate volume is reducing the volume of density gradients.

In cases of patients with retrograde ejaculation, where semen passes into the bladder instead of the passage of a normal ejaculation, the sperm are recovered from the urine. Before recovering the sample, the bladder must be neutralized through the uptake of sodium bicarbonate. Sperm are collected from post-ejaculatory urine analysis (PEUA) and recovered by washing and centrifugation and re-suspension to sperm wash media, in order to improve ambient sperm conditions [11].

In cases of testicular sperm extraction (TESE) biopsies, mechanical methods such as rough shredding, fine mincing, vortexing, squeezing, and crushing are used to mince the seminiferous tubules [12]. Consequently, the tissue is observed under the inverted microscope for the identification of spermatozoa, and the sample is processed by centrifugation at 750*g* for 5 min.

Electrophoresis and Zeta Potential Selection Method Sperm

Electrophoresis is a method that enables the separation of spermatozoa under an electric field, according to their surface charge. The presence of a negative charge of the spermatozoon appears to be linked to normal spermatogenesis and may be responsible for the transfer of glycosylphosphatidylinositol (GPI)-anchored CD52 to the sperm surface [13]. The DNA of positively charged sperm (PCS) has been found to be more damaged compared to negatively charged sperm (NCS) [14]. The suspensions derived from electrophoretic separation have been suggested to consist of morphologically normal spermatozoa with low DNA damage [15].

The zeta method is a simple and inexpensive non-invasive technique that applies the principles of electrophoresis. The plastic tube containing the sperm dilution is placed inside a latex glove up to the cap and then grasped by the cap, rotated for two of three turns and quickly removed from the glove [16]. The low voltage used by the zeta method makes this technique suitable for the isolation of sperm to be used in ART [16]. The zeta method is a valid alternative to conventional sperm preparation specifically in patient groups with oligoasthenospermia and/or high DNA fragmentation [17]. Additionally, the combination of density gradient and zeta method has been found to improve the quality of a sperm sample and, as a result, may facilitate the selection of a healthy sperm for intracytoplasmic sperm injection (ICSI) [18]. Micro-electrophoresis is a modified technique that has the advantage that it can be used in real-time during ICSI for sperm selection without altering or damaging the sperm [14].

The authors of a recent Cochrane review did not conclude that there is a benefit for patients when using Zeta sperm selection in terms of live birth, pregnancy, or miscarriage [19].

Macs

The integrity of sperm DNA is essential not only for proper embryonic development but also for implantation and gestation [20, 21]. That is why one of the most promising tests in the diagnosis of male infertility is the analysis of sperm DNA fragmentation [21, 22]. The Magnetic Activity Cell Sorting (MACS) technique consists of separating live sperm from apoptotic sperm, which suffer damage or fragmentation to their DNA [23]. Apoptotic spermatozoa are identified through phosphatidylserine (PS) residues externalized during the apoptosis process, which bind to nanoparticles conjugated with Annexin V [21, 24]. This technique, despite selecting sperm with intact DNA, does not discriminate concerning the type of motility, which is why MACS is recommended to be used in combination with some motile sperm separation techniques such as DGC or Swim-up [25, 26]. The use of MACS has been shown to improve pregnancy rates and, therefore, the success of ART cycles. However, since it is a technique that requires special equipment and its execution takes more time than conventional methods, it is less used in daily clinical practice [26].

Microfluidic Devices

Microfluidics is an application that mimics the in vivo processes for sperm selection occurring in the female reproductive tract. During incubation in a microfluidic device, spermatozoa with the highest progressive motility deviate to parallel streams through the micropore membrane, while sluggish or immotile sperm and debris remain in the initial streamline and remain as waste. The use of a microfluidic device has the advantage that the detrimental effects of centrifugation can be avoided. Thus, oxidative stress and DNA damage induced by these procedures are avoided. The first application of microfluidic technology in sperm sorting was reported in 2003 and was based on a steady flow maintained by microfluidic gravity and a capillary force-driven pump [27]. Since then, several microfluidic devices have been proposed and constructed either for conventional IVF [28] or ICSI procedures [29].

Sperm preparation with a microfluidic-based device diminished the proportion of sperm with double-stranded sperm DNA damage (dsSDF) compared to preparation with swim-up or non-processed sperm [30] (Fig. 15.1).

Moreover, the separation of sperm by the use of a microfluidic device results in the suspension of highly motile sperm with very low DNA fragmentation levels [31].

However, no benefit in terms of fertilization rate, embryo development, and pregnancy rate has been found in the general population undergoing IVF/ICSI when using the microfluidic device instead of the conventional sperm preparation through density gradients [32].

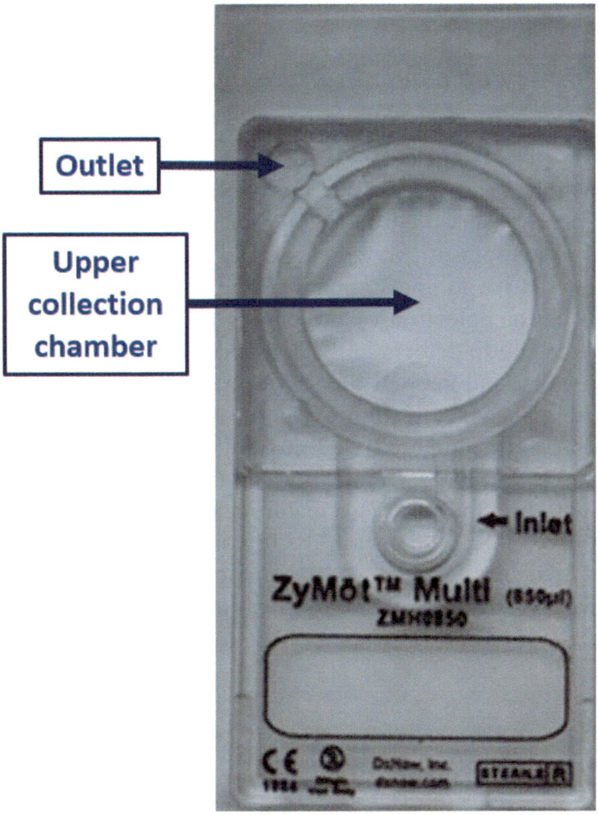

Fig. 15.1 Picture of a microfluidic device designed for sperm processing Sperm is injected through the inlet. Sperm wash solution is applied to the upper collection chamber. Sperm-containing fluid is aspirated by the outlet

Conventional Sperm Selection During ICSI

Intracytoplasmic sperm injection is an ART that allows fertilization and pregnancy to be carried out even with low-quality semen samples of low population, motility and/or morphology by injecting a sperm directly into a mature oocyte, which is why sperm retrieval and selection is essential. In conventional ICSI, sperm selection is mainly based on morphological and kinetic criteria of the spermatozoon o be micro-injected and relies largely on the experience of the embryologist for this selection [24, 33]. When performing ICSI under optical microscopy, spermatozoa with normal head shape and detectable acrosomal structure should be selected and viewed with good optical magnification [34]. The vitality of the sperm is considered through motility indications, which is another crucial factor as to the reason why highly motile sperm are preferred when selecting sperm for ICSI. Kinetic parameters, such as straight-line velocity (VSL) and curvilinear velocity (VCL), have prognostic value in predicting the spermatozoa fertilization potential. It has been reported that spermatozoa with VCL values less than 65 μm/s and a VSL less than 40 μm/s are recommended for ICSI instead of IVF, to increase the fertilization rates [35].

Advanced Techniques for Sperm Selection During ICSI

Intracytoplasmic Morphologically Selected Sperm Injection (IMSI)

Motile sperm organelle morphology examination (MSOME) is a method of sperm observation under high magnification in the range of 6000× to 10,000×. Intracytoplasmic morphologically selected sperm injection (IMSI) is a technique alternative to conventional ICSI that employs the MSOME method and facilitates the selection of morphologically normal sperm. Under these conditions, even subtle defects in the acrosome, nucleus mitochondria, tail, post-acrosomal lamina, and neck of the sperm may be seen (Fig. 15.2). Moreover, IMSI facilitates the visualization of sperm head vacuoles that have been associated with chromatin immaturity [36]. According to Boitrelle et al., the observation of a single and large vacuole seen on the sperm head is indicative of chromatin condensation failure [37], a feature that is linked to DNA fragmentation and compromised ICSI outcomes [38]. In contrast, some recent studies have reported that sperm head vacuoles are common physiological cellular features originating from nuclear-envelope invaginations [39].

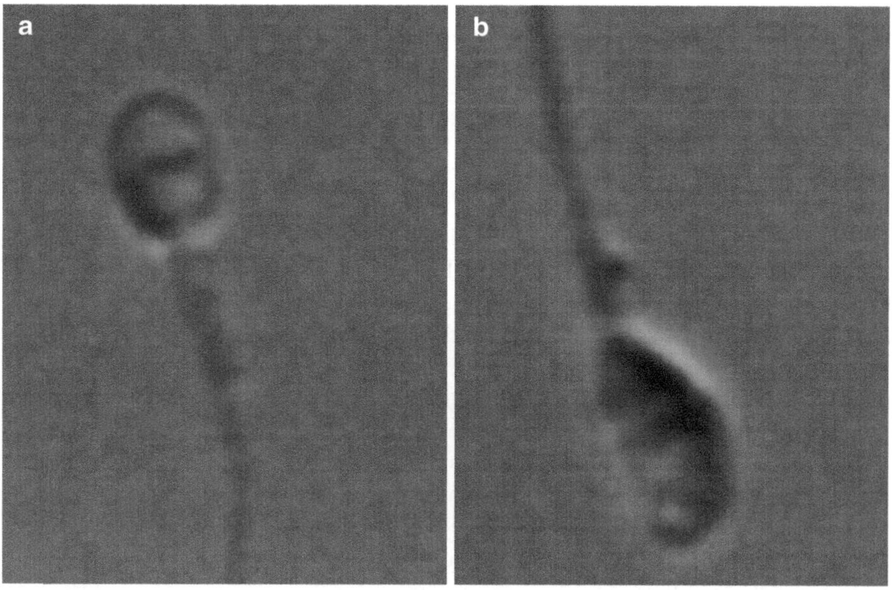

Fig. 15.2 IMSI. (**a**) A normal sperm head spermatozoon, observed under high magnification. (**b**) A vacuolated spermatozoon, observed under high magnification

A recent Cochrane systematic review did not find any robust evidence supporting the beneficial effects of IMSI over ICSI, due to the limitations of the included studies and inconsistency of results. The authors concluded that there is only low-quality evidence that IMSI increases the chances of a clinical pregnancy but data presented is uncertain about the chances of live birth or miscarriage [40].

Physiological Intracytoplasmic Sperm Injection (PICSI)

The physiological intracytoplasmic sperm injection (PICSI) technique employs the use of hyaluronic acid (HA) to immobilize and select the sperm [41]. Alternatively, drops of ICSI sperm selection medium containing HA can be used in a conventional ICSI dish. HA is a major component of the extracellular matrix surrounding the cumulus-oocyte complex [33, 42]. The principle of PICSI is based on the fact that only mature sperm express HA receptors, and therefore only mature spermatozoa can bind to HA. In this way, the selected spermatozoa are considered more likely to possess the physiologycal capacity to bind to and penetrate the zona pellucida of the oocyte [33, 43, 44]. PICSI allows the optimization of conventional ICSI by favoring the selection of sperm without DNA fragmentation and normal nuclei, thus improving fertilization rates [33, 44]. However, the discussion on the true benefits of this technique in the clinical field remains open. According to a 2019 Cochrane review on advanced sperm selection techniques, [19] hyaluronic acid binding has no or little effect on improving clinical pregnancies but may reduce miscarriages.

Birefringence

Sperm head birefringence is an easy, non-invasive, and cost-effective sperm sorting method that allows the selection of mature sperm with low DNA fragmentation [45]. In mature spermatozoa, birefringence is caused by the arrangement and orientation of nucleoprotein filaments and is assessed under an inverted microscope equipped with Hoffman contrast and polarizing lenses [46] (Fig. 15.3).

Recent studies demonstrate that there is a positive clinical impact in applying this simple method that can be used along with ICSI [47]. Another application of this technique is the detection of viable spermatozoa in complete asthenospermia samples. Immotile sperm with birefringence properties are more likely to be viable and lead to improved fertilization and embryo development rates without needing sophisticated or invasive techniques such as pentoxifylline [48].

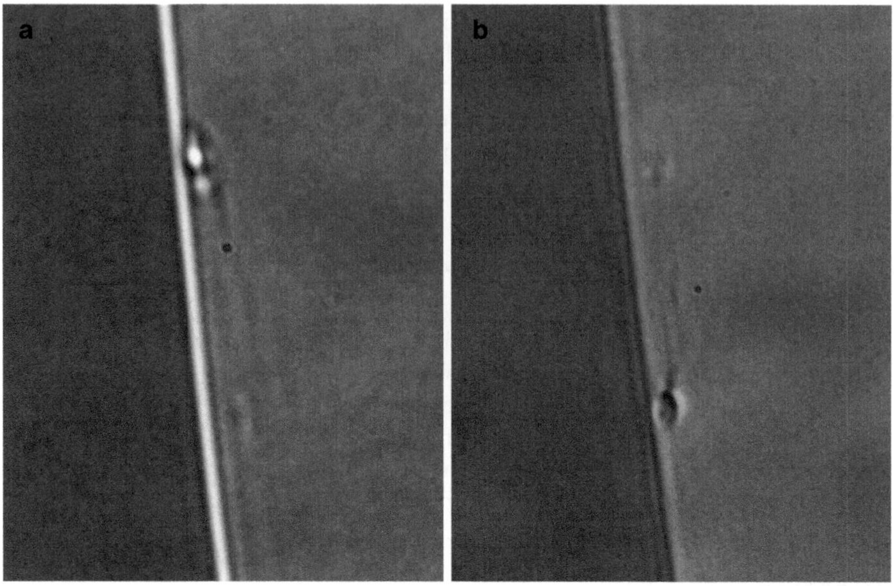

Fig. 15.3 Pictures of sperm selected by birefringence. (**a**) Birefrigent sperm. (**b**) Non-birefrigent sperm

Sperm Selection of Viable Sperm (HOST, Mechanical Touch, Use of Laser, Pentoxyfilline)

For samples that are recovered by testicular sperm extraction (TESE) or epididymal aspiration (MESA), it is important to evaluate cell viability, since spermatozoa may appear immotile, due to incomplete or interrupted maturation in the epididymis [33]. There are some advanced, less frequently used methods, that can help with sperm selection in ICSI procedures. One such method that has been proposed is the mechanical touch technique (MTT) for the selection of immotile sperm for ICSI [49]. This technique is based on the discrimination of viable sperm by its reaction when touching the tail with the ICSI pipette producing a small bend in the tail; if the sperm recovers the original tail position, it is considered viable [33, 49]. This technique does not require high implementation costs, while the key issue would be the embryologist's ability to perform it. Phosphodiesterase (PDE) inhibitors, such as pentoxifylline (PTX), are considered another method with great potential for ART due to their ability to induce activation of sperm motility by inducing the elevation of cAMP levels in this cell [50]. PTX use is controversial and is not yet used routinely since it can cause energetic depletion of the spermatozoa and early activation of essential events, such as the acrosomal reaction [33]. However, the use of modified versions of PTX, such as PTXm-1, with better pharmacological properties than PTX has been proposed to help sperm to improve its functions [50]. Another alternative sperm selection technique is the hypoosmotic swelling test (HOST), which evaluates the functional capacity of the sperm membrane that relates to viability [51]. When spermatozoa are introduced into a hypoosmotic environment, the tails of viable sperm swell and bend due to the activity of osmosensitive channels in the plasma membrane, allowing the integrity of the membrane and cell viability to be evaluated [33]. The HOST is recommended by the WHO sperm processing manual for sperm vitality analysis [52]. Another proposed intervention is the laser-assisted immotile sperm selection (LAISS) that be used to activate the motility of sperm that are initially immobile. Irradiation generates a slight movement of the tail in viable sperm [33, 53]. The main advantage of this method is that it is safe, does not produce side effects, and can also be used for any case of sperm immotility [53].

Artificial Intelligence

The introduction of artificial intelligence (AI) tools has been a breakthrough in the field of medicine, and more particularly in assisted reproduction technologies (ART). Early AI algorithms have been mainly used for semen analysis and have been suggested to be a valid alternative compared to the manual evaluation of sperm parameters [54]. Nevertheless, the evolution of such algorithms and the capability to process large sets of data in real-time could prove to be an invaluable tool that will potentially increase sperm selection efficiency and reliability during ICSI. In this framework, sperm selection is continuously evolving through machine deep learning, and training is conducted with data derived from fertilization parameters and their clinical results. Several studies have supported that deep learning networks can be trained by using data from sperm cells of known quality [55, 56].

A new automated sperm-individual identification system (SID: Sperm ID or identification) based on artificial intelligence (AI), possesses an algorithm that allows the selection of sperm during the ICSI procedure by evaluating motility parameters [57]. SID and other similar tools currently developed and assessed offer promising prospects for their use in a clinical context, as they can assist with sperm selection (viable and motile), in a real-time and more effective manner.

Embryo Selection Techniques

Classic Morphological Selection Methods

There is a consensus that embryonic development is evaluated and described for monitoring in vitro cultures in ART, which essentially focuses on morphological characteristics. The embryo and its developmental rate are conventionally evaluated by optical microscopy. 17 h post insemination, a normally fertilized oocyte should display two pronuclei (2PN) of similar size that are closely apposed and centrally located [58]. Istanbul consensus defines the rate of good quality embryos as the proportion of day 2 and 3 embryos with a high score or grade, depending on different variables, such as the number of cells and their size, fragmentation, and multinucleation. The cleavage rate reflects the ability of the culture system to support the cellular division of fertilized oocytes [59]. So, embryos are scored in four categories: A (superior quality), B (good quality; not for elective single embryo transfer), C (impaired embryonic quality), and D (not recommended for transfer). Since embryonic development can vary depending on the culture medium and conditions of each laboratory, the consensus recommends that each laboratory develop its own descriptions of embryos, based on the categories mentioned above and in the reported observations [58].

Time-Lapse Imaging and Morphokinetics

Although the conventional morphological evaluation is still valid and in most IVF clinics it remains the golden standard for embryo selection, time-lapse imaging has gained significant grounds by facilitating an in-depth understanding of embryo preimplantation development and offering numerous research opportunities. A time-lapse system (TLS) is based on the utilization of cameras that capture photos of embryo development every 5–15 min, thus monitoring dynamic changes of preimplantation embryo throughout embryo culture. With the advancement of time-lapse imaging, new parameters such as timing of cell division, duration of the cell cycle and time to blastulation and expansion have been introduced and are used to evaluate embryo quality.

Furthermore, abnormal features such as direct cleavage [60], reverse cleavage, [61] or multiple blastocyst collapses [62], all associated with embryo competence, were not previously assessed as these parameters would require multiple observations under the inverted microscope in a conventional setting (Figs. 15.4 and 15.5).

Until now, contradicting views have been presented on the efficiency and superiority of TLS over conventional morphological evaluation. According to a recent Cochrane systematic review, there is no evidence of a benefit in clinical outcomes for couples undergoing ART when using TLS [63].

Nevertheless, the value of existent TLS remains important and morphokinetics is a vast field to explore. The combination of time-lapse technology with the continuous advancement of artificial intelligence may lead to optimized and more efficient algorithms for embryo selection in the future.

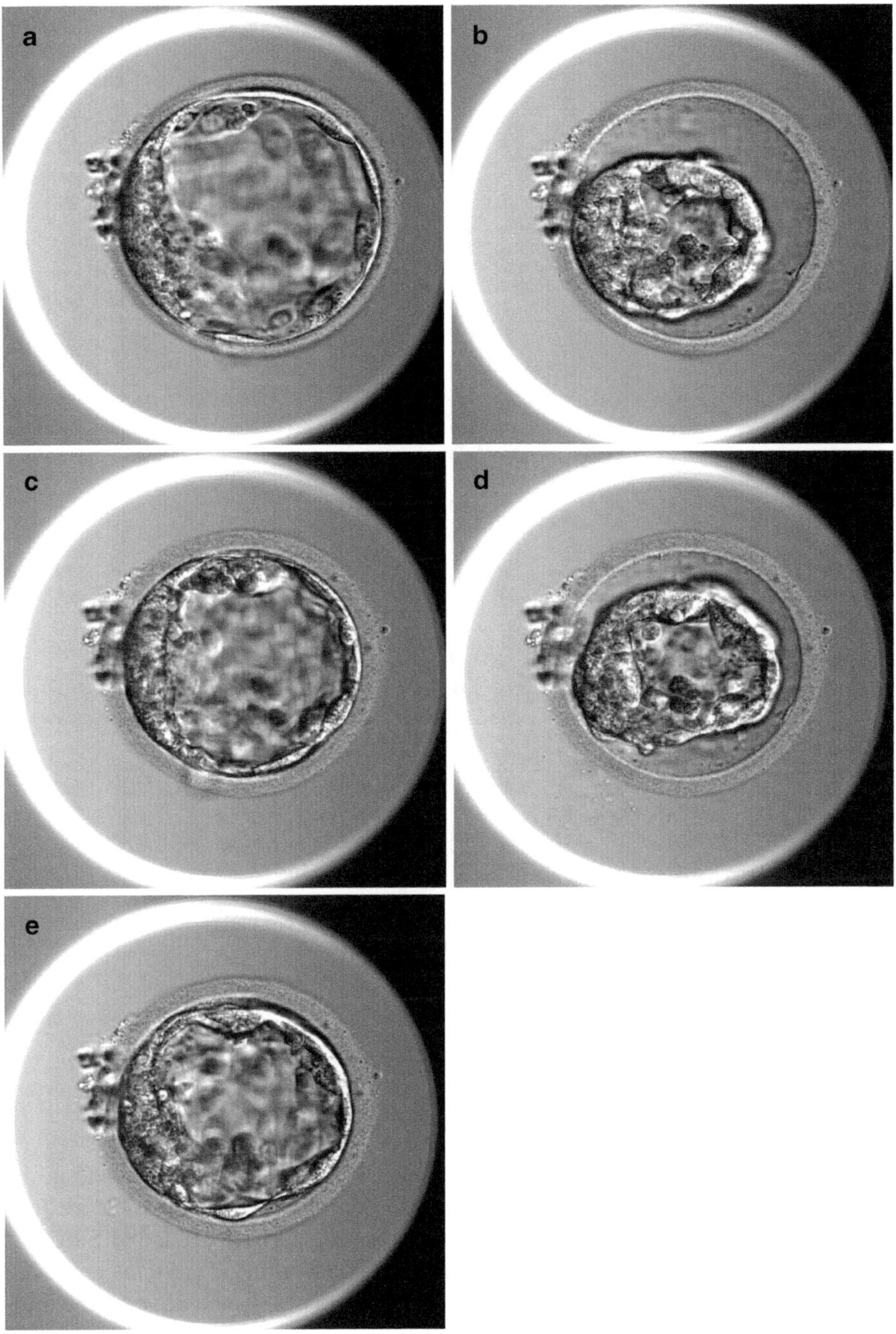

Fig. 15.4 Time-lapse monitoring of multiple collapses of a human blastosyst. (**a**) 112 h after insemination (**b**) 113 h after insemination (**c**) 114.5 h after insemination (**d**) 116 h after insemination (**e**) 117 h after insemination

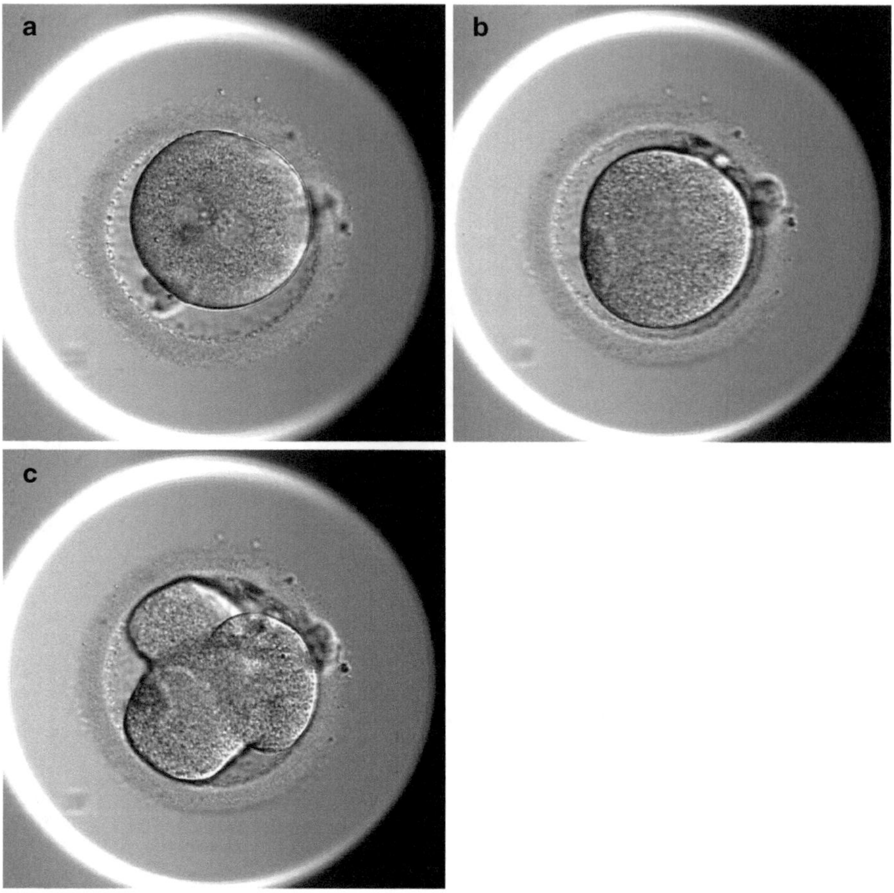

Fig. 15.5 Time-lapse monitoring of direct cleavage of a human preimplantation embryo. (**a**) At 18 h post insemination a normally fertilized 2PN embryo (**b**) At 32 h post insemination 1-cell embryo (**c**) At 33 h post insemination the embryo directly cleaved to 3-cells

Prediction of Embryo Competence Using Artificial Intelligence Models and Machine Learning

Artificial intelligence (AI) use in embryo competence has rapidly escalated in the last few years. Currently, various AI models such as iDAScore, KIDScore [64] (Invitrolife), genetics model [65], Life Whisperer [66], STORK [67], and EPA [68] models, have been developed using different machine learning algorithms grounded in embryo and blastocyst morphology and morphokinetics, which are employed for the prediction of implantation and the diagnosis of embryo ploidy. TLS combined with AI algorithms has demonstrated an improved accuracy in embryo ploidy prediction outperforming human grading [69, 70]. However, a clear understanding of the proposed models' limitations is crucial for embryo selection and the evolution of the AI algorithms [69]. Among AI models, STORK has shown promising potential since it has been adopted by different groups around the globe, thanks to its ease of interpretation and use of data [69]. The integration of AI algorithms into IVF laboratories and their platforms will enhance the adoption of the methodologies, promoting further development of algorithms that optimize clinical considerations to incorporate into research and increase the predictive capacity of AI in embryo quality and human blastocysts selection, reducing invasive procedures, clinical time and costs, and increasing ART success.

Preimplantation Genetic Testing (PGT)

Aneuploidies occur commonly in the embryos derived by both natural conception and ART. They are a main cause of infertility and miscarriage which carries a high physiological and psychological toll.

Embryo biopsy for PGT may be performed either at cleavage, or blastocyst stage. Trophectoderm (TE) biopsy, performed at the blastocyst stage allows the removal of more than one trophectoderm cells without disturbing the inner embryo cell mass, thus minimizing the impact on embryo competency (Fig. 15.6). Additionally, the chromosomal analysis conducted through next-generation sequencing (NGS) increases the sensitivity and mosaicism detection [71].

Several studies suggest that PGT-A employment increases pregnancy rates compared to conventional morphology evaluation alone [72, 73].

Despite the profound value of PGT-A in selecting euploid embryos, several limitations exist. In blastocyst biopsy for PGT-A, biopsy cells originate from the TE, while the inner cell mass (ICM) remains intact. Due to the high incidence

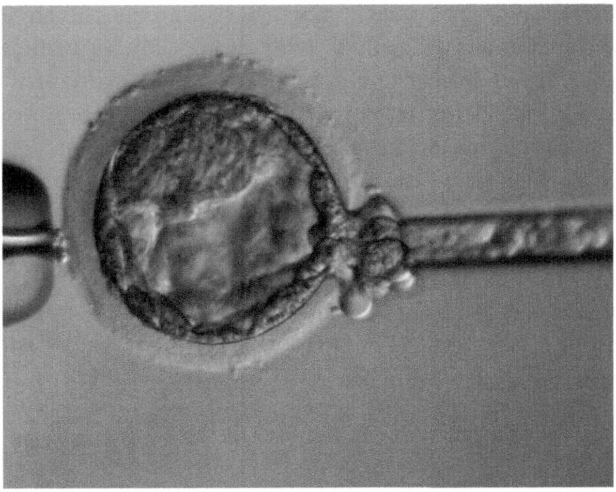

Fig. 15.6 Picture of a day-5 blastocyst trophectoderm biopsy

of mosaicism in the TE cell line, the genetic material analyzed may not be representative of the whole embryo and misdiagnosis is possible [74]. Moreover, according to the ESHRE guidelines on add-ons in reproductive medicine, PGT-A only slightly increases live birth rate (LBR), and the benefit of this method in reducing the abortion rate needs to be verified [75].

Non-invasive PGT (ni-PGT), a technique that uses cell-free DNA collected from either spent culture medium (SCM) or blastocoel fluid (BF), is an alternative approach to invasive PGT. The DNA analyzed is more representative of the whole embryo, as it derives from cellular processes from both the ICM and TE [76]. Additionally, it may offer an advantage in cases of advanced maternal age and poor-quality blastocysts, as no biopsy is needed, which could lower the chances of implantation. However, ni-PGT has its limitations, as the DNA collected in the culture medium may originate from aneuploid apoptotic cells expelled through a self-correction mechanism, thus leading to a false diagnosis of euploid blastocysts as aneuploid [77].

Other Methods (Oxygen Consumption, Metabolomics, Oxidative Stress)

Embryonic development dynamics and potential is influenced by the surrounding environment of the embryo, which is why oxidative stress and preimplantation metabolites are important markers for developmental monitoring during ART. The measurement of metabolite levels secreted by the embryo in the culture media, presents patterns that correlate with the formation of blastocysts and pregnancy, which has allowed the establishment of metabolic profiles that are associated with embryonic viability [78]. Fluorescence lifetime imaging microscopy is a useful tool to evaluate embryonic quality, and it can detect with high sensitivity associated metabolic variations with blastocyst development after fertilization [79]. However, there is still no clear evidence of the benefit of analyzing metabolomic profiles with respect to live birth or pregnancy rates on ART [80]. Another alternative method is the measurement of embryonic oxygen consumption during in vitro culture. The embryonic oxygen requirement remains constant from the formation of the zygote to the development of the blastocyst [81]. This has allowed several researchers to develop some systems such as a respirometric biochip [82] as well as an embryonic respiration monitor with a sensor chip [83], to measure the oxygen consumption of the embryo during in vitro development and before implantation; making these tools valuable for embryo monitoring. On the other hand, the assessment of oxidative stress in the culture medium, through tools such as thermochemiluminescence, provides a strategy to determine the susceptibility of embryos to oxidation [81].

Future Directions

The combination of different sperm selection methods has been employed towards optimization of clinical outcomes results. The application of interferometric phase microscopy (IPM) to microfluidics can facilitate sperm selection for ICSI according to both motility and morphology [84]. Additionally, when combining birefringence, MSOME, and vacuole observation for sperm selection the percentage of sperm with genetic integrity increased [45].

AI is a promising field that is expected to evolve rapidly and improve the current practices of sperm and embryo selection in the future. However, despite the preliminary promising results, major limitations exist currently as in most studies, data derives from single-center cohorts. Additional studies on a larger scale, paired with collaboration between centers may improve the existing algorithms and increase the predictive value of AI-based selection methods.

PGT-A is considered to be a technique that currently provides the most accurate results in terms of ploidy prediction. However, in many cases, the transfer of euploid blastocysts after trophectoderm biopsy does not result to pregnancy [85]. The main reasons for implantation failure of chromosomally normal blastocysts include low-quality blastocysts, advanced maternal age. and excessive embryo manipulation [85]. As a conclusion, ploidy status alone is insufficient as a predictive tool for a successful embryo transfer. On the contrary, the combination of embryo selection methods is beneficial in order to predict the embryo has the highest chance for a successful outcome. Furthermore, the application of non-invasive techniques such as conventional morphology, morphokinetics, or non-invasive PGT, may allow for increasing the efficacy of single embryo transfer SET without compromising the quality of the embryo.

Conclusion

Although sperm selection methods such as hyaluronic acid binding, Zeta sperm, or MACS have provided promising results, additional studies are needed to justify the routine use of the above techniques. IMSI, a method that allows detailed observation of the sperm morphology is not recommended for all ICSI cases as it is a time-consuming technique without proven clinical value.

However, sperm selection techniques may have a positive effect only on specific groups of patients. Given the negative impact of high SDF on embryo quality and miscarriage rates, sperm selection techniques such as MACS, microfluidics, and IMSI have a potential benefit for patients with persistently high SDF, as they allow the selection of spermatozoa with intact DNA [45] (Garrido, 2023). Moreover, the need for standardizing SDF assays and introducing them to routine clinical practice becomes more demanding.

Along with the standard morphological embryo evaluation that is routinely used in most IVF labs, morphokinetics combined with AI is gaining ground in embryo selection. STORK-A, a non-invasive AI method that combines maternal age, morphological, and morphokinetic data has demonstrated a strong ability to predict embryo ploidy status [70]. However, more large-scale multicenter studies are needed to design algorithms that would be universally accepted and to verify the predictive value of these methods.

Although PGT-A currently provides the highest accuracy in detecting embryo aneuploidies, ESHRE does not recommend biopsy for PGT-A for routine clinical use [75]. Patient groups that might benefit more from PGT-A employment are the ones facing RIF and/or RM and, at the same time, have a high number and high quality of blastocysts. On the contrary, low-quality embryos are more likely to be damaged because of extreme and unnecessary manipulations and as a result implantation chances may be diminished.

We can conclude that there is an abundance and variety of sperm and embryo selection methods, most of which are time-consuming, costly, and, in some cases, invasive (Table 15.1). As a consequence, it is highly important to choose the most proper selection method according to the specific indications and needs of each patient in order to maximize the success rates.

Table 15.1 Conventional and advanced techniques for sperm and embryo selection

Sperm selection techniques	Sperm preparation techniques	Conventional	Swim-up
			Density gradient
			Centrifugation
		Advanced	Electrophoresis
			Zeta potential
			MACS
			Microfluidics
	Sperm selection techniques during ICSI	Conventional	Morphological and kinetic criteria
		Advanced	PICSI
			IMSI
			Birefrigence
			Selection of viable sperm (HOST, MTT, LAISS, pentoxifylline)
			Artificial intelligence
Embryo selection techniques		Conventional	Embryo morphology evaluation
		Advanced	Morphokinetics
			Artificial intelligence
			PGT-A
			Oxygen consumption
			Metabolomics
			Oxidative stress

References

1. Byrd W, Ackerman GE, Carr BR, Edman CD, Guzick DS, McConnell JD. Treatment of refractory infertility by transcervical intrauterine insemination of washed spermatozoa. Fertil Steril. 1987;48(6):921–7. https://doi.org/10.1016/s0015-0282(16)59584-3. PMID: 3678511.
2. Wang S, Tan W, Huang Y, Mao X, Li Z, Zhang X, Wei P, Xue L. Sperm DNA fragmentation measured by sperm chromatin dispersion impacts morphokinetic parameters, fertilization rate and blastocyst quality in ICSI treatments. Zygote. 2022;30(1):72–9. https://doi.org/10.1017/S0967199421000332. PMID: 34034847.
3. Menezo Y, Dale B, Elder K. The negative impact of the environment on methylation/epigenetic marking in gametes and embryos: a plea for action to protect the fertility of future generations. Mol Reprod Dev. 2019;86(10):1273–82. https://doi.org/10.1002/mrd.23116. PMID: 30653787.
4. Amargant F, Pujol A, Ferrer-Vaquer A, Durban M, Martínez M, Vassena R, Vernos I. The human sperm basal body is a complex centrosome important for embryo preimplantation development. Mol Hum Reprod. 2021;27(11):gaab062. https://doi.org/10.1093/molehr/gaab062. PMID: 34581808; PMCID: PMC8561016.
5. Gordon JD, DiMattina M, Reh A, Botes A, Celia G, Payson M. Utilization and success rates of unstimulated in vitro fertilization in the United States: an analysis of the Society for Assisted Reproductive Technology database. Fertil Steril. 2013;100(2):392–5. https://doi.org/10.1016/j.fertnstert.2013.03.037. PMID: 23623475
6. Scholten I, Chambers GM, van Loendersloot L, van der Veen F, Repping S, Gianotten J, Hompes PG, Ledger W, Mol BW. Impact of assisted reproductive technology on the incidence of multiple-gestation infants: a population perspective. Fertil Steril. 2015;103(1):179–83. https://doi.org/10.1016/j.fertnstert.2014.09.033. PMID: 25439839
7. Henkel RR, Schill WB. Sperm preparation for ART. Reprod Biol Endocrinol. 2003;1:108. https://doi.org/10.1186/1477-7827-1-108. PMID: 14617368; PMCID: PMC293422.
8. Iván O-L, Sara R-D, Priscila R-I, Serafín P-C. Novel techniques of sperm selection for improving IVF and ICSI outcomes. Front Cell Dev Biol. 2019;7:298. https://doi.org/10.3389/fcell.2019.00298.
9. Mahadevan M, Baker G. Assessment and preparation of semen for in vitro fertilization. In: Wood C, Trounson A, editors. Clinical in vitro fertilization. London: Springer; 1984. p. 83–97. https://doi.org/10.1007/978-1-4471-3317-9_7.
10. Kiratli S, Yuncu M, Kose K, Ozkavukcu S. A comparative evaluation of migration sedimentation method for sperm preparation. Syst Biol Reprod Med. 2018;64:122–9. https://doi.org/10.1080/19396368.2017.1402100.
11. Gupta S, Sharma R, Agarwal A, Parekh N, Finelli R, Shah R, Kandil H, Saleh R, Arafa M, Ko E, Simopoulou M, Zini A, Rajmil O, Kavoussi P, Singh K, Ambar RF, Elbardisi H, Sengupta P, Martinez M, Boitrelle F, Alves MG, Khalafalla K, Roychoudhury S, Busetto GM, Gosalvez J, Tadros N, Palani A, Rodriguez MG, Anagnostopoulou C, Micic S, Rocco L, Mostafa T, Alvarez JG, Jindal S, Sallam H, Maldonado Rosas I, Lewis SEM, AlSaid S, Altan M, Park HJ, Ramsay J, Parekattil S, Sabbaghian M, Tremellen K, Vogiatzi P, Sadighi Gilani MA, Evenson DP, Colpi GM. A comprehensive guide to sperm recovery in infertile men with retrograde ejaculation. World J Mens Health. 2022;40(2):208–16. https://doi.org/10.5534/wjmh.210069. PMID: 34169680; PMCID: PMC8987146.
12. Verheyen G, Popovic-Todorovic B, Tournaye H. Processing and selection of surgically-retrieved sperm for ICSI: a review. Basic Clin Androl. 2017;27:6. https://doi.org/10.1186/s12610-017-0050-2. PMID: 28331619; PMCID: PMC5360083.
13. Schröter S, Derr P, Conradt HS, Nimtz M, Hale G, Kirchhoff C. Male-specific modification of human CD52. J Biol Chem. 1999;274(42):29862–73. https://doi.org/10.1074/jbc.274.42.29862. PMID: 10514467.

14. Simon L, Murphy K, Aston KI, Emery BR, Hotaling JM, Carrell DT. Micro-electrophoresis: a noninvasive method of sperm selection based on membrane charge. Fertil Steril. 2015;103(2):361–6.e3. https://doi.org/10.1016/j.fertnstert.2014.10.047. PMID: 25500020.
15. Ainsworth C, Nixon B, Aitken RJ. Development of a novel electrophoretic system for the isolation of human spermatozoa. Hum Reprod. 2005;20(8):2261–70. https://doi.org/10.1093/humrep/dei024. PMID: 15831507.
16. Chan PJ, Jacobson JD, Corselli JU, Patton WC. A simple zeta method for sperm selection based on membrane charge. Fertil Steril. 2006;85(2):481–6. https://doi.org/10.1016/j.fertnstert.2005.07.1302. PMID: 16595231.
17. Sefidgar Tehrani M, Amirian M, Jalali M, Attaranzadeh A, Fazel A, Ebrahimzadeh-Bideskan A. Role of the zeta method in intracytoplasmic sperm injection outcomes in high sperm DNA fragmentation in Oligoasthenozoospermic men. Galen Med J. 2018;7:e1107. https://doi.org/10.22086/gmj.v0i0.1107. PMID: 34466435; PMCID: PMC8343982.
18. Kheirollahi-Kouhestani M, Razavi S, Tavalaee M, Deemeh MR, Mardani M, Moshtaghian J, Nasr-Esfahani MH. Selection of sperm based on combined density gradient and zeta method may improve ICSI outcome. Hum Reprod. 2009;24(10):2409–16. https://doi.org/10.1093/humrep/dep088. PMID: 19553239.
19. Lepine S, McDowell S, Searle LM, Kroon B, Glujovsky D, Yazdani A. Advanced sperm selection techniques for assisted reproduction. Cochrane Database Syst Rev. 2019;7(7):CD010461. https://doi.org/10.1002/14651858.CD010461.pub3. PMID: 31425620; PMCID: PMC6699650.
20. Agarwal A, Majzoub A, Baskaran S, Panner Selvam MK, Cho CL, Henkel R, Finelli R, Leisegang K, Sengupta P, Barbarosie C, Parekh N, Alves MG, Ko E, Arafa M, Tadros N, Ramasamy R, Kavoussi P, Ambar R, Kuchakulla M, Robert KA, Iovine C, Durairajanayagam D, Jindal S, Shah R. Sperm DNA fragmentation: a new guideline for clinicians. World J Mens Health. 2020;38(4):412–71. https://doi.org/10.5534/wjmh.200128. PMID: 32777871; PMCID: PMC7502318.
21. Pacheco A, Blanco A, Bronet F, Cruz M, García-Fernández J, García-Velasco JA. Magnetic-activated cell sorting (MACS): a useful sperm-selection technique in cases of high levels of sperm DNA fragmentation. ClinMed. 2020;9(12):3976. https://doi.org/10.3390/jcm9123976.
22. Gil M, Sar-Shalom V, Sivira YM, Carreras R, Checa MA. Sperm selection using magnetic activated cell sorting (MACS) in assisted reproduction: a systematic review and meta-analysis. J Assist Reprod Genet. 2013;30(4):479–85. https://doi.org/10.1007/s10815-013-9962-8.
23. Lee TH, Liu CH, Shih YT, Tsao HM, Huang CC, Chen HH, Lee MS. Magnetic-activated cell sorting for sperm preparation reduces spermatozoa with apoptotic markers and improves the acrosome reaction in couples with unexplained infertility. Hum Reprod. 2010;25(4):839–46. https://doi.org/10.1093/humrep/deq009. PMID: 20150175
24. Nasr-Esfahani MH, Tavalaee M. New era in sperm selection for ICSI. Int J Androl. 2012;35(4):475–84. https://doi.org/10.1111/j.1365-2605.2011.01227.x.
25. Ješeta M, et al. Magnetic-activated cell sorting in combination with swim-up efficiency improve effectivity of spermatozoa separation. Med J Cell Biol. 2018;6(2):55–60. https://doi.org/10.2478/acb-2018-0010.
26. Vasilescu SA, Ding L, Parast FY, Nosrati R, Warkiani ME. Sperm quality metrics were improved by a biomimetic microfluidic selection platform compared to swim-up methods. Microsyst Nanoeng. 2023;9:37. https://doi.org/10.1038/s41378-023-00501-7. PMID: 37007605; PMCID: PMC10050147.
27. Schuster TG, Cho B, Keller LM, Takayama S, Smith GD. Isolation of motile spermatozoa from semen samples using microfluidics. Reprod Biomed Online. 2003;7(1):75–81. https://doi.org/10.1016/s1472-6483(10)61732-4. PMID: 12930579.
28. Huang HY, Lai YL, Yao DJ. Dielectrophoretic microfluidic device for in vitro fertilization. Micromachines (Basel). 2018;9(3):135. https://doi.org/10.3390/mi9030135.
29. Matsuura K, Uozumi T, Furuichi T, Sugimoto I, Kodama M, Funahashi H. A microfluidic device to reduce treatment time of intracytoplasmic sperm injection. Fertil Steril. 2013;99(2):400–7. https://doi.org/10.1016/j.fertnstert.2012.10.022. PMID: 23122951

30. Pujol A, García-Peiró A, Ribas-Maynou J, Lafuente R, Mataró D, Vassena R. A microfluidic sperm-sorting device reduces the proportion of sperm with double-stranded DNA fragmentation. Zygote. 2022;30(2):200–5. https://doi.org/10.1017/S0967199421000484. PMID: 34313213.
31. Quinn MM, Jalalian L, Ribeiro S, Ona K, Demirci U, Cedars MI, Rosen MP. Microfluidic sorting selects sperm for clinical use with reduced DNA damage compared to density gradient centrifugation with swim-up in split semen samples. Hum Reprod. 2018;33(8):1388–93. https://doi.org/10.1093/humrep/dey239. PMID: 30007319
32. Quinn MM, Ribeiro S, Juarez-Hernandez F, Simbulan RK, Jalalian L, Cedars MI, Rosen MP. Microfluidic preparation of spermatozoa for ICSI produces similar embryo quality to density-gradient centrifugation: a pragmatic, randomized controlled trial. Hum Reprod. 2022;37(7):1406–13. https://doi.org/10.1093/humrep/deac099. PMID: 35522187.
33. Baldini D, Ferri D, Baldini GM, Lot D, Catino A, Vizziello D, Vizziello G. Sperm selection for ICSI: do we have a winner? Cells. 2021;10(12):3566. https://doi.org/10.3390/cells10123566. PMID: 34944074; PMCID: PMC8700516.
34. Haddad M, Stewart J, Xie P, Cheung S, Trout A, Keating D, Parrella A, Lawrence S, Rosenwaks Z, Palermo GD. Thoughts on the popularity of ICSI. J Assist Reprod Genet. 2021;38(1):101–23. https://doi.org/10.1007/s10815-020-01987-0. PMID: 33155089; PMCID: PMC7823003.
35. Dcunha R, Hussein RS, Ananda H, Kumari S, Adiga SK, Kannan N, Zhao Y, Kalthur G. Current insights and latest updates in sperm motility and associated applications in assisted reproduction. Reprod Sci. 2022;29(1):7–25. https://doi.org/10.1007/s43032-020-00408-y. PMID: 33289064; PMCID: PMC7721202.
36. Perdrix A, Rives N. Motile sperm organelle morphology examination (MSOME) and sperm head vacuoles: state of the art in 2013. Hum Reprod Update. 2013;19(5):527–41. https://doi.org/10.1093/humupd/dmt021. PMID: 23825157
37. Boitrelle F, Ferfouri F, Petit JM, Segretain D, Tourain C, Bergere M, Bailly M, Vialard F, Albert M, Selva J. Large human sperm vacuoles observed in motile spermatozoa under high magnification: nuclear thumbprints linked to failure of chromatin condensation. Hum Reprod. 2011;26(7):1650–8. https://doi.org/10.1093/humrep/der129. PMID: 21536591
38. Greco E, Scarselli F, Fabozzi G, Colasante A, Zavaglia D, Alviggi E, Litwicka K, Varricchio MT, Minasi MG, Tesarik J. Sperm vacuoles negatively affect outcomes in intracytoplasmic morphologically selected sperm injection in terms of pregnancy, implantation, and live-birth rates. Fertil Steril. 2013;100(2):379–85. https://doi.org/10.1016/j.fertnstert.2013.04.033. PMID: 23706334
39. Gómez-Torres MJ, Luna-Romero J, Fernández-Colom PJ, Aizpurua J, Avilés M, Romero A. Human sperm head vacuoles are related to nuclear-envelope invaginations. Int J Mol Sci. 2023;24(12):10027. https://doi.org/10.3390/ijms241210027. PMID: 37373176; PMCID: PMC10298367.
40. Teixeira DM, Barbosa MA, Ferriani RA, Navarro PA, Raine-Fenning N, Nastri CO, Martins WP. Regular (ICSI) versus ultra-high magnification (IMSI) sperm selection for assisted reproduction. Cochrane Database Syst Rev. 2013;(7):CD010167. https://doi.org/10.1002/14651858.CD010167.pub2. Update in: Cochrane Database Syst Rev. 2020;2:CD010167. PMID: 23884963.
41. Simopoulou M, Gkoles L, Bakas P, Giannelou P, Kalampokas T, Pantos K, Koutsilieris M. Improving ICSI: a review from the spermatozoon perspective. Syst Biol Reprod Med. 2016;62(6):359–71. https://doi.org/10.1080/19396368.2016.1229365. PMID: 27646677.
42. Dandekar P, Aggeler J, Talbot P. Structure, distribution and composition of the extracellular matrix of human oocytes and cumulus masses. Hum Reprod. 1992;7(3):391–8. https://doi.org/10.1093/oxfordjournals.humrep.a137656. PMID: 1375234.
43. Huszar G, Ozkavukcu S, Jakab A, Celik-Ozenci C, Sati GL, Cayli S. Hyaluronic acid binding ability of human sperm reflects cellular maturity and fertilizing potential: selection of sperm

for intracytoplasmic sperm injection. Curr Opin Obstet Gynecol. 2006;18(3):260–7. https://doi.org/10.1097/01.gco.0000193018.98061.2f. PMID: 16735824.

44. Parmegiani L, Cognigni GE, Bernardi S, Troilo E, Ciampaglia W, Filicori M. "Physiologic ICSI": hyaluronic acid (HA) favors selection of spermatozoa without DNA fragmentation and with normal nucleus, resulting in improvement of embryo quality. Fertil Steril. 2010;93(2):598–604. https://doi.org/10.1016/j.fertnstert.2009.03.033. PMID: 19393999
45. Garolla A, Cosci I, Menegazzo M, De Palo R, Ambrosini G, Sartini B, Pizzol D, Foresta C. Sperm selected by both birefringence and motile sperm organelle morphology examination have reduced deoxyribonucleic acid fragmentation. Fertil Steril. 2014;101(3):647–52. https://doi.org/10.1016/j.fertnstert.2013.11.029. PMID: 24360607.
46. Gianaroli L, Magli MC, Collodel G, Moretti E, Ferraretti AP, Baccetti B. Sperm head's birefringence: a new criterion for sperm selection. Fertil Steril. 2008;90(1):104–12. https://doi.org/10.1016/j.fertnstert.2007.05.078. PMID: 18023436.
47. Ribeiro MA, Broi MGD, Rose MB, Garolla A, Foresta C, Bragheto AMDS, Hardy DGF. Sperm selection by birefringence: a promising non-invasive tool to improve ICSI outcomes. JBRA Assist Reprod. 2023;27(2):234–40. https://doi.org/10.5935/1518-0557.20220055. PMID: 36468799; PMCID: PMC10279423.
48. Magli MC, Crippa A, Perruzza D, Azzena S, Graziosi S, Coppola F, Tabanelli C, Ferraretti AP, Gianaroli L. Birefringence properties of human immotile spermatozoa and ICSI outcome. Reprod Biomed Online. 2023;46(3):597–606. https://doi.org/10.1016/j.rbmo.2022.11.015. PMID: 36642560.
49. de Oliveira NM, Vaca Sánchez R, Rodriguez Fiesta S, Lopez Salgado T, Rodríguez R, Bethencourt JC, Blanes ZR. Pregnancy with frozen-thawed and fresh testicular biopsy after motile and immotile sperm microinjection, using the mechanical touch technique to assess viability. Hum Reprod. 2004;19(2):262–5. https://doi.org/10.1093/humrep/deh083. PMID: 14747164.
50. Satish M, Kumari S, Deeksha W, Abhishek S, Nitin K, Adiga SK, Hegde P, Dasappa JP, Kalthur G, Rajakumara E. Structure-based redesigning of pentoxifylline analogs against selective phosphodiesterases to modulate sperm functional competence for assisted reproductive technologies. Sci Rep. 2021;11(1):12293. https://doi.org/10.1038/s41598-021-91636-y. PMID: 34112881; PMCID: PMC8192908.
51. Jeyendran RS, Van der Ven HH, Perez-Pelaez M, Crabo BG, Zaneveld LJ. Development of an assay to assess the functional integrity of the human sperm membrane and its relationship to other semen characteristics. J Reprod Fertil. 1984;70(1):219–28. https://doi.org/10.1530/jrf.0.0700219. PMID: 6694140
52. World Health Organization. WHO Laboratory manual for the examination and processing of human semen. 6th ed. Geneva: WHO Press; 2021.
53. Xue Y, Xiong Y, Cheng X, Li K. Applications of laser technology in the manipulation of human spermatozoa. Reprod Biol Endocrinol. 2023;21(1):93. https://doi.org/10.1186/s12958-023-01148-9. PMID: 37865766; PMCID: PMC10589983.
54. Finelli R, Leisegang K, Tumallapalli S, Henkel R, Agarwal A. The validity and reliability of computer-aided semen analyzers in performing semen analysis: a systematic review. Transl Androl Urol. 2021;10(7):3069–79. https://doi.org/10.21037/tau-21-276. PMID: 34430409; PMCID: PMC8350227.
55. McCallum C, Riordon J, Wang Y, Kong T, You JB, Sanner S, Lagunov A, Hannam TG, Jarvi K, Sinton D. Deep learning-based selection of human sperm with high DNA integrity. Commun Biol. 2019;2:250. https://doi.org/10.1038/s42003-019-0491-6. PMID: 31286067; PMCID: PMC6610103.
56. Iqbal I, Mustafa G, Ma J. Deep learning-based morphological classification of human sperm heads. Diagnostics (Basel). 2020;10(5):325. https://doi.org/10.3390/diagnostics10050325. PMID: 32443809; PMCID: PMC7277990.
57. Mendizabal-Ruiz G, Chavez-Badiola A, Aguilar Figueroa I, Martinez Nuño V, Flores-Saiffe Farias A, Valencia-Murilloa R, Drakeley A, Garcia-Sandoval JP, Cohen J. Computer

software (SiD) assisted real-time single sperm selection associated with fertilization and blastocyst formation. Reprod Biomed Online. 2022;45(4):703–11. https://doi.org/10.1016/j.rbmo.2022.03.036. PMID: 35989168.
58. Alpha Scientists in Reproductive Medicine and ESHRE Special Interest Group of Embryology. The Istanbul consensus workshop on embryo assessment: proceedings of an expert meeting. Hum Reprod. 2011;26(6):1270–83. 10.1093/humrep/der037
59. ESHRE Special Interest Group of Embryology and Alpha Scientists in Reproductive Medicine. Vienna consensus: report of an expert meeting on the development of art laboratory performance indicators. Hum Reprod Open. 2017;2017(2):hox011. https://doi.org/10.1093/hropen/hox011.
60. Athayde Wirka K, Chen AA, Conaghan J, Ivani K, Gvakharia M, Behr B, Suraj V, Tan L, Shen S. Atypical embryo phenotypes identified by time-lapse microscopy: high prevalence and association with embryo development. Fertil Steril. 2014;101(6):1637–48.e1–5. https://doi.org/10.1016/j.fertnstert.2014.02.050. PMID: 24726214.
61. Liu Y, Chapple V, Roberts P, Matson P. Prevalence, consequence, and significance of reverse cleavage by human embryos viewed with the use of the embryoscope time-lapse video system. Fertil Steril. 2014;102(5):1295–1300.e2. https://doi.org/10.1016/j.fertnstert.2014.07.1235. PMID: 25225070.
62. Sciorio R, Meseguer M. Focus on time-lapse analysis: blastocyst collapse and morphometric assessment as new features of embryo viability. Reprod Biomed Online. 2021;43(5):821–32. https://doi.org/10.1016/j.rbmo.2021.08.008. PMID: 34593324
63. Armstrong S, Bhide P, Jordan V, Pacey A, Marjoribanks J, Farquhar C. Time-lapse systems for embryo incubation and assessment in assisted reproduction. Cochrane Database Syst Rev. 2019;5(5):CD011320. https://doi.org/10.1002/14651858.CD011320.pub4. PMID: 31140578; PMCID: PMC6539473.
64. Berntsen J, Rimestad J, Lassen JT, Tran D, Kragh MF. Robust and generalizable embryo selection based on artificial intelligence and time-lapse image sequences. PLoS One. 2022;17(2):e0262661. https://doi.org/10.1371/journal.pone.0262661. PMID: 35108306; PMCID: PMC8809568.
65. Diakiw SM, Hall JMM, VerMilyea MD, Amin J, Aizpurua J, Giardini L, Briones YG, Lim AYX, Dakka MA, Nguyen TV, Perugini D, Perugini M. Development of an artificial intelligence model for predicting the likelihood of human embryo euploidy based on blastocyst images from multiple imaging systems during IVF. Hum Reprod. 2022;37(8):1746–59. https://doi.org/10.1093/humrep/deac131. PMID: 35674312; PMCID: PMC9340116.
66. VerMilyea M, Hall JMM, Diakiw SM, Johnston A, Nguyen T, Perugini D, Miller A, Picou A, Murphy AP, Perugini M. Development of an artificial intelligence-based assessment model for prediction of embryo viability using static images captured by optical light microscopy during IVF. Hum Reprod. 2020;35(4):770–84. https://doi.org/10.1093/humrep/deaa013. PMID: 32240301; PMCID: PMC7192535.
67. Khosravi P, Kazemi E, Zhan Q, et al. Deep learning enables robust assessment and selection of human blastocysts after in vitro fertilization. NPJ Digit Med. 2019;2:21. https://doi.org/10.1038/s41746-019-0096-y.
68. Huang B, Tan W, Li Z, et al. An artificial intelligence model (euploid prediction algorithm) can predict embryo ploidy status based on time-lapse data. Reprod Biol Endocrinol. 2021;19(1):185. https://doi.org/10.1186/s12958-021-00864-4.
69. Jiang VS, Bormann CL. Noninvasive genetic screening: current advances in artificial intelligence for embryo ploidy prediction. Fertil Steril. 2023;120(2):228–34. https://doi.org/10.1016/j.fertnstert.2023.06.025. PMID: 37394089.
70. Barnes J, Brendel M, Gao VR, Rajendran S, Kim J, Li Q, Malmsten JE, Sierra JT, Zisimopoulos P, Sigaras A, Khosravi P, Meseguer M, Zhan Q, Rosenwaks Z, Elemento O, Zaninovic N, Hajirasouliha I. A non-invasive artificial intelligence approach for the prediction of human blastocyst ploidy: a retrospective model development and validation study. Lancet Digit Health. 2023;5(1):e28–40. https://doi.org/10.1016/S2589-7500(22)00213-826.

71. Fragouli E, Munne S, Wells D. The cytogenetic constitution of human blastocysts: insights from comprehensive chromosome screening strategies. Hum Reprod Update. 2019;25(1):15–33. https://doi.org/10.1093/humupd/dmy036. PMID: 30395265
72. Munné S, Kaplan B, Frattarelli JL, Child T, Nakhuda G, Shamma FN, Silverberg K, Kalista T, Handyside AH, Katz-Jaffe M, Wells D, Gordon T, Stock-Myer S, Willman S, STAR Study Group. Preimplantation genetic testing for aneuploidy versus morphology as selection criteria for single frozen-thawed embryo transfer in good-prognosis patients: a multicenter randomized clinical trial. Fertil Steril. 2019;112(6):1071–1079.e7. https://doi.org/10.1016/j.fertnstert.2019.07.1346. PMID: 31551155.
73. Bhatt SJ, Marchetto NM, Roy J, Morelli SS, McGovern PG. Pregnancy outcomes following in vitro fertilization frozen embryo transfer (IVF-FET) with or without preimplantation genetic testing for aneuploidy (PGT-A) in women with recurrent pregnancy loss (RPL): a SART-CORS study. Hum Reprod. 2021;36(8):2339–44. https://doi.org/10.1093/humrep/deab117. PMID: 34027546.
74. Vera-Rodriguez M, Rubio C. Assessing the true incidence of mosaicism in preimplantation embryos. Fertil Steril. 2017;107(5):1107–12. https://doi.org/10.1016/j.fertnstert.2017.03.019. PMID: 28433370
75. ESHRE Add-ons Working Group, Lundin K, Bentzen JG, Bozdag G, Ebner T, Harper J, Le Clef N, Moffett A, Norcross S, Polyzos NP, Rautakallio-Hokkanen S, Sfontouris I, Sermon K, Vermeulen N, Pinborg A. Good practice recommendations on add-ons in reproductive medicine†. HumReprod. 2023;38(11):2062–104. https://doi.org/10.1093/humrep/dead184. PMID: 37747409; PMCID: PMC10628516.
76. Huang L, Bogale B, Tang Y, Lu S, Xie XS, Racowsky C. Noninvasive preimplantation genetic testing for aneuploidy in spent medium may be more reliable than trophectoderm biopsy. Proc Natl Acad Sci USA. 2019;116(28):14105–12. https://doi.org/10.1073/pnas.1907472116. PMID: 31235575; PMCID: PMC6628824.
77. Orvieto R, Shimon C, Rienstein S, Jonish-Grossman A, Shani H, Aizer A. Do human embryos have the ability of self-correction? Reprod Biol Endocrinol. 2020;18(1):98. https://doi.org/10.1186/s12958-020-00650-8. PMID: 33023576; PMCID: PMC7539487.
78. Uyar A, Seli E. Metabolomic assessment of embryo viability. Semin Reprod Med. 2014;32(2):141–52. https://doi.org/10.1055/s-0033-1363556. PMID: 24515909; PMCID: PMC4109799.
79. Venturas M, Shah JS, Yang X, Sanchez TH, Conway W, Sakkas D, Needleman DJ. Metabolic state of human blastocysts measured by fluorescence lifetime imaging microscopy. Hum Reprod. 2022;37(3):411–27. https://doi.org/10.1093/humrep/deab283. PMID: 34999823
80. Siristatidis C, Dafopoulos K, Papapanou M, Stavros S, Pouliakis A, Eleftheriades A, Sidiropoulou T, Vlahos N. Why has metabolomics so far not managed to efficiently contribute to the improvement of assisted reproduction outcomes? The answer through a review of the best available current evidence. Diagnostics (Basel). 2021;11(9):1602. https://doi.org/10.3390/diagnostics11091602. PMID: 34573944; PMCID: PMC8469471.
81. Anagnostopoulou C, Maldonado Rosas I, Singh N, Gugnani N, Chockalingham A, Singh K, Desai D, Darbandi M, Manoharan M, Darbandi S, Leonardi Diaz SI, Gupta S, Henkel R, Sallam HN, Boitrelle F, Wirka KA, Agarwal A. Oocyte quality and embryo selection strategies: a review for the embryologists, by the embryologists. Panminerva Med. 2022;64(2):171–84. https://doi.org/10.23736/S0031-0808.22.04680-8. PMID: 35179016.
82. O'Donovan C, Twomey E, Alderman J, Moore T, Papkovsky D. Development of a respirometric biochip for embryo assessment. Lab Chip. 2006;6(11):1438–44. https://doi.org/10.1039/b607622j. PMID: 17066167.
83. Kurosawa H, Utsunomiya H, Shiga N, Takahashi A, Ihara M, Ishibashi M, Nishimoto M, Watanabe Z, Abe H, Kumagai J, Terada Y, Igarashi H, Takahashi T, Fukui A, Suganuma R, Tachibana M, Yaegashi N. Development of a new clinically applicable device for embryo evaluation which measures embryo oxygen consumption. Hum Reprod. 2016;31(10):2321–30. https://doi.org/10.1093/humrep/dew187. PMID: 27609982.

84. Eravuchira PJ, Mirsky SK, Barnea I, Levi M, Balberg M, Shaked NT. Individual sperm selection by microfluidics integrated with interferometric phase microscopy. Methods. 2018;136:152–9. https://doi.org/10.1016/j.ymeth.2017.09.009. PMID: 28958952.
85. Cimadomo D, Rienzi L, Conforti A, Forman E, Canosa S, Innocenti F, Poli M, Hynes J, Gemmell L, Vaiarelli A, Alviggi C, Ubaldi FM, Capalbo A. Opening the black box: why do euploid blastocysts fail to implant? A systematic review and meta-analysis. Hum Reprod Update. 2023;29(5):570–633. https://doi.org/10.1093/humupd/dmad010. PMID: 37192834.

Part II
Male Sexual Dysfunction

Chapter 16
Hormonal Therapy for Late Male Hypogonadism: Controversies Revisited and Current Management Strategies

Manaf Al Hashimi, Christopher Chee Kong Ho, and Ates Kadıoglu

Hypogonadism Definition, Classifications, and Causes

Male hypogonadism is a condition characterized by inadequate testosterone production by the testes, leading to a range of physical and psychological symptoms. It can be categorized into three types: primary, secondary (central), or combined. Some classifications refer to primary and secondary hypogonadism as organic, while the combined type is termed functional [1].

Primary hypogonadism occurs when the testes themselves are defective and unable to produce sufficient testosterone, even though they receive standard signals from the pituitary gland. This condition leads to increased levels of gonadotropins—luteinizing hormone (LH) and Follicle Stimulating Hormone (FSH)—as the body tries to stimulate the testes to produce more testosterone. It can be triggered by various factors such as genetic conditions (e.g., Klinefelter syndrome), testicular trauma, infections, chemotherapy, or radiation therapy [2]. Secondary hypogonadism or central hypogonadism involves a dysfunction in the hypothalamus or pituitary gland, leading to reduced production of gonadotropins hormone (LH) and eventual inadequate testosterone production. It can be caused by hypothalamic or pituitary tumors, head trauma, certain medications, or systemic diseases affecting the pituitary-hypothalamic axis [3].

While the best representation of the collective classification (encompassing primary and secondary causes) is commonly referred to as LOH, it is also

M. Al Hashimi (✉)
Department of Urology, Burjeel Hospital-Abu Dhabi, Abu Dhabi, UAE

C. C. K. Ho
Department of Surgery, School of Medicine, Taylor's University, Subang Jaya, Selangor, Malaysia

A. Kadıoglu
Section of Andrology, Department of Urology, Istanbul School of Medicine, Istanbul, Turkey

E. Chung et al. (eds.), *Advances in Andrology*,
https://doi.org/10.1007/978-3-032-29112-7_16

sometimes termed age-related hypogonadism, Partial Androgen Deficiency in Aging Males (PADAM), Androgen Deficiency in the Aging Male (ADAM), or Testosterone Deficiency Syndrome. This condition primarily stems from various age-related changes that lead to decreased testosterone levels, such as reduced frequency and amplitude of LH pulses and diminished Leydig cell activity associated with atherosclerotic and degenerative aging processes. Additionally, aging can lead to a decline in testosterone activity due to elevated levels of sex hormone-binding globulin (SHBG), resulting in less free testosterone and increased aromatase activity, which converts testosterone to estradiol [4]. LOH is a clinical and biochemical state with advancing age, characterized by particular symptoms and a low serum testosterone level. LOH is the main focus of this study.

Prevalence and Demographics of LOH

There is a positive correlation between aging and hypogonadism prevalence, and numerous studies have supported this relationship, often correlated with decreases in testosterone levels or what is named testosterone deficiency (TD).

The Baltimore Aging Longitudinal Study found that around 10% of men aged 50–59 had low serum total testosterone concentrations, while this figure rose to 20% for men aged 60–69, and significantly increased to 70% for men aged 70–80 years old [5].

As individuals age, there's a gradual decline in total testosterone levels in the bloodstream, estimated to decrease by roughly 1–2% per year starting from around the third decade of life. This decline corresponds to an annual decrease of about 3.2–3.5 ng/dL (0.110–0.121 nmol/L). By the age of 75, men typically undergo a reduction of approximately 30% in their circulating testosterone levels compared to when they were 25 years old. Research indicates that TD in men over 60 is between 20% and 30%, with this occurrence progressively rising with age [6].

LOH is defined by EMAS study of over 3000 men ages 40–79 years, which demonstrated an overall prevalence of 2.1% when using a combination of 3 sexual symptoms (erectile dysfunction and decreased frequency of morning erections and sexual thoughts) and a low total testosterone concentration of less than 11 nmol/L [7]. There are many other studies that showed different prevalence rates based on their specific definition of TD and description of populations, as in Table 16.1.

Table 16.1 Prevalence of testosterone deficiency

Study	No. of patients	Definition of TD	Prevalence of TD
Harman et al., 2000 Baltimore longitudinal aging study (BLAS) [5]	890	TT < 325 ng/dl	50–59 years: 12% 60–69 years: 19% 70–79 years: 28% >80 years: 49%
Wu et al., 2010 European male aging study (EMAS) [7]	3219	TT < 317 ng/dl + 3 sexual symptoms	2.1% of study population
Araujo et al., 2004 Massachusetts male aging study (MMAS) [8]	1709 1156	TT < 200 ng/dl + 3 or more related symptoms	T1 40–49 years: 4.1% 50–59 years: 4.5% 60–70 years: 9.4% T2 40–49 years: 7.1% 50–59 years: 11.5% 60–70 years: 22.8%

Part-I: Controversies on Different LOH Perspectives

Clinical Evaluation of LOH

Controversies About the Significant Symptoms of LOH

The diagnosis of LOH requires meeting two essential criteria: displaying signs and symptoms of hypogonadism alongside biochemical proof of consistently low morning serum total testosterone levels on two occasions. However, a diverse array of symptoms, some of which may be mild and nonspecific, can pose challenges to diagnosis [9], as in Table 16.2. The most precise symptoms often related to TD are sexual, such as diminished libido, fewer spontaneous erections, and erectile dysfunction (ED). Conversely, the majority of other symptoms are nonspecific symptoms that encompass psychological and physical manifestations [9], as in Table 16.2.

Moreover, the variable manifestation of low testosterone symptoms may correspond to distinct testosterone levels, with certain symptoms become apparent at particular testosterone thresholds while others emerge at different levels [10], as illustrated in Fig. 16.1.

Table 16.2 Specific and nonspecific symptoms of LOH

	Specific symptoms	Non-specific symptoms
Sexual	Loss of libido Less morning erection Erectile dysfunction	Delayed ejaculation Reduced frequency of sex intercourse
Physical	Less vigorous activity Difficult walking long distances	Hot flushes Decreased energy Decreased physical capability
Psychological	Bad mood Less motivation Tiredness and weakness	Reduced concentration, memory, and cognitive function Sleep disturbances

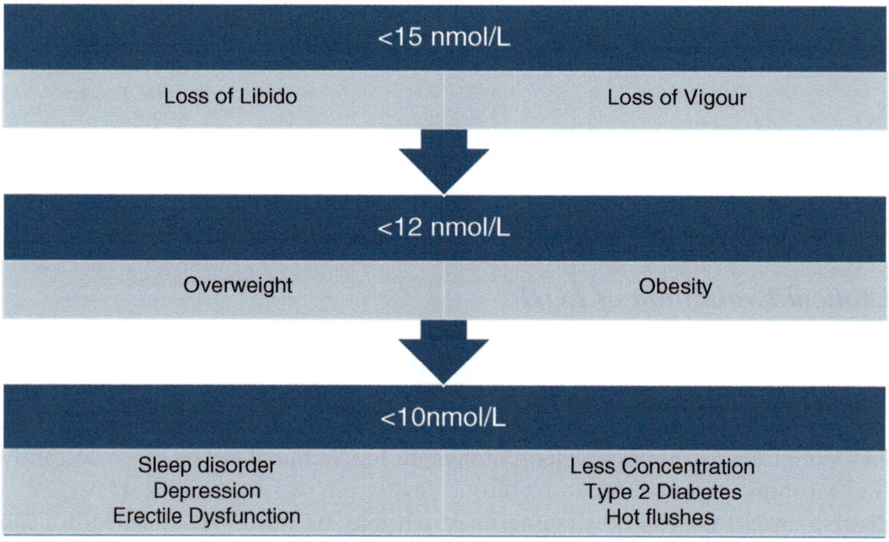

Fig. 16.1 Symptoms-specific testosterone thresholds in men

Table 16.3 Factors associated with an increased prevalence of TD

Andrological and endocrinological	Pharmacologic	Cardiovascular diseases	Other chronic diseases
Obesity Metabolic syndrome Type 2 diabetes Delayed puberty Cryptorchidism Pituitary disease Infertility Varicocele Testicular cancer plus associated therapy	Oral glucocorticoid treatment Regular opioid use Antipsychotic medications Androgen deprivation therapy Finasteride/dutasteride Methadone maintenance therapy Antiretroviral therapy Chemotherapy and radiation Anticonvulsant therapy Roaccutane therapy for acne	Hypertension Coronary artery disease Cerebrovascular disease Chronic heart failure Atrial fibrillation	Chronic obstructive pulmonary disease Obstructive sleep apnea End-stage renal disease Cirrhosis Osteoporosis Rheumatoid arthritis HIV infection Cancers Anemia Osteoporosis COVID19 infection

Although LOH is well correlated with aging, variabilities are excited between its incidence among individuals and the onset of symptoms. Some risk factors make individuals more likely to develop manifestations of LOH and should be considered during the clinical history [9], as in Table 16.3.

Controversies About the Significance of Diagnostic Questionnaires in LOH

Several structured questionnaires have been used for the diagnosis and screening of LOH and can help support the biochemical evidence of low testosterone, but generally, they are considered to have low specificity and supportive value rather than standards for the diagnosis. However, they can still offer a quantitative baseline evaluation of symptoms and gauge the clinical response to treatment. They can be helpful in showcasing symptom changes with TRT, particularly in cases where multiple physicians are managing a patient's care [11].

Signs of LOH

The general examination is considered valuable in detecting the physical associated signs of LOH, like obesity, especially central obesity, through the determination of body mass index (BMI) and the measurement of waist circumference. During a physical examination, findings that may suggest TD include pallor (anemia), diminished body hair, decreased size of the testicles, and the presence of gynecomastia; however, these signs are not consistently observed. In addition, prostate examination is mandatory before starting TRT to evaluate prostate size and exclude localized prostate lesions [9, 12].

Diagnostic Laboratory Tests

Testosterone Level Variations and Method Measurement

Testosterone levels fluctuate due to various factors such as age progression, cultural and geographical influences, lifestyle decisions (such as physical activity and obesity), and concurrent health conditions. These levels also demonstrate a daily rhythm and may change within individuals over time. Hence, it is recommended that testosterone levels be assessed in the morning (between 7 and 11 am) and a follow-up confirmatory test be conducted if the initial result indicates low levels [13].

Immunoassays and mass spectrometry (MS) are the predominant techniques for testosterone testing. While immunoassays are favored for their simplicity, ease of use, and widespread clinical adoption, MS is gaining popularity due to its high throughput, minimal sample preparation needs, and superior sensitivity and specificity across a range of testosterone concentrations [14, 15].

Testosterone Cutoff Values in LOH

Despite numerous studies exploring LOH, there remain several contentious issues, particularly regarding fundamental diagnostic aspects such as the testosterone cutoff value. Various guidelines, such as those from the American Urology Association (AUA) and the European Association of Urology (EAU), propose different values, with the AUA suggesting 10.4 nmol/L and the EUA recommending 12 nmol/L [16], as shown in Table 16.4.

Table 16.4 Cutoff value of TT and FT according to different societies

Society	Total testosterone nmol/L	Total testosterone ng/dl
American Urological Society, 2018	10.4	300
British Society for Sexual Medicine, 2017	12.0	346
Endocrine Society, 2018	9.2	265
Endocrine Society of Australia, 2016	6.6	190
European academy of andrology, 2020	12.0	346
European Association of Urology, 2024	12.0	346

Establishing a definitive biochemical threshold for diagnosing TD poses challenges due to various factors: limitations in measurement precision, variability in laboratory and immunoassay techniques, absence of age-specific reference norms, uncertainty regarding individual baseline testosterone levels, and differences in target organ receptor responsiveness to testosterone levels. Consequently, different societies may adopt distinct cutoff values based on diverse research findings. Collaborative efforts within international forums may facilitate the development of a consensus on this matter [17].

Free Testosterone (FT) and Sex Hormone Binding Globulin (SHBG)

The measurement of FT is of significant importance across various clinical scenarios, particularly when coupled with abnormal levels of SHBG. Approximately 40% of total testosterone (TT) is bound to SHBG, and the levels of this protein can be influenced by several conditions. Thus, it becomes essential to assess FT levels in patients presenting with conditions associated with either decreased concentrations of serum SHBG (such as obesity, diabetes, glucocorticoid usage, nephrotic syndrome, hypothyroidism, and acromegaly) or increased concentrations of serum SHBG (including aging, HIV disease, cirrhosis, hepatitis, and hyperthyroidism), as well as in those with borderline TT levels [3, 9, 18, 19].

FT can be assessed directly using equilibrium dialysis, which is the gold standard technique. It can also be measured indirectly through various established calculations and equations like the widely used (Vermeulen formula) and accessible through the International Society of sexual medicine (ISSM) website https://www.issam.ch/freetesto.htm [20].

Pituitary Hormones in LOH

Measurement of serum luteinizing hormone (LH) and follicle-stimulating hormone (FSH) levels are crucial to distinguish between primary (testicular) and secondary (pituitary-hypothalamic) hypogonadism when they are higher and lower than normal, respectively. While in LOH, they are usually normal. Evaluation of prolactin levels is vital in cases of low testosterone, especially with very low T (< 5.2 nmol/L) and low or low/normal LH, as hyperprolactinemia is frequently associated with hypogonadism [3, 9, 12].

Estradiol (E2)

The assessment of E2 and testosterone/estradiol ratio (T/E) is vital in obese men with LOH. This is because obesity stands out as perhaps the most prevalent factor leading to TD in developed regions, with more than half of men having a body mass index (BMI) exceeding 30 experiencing TD. E2 plays an important role also in the relationship between hypogonadism and obesity since the increased production of Estradiol within the fat tissue (due to an increase in aromatase activity) contributes to inhibiting LH secretion from the pituitary and reduces testosterone secretion from the testes. Additionally, the T/E2 ratio measurement during TRT is essential as an indicator of testosterone improvement and to avoid excessive levels and eventual conversion to E2 [6, 21].

Hemoglobin/Hematocrit (Hct) in LOH

Before initiating testosterone therapy, it is imperative to conduct a baseline assessment of Hct levels for all patients. If the Hct level exceeds 50%, TRT administration should be postponed until further investigation of the underlying cause. During TRT, if the Hct level exceeds 54%, appropriate measures such as dose adjustment or temporary cessation of treatment should be considered. While the comparative incidence of polycythemia between different testosterone modalities remains uncertain, research suggests that injectable testosterone is associated with the most pronounced elevations in hemoglobin/Hct levels due to treatment. Also, it is found that TRT individuals have a higher frequency of blood donation compared to the standard group [21, 22].

The Protocols for LOH Patient's Evaluation

Many societies recommended protocols to guide the practitioners in the best clinical practice of evaluating men with TD and LOH as the guidelines of EAU in Fig. 16.2 [9].

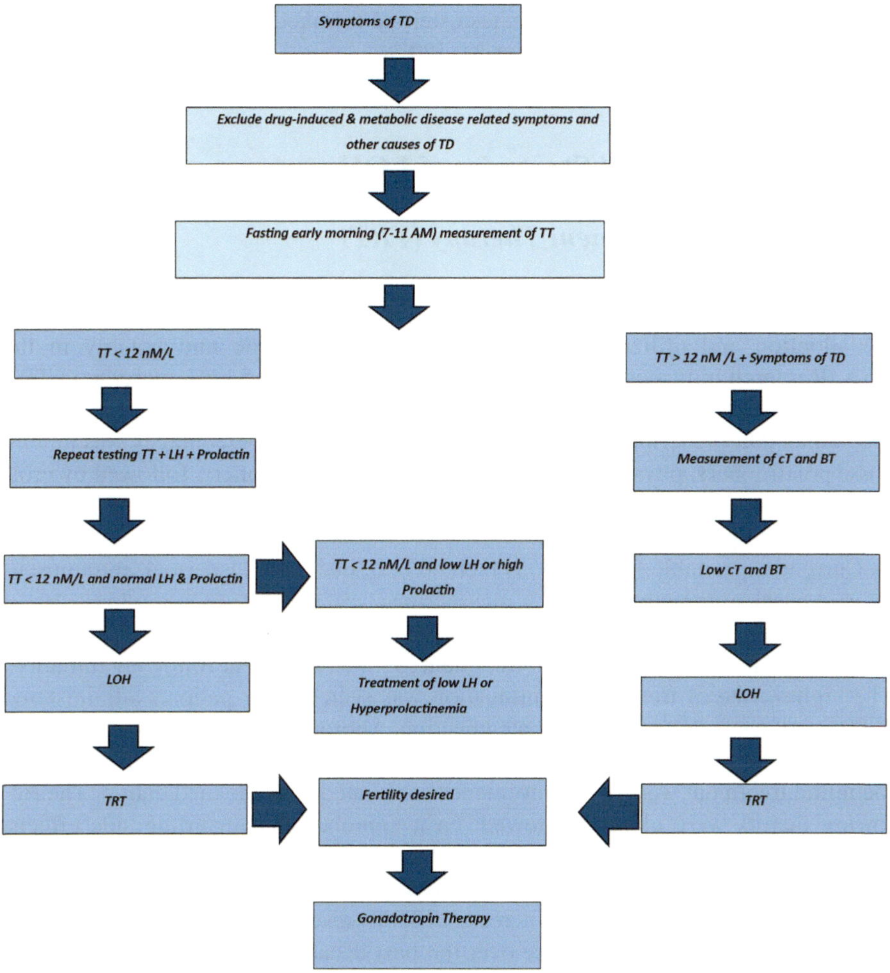

Fig. 16.2 Diagnostic evaluation of late-onset hypogonadism [9]. *TD* Testosterone deficiency, *TT* Total testosterone, *LH* Luteinizing hormone, *cT* Calculated Testosterone, *BT* Bioavailable Testosterone, *LOH* Late-onset hypogonadism

LOH and Associated Comorbidities

Many men with TD are liable to be affected by significant chronic morbidities, and it is essential to be evaluated along with the work-up of LOH patients. For men aged 45 years and older, the odds ratios reported for TD in conjunction with comorbid conditions were: obesity 2.38, diabetes 2.09, hypertension 1.84, dyslipidemia 1.47, chronic obstructive pulmonary disease (COPD) 1.40, and LUTS/BPH 1.20. Additionally, a notable deficiency in testosterone is linked to a heightened susceptibility to chronic anemia and osteoporosis [20].

Part-II: Management Strategies of LOH

Testosterone Replacement Therapy (TRT)

As related societies guidelines have evolved, there has been a significant uptick in the adoption and utilization of TRT, observed worldwide and notably in the USA. Research indicates a 28.6% rise in prescribers and a 54.6% increase in TRT claims from 2016 to 2019 [23]. The same study showed that there are nine main specialties that prescribe TRT, and the largest increase in percentages was among nurse practitioners, physician assistants, and family practitioners, followed by urologists and endocrinologists. These findings indicated the widespread of both prescriptions and prescribers of TRT.

Currently, available formulations include oral, buccal, transdermal, intramuscular, and nasal administration.

Most of the patients showed good compliance with TRT, and it was noted that 75.9% of patients maintained their treatment regimen for 1 year following initiation. The highest rate of treatment continuation was seen among patients administered 1000 mg of testosterone undecanoate injection. Approximately 65% of patients who ceased treatment later resumed it. The most prevalent cause cited for discontinuing the initial treatment was the inconvenience associated with the medication. The following factors were closely followed: cost, apprehension regarding side effects, lack of effectiveness, and the lack of symptoms improvement [24].

Diverse global variances exist in the prescription practices of TRT. Notably, the USA demonstrates a substantial increase in TRT prescriptions compared to the rest of the world, with a threefold rise over the past decade, particularly among eugonadal men. The majority of physicians administering TRT prioritize clinical symptomatology of TD over laboratory values, with as many as a quarter of their patients lacking serum testosterone levels [25] (Table 16.5).

Between 2000 and 2011, in a study encompassing 41 countries, the sales of testosterone worldwide saw a 12-fold increase, rising from $150 million to $1.8 billion. Driving this growth were Canada and the USA, the top two contributing countries [24]. Behind this increase are several new Direct-to-consumer online

Table 16.5 Different testosterone formulations used for the treatment of LOH

Formulation	Route	Examples/ brand names	Dosing frequency	Advantages	Limitations/side effects
Injectable—Short acting	Intramuscular (IM)	Testosterone propionate	Every 2–3 days	Rapid onset	Painful injections, frequent dosing, fluctuating levels
Injectable—Intermediate acting	IM	Testosterone enanthate (Delatestryl), testosterone cypionate (Depo-testosterone)	Every 1–2 weeks	Widely available, effective	Peaks and troughs, erythrocytosis, mood swings
Injectable—Long acting	IM (deep gluteal)	Testosterone undecanoate (Aveed, Nebido)	Every 10–14 weeks	Stable levels, fewer injections	Requires clinic administration, risk of POME*
Transdermal gel	Skin (shoulders, arms)	AndroGel, Testim, Fortesta	Daily	Steady levels, easy to apply	Risk of skin-to-skin transfer, skin irritation
Transdermal patch	Skin	Androderm	Daily	Mimics diurnal rhythm	Skin rash, adhesion problems
Buccal tablet	Oral mucosa	Striant	Twice daily	Avoids first-pass metabolism	Gum irritation, taste disturbance
Oral testosterone	Oral	Testosterone undecanoate (Jatenzo, Andriol)	Twice daily with fat	Convenient, no injection	Variable absorption, liver effects (older formulations)
Nasal gel	Intranasal	Natesto	2–3x daily	Rapid absorption, minimal skin transfer	Frequent dosing, nasal irritation
Subcutaneous pellets	Subdermal implant	Testopel	Every 3–6 months	Long duration, steady levels	Minor procedure required, extrusion risk

platforms that have surfaced, with some failing to meet the necessary clinical standards. A study showed that the initial assessment was carried out by a nurse practitioner, physician assistant, or other non-medically licensed personnel. Despite the individual reporting normal levels of total and free testosterone and expressing a desire for fertility, six out of seven platforms recommended testosterone therapy! Among these platforms, only one inquired about any recent cardiovascular events or the individual's future fertility intentions [26].

The Controversies on the Best-Used TRT Preparations

There Are Many Types of testosterone Preparation Available in the Market

Oral testosterone is known to undergo extensive first-pass metabolism; therefore supra-physiological doses are required to allow for the detection of measurable levels in the serum [27]. Modification of testosterone by alkylation at 17a yielded 17a methyl testosterone, which can bypass first-pass metabolism. Unfortunately, it causes significant liver toxicity and lowering of HDL cholesterol, and its use is prohibited [28]. Another attempt to bypass first-pass metabolism by esterification of carbon 17b produces testosterone undecanoate (TU). However, this formulation has low bioavailability and some adverse effects on the gastrointestinal tract [28].

Nevertheless, recent developments indicate a shift. A recent assessment conducted by Miller et al. revealed that oral testosterone undecanoate exhibited favorable tolerance among hypogonadal patients. This led to enhanced testosterone levels, increased height velocity, and alleviated sexual symptoms, all without notable hepatotoxicity, prostate enlargement, or exacerbation of hypertension [29]. This aligns with another study conducted by Ahmad et al., which concluded that oral administration offers similar benefits to other treatment methods for male hypogonadism. With further enhancements, oral administration has the potential to surpass injectables and transdermal testosterone to become the preferred treatment option [30].

Subdermal testosterone pellet was designed for consistent and prolonged release [31]. However, administration requires skin incision and local anesthesia. The dosing can be tailored according to age, diagnosis, patient's response, and adverse effects. The most common adverse event (10%) is pellet extrusion. Others are infection, bleeding, and fibrosis at the site of insertion. General dosing recommendations are 150 to 450 mg implanted at the hip area or other fatty area at 3–6-month intervals [32]. Potential advantages of pellet usage include the infrequency of dosing, guaranteed compliance, and lack of transference. Nevertheless, the administration process is invasive, necessitating a skin incision and local anesthesia. Moreover, there are apprehensions regarding pellet removal, particularly for patients encountering side effects related to androgen [33].

A transdermal patch like Androderm® is a transdermal patch containing testosterone, available in doses of 2 mg/day and 4 mg/day. The patch is applied nightly on clean, dry, unbroken skin on the back, abdomen, upper arms, or thighs only. For dosage adjustment, measure total serum testosterone levels in the early morning at least 2 weeks after starting therapy, following the previous evening's patch application. The target range for serum testosterone is between 400 and 930 ng/dL [34, 35].

Testosterone gel's numerous topical formulations are accessible, sharing similarities in indications, adverse effects, and contraindications. However, significant differences exist in dose adjustments and application sites, rendering them non-interchangeable. There is concern for testosterone gel or liquid being transferred to females and children who come into contact with a patient's skin after use. Patients should be reminded to wash their hands after application and to avoid skin contact with others. Recommended sites of application for these agents are areas that will be covered by clothing to minimize transfer. The potential advantages of testosterone transdermal gels and liquids include ease of application, less skin irritation than patches, and more consistent serum testosterone levels than other formulations, such as IM testosterone. The most common side effects are acne, erythema, and pruritus (7%), gynecomastia (4%). Discontinuation rates due to side effects are below 1%. There is no change in E2 and DHT levels during its use [36–38].

Nasal testosterone utilizes a metered dose pump applicator, allowing patients to self-administer into the nostrils. Each pump delivers 5.5 mg of testosterone, with the recommended dose of two pumps (one actuation per nostril) three times a day for a total daily dose of 33 mg. Doses should be separated by 6–8 h. Absorption occurs through the nasal mucosa, avoiding first-pass metabolism, and the C_{max} is reached within 40 min of administration [39].

In an open-label phase III trial assessing nasal testosterone usage in 306 hypogonadal men (testosterone <300 ng/dL) for 90 days, 90% achieved serum testosterone concentrations within the normal physiological range with a C_{avg} of 421 ng/dL, while 10% remained subtherapeutic. Treatment was well tolerated, with a low discontinuation rate of 3.7%. Adverse effects occurring in more than 3% of subjects included increased prostate-specific antigen (PSA), headache, rhinorrhea, nosebleed, nasal discomfort, upper respiratory tract infection, sinusitis, bronchitis, and nasal scab [40]. Testosterone nasal gel is another non-invasive alternative with simple administration, low total daily dose, and no concern for secondary transfer. Additionally, hypogonadal men undergoing long-acting forms of TRT who wish to resume spermatogenesis may opt to switch from their current long-acting TRT regimen to nasal testosterone, as it is associated with no negative impact on spermatogenesis and fertility, as stated in a recent study [41], although more studies with larger cohorts are needed to confirm this point.

Intramuscular (IM) Testosterone To overcome the short half-life of testosterone, current formulations have a prolonged duration of action as they are synthesized through esterification of the 17β carbon of natural testosterone, which increases the solubility of testosterone in oil, allowing slower release once injected into the muscle [38]. The different IM preparations are testosterone cypionate (TC), testosterone esters (TE), and testosterone undecanoate (TU). TU has a longer duration of action due to its longest carbon side chain [42, 43]. The Endocrine Society Clinical Practice Guidelines for testosterone therapy recommend measurements of serum testosterone levels 1 week after receiving a dose of TC or TE, targeting a therapeutic level of 400 to 700 ng/dL, whereas for TU, levels should be measured just before subsequent injections [44].

TC and other esters, due to their shorter lifespan, are linked to numerous adverse side effects. Research conducted on testosterone cypionate revealed significant variations in serum testosterone levels throughout 2 weeks. These fluctuations can produce mood swings or changes in libido. Other common side effects of TC use are local inflammation and pain at the site of injection. TC use is contraindicated in anyone with a known allergy to soy [45].

TE's associated adverse effects are similar to that of TC. It is dosed at 100 mg once weekly or 200 mg every 2 weeks, maintaining serum testosterone within the therapeutic range by the end of the dosing regimen. Due to TC and TE having different oil vehicles, they are not therapeutically equivalent [46, 47].

TU's open-label study showed that it does not demonstrate supratherapeutic peaks and trough levels are seen later after each injection, which is advantageous compared to TE and TC [48].

An adverse event known as pulmonary oil micro embolism (POME) can occur during or after any injection throughout therapy and includes symptoms such as the urge to cough, shortness of breath, throat tightening, chest pain, dizziness, and syncope. Other adverse effects reported are increased PSA, acne, and pain during injection [49].

What Is the Best Protocol for TRT Use?

Short-Acting vs Long-Acting

Short-acting testosterone closely imitates the physiological function as it maintains body testosterone near normal. Additionally, its method of delivery, such as nasal formulation, does not seem to affect 17-hydroxyprogesterone in the blood.

Diaz et al. (2002) concluded that short-acting testosterone is more beneficial for men who want to preserve their fertility [50]. Kavoussi et al. (2022) also stated that many men can maintain reproductive potential when they begin therapy with the latest short-acting intranasal androgen gel [42]. As a further matter, it has been shown that most men who switch from long-acting TRT to intranasal testosterone can maintain their testosterone production, maintain reduced E2 levels, and have increased libido.

Non-testosterone Preparations for Hypogonadism

Selective Estrogen Receptor Modulators (SERMs)

SERMs can elevate both testosterone and LH production by blocking the negative feedback of Estradiol (E2) on the hypothalamus. Examples of SERMs are Clomiphene Citrate (CC) and Tamoxifen. CC can effectively increase testosterone to a eugonadal level. CC can be prescribed at 25 mg alternate day to 50 mg daily based on testosterone response. A study by Moskovic et al. showed an elevation of testosterone level to a mean of 582 ± 227 ng/dL ($P < 0.001$), as well as distinctive improvements in ADAM questionnaire response ($P = 0.01$) and mean BMI ($P < 0.05$) [51]. Similarly, Taylor and Levine published that compared to testosterone gel therapy, CC treatment resulted in substantial improvements in testosterone levels at a fraction of the cost with significant improvements in ADAM questionnaire scores. In addition to that, no adverse effect on CC was reported; therefore, the patient compliance rate was high [52]. Ramasamy et al. have also demonstrated that quantitative ADAM scores were equivalent among patients treated with CC in comparison to those treated with testosterone gels or injections, with improvements in testosterone levels while on CC treatment to physiologic levels [53]. However, CC usage is still off-label due to the lack of long-term data regarding safety and efficacy.

Tamoxifen is a less desirable option for SERM. Other than its known effect to increase testosterone and gonadotrophin levels, it can also preserve spermatogenesis. Unfortunately, it is associated with greater side effects such as cardiovascular events, gastrointestinal distress, and venous thromboembolic events [54].

Aromatase Inhibitors (AIs)

Letrozole and Anastrozole are aromatase inhibitors that are well tolerated and act similarly to SERMs. In research done by Dias et al., testosterone levels significantly improved after 1 mg of Anastrozole prescribed daily for 12 months. However, the study of bone mineral density in these men showed to be lower when treated with AI as compared to those on testosterone therapy [55]. Therefore, AIs are not recommended for prolonged periods. Other than that, fasting glucose, insulin, and lipid levels are similar to those on testosterone therapy [56]. On the other hand, some studies have failed to show improvements in psychological and physiological parameters or symptoms of hypogonadism [57, 58]. Documented side effects of AIs include nausea, derangement of liver enzymes, headache, and hot flashes.

Gonadotrophin Injection

Gonadotropin replacement therapy includes gonadotropin-releasing hormone (GnRH) and hCG. GnRH requires a continuous infusion pump to be administered to titrate the GnRH levels to follow the pulsatile release of GnRH from the hypothalamus. hCG, an LH analog, binds to LH receptors to stimulate testosterone production. hCG can also be given with exogenous testosterone to maintain intratesticular testosterone levels and preserve spermatogenesis. The downside of hCG is that it is expensive and requires multiple injections per week [59].

Indications of Non-testosterone Preparations for Hypogonadism

These alternatives of testosterone are indicated in special group of patient as in the below clinical scenarios:

Clinical scenario	Preferred agent	Reference
Young man with secondary hypogonadism and desire for fertility	Clomiphene/hCG	[54]
Hypogonadism with obesity & high estrogen	AI ± SERM	[60]
Previous androgenic anabolic steroid use & post-cycle recovery	hCG ± Clomiphene	[61, 62]
Gynecomastia with low T, high E2	AI	[60]
Functional hypogonadism, borderline T	Clomiphene	[53]

Follow-Up Protocol

The following are recommendations from the AUA, EAU, Endocrine Society, and ISSM guidelines. For transdermal gel, testosterone concentrations should be evaluated 2–8 h and 1 week after application to ensure that serum concentrations are in the mid-to-normal range. On the other hand, concentrations should be assessed immediately before or after application for buccal formulations. Concentrations for pellets should be assessed at the end of the dosing interval. For oral testosterone undecanoate, it should be monitored 3–5 h after ingestion with a fat-containing meal. For IM testosterone undecanoate, serum concentrations of testosterone should be monitored at the end of the dosing interval just before the next injection.

For monitoring, patients on gel, patch, or intranasal formulations should be assessed 2–4 weeks after initiation. For those on short-acting IM or SC formulations, assessment should be made after at least 3–4 cycles. For those on long-acting IM formulations, assessment should be between the first two 10-week injections. Lastly, for those on long-acting SC pellets, evaluation should be at two intervals: first, at 2–4 weeks after initiation, followed by a second evaluation at 10–12 weeks. Close monitoring of hemoglobin and hematocrit during treatment is recommended by all guidelines. PSA also should also be monitored in men. One should also assess for signs and symptoms of testosterone deficiency at every follow-up visit, and testosterone therapy should be discontinued if there is no symptomatic improvement [9, 12, 63].

The Expected Benefits from TRT

Patient age, BMI, and diabetes status have been shown to not significantly affect the short-to-medium-term effectiveness of testosterone treatment in improving erectile dysfunction or quality of life [64]. Interestingly, in contrast to phosphodiesterase-5 inhibitors (PDE5i), besides erectile function, testosterone also enhances other aspects of sexual function, such as sexual desire [65].

Rodrigues, in his review, gave a comprehensive update on the effects of testosterone replacement therapy [66].

Testosterone replacement therapy was shown to have greater improvement in overall sexual activity, sexual desire, erectile function, and satisfaction with sexual experience than placebo. However, the improvements in erectile function are substantially less in older hypogonadal men on testosterone compared with PDE5i.

Testosterone treatment of young testosterone-deficient men has been shown to improve sexual daydreams, sexual thoughts, spontaneous erections, attentiveness to erotic stimuli, and frequency and duration of sleep-entrained penile erections. By restoring testosterone levels that are at or near the lower limit of the normal male range in healthy young testosterone-deficient men, sexual function is improved. However, in middle-aged and older men who have normal testosterone levels and no sexual symptoms, testosterone treatment does not improve sexual desire or erectile function. Similarly, in hypogonadal men with ejaculatory dysfunction, testosterone treatment has not been shown to improve ejaculatory function. Testosterone treatment also did not result in greater improvement in erectile function than placebo in men with erectile dysfunction and low testosterone levels, in whom the dose of sildenafil citrate was optimized.

Testosterone treatment increases skeletal muscle mass via hypertrophy of both type 1 and 2 skeletal muscle fibers. Testosterone treatment also improves physical performance, such as stair climbing speed and power in older men.

There was greater improvement in vertebral bone mineral density, volumetric bone density and estimated bone strength with better improvements seen in the spine than in the hip and also better in the trabecular than the peripheral bone. However, the effects of testosterone treatment on fracture risk in older hypogonadal men is still not known.

With regards to Major Depression Disorder (MDD), randomized controlled and placebo-controlled trials have failed to demonstrate consistent benefit of testosterone over placebo.

Testosterone replacement reduces whole-body adipose tissue mass. Hypogonadal men who had stopped testosterone replacement were found to be associated with the development of insulin resistance. Randomized trials of testosterone treatment in older men with type 2 diabetes and low testosterone levels have not found consistent improvement in glycemic control, although some studies have shown improvement in insulin resistance.

Data on the effects of testosterone on cognition, Alzheimer's Disease, verbal memory, and visuospatial skills are limited and have provided conflicting results.

Controversies of TRT in Special Patients' Populations

Patients with a History of or at Risk for Prostate Cancer

The recommendation from the AUA is for clinicians to inform patients that there is no evidence linking the use of testosterone therapy to the development of prostate cancer [67].

Currently, clinical guidelines advise against initiating testosterone therapy in patients with untreated prostate cancer, unevaluated palpable prostate nodule, induration, or an elevated age-adjusted PSA level. However, the choice to initiate testosterone therapy in patients with a history of prostate cancer should be discussed thoroughly with patients, as there is inadequate evidence to quantify the risk–benefit ratio of testosterone therapy in this population.

In men aged 40 years and above without a history of prostate cancer, PSA levels should be checked before starting testosterone therapy.

Long-term testosterone therapy in men with functional hypogonadism was found to improve urinary function with no associated increase in prostate cancer risk [68]. What was interesting to note was that when prostate cancer was detected, it was always reported within 18 months of starting testosterone therapy. This suggests that testosterone therapy may actually unmask prostate cancer that was present but previously undetectable.

TRT in men with hypogonadism, who were carefully screened for prostate cancer risk, does not increase the incidence of adverse prostate events compared to placebo. Large trials, particularly the TRAVERSE trial, showed that TRT did not raise the risk of prostate cancer, urinary retention, or procedures for benign prostatic hyperplasia. Proper screening and monitoring can ensure safety and early detection of significant prostate cancers during TRT [69].

Patients with Obesity or Type 2 Diabetes

Men with obesity (body mass index [BMI] ≥30 kg/m2), increased waist circumference (>40 inches), and type 2 diabetes should be evaluated for testosterone deficiency and have their testosterone levels checked [70]. Studies have demonstrated that low testosterone levels are almost five times more common in obese men than in non-obese men and are nearly twice as common in men with diabetes than in those without diabetes [71, 72]. Lifestyle modification should be counseled in these groups of patients as it can improve testosterone levels and may reduce the risk for CV disease.

Preliminary evidence implies that long-term testosterone therapy may delay diabetes progression, reduce BMI and waist circumference, improve glycemic and lipid control [73, 74]. It may also ameliorate the beneficial effects of supervised modification in diet and exercise on glycemic control and insulin sensitivity in hypogonadal men with type 2 diabetes [75, 76].

IM testosterone should be prescribed with caution in high-risk populations, including patients with obesity and type 2 diabetes, as there is an increased risk of erythrocytosis.

Usage of nasal testosterone gel in patients with hypogonadism with BMI > 35 kg/m2 can elevate total testosterone, free testosterone, dihydrotestosterone, and estradiol levels comparable to nonobese men [77]. Higher doses of transdermal testosterone preparation are required in obese patients due to its pharmacokinetic factor. The obese patient may also benefit from aromatase inhibitors, which can increase testosterone levels and maintain spermatogenesis. Aromatase inhibitors can be used as off-label as adipose tissue in obese patients contains aromatase, which converts testosterone to estrogen [78]. Unfortunately, AIs must be used with caution as they are associated with negative side effects, including decreased bone density and reductions in libido [79, 80].

Patients Seeking to Maintain Fertility

The decision to initiate testosterone therapy must be considered meticulously, as it may affect HPG axis function, spermatogenesis, and fertility. The majority of healthy men will recover sperm production after discontinuing exogenous testosterone if they have normal testosterone levels [81, 82]. However, no definitive studies have documented the recovery of spermatogenesis in either testosterone-deficient or infertile men who have used testosterone therapy, but the trial of nasal testosterone showed some promising data [83]. Consequently, the unknown long-term impact of testosterone therapy on spermatogenesis should be discussed with patients who seek to maintain reproductive potential.

All guidelines advised against testosterone initiation in testosterone-deficient patients who are interested in maintaining fertility. AUA guidelines suggest the use of either selective estrogen receptor modulators or aromatase inhibitors and acknowledge that testosterone deficiency is an off-label indication for the use of these agents. EAU guidelines also acknowledge that aromatase inhibitors are a possible treatment in the context of male infertility or secondary hypogonadism. However, the guidelines stated that more evidence is needed [9]. The Endocrine Society does not suggest specific treatment recommendations for patients wishing to maintain fertility [3]. Other non-suppressive treatment plans, such as simultaneous use of clomiphene citrate or human chorionic gonadotropin (hCG) or treatment with a shorter-acting testosterone formulation that is less likely to blunt the HPG axis can also be considered for cases of secondary hypogonadism. Other than that, FSH should be added to hCG as a standard therapy in patients with secondary hypogonadism [3, 9].

Patients with a History of Cardiovascular Disease

Testosterone deficiency has been shown to increase the incidence of major CV events, including myocardial infarction, stroke, and CV mortality, and an increased prevalence of CV risk factors. Extensive review suggests that initiation of appropriate doses of testosterone with appropriate monitoring is likely to be safe for men with CV disease and may even reduce CV events [84]. Nevertheless, patients should be informed that it cannot yet be stated definitively whether testosterone therapy increases or decreases the risk of CV events and that there is no definitive evidence linking testosterone therapy to a higher incidence of acute CV disease in patients with a history of CV events. AUA guidelines, however, endorsed against starting testosterone therapy in men who have had a major adverse CV event (MACE), including myocardial infarction or stroke, within the past 3–6 months. This recommendation was adopted in part because the studies cited in the guidelines excluded men with CV events during this time frame. The Endocrine Society has similarly advised against initiating testosterone therapy in men with a history of CV events in the past 6 months. The EAU does not mention a time frame but states that acute CV events are a relative contraindication.

In the recent TRAVERSE trial, testosterone-replacement therapy was found to be non-inferior to placebo with respect to the incidence of major adverse cardiac events in men with hypogonadism and preexisting or a high risk of cardiovascular disease [85].

Conclusions

LOH represents a well-established and significant medical condition that impacts somatic, sexual, and psychological aspects. Additionally, it correlates with an increased risk of type 2 diabetes, cardiovascular issues, and all-cause mortality. Recognizable clinical symptoms, particularly ED, loss of morning erections, and diminished sexual desire, should prompt evaluation, alongside addressing underlying risk factors and conducting further investigations as needed.

TRT, is supported by evidence, effective, and safe. Research indicates that achieving sustained normalization of serum testosterone levels through treatment correlates with reduced morbidity and mortality.

While TRT offers potential benefits in restoring testosterone levels and improving symptoms, its administration requires careful consideration of individual health factors, including age, fertility status, and comorbidities. Moreover, monitoring for adverse effects such as polycythemia, prostate issues, and cardiovascular events is essential. Given these complexities, a tailored and vigilant approach is imperative to optimize outcomes and mitigate risks associated with TRT in late-onset hypogonadism.

The Future of TRT

The future of testosterone replacement therapy (TRT) holds promise in several areas, including:

- Alternative Delivery Routes: In addition to traditional routes of administration (e.g., injections, patches, gels), future research may explore alternative delivery routes for TRT, such as intranasal sprays, buccal tablets, or sublingual formulations. These approaches could offer advantages in terms of convenience, compliance, and absorption kinetics.
- Regulatory Considerations: As TRT continues to evolve, regulatory agencies will play a crucial role in ensuring the safety, efficacy, and quality of emerging therapies. Regulatory frameworks may need to adapt to accommodate novel formulations, personalized medicine approaches, and advances in digital health technologies.
- Precision Medicine Approach: There's growing interest in personalized medicine, including TRT. Genetic factors, lifestyle, and individual health conditions may influence the effectiveness and safety of TRT. Future developments may involve tailored treatment plans based on genetic markers or other personalized factors to optimize outcomes and minimize risks.
- Telemedicine and Remote Monitoring: The integration of telemedicine platforms and remote monitoring technologies could improve access to TRT and enhance patient care. Remote consultations, home testosterone testing kits, and digital health apps may streamline the TRT process and facilitate ongoing monitoring of treatment efficacy and safety.

References

1. Grossmann M, Matsumoto AM. A perspective on middle-aged and older men with functional hypogonadism: focus on holistic management. J Clin Endocrinol Metab. 2017;102(3):1067–75.
2. Rey RA, et al. an extended classification based on a developmental, endocrine physiology-based approach. Andrology. 2013;1(1):3–16.
3. Bhasin S, Brito JP, Cunningham GR, Hayes FJ, Hodis HN, Matsumoto AM, Snyder PJ, Swerdloff RS, Wu FC, Yialamas MA. Testosterone therapy in men with hypogonadism: an endocrine society clinical practice guideline. J Clin Endocrinol Metab. 2018;103(5):1715–44.
4. Dudek P, Kozakowski J, Zgliczyński W. Late-onset hypogonadism. Prz Menopauzalny. 2017;16(2):66–9.
5. Harman SM, Metter EJ, Tobin JD, Pearson J, Blackman MR, Baltimore Longitudinal Study of Aging. Longitudinal effects of aging on serum total and free testosterone levels in healthy men. Baltimore Longitudinal Study of Aging. J Clin Endocrinol Metab. 2001;86(2):724–31.
6. Decaroli MC, Rochira V. Aging and sex hormones in males. Virulence. 2017;8(5):545–70.
7. Wu FC, et al. Identification of late-onset hypogonadism in middle-aged and elderly men. N Engl J Med. 2010;363(2):123–35.
8. Araujo AB, O'Donnell AB, Brambilla DJ, Simpson WB, Longcope C, Matsumoto AM, McKinlay JB. Prevalence and incidence of androgen deficiency in middle-aged and older

men: estimates from the Massachusetts Male Aging Study. J Clin Endocrinol Metab. 2004;89(12):5920–6.
9. Mulhall JP, Trost LW, Brannigan RE, Kurtz EG, Redmon JB, Chiles KA, Lightner DJ, Miner MM, Murad MH, Nelson CJ, Platz EA, Ramanathan LV, Lewis RW. Evaluation and management of testosterone deficiency: AUA guideline. J Urol. 2018;200(2):423–32.
10. Salonia A, Bettocchi C, Carvalho J, et al. EUA guidelines on sexual and reproductive health; 2024. Available from: EAU guidelines on sexual and reproductive health, 2024. http://www.uroweb.org/guideline/sexual-and-reproductive-health/.
11. Lunenfeld B, Mskhalaya G, Zitzmann M, Arver S, Kalinchenko S, Tishova Y, Morgentaler A. Recommendations on the diagnosis, treatment, and monitoring of hypogonadism in men. Aging Male. 2015;18(1):5–15.
12. Khera M, Adaikan G, Buvat J, Carrier S, El-Meliegy A, Hatzimouratidis K, McCullough A, Morgentaler A, Torres LO, Salonia A. Diagnosis and treatment of testosterone deficiency: recommendations from the Fourth International Consultation for Sexual Medicine (ICSM 2015). J Sex Med. 2016;13(12):1787–804.
13. Hackett G, Kirby M, Rees RW, Jones TH, Muneer A, Livingston M, Ossei-Gerning N, David J, Foster J, Kalra PA, Ramachandran S. The British Society for Sexual Medicine guidelines on male adult testosterone deficiency, with statements for practice. World J Mens Health. 2023;41(3):508–37.
14. Millar AC, Lau ANC, Tomlinson G, Kraguljac A, Simel DL, Detsky AS, Lipscombe LL. Predicting low testosterone in aging men: a systematic review. CMAJ. 2016;188(13):E321–30.
15. Trost LW, Mulhall JP. Challenges in testosterone measurement, data interpretation, and methodological appraisal of interventional trials. J Sex Med. 2016;13(7):1029–46. https://doi.org/10.1016/j.jsxm.2016.04.068. Epub 2016 May 18
16. Carvalho VM. The coming of age of liquid chromatography coupled to tandem mass spectrometry in the endocrinology laboratory. J Chromatogr B Analyt Technol Biomed Life Sci. 2012;883–884:50–8.
17. Giagulli VA, Castellana M, Lisco G, Triggiani V. Critical evaluation of different available guidelines for late-onset hypogonadism. Andrology. 2020;8(6):1628–41.
18. Grober ED, Krakowsky Y, Khera M, Holmes DT, Lee JC, Grantmyre JE, Patel P, Bebb RA, Fitzpatrick R, Campbell JD, Carrier S, Morgentaler A. Canadian Urological Association guideline on testosterone deficiency in men: evidence-based Q&A. Can Urol Assoc J. 2021;15(5):E234–43.
19. Park HJ, Ahn ST, Moon DG. Evolution of guidelines for testosterone replacement therapy. J Clin Med. 2019;8(3):410.
20. Morgentaler A, Traish A, Geoffrey Hackett T, Jones H, Ramasamy R. Diagnosis and treatment of testosterone deficiency: updated recommendations from the Lisbon 2018 International Consultation for Sexual Medicine. Sex Med Rev. 2019;7(4):636–49.
21. Dalmiglio C, Bombardieri A, Mattii E, Sestini F, Fioravanti C, Castagna MG, Fiorini M, Dotta F, Cantara S. Analytical performance of free testosterone calculated by direct immunoluminometric method compared with the Vermeulen equation: results from a clinical series. Hormones (Athens). 2024;
22. Keihani S, Alder NJ, Cheng PJ, Stoddard GJ, Pastuszak AW, Hotaling JM. Obesity and baseline estradiol levels are independent predictors for initiation of anastrozole in hypogonadal men on clomiphene citrate. World J Mens Health. 2020;38(4):582–90.
23. Buvat J, Maggi M, Guay A, Torres LO. Testosterone deficiency in men: systematic review and standard operating procedures for diagnosis and treatment. J Sex Med. 2013;10:245–84.
24. Hazegh K, Bravo MD, Kamel H, Dumont L, Kanias T. The prevalence and demographic determinants of blood donors receiving testosterone replacement therapy at a large USA blood service organization. Transfusion. 2020;60(5):947–54.
25. Sellke N, Omil-Lima D, Sun HH, Tay K, Rhodes S, Loeb A, Thirumavalavan N. Trends in testosterone prescription during the release of society guidelines. Int J Impot Res. 2023:1–5.

26. Anaissie J, DeLay KJ, Wang W, Hatzichristodoulou G, Hellstrom WJ. Testosterone deficiency in adults and corresponding treatment patterns across the globe. Transl Androl Urol. 2017;6(2):183–91.
27. Handelsmanv DJ. Global trends in testosterone prescribing, 2000–2011: expanding the spectrum of prescription drug misuse. Med J Aust. 2013;199:548–51.
28. Dubin JM, Jesse E, Fantus RJ, Bennett NE, Brannigan RE, Thirumavalavan N, Halpern JA. Guideline-discordant care among direct-to-consumer testosterone therapy platforms. JAMA Intern Med. 2022;182(12):1321–3.
29. Daggett PR, Wheeler MJ, Nabarro JD. Oral testosterone, a reappraisal. Horm Res. 1978;9:121–9.
30. Miller JA, Nguyen TT, Loeb C, Khera M, Yafi FA. Oral testosterone therapy: past, present, and future. Sex Med Rev. 2023;11(2):124–38.
31. Ahmad SW, Molfetto G, Montoya D, Camero A. Is oral testosterone the new frontier of testosterone replacement therapy? Cureus. 2022;14(8):e27796. https://doi.org/10.7759/cureus.27796.
32. Bagatell CJ, Bremner WJ. Androgen and progestagen effects on plasma lipids. Prog Cardiovasc Dis. 1995;38:255–71.
33. Nieschlag E, Behre HM, Bouchard P, et al. Testosterone replacement therapy: current trends and future directions. Hum Reprod Update. 2004;10:409–19.
34. Yoshida EM, Erb SR, Scudamore CH, et al. Severe cholestasis and jaundice secondary to an esterified testosterone, a non-C17 alkylated anabolic steroid. J Clin Gastroenterol. 1994;18:268–70.
35. Behre HM, Wang CC, Handelsman DJ, et al. Pharmacology of testosterone preparations. Available online: https://www.researchgate.net/publication/264848721_Pharmacology_of_testosterone_preparations
36. Testopel® [package insert]. Malvern: Auxilium Pharmaceuticals Inc.; 2015.
37. Ullah MI, Riche DM, Koch CA. Transdermal testosterone replacement therapy in men. Drug Des Devel Ther. 2014;8:101–12.
38. Abadilla KA, Dobs AS. Topical testosterone supplementation for the treatment of male hypogonadism. Drugs. 2012;72:1591–603.
39. Swerdloff RS, Wang C, Cunningham G, Dobs A, Iranmanesh A, Matsumoto AM, Snyder PJ, Weber T, Longstreth J, Berman N. Long-term pharmacokinetics of transdermal testosterone gel in hypogonadal men. J Clin Endocrinol Metabol. 2000;85(12):4500–10.
40. Shoskes JJ, Wilson MK, Spinner ML. Pharmacology of testosterone replacement therapy preparations. Transl Androl Urol. 2016;5(6):834–43.
41. Mattern C, Hoffmann C, Morley JE, et al. Testosterone supplementation for hypogonadal men by the nasal route. Aging Male. 2008;11:171–8.
42. Gronski MA, Grober ED, Gottesman IS, Ormsby RW, Bryson N. Efficacy of nasal testosterone gel (Natesto®) stratified by baseline endogenous testosterone levels. J Endocr Soc. 2019;3(9):1652–62.
43. Kavoussi PK, Machen GL, Chen SH, Gilkey MS, Chen J, Hamzeh Y, Aston KI, Kavoussi SK. Direct conversion from long-acting testosterone replacement therapy to Natesto allows for spermatogenesis resumption: proof of concept. Andrologia. 2022;54(8):e14453.
44. Byrne M, Nieschlag E. Testosterone replacement therapy in male hypogonadism. J Endocrinol Investig. 2003;26:481–9.
45. Edelstein D, Basaria S. Testosterone undecanoate in the treatment of male hypogonadism. Expert Opin Pharmacother. 2010;11:2095–106.
46. Bhasin S, Cunningham GR, Hayes FJ, et al. Testosterone therapy in men with androgen deficiency syndromes: an Endocrine Society clinical practice guideline. J Clin Endocrinol Metab. 2010;95:2536–59.
47. Nankin HR. Hormone kinetics after intramuscular testosterone cypionate. Fertil Steril. 1987;47:1004–9.
48. Snyder PJ, Lawrence DA. Treatment of male hypogonadism with testosterone enanthate. J Clin Endocrinol Metab. 1980;51:1335–9.

49. United States Food and Drug Administration Orange Book [Internet]. Silver Spring: United States Food and Drug Administration; 2016 [updated 2016 April; cited 2016 May 13]. Available online: http://www.accessdata.fda.gov/scripts/cder/ob/docs/tempai.cfm
50. Wang C, Harnett M, Dobs AS, et al. Pharmacokinetics and safety of long-acting testosterone undecanoate injections in hypogonadal men: an 84-week phase III clinical trial. J Androl. 2010;31:457–65.
51. Diaz P, Reddy R, Blachman-Braun R, Zucker I, Dullea A, Gonzalez DC, Kresch E, Ramasamy R. Comparison of intratesticular testosterone between men receiving nasal, intramuscular, and subcutaneous pellet testosterone therapy: evaluation of data from two single-center randomized clinical trials. World J Men's Health. 2022; https://doi.org/10.5534/wjmh.210261. Epub ahead of print
52. Moskovic DJ, Katz DJ, Akhavan A, et al. Clomiphene citrate is safe and effective for long-term management of hypogonadism. BJU Int. 2012;110:1524–8.
53. Taylor F, Levine L. Clomiphene citrate and testosterone gel replacement therapy for male hypogonadism: efficacy and treatment cost. J Sex Med. 2010;7:269–76.
54. Ramasamy R, Scovell JM, Kovac JR, et al. Testosterone supplementation versus clomiphene citrate for hypogonadism: an age matched comparison of satisfaction and efficacy. J Urol. 2014;192:875–9.
55. Wibowo E, Pollock PA, Hollis N, et al. Tamoxifen in men: a review of adverse events. Andrology. 2016;4:776–88.
56. Dias JP, Melvin D, Simonsick EM, et al. Effects of aromatase inhibition vs. testosterone in older men with low testosterone: randomized-controlled trial. Andrology. 2016;4:33–40.
57. Dias JP, Shardell MD, Carlson OD, et al. Testosterone vs. aromatase inhibitor in older men with low testosterone: effects on cardiometabolic parameters. Andrology. 2017;5:31–40.
58. Loves S, de Jong J, van Sorge A, et al. Somatic and psychological effects of low-dose aromatase inhibition in men with obesity-related hypogonadotropic hypotestosteronemia. Eur J Endocrinol. 2013;169:705–14.
59. Helo S, Ellen J, Mechlin C, et al. A randomized prospective double-blind comparison trial of clomiphene citrate and anastrozole in raising testosterone in hypogonadal infertile men. J Sex Med. 2015;12:1761–9.
60. Lo EM, Rodriguez KM, Pastuszak AW, Khera M. Alternatives to testosterone therapy: a review. Sex Med Rev. 2018;6(1):106–13. https://doi.org/10.1016/j.sxmr.2017.09.004. Epub 2017 Nov 27. PMID: 29174957
61. Al Hashimi M. The deleterious effects of anabolic androgenic steroid abuse on sexual and reproductive health and comparison of recovery between treated and untreated patients: single-center prospective randomized study. Andrologia. 2022;54(11):e14576. https://doi.org/10.1111/and.14576. Epub 2022 Sep 5. PMID: 36065528; PMCID: PMC10078442
62. Al Hashimi M, Farahat Y, Kandil H, Al Khalidi I. Androgenic-anabolic steroid abuse trend and management: a prospective, cross-sectional, questionnaire-based survey. Health Sci Rep. 2023;6(1):e1032. https://doi.org/10.1002/hsr2.1032. PMID: 36628108; PMCID: PMC9827233
63. Tatem AJ, Beilan J, Kovac JR, et al. Management of anabolic steroid-induced infertility: novel strategies for fertility maintenance and recovery. World J Mens Health. 2019;38(2):141–50.
64. Dobs AS, Campbell KJ. An individualized approach to managing testosterone therapy in the primary care setting. Int J Gen Med. 2022;15:7719–33. https://doi.org/10.2147/IJGM.S364189.
65. Hudson J, Cruickshank M, Quinton R, et al. Symptomatic benefits of testosterone treatment in patient subgroups: a systematic review, individual participant data meta-analysis, and aggregate data meta-analysis. Lancet Healthy Longev. 2023;4:e561–72.
66. Deng L, Shi Q. Testosterone treatment: who will benefit the most? Lancet Healthy Longev. 2023;4(10):e524–5. https://doi.org/10.1016/S2666-7568(23)00191-5.
67. Rodrigues Dos Santos M, Bhasin S. Benefits and risks of testosterone treatment in men with age-related decline in testosterone. Annu Rev Med. 2021;72:75–91.
68. Mulhall JP, Trost LW, Brannigan RE, et al. Evaluation and management of testosterone deficiency: AUA guideline. J Urol. 2018;200(2):423–32.

69. Bhasin S, Thompson IM. Prostate risk and monitoring during testosterone replacement therapy. J Clin Endocrinol Metab. 2024;109(8):1975–83. https://doi.org/10.1210/clinem/dgae334. PMID: 38753865
70. Haider A, Haider KS, Doror G, Traish A. Urinary function and prostate safety of long-term testosterone therapy (TTH) in men with functional hypogonadism in a urological registry study. J Urol. 2021;206(suppl 3):e639. https://doi.org/10.1097/JU.0000000000002045.09.
71. Hackett G. Metabolic effects of testosterone therapy in men with type 2 diabetes and metabolic syndrome. Sex Med Rev. 2019;7(3):476–90.
72. Corona G, Mannucci E, Petrone L, et al. Association of hypogonadism and type II diabetes in men attending an outpatient erectile dysfunction clinic. Int J Impot Res. 2006;18(2):190–7. https://doi.org/10.1038/sj.ijir.3901391. [PubMed] [CrossRef] [Google Scholar]
73. Dohle GR, Arver S, Bettocchi C, Jones TH, Kliesch S. EAU guidelines on male hypogonadism. In: Presented at: EAU Annual Congress. Barcelona; 2019.
74. Yassin A, Haider A, Haider KS, et al. Testosterone therapy in men with hypogonadism prevents progression from prediabetes to type 2 diabetes: eight-year data from a registry study. Diabetes Care. 2019;42(6):1104–11.
75. Abourmarzouk O, Al-Qudimat A, Alwani M, et al. Glycemic control and insulin resistance in hypogonadal men with type 2 diabetes (T2DM) with long-term testosterone therapy (TTH): 15-year data from a prospective controlled registry study. J Urol. 2021;206(suppl3):e477–8.
76. Heufelder AE, Saad F, Bunck MC, Gooren L. Fifty-two-week treatment with diet and exercise plus transdermal testosterone reverses the metabolic syndrome and improves glycemic control in men with newly diagnosed type 2 diabetes and subnormal plasma testosterone. J Androl. 2009;30(6):726–33.
77. Lee J, Brock G, Barkin J, Bryson N, Gronski MA, Ormsby R. MY-T study: symptom-based titration decisions when using testosterone nasal gel, Natesto®. Can Urol Assoc J. 2019;13(10):301–6.
78. Winters SJ, Shkurovic S, Bedford B, Sorli C. Testosterone nasal gel in hypogonadal men with extreme obesity. In: Presented at: Western Section AUA Annual Meeting. Indian Wells; 2021.
79. Cohen J, Nassau DE, Patel P, Ramasamy R. Low testosterone in adolescents and young adults. Front Endocrinol (Lausanne). 2019;10:916.
80. Alder NJ, Keihani S, Stoddard GJ, Myers JB, Hotaling JM. Combination therapy with clomiphene citrate and Anastrozole is a safe and effective alternative for hypoandrogenic subfertile men. BJU Int. 2018;122(4):688–94.
81. Dadhich P, Ramasamy R, Scovell J, Wilken N, Lipshultz L. Testosterone versus clomiphene citrate in managing symptoms of hypogonadism in men. Indian J Urol. 2017;33(3):236–40.
82. Grimes DA, Lopez LM, Gallo MF, Halpern V, Nanda K, Schulz KF. Steroid hormones for contraception in men. Cochrane Database Syst Rev. 2012;3:CD004316.
83. Masterson T, Molina M, Ibrahim E, Ramasamy R. Natesto effects on reproductive hormones and semen parameters: results from an ongoing single-center, investigator-initiated Phase IV clinical trial. Eur Urol Focus. 2018;4(3):333–5.
84. Al-Qudimat A, Alwani M, Al-Zoubi RM, et al. Less mortality and less major adverse events (MACE) under long-term testosterone therapy (TTH): 15-year data from a prospective controlled registry study. J Urol. 2021;206(suppl3):e992–3.
85. Lincoff AM, Bhasin S, Flevaris P, Mitchell LM, TRAVERSE Study Investigators, et al. Cardiovascular safety of testosterone-replacement therapy. N Engl J Med. 2023;389(2):107–17.

Chapter 17
Cellular Regenerative and Gene Therapy for Male Sexual Dysfunction: A Reality?

Manh Truong Nguyen, Hiva Alipour, and Akmal Taher

Introduction

Definition and Prevalence of Male Sexual Dysfunction

Male sexual dysfunction (MSD) generally entails an alteration in at least one of the basic sexual functions (desire, erection, orgasm, and ejaculation). The most common MSD-related complaints are hypoactive sexual desire disorder, erectile dysfunction (ED), anorgasmia or difficulties in reaching orgasm, premature ejaculation (PE), delayed ejaculation, and Peyronie disease [128]. Pain during sexual activities and dissatisfaction with sexual life have also been considered MSD in some references [111]. It can be challenging to compare findings due to differences in defining sexual dysfunctions, patient demographics, and medical history [69].

The prevalence of sexual dysfunction is relatively high, with over 50% of males aged 40–70 experiencing some degree of ED [8], exhibiting a higher incidence with advancing age [141].

M. T. Nguyen (✉)
Fertility Centre, Hanh Phuc International Hospital, Ho Chi Minh City, Vietnam

Department of Urology, School of Medicine, University of Medicine and Pharmacy, Ho Chi Minh City, Vietnam

Men's Health Centre, Ho Chi Minh City, Vietnam

H. Alipour
Regenerative Medicine, Department of Health Science and Technology, Faculty of Medicine, Aalborg University, Aalborg, Denmark
e-mail: hiva@hst.aau.dk

A. Taher
Department of Urology, Faculty of Medicine, Universitas Indonesia, Jakarta, Indonesia

Dr. Cipto Mangunkusumo Hospital, Jakarta, Indonesia

E. Chung et al. (eds.), *Advances in Andrology*,
https://doi.org/10.1007/978-3-032-29112-7_17

Overview of the Current Landscape: Existing Treatments and Their Limitations

Depending on the underlying conditions or medications causing the sexual dysfunction, current treatment options can be divided into the categories of cognitive/behavioral, pharmacotherapy, and surgical approaches [8].

Significance of Cellular Regenerative and Gene Therapy in Addressing Male Sexual Dysfunction

The currently available pharmacological therapies for MSD are primarily focused on alleviating symptoms and do not resolve the cause of the dysfunction, making them a temporary solution [10]. These treatments have shown consistent discontinuation rates, including 4.4% to 76% for phosphodiesterase type 5 inhibitors (PDE5Is), 18.6% to 79.9% for intraurethral alprostadil and intracavernosal injections (ICIs), 32% to 69.2% for urethral suppositories, and 50% to 64% for vacuum erection device [17].

Furthermore, the lack of response or consistency in the on-demand effectiveness of pharmacological therapies for male sexual dysfunction, especially in patients with severe vascular or neurogenic ED, such as diabetes, cardiovascular disease, and metabolic syndrome, secondary to the presence of other pathologies, lesions of pelvic and cavernous nerves as a consequence of surgical interventions at the pelvic level (i.e., partial or radical prostatectomy and radiotherapy for cancer control), or trauma of the pelvic cavernous nerves and/or the vascular system of the genital apparatus, has necessitated the testing and utilization of various new approaches [26].

Some new approaches under evaluation for treating MSD include platelet-rich plasma, protein therapy, low-intensity shockwave therapy, and regenerative therapy [10, 26]. In response to the growing population of difficult-to-treat patients with ED, various regenerative medicine strategies have been investigated over the past two decades [10].

Current research is exploring novel therapeutic approaches such as stem cells and platelet-rich plasma (PRP) for the treatment of ED, with several studies assessing the efficacy of ICIs of stem cells derived from the human placenta, bone marrow, and adipose tissue in repairing the damaged cavernous nerve associated with ED [92, 127]. Stem cell-based regenerative therapy has been shown to be effective in men experiencing ED following radical prostatectomy for prostate cancer treatment or as a result of diabetes mellitus [7, 63]. The American Urological Association (AUA) currently considers ICI with SC therapy "investigational" and a grade C recommendation for men with ED [20]. Human and rodent-model studies suggest nerve regeneration as the potential mechanism of action of PRP injection therapy in ED [92, 127].

Platelets impact tissue regeneration via insulin-like growth factor, transforming growth factor-beta, and platelet-derived growth factor. These growth factors may result in connective tissue regeneration and enhanced erectile function [92]. The AUA currently considers PRP for ED to be "experimental" [20].

These innovative approaches target specific genetic factors contributing to ED by introducing genetic material into cells to compensate for abnormal genes or to produce beneficial proteins. Their approach aims to provide a more permanent solution by correcting the genetic causes of ED. Current research is exploring various gene therapy strategies, although these are still in experimental stages and require further clinical validation. In contrast to conventional ED treatments which offer immediate but temporary symptom relief, cellular regenerative and gene therapies focus on repairing underlying tissue damage and addressing genetic causes, potentially providing more durable and long-term solutions for ED patients [20, 92, 127].

Cellular Regenerative Therapies

Stem Cell Therapy

Overview of Stem Cells and Their Potential in Regenerating Damaged Tissues

Stem cells are unspecialized cells of the human body with the potential to self-renew, colonize, and differentiate into a variety of specialized mature cell types of an organism, enabling them to produce and regenerate tissues and organs [169].

Stem cells can be divided into embryonic stem cells, mesenchymal stem cells, and induced pluripotent stem cells based on their origin:

- *Embryonic Stem Cells (ESCs)*: ESCs are pluripotent cells comprising the inner cell mass of a blastocyst. The isolation of human embryonic stem cells (hESC) with the ability to differentiate into different precursor cells started a new era for regenerative medicine in the late 1990s [55]. Although these cells have the potential to differentiate into any cell type in the body, their use in regenerative medicine remains limited by the need for lifelong immunosuppressive therapy, limited effectiveness, tumorigenic potential, and ethical concern [55].
- *Mesenchymal Stem Cells (MSCs)*: MSCs are multipotent progenitor cells found in bone marrow, peripheral blood, muscle, adipose, placenta, fetal tissue, umbilical cord, and amniotic fluid [18]. These cells have been differentiated into adipogenic, chondrogenic, and osteogenic lineages in vitro [18], and have been used in regenerative medicine for bone regeneration and repair [68], as well as in the treatment of periodontitis [91]. Similar to hESCs, ethical concerns and the risk of tumor formation are also limiting factors in using MSCs in regenerative medicine [18].

- *Induced Pluripotent Stem Cells (iPSCs)*: iPSCs are generated by reprogramming adult cells, such as skin or blood cells, into a pluripotent state using specific genes [18]. They have the potential to differentiate into any cell type in the body and can be used for regenerative medicine. However, their use is still in the early stages of research and development [18].

The ability of stem cells to self-renew and differentiate into specialized cell types underpins their role in regenerative medicine, which aims to repair, regenerate, or replace damaged cells, tissues, and organs [29].

Current Research and Developments in Using Stem Cells for ED, PE, and Other Sexual Dysfunctions

Stem cell therapy (SCT) has received increasing interest as a potential treatment strategy for ED. Stem cells have the ability to differentiate into various cell types, such as neuronal, smooth muscle, and endothelial cells [112]. This process makes them a potential candidate to aid in the regeneration and repair of the damaged corpus cavernosal nerve, as well as mitigate the effects of trauma, tobacco use, and neuropathic diseases (e.g., diabetes) that adversely affect the nervous system [1].

In addition, paracrine signaling may recruit other cells to help repair damaged penile tissue in ED. During this process, the endogenous repair systems are stimulated by the release of cell-repair cytokines, allowing stem cells that do not directly interact with the target to perform healing functions nevertheless [144]. The paracrine effect stimulates nervous and vascular tissue repair using anti-apoptotic and pro-angiogenic molecules, revealing that direct stem cell incorporation is not necessarily required for an effective therapy [144].

Many types of stem cells, including mesenchymal stem cells, placental matrix-derived stem cells, mesenchymal stem cell-derived exosomes, adipose-derived stem cells (ADSCs), bone marrow-derived mononuclear stem cells, umbilical cord tissue or blood stem cells, and urine-derived stem cells, have been used in most studies that use regenerative treatments for ED [10]. Table 17.1 presents a selection of studies evaluating the potential of diverse stem cell types for treating and managing ED.

Stem cell therapy for ED primarily relies on ADSCs and MSCs, while USCs, PSCs, and MDSCs play a smaller role. Despite all the progress in this field, current stem cell treatments can still only partially restore erectile function. As most stem cells need to be modified further before they can be used to treat ED, there is an increasing demand for more potent or engineered stem cells to effectively address ED caused by various factors.

Cavernous pericytes have recently come to be understood to play a key role in neurovascular regeneration and vascular maintenance in ED patients [162, 167]. Pericytes exhibit stem cell-like characteristics and can differentiate into chondrocytes, adipocytes, granulocytes, and osteoblasts [2]. These characteristics open the possibility that pericytes, or pericyte-differentiated cells, have the potential to improve ED treatment.

Table 17.1 Source and type of stem cells and the parameter of therapy in selected preclinical studies evaluating the potential of stem cells for treating and managing erectile dysfunction (ED) [26]

Cell type	Source of stem cell	Type of ED	Parameter of therapy	References
ADSCs	Bilateral groin, inguinal area, epididymal adipose tissue, human adipose tissues	Type 1 diabetic ED, CNI-ED, age-associated ED	ICP-MAP, smooth muscle, nNOS, cavernosum pyroptosis, VEGFA, eNOS, growth factor	[22, 24, 45, 64, 172]
MSCs	Human umbilical cord, human gingiva, bone marrow	Type 1 diabetic ED, type 2 diabetic ED, CNI-ED, age-associated ED	ICP-MAP, microRNA sequencing, growth factor, eNOS. nNOS, TGF-β, smooth muscle, collagen	[45, 74, 93, 142, 154, 155]
USCs	Urine	Type 2 diabetic ED, CNI-ED	ICP-MAP, morphometric assessment, smooth muscle, nNOS, collagen	[51, 159]
PSCs	Human placental	CNI-ED	ICP-MAP, nNOS, eNOS, MPG fluorescence	[37, 57]
MDSCs	Gastrocnemius, abdominal muscles	Type 2 diabetic ED	Tunel assay, smooth muscle, urethral pressure profile measurement, blood vessel formation, angiogenic capacity	[100, 110]

ED erectile dysfunction, *ADSC* adipose-derived stem cell, *MSC* mesenchymal stem cell, *USC* urine-derived stem cell, *PSC* placental stem cell, *MDSC* muscle-derived stem cell, *CNI* cavernous nerve injury, *ICP-MAP* intracavernosal pressure-mean arterial pressure, *VEGFA* vascular endothelial growth factor A, *eNOS* endothelial nitric oxide synthase, *nNOS* neuronal nitric oxide synthase, *TGF-β* transforming growth factor-beta, *MPG* major pelvic ganglion

Platelet-Rich Plasma Therapy

Overview of PRP Therapy

Platelet-rich plasma is an autologous derivative of whole blood containing higher-than-average platelet concentrations and platelet-related growth factors. Platelets, or thrombocytes, are derived from megakaryocytic cells in the bone marrow and circulate in the bloodstream at concentrations ranging from 150,000 to 400,000 platelets/uL [60]. These cells participate in inflammation, cell proliferation, angiogenesis, and wound healing while also responsible for aggregation [60]. Since PRP therapy was first introduced in hematology in the 1970s to treat thrombocytopenia [60], it has been used for various indications, and its broad potential as a regenerative therapy has drawn great interest from scientists. Table 17.2 provides a selected list of PRP-based growth factors and platelet cytokines, along with their cell sources.

PRP is a therapeutic option that can be used alone or in conjunction with other procedures. Numerous studies in various medical fields, including sports medicine, cosmetology, ophthalmology, cardiology, tissue engineering, plastic surgery,

Table 17.2 A partial list of PRP-based growth factors and platelet cytokines and their cell sources

PGF and cytokines	Cell sources	Function and effects
PDGF (AA-BB-AB)	Platelets, endothelial Cells, macrophages, smooth muscle cells	Mitogenic for mesenchymal cells and osteoblasts Stimulates chemotaxis and mitogenesis in fibroblast/glial/smooth muscle cells; regulates collagenase secretion and collagen synthesis; stimulates macrophage and neutrophil chemotaxis
TGF (α–β)	Macrophages, T lymphocytes, keratinocytes	Stimulates undifferentiated mesenchymal cell proliferation; regulates endothelial, fibroblastic, and osteoblastic mitogenesis; regulates collagen synthesis and collagenase secretion; regulates mitogenic effects of other growth factors; stimulates endothelial chemotaxis and angiogenesis; inhibits macrophage and lymphocyte proliferation
VEGF	Platelets, macrophages, keratinocytes, endothelial cells	Increases angiogenesis and vessel permeability; stimulates mitogenesis for endothelial cells
EGF	Platelets, macrophages, monocytes	Proliferation of keratinocytes, fibroblasts, stimulates mitogenesis for endothelial cells
(a-b)-FGF	Platelets, macrophages, mesenchymal cells, chondrocytes, osteoblasts	Promotes growth and differentiation of chondrocytes and osteoblasts; mitogenic for mesenchymal cells, chondrocytes, and osteoblasts
CTGF	Platelets, fibroblasts	Promotes angiogenesis, cartilage regeneration, fibrosis, and platelet adhesion
IGF-1	Platelets, plasma, epithelial cells, endothelial cells, fibroblasts, osteoblasts, bone matrix	Chemotactic for fibroblasts and stimulates protein synthesis. Enhances bone formation by proliferation and differentiation of osteoblasts
HGF	Platelets, mesenchymal cells	Regulates cell growth and motility in epithelial/endothelial cells, supporting epithelial repair and neovascularization during wound healing
KGF	Fibroblasts, mesenchymal cells	Regulates epithelial migration and proliferation
Ang-1	Platelets, neutrophils	Induces angiogenesis stimulating migration and proliferation of endothelial cells. Supports and stabilizes blood vessel development via the recruitment of pericyte
PF4	Platelets	Calls leucocytes and regulates their activation. Microbiocidal activities

(continued)

Table 17.2 (continued)

PGF and cytokines	Cell sources	Function and effects
SDF-1α	Platelets, endothelial cells, fibroblasts	Calls CD34+ cells, induces their homing, proliferation and differentiation into endothelial progenitor cells stimulating angiogenesis. Calls mesenchymal stem cells and leucocytes
TNF	Macrophages, mast cells, T lymphocytes	Regulates monocyte migration, fibroblast proliferation, macrophage activation, angiogenesis

Adapted from [54, 119]

Abbreviations: *PDGF* platelet-derived growth factors, *TGF* transforming growth factor, *VEGF* vascular endothelial growth factor, *EGF* epidermal growth factor, *FGF* fibroblast growth factor, *CTCG* connective tissue growth factor, *IGF* insulin-like growth factor, *HGF* hepatocyte growth factor, *KGF* keratinocyte growth factor, *Ang-1* angiopoietin-1, *PF4* platelet factor 4, *SDF* stromal cell-derived factor, *TNF* tumor necrosis factor

trauma surgery, nerve and nerve trunk restoration, and the treatment of type 2 diabetes mellitus and its complications, have demonstrated the safety and efficiency of PRP therapy.

The regenerative capacity of a diverse biologically active PRP cellular cocktail has shown promising results for treating musculoskeletal disorders (orthobiologics). PRP therapies are currently considered a viable treatment option with clinical benefits, backed up by encouraging reports of patient outcomes [12, 157].

The efficacy and safety of PRP have been demonstrated in various medical conditions. However, there is still a lack of sufficient randomized clinical trials to provide a complete understanding of the potential complexities of PRP therapy on the body's healing processes. It is important to note that while PRP therapy is gaining popularity, the complexity of the physiological pathways cannot be overstated. The limited knowledge about the mechanism of action of PRP, the scarcity of large-scale studies, and the most rudimentary theories must be acknowledged. When analyzing studies, the authors considered the lack of standardization in preparation methods and the variability in PRP context and product quality. Various blood cell concentrations, such as leukocytes, platelets, and red blood cells, are common, making it difficult to study PRP products' correct biological properties and efficacy. Some of the clinical trials available did not use standardized terminology.

In conclusion, PRP therapy, derived from autologous blood, has advanced from its original application in hematology to become a versatile regenerative option. Studies across several medical domains, including musculoskeletal disorders and diabetes mellitus, support the safety and potential clinical benefits of PRP therapy. Nevertheless, the present scenario highlights the importance of caution due to the incomplete comprehension of its mechanisms, absence of standardization, and inconsistencies in product quality. Despite its potential, a comprehensive understanding of PRP's influence on healing processes necessitates additional investigation through robust randomized clinical trials and standardized protocols.

Current Research and Developments in Using PRP Therapy for ED, PE, and Other Sexual Dysfunctions

In recent years, PRP therapy has emerged as a promising non-surgical treatment option for ED [41]. Epifanova et al. laid the groundwork by investigating the mechanisms of PRP [21]. Building on this, a randomized clinical study conducted by Epifanova and Chalyj demonstrated statistically significant improvements in Peak Systolic Velocity and International Index of Erectile Function (IIEF-5) scores after PRP administration [39]. However, the absence of a true placebo group and limited long-term results tempered the impact of their study.

Alkhayal and Lourdes expanded the scope by administering intracavernosal PRP injections to men with ED, reporting significant improvements in IIEF-5 and successful intercourse rates [5]. Nevertheless, the study faced limitations such as unclear procedures and the absence of a placebo group.

Tas et al. delved into the effectiveness of autologous PRP application in ED patients with metabolic syndrome, showing a significant increase in mean IIEF-EF scores. Despite this, the median value remained within the mild-moderate classification, indicating minimal clinical improvement. Concerns about the lack of a placebo group and a small cohort size emphasize the need for more extensive and blinded trials before validating PRP as an ED treatment modality [143].

Matz et al. prioritized safety in their study, using Platelet-Rich Fibrin-Matrix (PRFM) injections for both ED and PE. The study demonstrated no decrease in IIEF-5 evaluations and reported minor adverse events, such as mild penile bruising, in a small cohort [103]. However, the study faced limitations like the absence of a control group and a small sample size.

The field took a significant leap with the first randomized controlled trial (RCT) evaluating PRP for ED [124]. This double-blinded placebo-controlled study, involving two groups of 30 patients each, demonstrated that 76% of PRP patients achieved minimal clinically important difference at 1 month compared to 25% in the control group. The study reported short-term improvements in erectile function and supported further investigation of PRP, given its exclusion of more severe ED cases and surgical causes.

A recent prospective, randomized, double-blind, placebo-controlled clinical trial found no difference in the percentage of men meeting minimum clinically important difference 1 month after treatment or any changes in penile Doppler parameters from baseline to 6 months of treatment with PRP vs the placebo group [101]. In contrast, another recent placebo-controlled study on platelet-rich plasma in the treatment of ED found the patients' overall and intercourse satisfaction levels were higher in the PRP group than the placebo group, as demonstrated by higher IIEF scores, with maximum improvement at the 3-month follow-up. There were no reports of plaque formation, subcutaneous bruising, or any other major side effects among participants, suggesting PRP is a safe and promising method for the improvement of mild to moderate erectile dysfunction [134].

In conclusion, the available evidence suggests that PRP is a safe treatment option for ED, but its pathogenic basis and exact mechanisms are unknown. The available RCTs provide valuable data, emphasizing the need for ongoing studies to address the heterogeneity among current works and fully elucidate PRP's therapeutic potential in ED and PE.

Studies on PRP therapy for Peyronie's Disease (PD) face limitations, often characterized by small cohorts and a lack of placebo controls. A case report by Marcovici in 2018 showcased improved penile curvature with PRP combined with daily penile pump use [99].

The first clinical studies confirming the safety of "PRP for PD" date back to 2014 [32]. In a preclinical study, Culha and colleagues utilized a rat model, injecting TGF-β1 to create PD-like conditions. The study concluded that PRP therapy may not be effective for PD and could induce fibrosis, highlighting limitations such as the lack of qualitative and quantitative analysis of growth factors in PRP [32].

Marcovici's clinical case described two PRP injections at the point of maximum penile curvature, coupled with daily penile pump use, resulting in a significant reduction in curvature angle after 2 months [99]. However, the study lacked a penile ultrasound scan, documentation of calcifications, and the use of PDQ and IIEF-5 assessments.

Matz et al. [103] evaluated the effects of PRFM injections in PD treatment, reporting an increase in IIEF-5 score and a decrease in penile curvature angle for 80% of patients [103]. However, limitations included varying injection numbers among patients and the absence of a placebo group.

While PRP is biologically plausible and appears to be safe for ED and PD, its exact mechanisms remain elusive. The literature review by Epifanova et al. [41] emphasized the need for large, placebo-controlled, multicenter studies to confirm or deny the effectiveness of PRP [41].

A recent study in 2024 evaluated the feasibility, efficacy, and safety of a combined treatment approach for PD involving percutaneous needle tunneling, penile modeling, and PRP injection in thirty-six patients with PD. The results showed a significant improvement in curvature angle, with a mean improvement difference of 16.85 degrees and a mean improvement percentage of 47.7%. The treatment was well tolerated, with no major complications reported. However, the study had limitations, such as a small sample size and the lack of a placebo group. Further research is needed to validate these findings in larger studies [6].

Given the heterogeneity of PRP preparation and treatment protocols, as well as the potential need for repeated injections to maintain local growth factor activity, the optimal injection volume, interval, and frequency for ED and PD remain undefined [41]. Determining the safe and effective adjustment of ED and PD degrees with PRP, identifying contraindications, and assessing age-related outcomes are additional challenges that warrant further investigation.

Protein Therapy

Overview of Protein Therapy

Since the introduction of the first recombinant protein therapeutic drug (human insulin) in 1978, the United States Food and Drug Administration (FDA) has approved and used approximately 239 protein therapeutic drugs [83, 148]. Protein therapies were previously used infrequently, but their use and frequency have recently increased dramatically [96], with many therapeutic proteins currently in clinical trials. Protein therapy has numerous advantages; due to its high specificity, autologously produced proteins are well tolerated and less likely to elicit an immune response, making them an alternative to gene therapy for diseases with gene mutations or deletions [83]. As a result, protein therapy has found a place as a key therapeutic agent in almost every field of medicine. Furthermore, the FDA has approved roughly 79 therapeutic monoclonal antibodies (mAbs), the primary form of therapeutic protein [3, 97]. Table 17.3 summarizes selected preclinical protein- and antibody-based therapeutic candidates investigated in experimental models of ED, categorized according to their proposed roles in angiogenesis and nerve regeneration.

Recombinant Protein Therapy for ED, PE, and Other Sexual Dysfunctions

Table 17.3 showcases select preclinical research outcomes of protein therapy for ED, summarizing 15 currently prescribed proteins or mAbs and organizing them based on their respective contributions to angiogenesis and nerve regeneration. Recombinant protein is a class of protein medication derived from recombinant DNA or recombinant RNA technology. It offers reduced toxicity, fewer side effects, and a more notable curative effect [82]. Recombinant protein therapies for ED are still in their infancy, according to a comprehensive review of the literature that we conducted.

Numerous studies have explored the efficacy of protein therapies utilizing angiogenic growth factors and neurotrophic factors in addressing ED. Initial demonstrations have revealed the significant restoration of erectile function in rat models of vasculogenic and neurogenic ED using recombinant VEGF or a combination of VEGF plus BDNF protein [130].

Further investigations explored the restoration of erectile function through repeated ICIs of angiopoietins, such as angiopoietin-1, COMP-angiopoietin-1, angiopoietin-4, and hepatocyte growth factor, in diabetic ED mice highlighted the induction of cavernous angiogenesis, NO-cGMP activity, tight junction expression, and reduction in reactive oxygen species (ROS) production [26].

The sonic hedgehog (Shh) cascade emerged as a critical regulator of erectile function, notably reduced in diabetic and neurogenic ED conditions. The Podlasek CA group extensively studied the Shh signaling pathway in 23 related studies on ED treatment [25]. Pro-angiogenic proteins, including DKK2 and LRG1 recombinant

Table 17.3 Preclinical protein therapy on ED biotherapeutics

Protein type	Protein names	Type of ED	Target signaling	References
Recombinant protein	HEBP1	Type 1 diabetic ED	Angiogenesis, ROS, PI3K/AKT/eNOS	[162]
	VEGF	Vasculogenic ED, age-associated ED, CNI-ED	Angiogenesis, smooth muscle integrity	[67, 117, 130]
	Angiopoietin-1	Type 2 diabetic ED	Angiogenesis, eNOS phosphorylation	[72]
	COMP-angiopoietin-1	Type 1 diabetic ED, high-cholesterol ED	Angiogenesis, NO-cGMP, ROS, tight junction	[73, 131]
	Angiopoietin-4	Type 1 diabetic ED	Angiogenesis, Tie2, eNOS phosphorylation	[79]
	HGF	Type 1 diabetic ED	Angiogenesis, ROS, smooth muscle integrity	[33, 95]
	Sonic hedgehog	CNI-ED, age-associated ED	Nerve regeneration, neurotrophic factors	[25, 122, 123]
	DKK2	Type 1 diabetic ED, CNI-ED	Angiogenesis, nerve regeneration, Ang1-Tie2, eNOS phosphorylation, ROS, neurotrophic factors	[52, 164]
	Apelin	Type 1 diabetic ED, CNI-ED	Angiogenesis, NO-cGMP, ROS	[79]
	LRG1	Type 1 diabetic ED	Angiogenesis, nerve regeneration, tight junction, eNOS phosphorylation, ROS, PI3K/AKT/NFkB	[165]
	BDNF	CNI-ED, age-associated ED	Angiogenesis, nerve regeneration, nNOS, cGMP	[67, 89]
Monoclonal antibody	TrkA	CNI-ED	Nerve regeneration, nNOS, smooth muscle integrity	[88]
	Ninjurin 1	Type 1 diabetic ED, CNI-ED	Angiogenesis, Ang1-Tie2, eNOS phosphorylation, ROS, neurotrophic factors	[163, 166]
Polyclonal antibody	proNGF	CNI-ED	Angiogenesis, nerve regeneration, nNOS, eNOS phosphorylation cGMP	[27]

ED erectile dysfunction, *VEGF* vascular endothelial growth factor, *COMP* cartilage oligomeric matrix protein, *HGF* hepatocyte growth factor, *BDNF* brain-derived neurotrophic factor, *DKK2* dickkopf WNT signaling pathway inhibitor 2, *HEBP1* heme-binding protein 1, *LRG1* leucine-rich alpha-2-glycoprotein 1, *TrkA* tyrosine receptor kinases, *proNGF* precursor for nerve growth factor, *CNI* cavernous nerve injury, *eNOS* endothelial nitric oxide synthase, *NO* nitric oxide, *cGMP* cyclic guanosine monophosphate, *ROS* reactive oxygen species, *PI3K* phosphoinositide 3-kinase, *AKT* protein kinase B, *NFkB* nuclear factor kappa B, *nNOS* neuronal nitric oxide synthase proteins, have been demonstrated to have the potential to promote the regeneration of penile blood vessels and nerves, reduce ROS production, and restore erectile function in different ED models [26].

It is evident from these studies that therapeutic candidate proteins predominantly belong to the category of angiogenic and neurotrophic factors [89]. However, limitations in protein therapeutics, such as high production costs and challenges in effective tissue penetration, have kept most of them in the preclinical stage. The need for developing more candidate proteins in the future is emphasized, as this would contribute significantly to understanding ED mechanisms and advancing therapeutic drug development.

Antibody Therapy for ED, PE, and Other Sexual Dysfunctions

Neutralizing mAbs, recognized as recombinant proteins derived from B cells, have gained prominence in the biopharmaceutical market due to their heightened safety, lower toxicity, higher specificity, and singular biological function [147]. Despite their widespread use in various medical fields, such as cancer, asthma, arthritis, transplant rejection, and infectious diseases, their application in treating ED has been limited, with only three studies published.

ICIs of tyrosine kinase receptor type 1 mAbs (TrkA-mAbs) were shown to significantly inhibit sympathetic nerve regeneration and stimulate parasympathetic nerve regeneration in CNI-induced ED rats [88]. This ultimately led to the promotion of erectile function. Yin et al. [163] discovered that intracavernosal blocking of ninjurin 1 expression in diabetic and CNI-induced ED mice rescued erectile function by inducing Ang1-Tie2 signaling, increasing neurotrophic factors expression, and reducing ROS production. Chung et al. [27] demonstrated that neutralizing antibodies to proNGF could also rescue erectile function by regulating neurotrophic and angiogenic factors in CNI-induced ED mice.

Despite the promising outcomes of these studies, it is important to note that mAb preparation is time-consuming (taking 6–9 months) and expensive. Additionally, the production system is currently applicable only to mice and rats. As antibody-based drug therapy for ED is still in its early stages, the identification of new target antigens becomes crucial for the future development of effective antibody-based therapeutic drugs [147].

Low-Intensity Shockwave Therapy (LISWT)

Mechanisms of Low-Intensity Shockwave Therapy in Tissue Regeneration

Low-intensity extracorporeal shockwave therapy (Li-ESWT) is a non-invasive technique utilizing targeted acoustic waves to induce a stress effect. The shockwaves exert stress through direct mechanical force and cavitation bubble-related mechanisms [46]. Cavitation impact is more likely to affect blood vessels, potentially causing lesions, while microbubbles from bubble implosion contribute to endothelium disruption, promoting neoangiogenesis [34]. Microbubble collapse induces shear stress, simulating endothelial nitric oxide production, and may enhance Schwann-cell-mediated nitrergic-nerve repair after injury [46]. However, the precise mechanism of Li-ESWT for ED remains not fully understood, including factors influencing treatment success.

In recent years, Li-ESWT has emerged as a promising treatment for vasculogenic ED, offering a potential cure, the most desired outcome for ED sufferers [17]. Studies in vitro and in animals have explored the effects of low-intensity shockwaves, indicating positive outcomes in nerve, endothelium, and smooth muscle regeneration [87, 126]. Reviews have hypothesized that shockwave-induced microtrauma leads to angiogenic neovascularization, improving penile blood flow [116]. Systematic reviews and meta-analyses on Li-ESWT for human ED treatment have been conducted, acknowledging the wide heterogeneity of evaluated variables in the literature.

Recent reviews highlight Li-ESWT as a valid option for ED treatment, particularly for patients with poor responses to oral medications and aversion to invasive procedures [17]. The IIEF-5 score and Erectile Hardness Score (EHS) improved in treated patients, with sustained results at 12 months of follow-up, emphasizing treatment effectiveness. Few studies reported low-grade complications, indicating the procedure's safety [17]. Further research is crucial to identify patients who will benefit most from Li-ESWT and establish optimal treatment protocols.

Current Research and Developments in Using LISWT for ED, PE, and Other Sexual Dysfunctions

Extracorporeal shockwave therapy (ESWT) has been gaining recognition as an effective treatment for ED, especially in non-responders to PDE5is [115, 146]. Several clinical trials and studies have confirmed that Li-ESWT significantly improved erectile function and penile hemodynamics using focused ESWT without adverse effects [56, 140]. Comparative studies of focused, unfocused, and radial shockwave modalities for ED have reported variable findings, and treatment protocols remain heterogeneous. Eryilmaz et al. reported improvements after both focused and unfocused ESWT, with greater improvement in the unfocused group [42], whereas sham-controlled studies of radial pressure wave therapy have not consistently demonstrated superiority over placebo in men with mild-to-moderate ED [132].

The use of ESWT for PD has appeared to generate beneficial effects, including but not necessarily limited to pain relief. However, the mechanism remains uncertain, and various schools of thought exist. ESWT may directly damage and remodel the plaque and may also increase local circulation due to the heat of ESWT. This heat promotes inflammation and increased macrophage activity, culminating in plaque destruction and resorption [34].

The potent mix of platelet growth factors and cytokines may diminish PD plaques and improve penile curvature. Platelet molecules include PDGF, VEGF, TGF-b, IGF, FGF, and others that can lead to vigorous tissue repair by inducing the inflammatory and proliferative phases of wounds. These molecules regulate cell growth and division and stimulate extracellular matrix production in tissue healing. Additionally, the plasma contains proteins such as fibrinogen, vitronectin, and fibronectin that play integral roles in regulating cell-cell interactions and the spatial organization of cell healing [150].

Research on Li-ESWT for ED has revealed promising outcomes, particularly in various rat models and clinical studies. Li-ESWT was demonstrated to have the ability to partially ameliorate ED in type 1 diabetic rats with increased endothelial cell regeneration and reduced smooth muscle atrophy, correlating with elevated expressions of nNOS, eNOS, and VEGF signaling pathways. This effect was attributed to the recruitment of endogenous MSCs and the potential induction of nerve regeneration, endothelial cell proliferation, and increased smooth muscle content in the penis [71].

Further investigations extended to neurovascular ED models and aging-induced ED models demonstrated that Li-ESWT induced angiogenesis and tissue regeneration in damaged penile areas. The treatment recruited endogenous progenitor cells and proliferated Schwann cells, ultimately improving erectile function [26].

Transitioning to clinical studies, positive outcomes in patients with vasculogenic ED included increased IIEF scores after Li-ESWT treatment. However, the lack of standardized treatment protocols resulted in varied research approaches. Conflicting results were reported, with some studies questioning the long-term effectiveness of Li-ESWT. To reconcile these conflicting results, meta-analyses of RCTs have shown significantly improved IIEF and EHS scores in patients treated with Li-ESWT compared to controls. Subsequent meta-analyses continued to present varied results, emphasizing the need for standardized treatment protocols [26].

While most studies have focused on vasculogenic ED and Peyronie's disease, a pilot study of Li-ESWT after bilateral nerve-sparing radical prostatectomy reported potential benefit in erectile function recovery, with modest improvements in IIEF-5 scores [49]. Subsequent meta-analytic evidence suggests a possible early benefit in post-prostatectomy ED recovery, although long-term outcomes remain inconclusive [26].

In summary, Li-ESWT presents itself as a promising alternative treatment for ED, with evidence supporting its efficacy in preclinical and clinical studies. However, the lack of standardized treatment protocols and the variation in patient populations contribute to the ongoing debate over its long-term effectiveness. Despite these controversies, Li-ESWT remains a viable and safe short-term alternative for ED treatment. Further research, particularly in refining treatment protocols and exploring specific signaling pathways, is essential for establishing stronger evidence in its favor.

Combination Regenerative Therapy

Various studies have highlighted the significant activation of human ADSCs, bone marrow-derived MSCs, and human MSCs proliferation and differentiation through Li-ESWT treatment [86]. Thus, Li-ESWT has the potential to enhance the quality of ADSCs for cell therapy in regenerative medicine applications. Investigations into the combined effect of Li-ESWT with stem cell therapy for ED treatment have reported that combining Li-ESWT with ADSCs therapy outperformed individual treatments in restoring damaged nerves and improving corpus cavernosum angiogenesis. For example, Li-ESWT combined with bone marrow-derived MSC therapy significantly improved erectile function and penile blood flow compared to monotherapy [135]. However, it is crucial to acknowledge that research on the combined treatment of ED with Li-ESWT and stem cells is still in its early stages, and extensive research data are required to determine the optimal regimen for maximizing therapeutic effects. Larger clinical trials with extended follow-up periods are essential to assess efficacy, safety, and long-term outcomes.

In Peyronie's disease, PRP-based approaches have been explored as potential regenerative treatments because platelet-derived growth factors may contribute to angiogenesis, cell proliferation, extracellular matrix remodeling, and tissue repair. Small clinical studies and case reports have reported improvements in penile curvature or erectile function after PRP- or PRFM-based injections, sometimes in combination with hyaluronic acid or penile pump therapy. However, the available evidence remains limited by small sample sizes, heterogeneous protocols, short follow-up, and the lack of robust placebo-controlled trials [39].

In a small pilot study, Lander et al. evaluated autologous stromal vascular fraction (SVF) isolated from lipoaspirate and injected into Peyronie's plaques in combination with penile shock wave therapy. At 6 months, patients reported subjective reductions in plaque size and penile curvature, and 7 of 11 patients reported improved erectile function. However, these findings should be interpreted cautiously because the study was limited by its small sample size, subjective outcome measures, and lack of a placebo or sham-control group [81].

Gene Therapy

In the context of current treatment options with low response rates, gene therapy is being investigated as a potential therapeutic strategy for male sexual dysfunction, particularly ED, PE, and related diseases.

Gene Editing

Overview of Gene Editing

Gene editing involves modifying the genetic material of a living organism through actions like removing, replacing, inverting, translocating, or inserting DNA sequences. In the realm of biomedical research, gene editing serves purposes such as unraveling gene functionality, simulating human diseases, delving into disease development, and potentially rectifying or averting human disorders. It opens new therapeutic possibilities for cases related to genetic alterations. Some common genome editing methods include clustered regularly interspaced short palindromic repeat-Cas protein (CRISPR-Cas), zinc-finger nucleases (ZFNs), and transcription-activating nucleases (TALENs), which offer precise modification capabilities targeting genes associated with diseases [105].

The CRISPR-Cas9 system is the most renowned gene editing tool among many approaches. Yoshizumi Ishino et al. [70] discovered an unusual repetitive DNA sequence, later identified as CRISPR, found in the gene cluster of Escherichia coli during the analysis of genes responsible for the isozyme conversion of alkaline phosphatase [70]. The CRISPR-Cas9 technology allows for nucleic acid modifications; through the mechanism of gene cutting and stitching, damaged DNA loci can be identified and replaced with functional sequences, aiding in gene function restoration.

In December 2023, Casgevy, a therapeutic intervention utilizing CRISPR-Cas9 gene editing technology, became the first FDA-approved treatment for patients with sickle cell disease (SCD) aged 12 and above [44, 120]. Previously, Casgevy was approved in the UK for treating transfusion-dependent β-thalassemia in patients aged ≥12 years for whom hematopoietic stem cell (HSC) transplantation is appropriate and a human leukocyte antigen matched related HSC donor is not available and SCD in patients aged ≥12 years with recurrent vasoocclusive crises (VOCs) who have the βS/βS, βS/β+, or βS/β0 genotype for whom HSC transplantation is appropriate and a human leukocyte antigen matched related HSC donor is not available.

Furthermore, integrating the CRISPR-Cas9 system with biological carriers like lipid nanoparticles or viral vectors for gene delivery exhibits promising prospects in disease therapies [40]. The advantages of CRISPR-Cas9 technology are combined with the protective qualities of biological materials in this comprehensive method, making precise and efficient gene manipulation possible while enhancing safety precautions. In addition to patient gene editing, the CRISPR-Cas9 technique is intended to regulate antimicrobial-resistance microbes by modifying the bacterial disease-causing gene sequence [30].

Current Research and Developments in Using Gene Editing for ED, PE, and Other Sexual Dysfunctions

Numerous gene mutations or polymorphisms have been identified as being connected with male sexual dysfunction diseases. For instance, polymorphisms such as MTHFR 677TT, eNOS intron 4 VNTR, G894T, T786C, rs2682826, and Pea3 (Pea3 null) are considered to be related to erectile dysfunction occurrences [9, 11, 109, 118, 152, 161].

Polymorphisms in genes like SLC6A4, dopamine transporter gene (SLC6A3, DAT1), the 5-hydroxytryptamine (5-HT) system, and androgen receptor are associated with premature ejaculation [77, 108, 133, 149, 151]. Furthermore, it has been found that a number of genes are connected to the underlying causes of ailments, including diabetes, hypertension, dyslipidemia, pituitary gland diseases, and several other illnesses that are connected to male sexual dysfunction [173]. Zhang et al. [171] used CRISPR/Cas9 technology delivered via a lentiviral vector to knock out TEAD1 in corpus cavernosum smooth muscle cells derived from diabetic rats with ED. TEAD1 knockout induced phenotypic modulation of CCSMCs from a synthetic toward a contractile phenotype, as reflected by increased SMMHC and calponin expression and reduced PCNA expression.

While the potential of editing genes, especially those passed to future generations (germline editing), is exciting, ethical and legal hurdles need careful consideration. The intricate nature of genes and the difficulty of ensuring complete safety add another layer of complexity. These challenges are further compounded by the risk of unintended consequences (off-target effects) and the high costs involved. Researchers are addressing these issues with innovative solutions. They are developing improved methods, including enhanced nucleases, sophisticated delivery mechanisms, and advanced bioinformatics tools, to accomplish more precise editing while also predicting and minimizing unexpected consequences. Despite these challenges, the potential for precise gene editing in gene therapy remains promising. Continued research and innovation are expected to refine existing techniques and unlock new disease treatment possibilities [38, 113, 137].

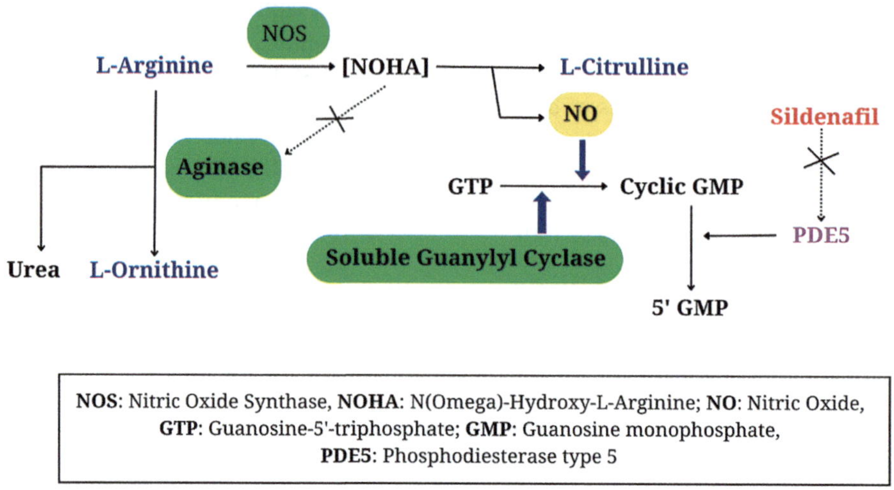

Fig. 17.1 Schema of l-arginine and nitric oxide synthase (NOS) catabolism [102]

Modulation of the Nitrergic System

Overview of NOS Gene Therapy and Other Gene Therapies Targeting the Nitrergic Mechanisms

Nitric oxide (NO) is a powerful vasodilator produced when L-arginine is oxidized to L-citrulline by the enzyme nitric oxide synthase (NOS) (Fig. 17.1). It plays an important function in achieving a penile erection by relaxing the smooth muscle tissues of the arteries and cavernosal bodies, increasing blood flow to the penis. Different isoforms of NOS, such as neuronal NOS (nNOS) in the non-adrenergic and non-cholinergic nerves, endothelial NOS (eNOS) in the penile arteries' endothelium, and inducible NOS (iNOS), contribute to penile erection. Reduced NO production due to decreased NOS expression may occur in patients with diabetes, cardiovascular diseases, high-cholesterol levels, or aging, often associated with ED [16].

Elevated endogenous NOS inhibitors and increased arginase activity may lead to NO deficiency. Gene therapy aimed at enhancing the expression of eNOS, nNOS, iNOS isoforms, or optimizing other factors related to nitrergic mechanisms, such as protein inhibitor of NOS, cGMP-dependent protein kinase G1 (PKG1), and anti-arginase, could enhance NO production or optimize signaling pathways mediated by NO intermediates [145, 168].

Current Research and Developments in Using Gene Therapies Targeting the Nitrergic Mechanisms for ED, PE, and Other Sexual Dysfunctions

Research on diabetic or elderly mouse models has shown promising outcomes for treating male sexual dysfunction, particularly erectile dysfunction. Xu et al. [156] demonstrated the role of iNOS and the effect of angiotensin 1-7 (Ang-[1-7]) on NOS levels in the pathogenesis mechanism of diabetes-induced erectile dysfunction (DMED). In the experiment by Silva et al. [136] using a diabetic mouse model with erectile dysfunction, the synthetic peptide PnPP-19 enhanced erectile function by activating nNOS and iNOS through the NO-activated cGMP pathway. The activity of PKG1 is reduced in the corporal tissue of diabetic mice with ED. Bivalacqua, Kendirci, et al. [15] demonstrated that in vivo gene transfer of PKG-1α into the penile corpus cavernosum in diabetic mouse models restored PKG activity and improved erectile function during nerve stimulation. In the same year, another study by Bivalacqua, Burnett, et al. [14] was conducted on B6/129 mouse models with age-related erectile dysfunction. Adenoviral gene transfer of anti-arginase reduced arginase protein and mRNA in the aged mouse penile tissue, enhancing eNOS activity and penile cGMP levels, thereby restoring erectile function. Arginase may be a novel molecular therapeutic target for age-related ED (ED due to vascular factors).

Furthermore, decreased NO levels seem to be linked with individuals experiencing PE. According to Otunctemur [114], after treatment with SSRIs like fluoxetine, paroxetine, and sertraline, NO may help prolong ejaculation time [114]. However, additional research is required to confirm the hypothesis and the role of NO in the physiology of the disease and PE treatment.

Gene therapy targeting the NO system is a new treatment approach being actively researched to improve male sexual function. Although preliminary preclinical research has shown encouraging results, more human-subject clinical research is required to evaluate its efficacy and safety.

Growth Factors

Overview of Growth Factors

Neurological damage due to spinal cord injury, pelvic or retroperitoneal surgery or trauma, and diabetic autonomic neuropathy may cause erectile dysfunction and ejaculatory dysfunction, including retrograde ejaculation, anejaculation, delayed ejaculation, reduced ejaculate volume, and infertility [47].

Therefore, restoring damaged cavernous nerve sites may facilitate the restoration of erectile function and sensory transmission. Some identified growth factors include fibroblast growth factor 21 (FGF21), neurotrophin-3 (NT3), glial cell-derived neurotrophic factor (GDNF), and neurturin (NTN), insulin-like growth factor-1 (IGF-1), brain-derived neurotrophic factor (BDNF), vascular endothelial-derived growth factor (VEGF), and many others [21].

Current Research and Developments in Using Growth Factors for ED, PE, and Other Sexual Dysfunctions

In Yang et al.'s study [160], it was demonstrated that there is a relationship between FGF21 and ED in populations with T2DM and in mouse models with diabetes. Bennett and colleagues reported that gene therapy to deliver NT3 via herpes simplex virus (HSV) intermediates in treating diabetes-induced ED yielded feasible results in animal models [13]. GDNF and NTN are essential for cavernous nerve survival and regeneration. Kato et al. [76] provided NTN factor through HSV vector intermediates in a mouse model of nerve injury-induced ED, resulting in significantly increased intracavernous pressure/arterial pressure compared to the control group [76]. Pu et al. [125] reported study results of gene transfer through adenovirus vector intermediates of IGF-1 into cavernous bodies in diabetic mice, which improved erectile function along with increased expression of IGF-1 mRNA and protein in cavernous tissues [125]. Gholami et al. [53] reported study results evaluating VEGF and BDNF through adeno-associated virus (AAV) intermediates in a mouse model of nerve and blood vessel-related ED associated with high cholesterol [53]. Gene therapy through growth factors is a promising direction that may help restore erectile function when cavernous nerves are damaged.

Ion Channels

Overview of Modulation of K+ Channels

Ion channels such as Ca2+, K+, Cl, and Na+ play an important role in relaxing smooth muscle tissues of the penis and causing penile erection by stabilizing cell membrane potential and reducing nerve and muscle cell sensitivity. Among these, the large-conductance Ca2+-activated potassium channel (BK or Maxi-K) and ATP-sensitive K+ channels (KATP) are studied for treating ED [78].

Current Research and Developments in Using Modulation of K+ Channels for ED, PE and Other Sexual Dysfunctions

In 2006, Arnold Melman and colleagues conducted a phase 1 clinical safety trial by injecting hMaxi-K into the penis to treat ED in 11 patients, showing initial improvement in erectile function (EF) [104]. This was the first human clinical trial of gene therapy for ED; although the results were promising, the lack of a control group prevented conclusive findings. Therefore, further study is needed to assess this approach's safety and effectiveness.

In a study by So et al. [138], naked K(ATP) channel cDNA was injected into aging-related ED mice. The results showed increased intracavernosal pressure (ICP) in response to cavernous nerve stimulation compared to age-matched control mice, associated with elevated levels of KATP channel mRNA (Kir 6.1 and 6.2) in the penis.

Additionally, the piezo-type mechanosensitive ion channel component 2 (PIEZO2) ion channel has been found to play a role in peripheral nerve sensitivity, which could be applied in treating PE using molecular biology and electrophysiology methods [23].

Gene Delivery Systems

Overview of Non-viral Vector and Viral Vectors

Gene therapy involves introducing specific genetic material that can alter cell function into a patient, in order to treat a genetic disease.

Gene replacement, which involves delivering a functional gene to replace a non-functional gene; gene silencing, which involves inactivating a mutated gene that has become toxic to cells; gene addition, which involves overexpressing a "foreign" or exogenous gene to affect cellular function; and gene editing, which involves permanently altering a gene in a patient's genome. These are the four main approaches to gene therapy.

The success and effectiveness of gene therapy partly depend on efficient gene delivery systems into the target tissue or cells. This crucial step is carried out using either viral or non-viral vectors. Viral vector-based gene therapy is carried out by in vivo delivery of the therapeutic gene to the patient using retroviruses-based vectors, adenoviruses (Ads), or adeno-associated viruses (AAVs). Alternatively, the delivery of the therapeutic transgene can be carried out ex-vivo by adding it to the patient's cells which have been removed and cultured outside of the body. The altered cells will then be reintroduced back into the patient [19].

Non-viral vectors include electroporation, chemical transfection, mechanical transduction, and fusion of cas9 with cell-penetrating peptides and other vectors.

Each system has its own advantages and challenges, affecting its applicability in different gene therapies. Viral vectors have a greater immune response and various degrees of alteration, while non-viral vectors have lower immunogenicity. Viral vectors are more efficient in gene delivery and distributing genetic characteristics across multiple cell generations, whereas non-viral vectors often exhibit short-term gene expression due to limited maintenance of delivery vehicles in loaded cells. Another advantage of viral vectors is their easier refinement and production than non-viral vectors. However, using viral vectors also carries risks, such as endogenous viral recombination, cancer development, and immunological reactions.

Current Research and Developments in Using Gene Delivery Systems for ED, PE, and Other Sexual Dysfunctions

Combining gene delivery systems with various gene therapies, especially the CRISPR-Cas9 system, brings significant potential and new treatment directions for many diseases such as β-Thalassemia, sickle cell anemia, cystic fibrosis, HIV infection, Duchenne muscular dystrophy, cancer, etc. [40].

In addition to Casgevy therapy, Lyfgenia was also FDA-approved in December 2023 [44]. Lyfgenia is a cell-based gene therapy that uses a lentiviral vector to genetically modify autologous hematopoietic stem cells to produce HbA^T87Q and is approved for patients aged 12 years and older with sickle cell disease and a history of vaso-occlusive events.

Using CRISPR/Cas9 technology delivered via a lentiviral vector, Zhang et al. knocked out TEAD1 in corpus cavernosum smooth muscle cells derived from diabetic rats with erectile dysfunction and showed that TEAD1 knockout induced phenotypic modulation from the synthetic to the contractile type [171] Kato et al. [76] used herpes simplex vector to deliver neurturin to treat ED caused by cavernous nerve injury [76].

Combining Cellular Regenerative and Gene Therapy

Current research findings on the synergies between cellular regenerative and gene therapy in male sexual dysfunction have provided fascinating insights into novel treatment approaches for ED. Combining the regenerative potential of cell therapy with gene therapy offers a new frontier for research into treating male sexual dysfunctions. A study by Lee et al. [84] demonstrated the use of a gene expression system driven by a specific promoter for gene therapy in rats with cholesterol-induced ED, showcasing the potential of genetic interventions in treating vasculogenic ED [84]. A study by Hakim et al. [62] highlighted the emergence of novel treatment approaches for ED, aiming at curing and restoring the condition's underlying causes [62]. This emphasis on cure aligns with the current trend toward combining cellular regenerative and gene therapy in tackling male sexual dysfunction.

Additionally, Soebadi et al. [139] showcased the potential of stem cells as a curative treatment for ED through preclinical studies and early-phase clinical trials, indicating a promising direction for integrating cellular regenerative therapies into the treatment landscape of male sexual dysfunction. Moreover, the research by La Favor et al. [80] on hydrogen sulfide therapy reversing erectile dysfunction in Western diet-fed mice highlights the importance of innovative therapeutic approaches in addressing sexual dysfunctions [80]. This study underscores the potential of novel therapies, such as hydrogen sulfide treatment, to effectively combat the physiological challenges contributing to male sexual dysfunction.

A study by Liu et al. demonstrated the association between ED and impaired endothelial function and disruption of the VEGF signaling pathway. The study also promoted the recovery of erectile function by enhancing endothelial function and increasing smooth muscle content using ADSCs modified by the VEGF gene, showing their superiority in improving erectile function in DMED rats compared to unmodified ADSCs [90]. However, transgenic technology has limited clinical application due to the risk of integrating exogenous genes into the host genome. EPCs can produce mature endothelial cells both in vitro and in vivo, and they are crucial for the regeneration of damaged blood vessels in vivo [153]. Paracrine stromal cell-derived factor-1 (SDF-1) from ADSCs was shown to enhance the "value-added" differentiation of EPCs and enhance cavernous smooth muscle and nNOS expression [158].

Additionally, SDF-1 demonstrated a synergistic effect of the combined transplantation of ADSCs and EPCs on the repair of the endothelial function. This approach presented as significantly more therapeutic effect than either treatment alone, opening up new avenues of treatment for patients with type 2 diabetes [158]. Luo and colleagues found that shNLRP3 lentivirus can protect the paracrine function of ADSCs. They enhanced their ability to improve diabetic ED in a hyperglycemic state by reducing cavernous endothelial dysfunction and smooth muscle cell injury through anti-apoptotic and anti-ROS deposition mechanisms [98]. Furthermore, overexpression or knockdown of certain genes, such as NRIP1 and HIF 1α in stem cells, increased their response to a hyperglycemic hypoxic environment [98].

Overall, the current research findings on the synergies between cellular regenerative and gene therapy provide a glimpse into the promising future of male sexual dysfunction treatment. By integrating these two therapeutic approaches, researchers are moving closer to developing comprehensive and effective strategies to enhance male sexual health and function.

Ethical and Legal Considerations

Ethical considerations are paramount in the development and application of any innovative therapy. The field of cellular regenerative and gene therapy for male sexual dysfunction involves a complex interplay of ethical and legal considerations.

With the focus often on efficacy and safety, the ethical implications of cellular regenerative and gene therapies cannot be overlooked. Stem cell therapy raises various bioethical, legal, and societal concerns that necessitate a thoughtful approach by researchers, legal authorities, and social activists [106].

As researchers focus more on the molecular mechanisms and gene expression systems related to sexual dysfunction, it becomes imperative to address the ethical dimensions of using these technologies in clinical settings as well. For instance, the study on antiretroviral-free HIV-1 remission after allogeneic stem cell transplantation delves into ethical implications by closely monitoring the achieved viral remission, highlighting the importance of ethical implications of such therapies [65]. Furthermore, the paper on nephropathic cystinosis in adults emphasizes oral cysteamine therapy's natural history and effects [50]. While not directly related to male sexual dysfunction, this study underscores the significance of long-term therapy in mitigating complications, which could be a vital consideration in the context of regenerative therapies for sexual dysfunction.

Patients undergoing these innovative treatments must be fully informed about the procedures, potential risks, benefits, and alternatives. Studies emphasize the importance of patient education and awareness to enable individuals to make well-informed decisions regarding their treatment options [28]. This sheds light on the importance of informed consent and patient awareness before undertaking any therapeutic intervention, aligning with the ethical considerations in the field.

Moreover, the future of male infertility management and assisted reproduction technology paper alludes to the need for careful diagnosis, patient education, and obtaining informed consent before commencing treatment [107]. Studies have emphasized the need for clear guidelines to govern the application of stem cells and gene therapies in clinical practice for cellular regenerative and gene therapies for male sexual dysfunction [61], where regulatory frameworks and international standards come into play to ensure ethical practices and patient safety. At the time of this publication, the NHS "Clinical Commissioning Policy" for Erectile dysfunction [31] referred to the study by Karakus and Burnett and state that, due to insufficient data to support long-term safety and efficacy of all novel therapies for sexual dysfunction (apart from penile implants), including intracavernosal stem cell therapies, shockwave therapy, and penile vascular surgery should be regarded as investigational [75].

On another note, there is currently a lack of global uniformity in the regulations governing cell and gene therapy reimbursement and pricing. Regulatory barriers can, in practice, slow down technological advancements and prevent novel medications from entering the market. As an example, while Americans and Germans have access to 87% and 63% of new drugs, respectively, South Koreans have access to only 35% of new drugs on average [121]. To support the expansion of the market for gene and cell therapies, authorities have attempted to construct some forward-looking regulatory guidelines to lay the ground for regulatory harmonization. Attempts toward coordinating pricing and reimbursement (P&R) and regulatory processes have also initiated various forms of harmonizing movements and "horizon-scanning" initiatives [85].

In conclusion, the literature review reveals a multifaceted landscape where ethical implications, patient awareness, and regulatory frameworks converge in the realm of cellular regenerative and gene therapy for male sexual dysfunction.

Challenges and Future Directions

Challenges in Implementing Cellular Regenerative and Gene Therapies

Although cellular regenerative and gene therapies have shown promise in identifying and treating various diseases, they also carry risks and challenges, including unintended mutations, tumor formation, long-term health impacts on patients, and cost-effectiveness.

One of the significant challenges is the risk of unintended mutations or cancer cell contamination in cancer patients [58, 59]. These methods may have short-term benefits, but their long-term usefulness and safety for future patient health are unknown. Gene editing could introduce unpredictable genetic changes, potentially impacting future generations. This raises concerns about the lasting consequences of gene therapies and regenerative medicine for human health.

Another risk is the occurrence of adverse immune reactions during stem cell transplantation and gene editing. To mitigate negative immune reactions and enhance their safety, biocompatible materials combined with gene editing techniques such as CRISPR/Cas9 aim to ensure biological compatibility, avoiding immune reactions, inflammation, or cell toxicity [39]. Furthermore, bioengineered materials can be surface-modified and formulated with immune modulators, helping to limit immune cell activation and prevent adverse immune reactions [43].

Additionally, biocompatible materials can only target certain types of cells or specific tissues for gene editing. Therefore, precise targeting techniques are required to minimize off-target effects, allowing biocompatible materials to detect and attach to target cells or tissues [174].

Treatment costs are also a consideration. Gene editing and regenerative medicine techniques are modern methods that utilize advanced technologies and machinery, making the implementation costs relatively high. Therefore, finding ways to reduce costs is crucial, ensuring that more people can access these therapies [35].

Future Technological Advancements and Innovations

Nanomedicine Targeted Drug Delivery

One significant and promising advancement for the future application in treating male sexual disorders is nanotechnology [94]. Nanotechnology can precisely and efficiently deliver drugs to the necessary sites in the body, minimizing side effects and enhancing treatment efficacy. Hosny and Aljaeid used nanoparticles containing sildenafil in the treatment of ED in their study on rabbit models, reported higher bioavailability and sustained action of sildenafil [66]. In the study by Cheng et al. [24], the Neuregulin-1 gene was transferred into ADSCs using superparamagnetic iron oxide nanoparticles to further enhance the therapeutic efficacy of ADSCs by locally retaining ADSCs in the corpus cavernosum and exerting the effects of stem cell therapy on ED patients.

Dapoxetine is heavily metabolized in the liver, resulting in poor oral bioavailability. In Fouad et al.'s study [48], an instantly-dispersible nanocarrier powder system (IDNPs) was developed to deliver dapoxetine intranasally in rabbit models [48]. The improved permeation and bioavailability suggest that IDNPs could be a promising model for delivering drugs through the intranasal route, bypassing first-pass hepatic metabolism.

Personalized Therapies Based on Genetic Profiling

Genetic profiling helps clinicians understand the genetic makeup of each individual and design tailored treatment strategies for diagnosis and treatment. In recent years, personalized medicine combined with nanotechnology has improved biological availability and provided better compatibility, resulting in maximum treatment efficacy with controlled drug release mechanisms to ensure that the drug reaches the target accurately and at the right time. Both nanotechnology and personalized medicine based on genetic profiling are considered promising medical directions [4].

Integration of AI and Machine Learning

Recent studies on artificial intelligence (AI) and machine learning have shown promising potential in optimizing treatment processes, predicting occurring reactions, and selecting effective treatment methods to support medical research. However, these systems are developed based on a large amount of high-quality initial data to ensure the accuracy and reliability of predictions. When combined with gene editing, regenerative medicine, and precision medicine, allowing personalized treatment methods based on genetic profiling helps optimize treatment outcomes and minimize the risk of unintended adverse effects [36]. Furthermore, in the field of reproductive support, AI and machine learning assist in sperm selection for IVF/

ICSI, oocyte collection, gamete quality assessment, assisting protocols for controlled ovarian hyperstimulation, donor matching, or selecting and ranking embryos for transfer and cryopreservation [170]. Additionally, clear regulations and assessment procedures are necessary to ensure these systems are developed and implemented safely and reliably [129].

Conclusion

Although male sexual dysfunction is becoming increasingly prevalent, current treatment methods still have many limitations, so finding new treatment methods is necessary. Currently, regenerative medicine and gene editing therapies are promising new treatment avenues for their potential applications in treating various diseases, including male sexual dysfunction.

Recent studies suggest that SCT, PRP therapy, protein therapy, and Li-ESWT may contribute to tissue regeneration and improvements in male sexual function. These approaches may offer new therapeutic opportunities for conditions such as ED and PE, although further clinical validation is required before their broader clinical application.

Additionally, gene therapy is gaining popularity, with gene editing methods like CRISPR/CAS9 or targeting the nitrergic system, growth factors, K+ channels, and gene delivery systems being utilized to modify gene variants related to male sexual dysfunction. This offers new potential for treating and preventing these conditions. Furthermore, the proposed combination of cellular regeneration and gene therapy may provide significant benefits by increasing treatment efficacy and improving patient outcomes.

Although results from initial experiments on animal models and preliminary clinical trials show positive outcomes, integrating regenerative medicine and gene therapy also presents many challenges and potential risks. From regulatory barriers to social and ethical issues and legal regulations to the risk of off-target mutations, adverse immune reactions, cancer development, long-term health impacts, complex technical machinery, and expensive treatment costs, all must be carefully controlled and further researched before clinical application.

Recently, with advances in nanotechnology, personalized medicine based on genetic profiles, and the integration of artificial intelligence and machine learning, some of these challenges can be addressed, and new potential for the treatment of male sexual dysfunction can be opened up.

In conclusion, despite the remaining challenges and risks, cellular regeneration and gene therapy approaches are opening new prospects for improving the quality of life for patients with male sexual dysfunctions. Continued research and collaboration, as well as ensuring ethics in the development process, are essential to ensure that these methods can become a reality in the near future.

References

1. Abidu-Figueiredo M, Ribeiro IC, Chagas MA, Cardoso LE, Costa WS, Sampaio FJ. The penis in diabetes: structural analysis of connective tissue and smooth muscle alterations in a rabbit model. BJU Int. 2011;108(3):400–4. https://doi.org/10.1111/j.1464-410X.2010.09944.x.
2. Ahmed TA, El-Badri N. Pericytes: the role of multipotent stem cells in vascular maintenance and regenerative medicine. Adv Exp Med Biol. 2018;1079:69–86. https://doi.org/10.1007/5584_2017_138.
3. Alfaleh MA, Alsaab HO, Mahmoud AB, Alkayyal AA, Jones ML, Mahler SM, Hashem AM. Phage display derived monoclonal antibodies: from bench to bedside. Front Immunol. 2020;11:1986. https://doi.org/10.3389/fimmu.2020.01986.
4. Alghamdi MA, Fallica AN, Virzì N, Kesharwani P, Pittalà V, Greish K. The promise of nanotechnology in personalized medicine. J Pers Med. 2022;12(5) https://doi.org/10.3390/jpm12050673.
5. Alkhayal S, Lourdes M. PO-01–091 Platelet rich plasma penile rejuvenation as a treatment for erectile dysfunction: an update. J Sex Med. 2019;16(5):S71.
6. Alshuaibi M, Zugail AS, Lombion S, Beley S. New protocol in the treatment of Peyronie's disease by combining platelet-rich plasma, percutaneous needle tunneling, and penile modeling: preliminary results. Fr J Urol. 2024;34(1):102526. https://doi.org/10.1016/j.purol.2023.09.013.
7. Alwaal A, Zaid UB, Lin CS, Lue TF. Stem cell treatment of erectile dysfunction. Adv Drug Deliv Rev. 2015;82–83:137–44. https://doi.org/10.1016/j.addr.2014.11.012.
8. Anderson D, Laforge J, Ross MM, Vanlangendonck R, Hasoon J, Viswanath O, Kaye AD, Urits I. Male sexual dysfunction. Health Psychol Res. 2022;10(3):37533. https://doi.org/10.52965/001c.37533.
9. Arda E, Ay A, Akdere H, Akdeniz E. The association of Intron 4 VNTR and Glu298Asp polymorphisms of the nitric oxide synthetase 3 gene and vasculogenic erectile dysfunction in Turkish men. Syst Biol Reprod Med. 2019;65(5):383–9. https://doi.org/10.1080/19396368.2019.1601792.
10. Argiolas A, Argiolas FM, Argiolas G, Melis MR. Erectile dysfunction: treatments, advances and new therapeutic strategies. Brain Sci. 2023;13(5) https://doi.org/10.3390/brainsci13050802.
11. Bai S, Li MZ, Wan YY, Hu XC, Liu YX, Tong XH, Guo TH, Zong L, Liu R, Zhao YQ, Xiang P, Xu B, Jiang XH. Association between MTHFR c.677C>T variant and erectile dysfunction among males attending fertility clinic. Asian J Androl. 2023;26(1):41–5. https://doi.org/10.4103/aja202335.
12. Belk JW, Kraeutler MJ, Houck DA, Goodrich JA, Dragoo JL, McCarty EC. Platelet-rich plasma versus hyaluronic acid for knee osteoarthritis: a systematic review and meta-analysis of randomized controlled trials. Am J Sports Med. 2021;49(1):249–60. https://doi.org/10.1177/0363546520909397.
13. Bennett NE, Kim JH, Wolfe DP, Sasaki K, Yoshimura N, Goins WF, Huang S, Nelson JB, de Groat WC, Glorioso JC, Chancellor MB. Improvement in erectile dysfunction after neurotrophic factor gene therapy in diabetic rats. J Urol. 2005;173(5):1820–4. https://doi.org/10.1097/01.ju.0000158056.66236.1f.
14. Bivalacqua TJ, Burnett AL, Hellstrom WJ, Champion HC. Overexpression of arginase in the aged mouse penis impairs erectile function and decreases eNOS activity: influence of in vivo gene therapy of anti-arginase. Am J Physiol Heart Circ Physiol. 2007;292(3):H1340–51. https://doi.org/10.1152/ajpheart.00121.2005.
15. Bivalacqua TJ, Kendirci M, Champion HC, Hellstrom WJ, Andersson KE, Hedlund P. Dysregulation of cGMP-dependent protein kinase 1 (PKG-1) impairs erectile function in diabetic rats: influence of in vivo gene therapy of PKG1alpha. BJU Int. 2007;99(6):1488–94. https://doi.org/10.1111/j.1464-410X.2007.06794.x.

16. Bivalacqua TJ, Musicki B, Usta MF, Champion HC, Kadowitz PJ, Burnett AL, Hellstrom WJ. Endothelial nitric oxide synthase gene therapy for erectile dysfunction. Curr Pharm Des. 2005;11(31):4059–67. https://doi.org/10.2174/138161205774913345.
17. Bocchino AC, Pezzoli M, Martínez-Salamanca JI, Russo GI, Lo Giudice A, Cocci A. Low-intensity extracorporeal shock wave therapy for erectile dysfunction: myths and realities. Investig Clin Urol. 2023;64(2):118–25. https://doi.org/10.4111/icu.20220327.
18. Brown C, McKee C, Bakshi S, Walker K, Hakman E, Halassy S, Svinarich D, Dodds R, Govind CK, Chaudhry GR. Mesenchymal stem cells: cell therapy and regeneration potential. J Tissue Eng Regen Med. 2019;13(9):1738–55. https://doi.org/10.1002/term.2914.
19. Bulcha JT, Wang Y, Ma H, Tai PWL, Gao G. Viral vector platforms within the gene therapy landscape. Signal Transduct Target Ther. 2021;6(1):53. https://doi.org/10.1038/s41392-021-00487-6.
20. Burnett AL, Nehra A, Breau RH, Culkin DJ, Faraday MM, Hakim LS, Heidelbaugh J, Khera M, McVary KT, Miner MM, Nelson CJ, Sadeghi-Nejad H, Seftel AD, Shindel AW. Erectile dysfunction: AUA guideline. J Urol. 2018;200(3):633–41. https://doi.org/10.1016/j.juro.2018.05.004.
21. Campbell JD, Burnett AL. Neuroprotective and nerve regenerative approaches for treatment of erectile dysfunction after cavernous nerve injury. Int J Mol Sci. 2017;18(8) https://doi.org/10.3390/ijms18081794.
22. Chen X, Yang Q, Xie Y, Deng C, Liu G, Zhang X. Comparative study of different transplantation methods of adipose tissue-derived stem cells in the treatment of erectile dysfunction caused by cavernous nerve injury. Andrologia. 2021;53(4):e13950. https://doi.org/10.1111/and.13950.
23. Chen Z, Yuan M, Ma Z, Wen J, Wang X, Zhao M, Liu J, Zhang X, Zhao S, Guo L. Significance of piezo-type mechanosensitive ion channel component 2 in premature ejaculation: an animal study. Andrology. 2020;8(5):1347–59. https://doi.org/10.1111/andr.12779.
24. Cheng J, Zheng Z, Tang W, Shao J, Jiang H, Lin H. A new strategy for stem cells therapy for erectile dysfunction: adipose-derived stem cells transfect Neuregulin-1 gene through superparamagnetic iron oxide nanoparticles. Investig Clin Urol. 2022;63(3):359–67. https://doi.org/10.4111/icu.20220016.
25. Choe S, Kalmanek E, Bond C, Harrington DA, Stupp SI, McVary KT, Podlasek CA. Optimization of sonic hedgehog delivery to the penis from self-assembling nanofiber hydrogels to preserve penile morphology after cavernous nerve injury. Nanomedicine. 2019;20:102033. https://doi.org/10.1016/j.nano.2019.102033.
26. Chung DY, Ryu JK, Yin GN. Regenerative therapies as a potential treatment of erectile dysfunction. Investig Clin Urol. 2023;64(4):312–24. https://doi.org/10.4111/icu.20230104.
27. Chung DY, Song KM, Choi MJ, Limanjaya A, Ghatak K, Ock J, Yin GN, Hong CH, Hong SS, Suh JK, Ryu JK. Neutralizing antibody to proNGF rescues erectile function by regulating the expression of neurotrophic and angiogenic factors in a mouse model of cavernous nerve injury. Andrology. 2021;9(1):329–41. https://doi.org/10.1111/andr.12873.
28. Chung E. Regenerative technology to restore and preserve erectile function in men following prostate cancer treatment: evidence for penile rehabilitation in the context of prostate cancer survivorship. Ther Adv Urol. 2021;13:17562872211026421. https://doi.org/10.1177/17562872211026421.
29. Ciccocioppo R, Cantore A, Chaimov D, Orlando G. Regenerative medicine: the red planet for clinicians. Intern Emerg Med. 2019;14(6):911–21. https://doi.org/10.1007/s11739-019-02126-z.
30. Citorik RJ, Mimee M, Lu TK. Sequence-specific antimicrobials using efficiently delivered RNA-guided nucleases. Nat Biotechnol. 2014;32(11):1141–5. https://doi.org/10.1038/nbt.3011.
31. Consultant in Public Health, N. M. a. L. Clinical Commissioning Policy: Erectile Dysfunction—secondary care referral. (CMICB_Clin110), 2024. NHS Retrieved from https://www.wirralccg.nhs.uk/media/j4pcd1gu/pol-clin110-erectiledys-v1-final.pdf#page=1.07.

32. Culha MG, Erkan E, Cay T, Yücetaş U. The effect of platelet-rich plasma on Peyronie's disease in Rat Model. Urol Int. 2019;102(2):218–23. https://doi.org/10.1159/000492755.
33. Das ND, Yin GN, Choi MJ, Song KM, Park JM, Limanjaya A, Ghatak K, Minh NN, Ock J, Park SH, Kim HM, Ryu JK, Suh JK. Effectiveness of intracavernous delivery of recombinant human hepatocyte growth factor on erectile function in the Streptozotocin-induced diabetic mouse. J Sex Med. 2016;13(11):1618–28. https://doi.org/10.1016/j.jsxm.2016.09.017.
34. Di Mauro M, Russo GI, Della Camera PA, Di Maida F, Cito G, Mondaini N, Capece M, Falcone M, Sessa F, Mari A, Campi R, Sabini C, Serni S, Gacci M, Minervini A, Carini M, Cimino S, Morelli G, Cocci A. Extracorporeal shock wave therapy in Peyronie's disease: clinical efficacy and safety from a single-arm observational study. World J Mens Health. 2019;37(3):339–46. https://doi.org/10.5534/wjmh.180100.
35. Di Minno G, Miesbach W, Castaman G, Peyvandi F. Next-generation strategies to improve safety and efficacy of adeno-associated virus-based gene therapy for hemophilia: lessons from clinical trials in other gene therapies. Haematologica. 2024; https://doi.org/10.3324/haematol.2023.284622.
36. Dixit S, Kumar A, Srinivasan K, Vincent P, Ramu Krishnan N. Advancing genome editing with artificial intelligence: opportunities, challenges, and future directions. Front Bioeng Biotechnol. 2023;11:1335901. https://doi.org/10.3389/fbioe.2023.1335901.
37. Dou L, Matz EL, Gu X, Shu F, Paxton J, Song J, Yoo J, Atala A, Jackson J, Zhang Y. Non-invasive cell tracking with brighter and Red-Transferred Luciferase for potential application in stem cell therapy. Cell Transplant. 2019;28(12):1542–51. https://doi.org/10.1177/0963689719885078.
38. Doudna JA. The promise and challenge of therapeutic genome editing. Nature. 2020;578(7794):229–36. https://doi.org/10.1038/s41586-020-1978-5.
39. Dubey AK, Kumar Gupta V, Kujawska M, Orive G, Kim NY, Li CZ, Kumar Mishra Y, Kaushik A. Exploring nano-enabled CRISPR-Cas-powered strategies for efficient diagnostics and treatment of infectious diseases. J Nanostructure Chem. 2022;12(5):833–64. https://doi.org/10.1007/s40097-022-00472-7.
40. Dubey AK, Mostafavi E. Biomaterials-mediated CRISPR/Cas9 delivery: recent challenges and opportunities in gene therapy. Front Chem. 2023;11:1259435. https://doi.org/10.3389/fchem.2023.1259435.
41. Epifanova MV, Gvasalia BR, Durashov MA, Artemenko SA. Platelet-rich plasma therapy for male sexual dysfunction: myth or reality? Sex Med Rev. 2020;8(1):106–13. https://doi.org/10.1016/j.sxmr.2019.02.002.
42. Eryilmaz R, Kaplan Ş, Aslan R, Demir M, Taken K. Comparison of focused and unfocused ESWT in treatment of erectile dysfunction. Aging Male. 2020;23(3):206–9. https://doi.org/10.1080/13685538.2019.1610377.
43. Ewaisha R, Anderson KS. Immunogenicity of CRISPR therapeutics-critical considerations for clinical translation. Front Bioeng Biotechnol. 2023;11:1138596. https://doi.org/10.3389/fbioe.2023.1138596.
44. FDA. FDA approves first gene therapies to treat patients with Sickle cell disease, 2023. https://www.fda.gov/news-events/press-announcements/fda-approves-first-gene-therapies-treat--patients-sickle-cell-disease.
45. Feng H, Liu Q, Deng Z, Li H, Zhang H, Song J, Liu X, Liu J, Wen B, Wang T. Human umbilical cord mesenchymal stem cells ameliorate erectile dysfunction in rats with diabetes mellitus through the attenuation of ferroptosis. Stem Cell Res Ther. 2022;13(1):450. https://doi.org/10.1186/s13287-022-03147-w.
46. Fode M, Hatzichristodoulou G, Serefoglu EC, Verze P, Albersen M. Low-intensity shockwave therapy for erectile dysfunction: is the evidence strong enough? Nat Rev Urol. 2017;14(10):593–606. https://doi.org/10.1038/nrurol.2017.119.
47. Fode M, Krogh-Jespersen S, Brackett NL, Ohl DA, Lynne CM, Sønksen J. Male sexual dysfunction and infertility associated with neurological disorders. Asian J Androl. 2012;14:61–68. https://doi.org/10.1038/aja.2011.70.

48. Fouad SA, Shamma RN, Basalious EB, El-Nabarawi MM, Tayel SA. Novel instantly-dispersible nanocarrier powder system (IDNPs) for intranasal delivery of dapoxetine hydrochloride: in-vitro optimization, ex-vivo permeation studies, and in-vivo evaluation. Drug Dev Ind Pharm. 2018;44(9):1443–50. https://doi.org/10.1080/03639045.2018.1459675.
49. Frey A, Sønksen J, Fode M. Low-intensity extracorporeal shockwave therapy in the treatment of postprostatectomy erectile dysfunction: a pilot study. Scand J Urol. 2016;50(2):123–7. https://doi.org/10.3109/21681805.2015.1100675.
50. Gahl WA, Balog JZ, Kleta R. Nephropathic cystinosis in adults: natural history and effects of oral cysteamine therapy. Ann Intern Med. 2007;147(4):242–50. https://doi.org/10.7326/0003-4819-147-4-200708210-00006.
51. Galhom RA, Korayem HE, Ibrahim MA, Abd-Eltawab Tammam A, Khalifa MM, Rashwan EK, Al Badawi MH. Urine-derived stem cells versus their lysate in ameliorating erectile dysfunction in a Rat Model of type 2 diabetes. Front Physiol. 2022;13:854949. https://doi.org/10.3389/fphys.2022.854949.
52. Ghatak K, Yin GN, Choi MJ, Limanjaya A, Minh NN, Ock J, Song KM, Kang DH, Kwon YG, Kim HM, Ryu JK, Suh JK. Dickkopf2 rescues erectile function by enhancing penile neurovascular regeneration in a mouse model of cavernous nerve injury. Sci Rep. 2017;7(1):17819. https://doi.org/10.1038/s41598-017-17862-5.
53. Gholami SS, Rogers R, Chang J, Ho HC, Grazziottin T, Lin CS, Lue TF. The effect of vascular endothelial growth factor and adeno-associated virus mediated brain derived neurotrophic factor on neurogenic and vasculogenic erectile dysfunction induced by hyperlipidemia. J Urol. 2003;169(4):1577–81. https://doi.org/10.1097/01.ju.0000055120.73261.76.
54. Giusti I, D'Ascenzo S, Macchiarelli G, Dolo V. In vitro evidence supporting applications of platelet derivatives in regenerative medicine. Blood Transfus. 2020;18(2):117–29. https://doi.org/10.2450/2019.0164-19.
55. Golchin A, Chatziparasidou A, Ranjbarvan P, Niknam Z, Ardeshirylajimi A. Embryonic stem cells in clinical trials: current overview of developments and challenges. Adv Exp Med Biol. 2021;1312:19–37. https://doi.org/10.1007/5584_2020_592.
56. Gruenwald I, Appel B, Kitrey ND, Vardi Y. Shockwave treatment of erectile dysfunction. Ther Adv Urol. 2013;5(2):95–9. https://doi.org/10.1177/1756287212470696.
57. Gu X, Thakker PU, Matz EL, Terlecki RP, Marini FC, Allickson JG, Lue TF, Lin G, Atala A, Yoo JJ, Zhang Y, Jackson JD. Dynamic changes in erectile function and histological architecture after intracorporal injection of human placental stem cells in a pelvic neurovascular injury Rat Model. J Sex Med. 2020;17(3):400–11. https://doi.org/10.1016/j.jsxm.2019.12.002.
58. Gul M, Hildorf S, Dong L, Thorup J, Hoffmann ER, Jensen CFS, Sønksen J, Cortes D, Fedder J, Andersen CY, Goossens E. Review of injection techniques for spermatogonial stem cell transplantation. Hum Reprod Update. 2020;26(3):368–91. https://doi.org/10.1093/humupd/dmaa003.
59. Guo C, Ma X, Gao F, Guo Y. Off-target effects in CRISPR/Cas9 gene editing. Front Bioeng Biotechnol. 2023;11:1143157. https://doi.org/10.3389/fbioe.2023.1143157.
60. Gupta S, Paliczak A, Delgado D. Evidence-based indications of platelet-rich plasma therapy. Expert Rev Hematol. 2021;14(1):97–108. https://doi.org/10.1080/17474086.2021.1860002.
61. Gur S, Abdel-Mageed AB, Sikka SC, Hellstrom WJG. Advances in stem cell therapy for erectile dysfunction. Expert Opin Biol Ther. 2018;18(11):1137–50. https://doi.org/10.1080/14712598.2018.1534955.
62. Hakim L, Van der Aa F, Bivalacqua TJ, Hedlund P, Albersen M. Emerging tools for erectile dysfunction: a role for regenerative medicine. Nat Rev Urol. 2012;9(9):520–36. https://doi.org/10.1038/nrurol.2012.143.
63. Hansen ST, Lund M, Ostergaard LD, Lund L. Role of regenerative therapies on erectile dysfunction after radical prostatectomy. Int J Impot Res. 2021;33(4):488–96. https://doi.org/10.1038/s41443-020-00406-3.

64. He L, Yu T, Xiao Y, Huang Y, Guan Y, Zhao F, Ma L. Co-overexpression of VEGF and Smad7 improved the therapeutic effects of adipose-derived stem cells on neurogenic erectile dysfunction in the rat model. Andrologia. 2022;54(10):e14538. https://doi.org/10.1111/and.14538.
65. Henrich TJ, Hanhauser E, Marty FM, Sirignano MN, Keating S, Lee TH, Robles YP, Davis BT, Li JZ, Heisey A, Hill AL, Busch MP, Armand P, Soiffer RJ, Altfeld M, Kuritzkes DR. Antiretroviral-free HIV-1 remission and viral rebound after allogeneic stem cell transplantation: report of 2 cases. Ann Intern Med. 2014;161(5):319–27. https://doi.org/10.7326/m14-1027.
66. Hosny KM, Aljaeid BM. Sildenafil citrate as oral solid lipid nanoparticles: a novel formula with higher bioavailability and sustained action for treatment of erectile dysfunction. Expert Opin Drug Deliv. 2014;11(7):1015–22. https://doi.org/10.1517/17425247.2014.912212.
67. Hsieh PS, Bochinski DJ, Lin GT, Nunes L, Lin CS, Lue TF. The effect of vascular endothelial growth factor and brain-derived neurotrophic factor on cavernosal nerve regeneration in a nerve-crush rat model. BJU Int. 2003;92(4):470–5. https://doi.org/10.1046/j.1464-410x.2003.04373.x.
68. Iaquinta MR, Mazzoni E, Bononi I, Rotondo JC, Mazziotta C, Montesi M, Sprio S, Tampieri A, Tognon M, Martini F. Adult stem cells for bone regeneration and repair. Front Cell Dev Biol. 2019;7:268. https://doi.org/10.3389/fcell.2019.00268.
69. Irfan M, Hussain NHN, Noor NM, Mohamed M, Sidi H, Ismail SB. Epidemiology of male sexual dysfunction in Asian and European regions: a systematic review. Am J Mens Health. 2020;14(4):1557988320937200. https://doi.org/10.1177/1557988320937200.
70. Ishino Y, Shinagawa H, Makino K, Amemura M, Nakata A. Nucleotide sequence of the iap gene, responsible for alkaline phosphatase isozyme conversion in Escherichia coli, and identification of the gene product. J Bacteriol. 1987;169(12):5429–33. https://doi.org/10.1128/jb.169.12.5429-5433.1987.
71. Jeong HC, Jeon SH, Qun ZG, Kim KS, Choi SW, Bashraheel F, Bae WJ, Kim SJ, Cho HJ, Ha US, Hong SH, Lee JY, Moon DG, Kim SW. Effects of next-generation low-energy extracorporeal shockwave therapy on erectile dysfunction in an animal model of diabetes. World J Mens Health. 2017;35(3):186–95. https://doi.org/10.5534/wjmh.17024.
72. Jin HR, Kim WJ, Song JS, Piao S, Choi MJ, Tumurbaatar M, Shin SH, Yin GN, Koh GY, Ryu JK, Suh JK. Intracavernous delivery of a designed angiopoietin-1 variant rescues erectile function by enhancing endothelial regeneration in the streptozotocin-induced diabetic mouse. Diabetes. 2011;60(3):969–80. https://doi.org/10.2337/db10-0354.
73. Jin HR, Kim WJ, Song JS, Piao S, Tumurbaatar M, Shin SH, Choi MJ, Tuvshintur B, Song KM, Kwon MH, Yin GN, Koh GY, Ryu JK, Suh JK. Intracavernous delivery of synthetic angiopoietin-1 protein as a novel therapeutic strategy for erectile dysfunction in the type II diabetic db/db mouse. J Sex Med. 2010;7(11):3635–46. https://doi.org/10.1111/j.1743-6109.2010.01925.x.
74. Kang J, Song Y, Zhang Z, Wang S, Lu Y, Liu X. Identification of key microRNAs in diabetes mellitus erectile dysfunction rats with stem cell therapy by bioinformatic analysis of deep sequencing data. World J Mens Health. 2022;40(4):663–77. https://doi.org/10.5534/wjmh.210147.
75. Karakus S, Burnett AL. The medical and surgical treatment of erectile dysfunction: a review and update. Can J Urol. 2020;27(S3):28–35.
76. Kato R, Wolfe D, Coyle CH, Wechuck JB, Tyagi P, Tsukamoto T, Nelson JB, Glorioso JC, Chancellor MB, Yoshimura N. Herpes simplex virus vector-mediated delivery of neurturin rescues erectile dysfunction of cavernous nerve injury. Gene Ther. 2009;16(1):26–33. https://doi.org/10.1038/gt.2008.132.
77. Khan HL, Bhatti S, Abbas S, Khan YL, Gonzalez RMM, Aslamkhan M, Gonzalez GR, Aydin HH. Serotonin transporter (5-HTTLPR) genotypes and trinucleotide repeats of androgen receptor exert a combinatorial effect on hormonal milieu in patients with lifelong premature ejaculation. Andrology. 2018;6(6):916–26. https://doi.org/10.1111/andr.12518.
78. Király I, Pataricza J, Bajory Z, Simonsen U, Varro A, Papp JG, Pajor L, Kun A. Involvement of large-conductance Ca(2+) -activated K(+) channels in both nitric oxide and endothelium-derived hyperpolarization-type relaxation in human penile small arteries. Basic Clin Pharmacol Toxicol. 2013;113(1):19–24. https://doi.org/10.1111/bcpt.12059.

79. Kwon MH, Ryu JK, Kim WJ, Jin HR, Song KM, Kwon KD, Batbold D, Yin GN, Koh GY, Suh JK. Effect of intracavernous administration of angiopoietin-4 on erectile function in the streptozotocin-induced diabetic mouse. J Sex Med. 2013;10(12):2912–27. https://doi.org/10.1111/jsm.12278.
80. La Favor J, Rhein P, Pierre C, Azeez T, Burnett A. (090) Hydrogen Sulfide therapy stimulates cellular antioxidant defense and reverses erectile dysfunction in Western Diet-fed Mice. J Sex Med. 2023;20(Supplement_1) https://doi.org/10.1093/jsxmed/qdad060.085.
81. Lander EB, Berman MH, See JR. Stromal Vascular Fraction Combined with Shock Wave for the Treatment of Peyronie's Disease. Plast Reconstr Surg Glob Open. 2016;4(3):e631. https://doi.org/10.1097/GOX.0000000000000622.
82. Lau JL, Dunn MK. Therapeutic peptides: historical perspectives, current development trends, and future directions. Bioorg Med Chem. 2018;26(10):2700–7. https://doi.org/10.1016/j.bmc.2017.06.052.
83. Leader B, Baca QJ, Golan DE. Protein therapeutics: a summary and pharmacological classification. Nat Rev Drug Discov. 2008;7(1):21–39. https://doi.org/10.1038/nrd2399.
84. Lee M, Ryu JK, Piao S, Choi MJ, Kim HA, Zhang LW, Shin HY, Jung HI, Kim IH, Kim SW, Suh JK. Efficient gene expression system using the RTP801 promoter in the corpus cavernosum of high-cholesterol diet-induced erectile dysfunction rats for gene therapy. J Sex Med. 2008;5(6):1355–64. https://doi.org/10.1111/j.1743-6109.2008.00771.x.
85. Lee S, Lee JH. Cell and gene therapy regulatory, pricing, and reimbursement framework: with a focus on South Korea and the EU. Front Public Health. 2023;11:1109873. https://doi.org/10.3389/fpubh.2023.1109873.
86. Leone L, Raffa S, Vetrano M, Ranieri D, Malisan F, Scrofani C, Vulpiani MC, Ferretti A, Torrisi MR, Visco V. Extracorporeal Shock Wave Treatment (ESWT) enhances the in vitro-induced differentiation of human tendon-derived stem/progenitor cells (hTSPCs). Oncotarget. 2016;7(6):6410–23. https://doi.org/10.18632/oncotarget.7064.
87. Li H, Matheu MP, Sun F, Wang L, Sanford MT, Ning H, Banie L, Lee YC, Xin Z, Guo Y, Lin G, Lue TF. Low-energy shock wave therapy ameliorates erectile dysfunction in a pelvic neurovascular injuries Rat Model. J Sex Med. 2016;13(1):22–32. https://doi.org/10.1016/j.jsxm.2015.11.008.
88. Lin G, Li H, Zhang X, Wang J, Zaid U, Sanford MT, Tu V, Wu A, Wang L, Tian F, Kotanides H, Krishnan V, Wang G, Ning H, Banie L, Lin CS, Deng GG, Lue TF. Novel therapeutic approach for neurogenic erectile dysfunction: effect of neurotrophic tyrosine kinase receptor type 1 monoclonal antibody. Eur Urol. 2015;67(4):716–26. https://doi.org/10.1016/j.eururo.2014.10.013.
89. Lin G, Shindel AW, Fandel TM, Bella AJ, Lin CS, Lue TF. Neurotrophic effects of brain-derived neurotrophic factor and vascular endothelial growth factor in major pelvic ganglia of young and aged rats. BJU Int. 2010;105(1):114–20. https://doi.org/10.1111/j.1464-410X.2009.08647.x.
90. Liu G, Sun X, Bian J, Wu R, Guan X, Ouyang B, Huang Y, Xiao H, Luo D, Atala A, Zhang Y, Deng C. Correction of diabetic erectile dysfunction with adipose derived stem cells modified with the vascular endothelial growth factor gene in a rodent diabetic model. PLoS One. 2013;8(8):e72790. https://doi.org/10.1371/journal.pone.0072790.
91. Liu J, Ruan J, Weir MD, Ren K, Schneider A, Wang P, Oates TW, Chang X, Xu HHK. Periodontal bone-ligament-cementum regeneration via Scaffolds and stem cells. Cells. 2019;8(6) https://doi.org/10.3390/cells8060537.
92. Liu MC, Chang ML, Wang YC, Chen WH, Wu CC, Yeh SD. Revisiting the regenerative therapeutic advances towards erectile dysfunction. Cells. 2020;9(5) https://doi.org/10.3390/cells9051250.
93. Liu Q, Cui Y, Lin H, Hu D, Qi T, Wang B, Huang Z, Chen J, Li K, Xiao H. MicroRNA-145 engineered bone marrow-derived mesenchymal stem cells alleviated erectile dysfunction in aged rats. Stem Cell Res Ther. 2019;10(1):398. https://doi.org/10.1186/s13287-019-1509-1.
94. Liu SZ, Feng DC, Liu ZH, Liang JY, Ren ZJ, Zhou C, Wu K, Zhang FX, Zhang F, Lu YP, Wang XD. Development of nanotechnology in andrology. Transl Androl Urol. 2020;9(2):702–8. https://doi.org/10.21037/tau.2020.01.18.

95. Liu T, Peng Y, Jia C, Fang X, Li J, Zhong W. Hepatocyte growth factor-modified adipose tissue-derived stem cells improve erectile function in streptozotocin-induced diabetic rats. Growth Factors. 2015;33(4):282–9. https://doi.org/10.3109/08977194.2015.1077825.
96. Lu H, Zhou Q, He J, Jiang Z, Peng C, Tong R, Shi J. Recent advances in the development of protein-protein interactions modulators: mechanisms and clinical trials. Signal Transduct Target Ther. 2020;5(1):213. https://doi.org/10.1038/s41392-020-00315-3.
97. Lu RM, Hwang YC, Liu IJ, Lee CC, Tsai HZ, Li HJ, Wu HC. Development of therapeutic antibodies for the treatment of diseases. J Biomed Sci. 2020;27(1):1. https://doi.org/10.1186/s12929-019-0592-z.
98. Luo C, Peng Y, Zhou X, Fan J, Chen W, Zhang H, Wei A. NLRP3 downregulation enhances engraftment and functionality of adipose-derived stem cells to alleviate erectile dysfunction in diabetic rats. Front Endocrinol (Lausanne). 2022;13:913296. https://doi.org/10.3389/fendo.2022.913296.
99. Marcovici I. PRP and correction of penile curvature (Peyronie's disease). Am J Cosmet Surg. 2018;36:074880681879828. https://doi.org/10.1177/0748806818798280.
100. Masouminia M, Gelfand R, Kovanecz I, Vernet D, Tsao J, Salas R, Castro K, Loni L, Rajfer J, Gonzalez-Cadavid NF. Dyslipidemia is a major factor in stem cell damage induced by uncontrolled long-term type 2 diabetes and obesity in the rat, as suggested by the effects on stem cell culture. J Sex Med. 2018;15(12):1678–97. https://doi.org/10.1016/j.jsxm.2018.09.019.
101. Masterson TA, Molina M, Ledesma B, Zucker I, Saltzman R, Ibrahim E, Han S, Reis IM, Ramasamy R. Platelet-rich plasma for the treatment of erectile dysfunction: a prospective, randomized, double-blind, placebo-controlled clinical trial. J Urol. 2023;210(1):154–61. https://doi.org/10.1097/ju.0000000000003481.
102. Masuda H. Significance of nitric oxide and its modulation mechanisms by endogenous nitric oxide synthase inhibitors and arginase in the micturition disorders and erectile dysfunction. Int J Urol. 2008;15(2):128–34. https://doi.org/10.1111/j.1442-2042.2007.01973.x.
103. Matz EL, Pearlman AM, Terlecki RP. Safety and feasibility of platelet rich fibrin matrix injections for treatment of common urologic conditions. Investig Clin Urol. 2018;59(1):61–5. https://doi.org/10.4111/icu.2018.59.1.61.
104. Melman A, Bar-Chama N, McCullough A, Davies K, Christ G. hMaxi-K gene transfer in males with erectile dysfunction: results of the first human trial. Hum Gene Ther. 2006;17(12):1165–76. https://doi.org/10.1089/hum.2006.17.1165.
105. Mittal RD. Gene editing in clinical practice: where are we? Indian J Clin Biochem. 2019;34(1):19–25. https://doi.org/10.1007/s12291-018-0804-4.
106. Moradi S, Mahdizadeh H, Šarić T, Kim J, Harati J, Shahsavarani H, Greber B, Moore JB. Research and therapy with induced pluripotent stem cells (iPSCs): social, legal, and ethical considerations. Stem Cell Res Ther. 2019;10(1):341. https://doi.org/10.1186/s13287-019-1455-y.
107. Mortimer D. The future of male infertility management and assisted reproduction technology. Hum Reprod. 2000;15(Suppl 5):98–110. https://doi.org/10.1093/humrep/15.suppl_5.98.
108. Mostafa T, Abdel-Hamid IA, Taymour M, Ali OI. Gene variants in premature ejaculation: systematic review and future directions. Sex Med Rev. 2020;8(4):586–602. https://doi.org/10.1016/j.sxmr.2020.07.002.
109. Mostafa T, Hassan A, Alghobary MF, Abdelrahman SH. Effect of genetic polymorphism on the response to PDE5 inhibitors in patients with erectile dysfunction: a systematic review and a critical appraisal. Sex Med Rev. 2020;8(4):573–85. https://doi.org/10.1016/j.sxmr.2020.05.005.
110. Nakajima N, Tamaki T, Hirata M, Soeda S, Nitta M, Hoshi A, Terachi T. Purified human skeletal muscle-derived stem cells enhance the repair and regeneration in the damaged urethra. Transplantation. 2017;101(10):2312–20. https://doi.org/10.1097/tp.0000000000001613.
111. Ni Lochlainn M, Kenny RA. Sexual activity and aging. J Am Med Dir Assoc. 2013;14(8):565–72. https://doi.org/10.1016/j.jamda.2013.01.022.
112. Ning H, Lin G, Lue TF, Lin CS. Neuron-like differentiation of adipose tissue-derived stromal cells and vascular smooth muscle cells. Differentiation. 2006;74(9–10):510–8. https://doi.org/10.1111/j.1432-0436.2006.00081.x.

113. Ormond KE, Bombard Y, Bonham VL, Hoffman-Andrews L, Howard H, Isasi R, Musunuru K, Riggan KA, Michie M, Allyse M. The clinical application of gene editing: ethical and social issues. Per Med. 2019;16(4):337–50. https://doi.org/10.2217/pme-2018-0155.
114. Otunctemur A, Ozbek E, Kirecci SL, Ozcan L, Dursun M, Cekmen M, Ozdogan HK. Relevance of serum nitric oxide levels and the efficacy of selective serotonin reuptake inhibitors treatment on premature ejaculation: decreased nitric oxide is associated with premature ejaculation. Andrologia. 2014;46(9):951–5. https://doi.org/10.1111/and.12179.
115. Palmieri A, Arcaniolo D, Palumbo F, Verze P, Liguori G, Mondaini N, Falcone M, Scroppo FI, Salonia A, Cai T. Low intensity shockwave therapy in combination with phosphodiesterase-5 inhibitors is an effective and safe treatment option in patients with vasculogenic ED who are PDE5i non-responders: a multicenter single-arm clinical trial. Int J Impot Res. 2021;33(6):634–40. https://doi.org/10.1038/s41443-020-0332-7.
116. Pan MM, Raees A, Kovac JR. Low-intensity extracorporeal shock wave as a novel treatment for erectile dysfunction. Am J Mens Health. 2016;10(2):146–8. https://doi.org/10.1177/1557988315574511.
117. Park K, Ahn KY, Kim MK, Lee SE, Kang TW, Ryu SB. Intracavernosal injection of vascular endothelial growth factor improves erectile function in aged rats. Eur Urol. 2004;46(3):403–7. https://doi.org/10.1016/j.eururo.2004.04.032.
118. Perticarrara Ferezin L, Kayzuka C, Rondon Pereira VC, Ferreira de Andrade M, Molina CAF, Tucci S Jr, Tanus-Santos JE, Lacchini R. The rs2682826 polymorphism of the NOS1 gene is associated with the degree of disability of erectile dysfunction. Life (Basel). 2023;13(5) https://doi.org/10.3390/life13051082.
119. Peter AE. Autologous platelet-rich plasma and mesenchymal stem cells for the treatment of chronic wounds. In: Kamil Hakan D, editor. Wound healing (pp. Ch. 9). IntechOpen; 2018. https://doi.org/10.5772/intechopen.80502.
120. Philippidis A. CASGEVY makes history as FDA approves first CRISPR/Cas9 genome edited therapy. Hum Gene Ther. 2024;35(1–2):1–4. https://doi.org/10.1089/hum.2023.29263.bfs.
121. PhRMA. The United States vs. other countries: availability of new medicines varies, 2020. Retrieved October 01 from https://www.phrma.org/medicare/the-united-states-vs-other-countries-availability-of-new-medicines-varies.
122. Podlasek CA. Sonic hedgehog, apoptosis, and the penis. J Sex Med. 2009;6 Suppl 3(Suppl 3):334–9. https://doi.org/10.1111/j.1743-6109.2008.01192.x.
123. Podlasek CA, Zelner DJ, Jiang HB, Tang Y, Houston J, McKenna KE, McVary KT. Sonic hedgehog cascade is required for penile postnatal morphogenesis, differentiation, and adult homeostasis. Biol Reprod. 2003;68(2):423–38. https://doi.org/10.1095/biolreprod.102.006643.
124. Poulios E, Mykoniatis I, Pyrgidis N, Zilotis F, Kapoteli P, Kotsiris D, Kalyvianakis D, Hatzichristou D. Platelet-Rich Plasma (PRP) improves erectile function: a double-blind, randomized, placebo-controlled clinical trial. J Sex Med. 2021;18(5):926–35. https://doi.org/10.1016/j.jsxm.2021.03.008.
125. Pu XY, Hu LQ, Wang HP, Luo YX, Wang XH. Improvement in erectile dysfunction after insulin-like growth factor-1 gene therapy in diabetic rats. Asian J Androl. 2007;9(1):83–91. https://doi.org/10.1111/j.1745-7262.2007.00215.x.
126. Qiu X, Lin G, Xin Z, Ferretti L, Zhang H, Lue TF, Lin CS. Effects of low-energy shockwave therapy on the erectile function and tissue of a diabetic rat model. J Sex Med. 2013;10(3):738–46. https://doi.org/10.1111/jsm.12024.
127. Raheem OA, Natale C, Dick B, Reddy AG, Yousif A, Khera M, Baum N. Novel treatments of erectile dysfunction: review of the current literature. Sex Med Rev. 2021;9(1):123–32. https://doi.org/10.1016/j.sxmr.2020.03.005.
128. Rew KT. Men's health: male sexual dysfunction. FP Essent. 2021;503:28–33.
129. Riegler MA, Stensen MH, Witczak O, Andersen JM, Hicks SA, Hammer HL, Delbarre E, Halvorsen P, Yazidi A, Holst N, Haugen TB. Artificial intelligence in the fertility clinic: status, pitfalls and possibilities. Hum Reprod. 2021;36(9):2429–42. https://doi.org/10.1093/humrep/deab168.

130. Rogers RS, Graziottin TM, Lin CS, Kan YW, Lue TF. Intracavernosal vascular endothelial growth factor (VEGF) injection and adeno-associated virus-mediated VEGF gene therapy prevent and reverse venogenic erectile dysfunction in rats. Int J Impot Res. 2003;15(1):26–37. https://doi.org/10.1038/sj.ijir.3900943.
131. Ryu JK, Kim WJ, Koh YJ, Piao S, Jin HR, Lee SW, Choi MJ, Shin HY, Kwon MH, Jung K, Koh GY, Suh JK. Designed angiopoietin-1 variant, COMP-angiopoietin-1, rescues erectile function through healthy cavernous angiogenesis in a hypercholesterolemic mouse. Sci Rep. 2015;5:9222. https://doi.org/10.1038/srep09222.
132. Sandoval-Salinas C, Saffon JP, Martínez JM, Corredor HA, Gallego A. Are radial pressure waves effective for the treatment of moderate or mild to moderate erectile dysfunction? A randomized sham therapy controlled clinical trial. J Sex Med. 2022;19(5):738–44. https://doi.org/10.1016/j.jsxm.2022.02.010.
133. Santtila P, Jern P, Westberg L, Walum H, Pedersen CT, Eriksson E, Kenneth Sandnabba N. The dopamine transporter gene (DAT1) polymorphism is associated with premature ejaculation. J Sex Med. 2010;7(4 Pt 1):1538–46. https://doi.org/10.1111/j.1743-6109.2009.01696.x.
134. Shaher H, Fathi A, Elbashir S, Abdelbaki SA, Soliman T. Is platelet rich plasma safe and effective in treatment of erectile dysfunction? Randomized controlled study. Urology. 2023;175:114–9. https://doi.org/10.1016/j.urology.2023.01.028.
135. Shin D, Jeon SH, Tian WJ, Kwon EB, Kim GE, Bae WJ, Cho HJ, Hong SH, Lee JY, Kim SW. Extracorporeal shock wave therapy combined with engineered mesenchymal stem cells expressing stromal cell-derived factor-1 can improve erectile dysfunction in streptozotocin-induced diabetic rats. Transl Androl Urol. 2021;10(6):2362–72. https://doi.org/10.21037/tau-21-79.
136. Silva CND, Pedrosa KN, Silva GCD, Cunha PDS, Diniz TF, Maia LMS, Almeida FM, Gomez RS, Lemos VS, Gomes DA, de Lima ME. The synthetic peptide PnPP-19 potentiates erectile function via nNOS and iNOS. Nitric Oxide. 2021;113–114:23–30. https://doi.org/10.1016/j.niox.2021.04.007.
137. Singh K, Bhushan B, Kumar S, Singh S, Macadangdang RR Jr, Pandey E, Varma AK, Kumar S. Precision genome editing techniques in gene therapy: current state and future prospects. Curr Gene Ther. 2024; https://doi.org/10.2174/0115665232279528240115075352.
138. So I, Chae MR, Lee SW. Gene transfer of the K(ATP) channel restores age-related erectile dysfunction in rats. BJU Int. 2007;100(5):1154–60. https://doi.org/10.1111/j.1464-410X.2007.07050.x.
139. Soebadi MA, Moris L, Castiglione F, Weyne E, Albersen M. Advances in stem cell research for the treatment of male sexual dysfunctions. Curr Opin Urol. 2016;26(2):129–39. https://doi.org/10.1097/mou.0000000000000255.
140. Sramkova T, Motil I, Jarkovsky J, Sramkova K. Erectile dysfunction treatment using focused linear low-intensity extracorporeal shockwaves: single-blind, sham-controlled, randomized clinical trial. Urol Int. 2020;104(5–6):417–24. https://doi.org/10.1159/000504788.
141. Stringer JD. Gender and sexual health: sexual dysfunction. FP Essent. 2016;449:18–26.
142. Sun X, Luo L, Li J. LncRNA MALAT1 facilitates BM-MSCs differentiation into endothelial cells via targeting miR-206/VEGFA axis. Cell Cycle. 2020;19(22):3018–28. https://doi.org/10.1080/15384101.2020.1829799.
143. Taş T, Çakıroğlu B, Arda E, Onuk Ö, Nuhoğlu B. Early clinical results of the tolerability, safety, and efficacy of autologous platelet-rich plasma administration in erectile dysfunction. Sex Med. 2021;9(2):100313. https://doi.org/10.1016/j.esxm.2020.100313.
144. Tögel F, Hu Z, Weiss K, Isaac J, Lange C, Westenfelder C. Administered mesenchymal stem cells protect against ischemic acute renal failure through differentiation-independent mechanisms. Am J Physiol Renal Physiol. 2005;289(1):F31–42. https://doi.org/10.1152/ajprenal.00007.2005.
145. Toque HA, Caldwell RW. New approaches to the design and discovery of therapies to prevent erectile dysfunction. Expert Opin Drug Discov. 2014;9(12):1447–69. https://doi.org/10.1517/17460441.2014.949234.
146. Tsai CC, Wang CJ, Lee YC, Kuo YT, Lin HH, Li CC, Wu WJ, Liu CC. Low-intensity extracorporeal shockwave therapy can improve erectile function in patients who failed to respond to

phosphodiesterase type 5 inhibitors. Am J Mens Health. 2017;11(6):1781–90. https://doi.org/10.1177/1557988317721643.
147. Tsumoto K, Isozaki Y, Yagami H, Tomita M. Future perspectives of therapeutic monoclonal antibodies. Immunotherapy. 2019;11(2):119–27. https://doi.org/10.2217/imt-2018-0130.
148. Usmani SS, Bedi G, Samuel JS, Singh S, Kalra S, Kumar P, Ahuja AA, Sharma M, Gautam A, Raghava GPS. THPdb: database of FDA-approved peptide and protein therapeutics. PLoS One. 2017;12(7):e0181748. https://doi.org/10.1371/journal.pone.0181748.
149. van Raaij JJ, Janssen PKC. The rs6296 polymorphism in the 5-HT1b receptor in Dutch men with lifelong premature ejaculation: a genetic case-control association study. J Sex Med. 2024;21(2):122–8. https://doi.org/10.1093/jsxmed/qdad159.
150. Virag R, Sussman H, Lambion S, Fourmestraux V. Evaluation of the benefit of using a combination of autologous platelet rich-plasma and hyaluronic acid for the treatment of Peyronie's disease. Sex Health Issues. 2017;1 https://doi.org/10.15761/SHI.1000102.
151. Wang F, Luo D, Chen J, Pan C, Wang Z, Fu H, Xu J, Yang M, Mo S, Zhuang L, Wang W. Rs9303628 and rs2054847 of SLC6A4 are protective factors for the onset of lifelong premature ejaculation among the Chinese population. Andrologia. 2021;53(1):e13650. https://doi.org/10.1111/and.13650.
152. Weinrich JAP, Tyagi A, Kenney MC, DiCasoli RJ, Kaltschmidt JA. Transcription factor gene Pea3 regulates erectile function during copulation in mice. PLoS One. 2022;17(10):e0276069. https://doi.org/10.1371/journal.pone.0276069.
153. Wils J, Favre J, Bellien J. Modulating putative endothelial progenitor cells for the treatment of endothelial dysfunction and cardiovascular complications in diabetes. Pharmacol Ther. 2017;170:98–115. https://doi.org/10.1016/j.pharmthera.2016.10.014.
154. Wu J, Chen Z, Zhong F, Yang W, Ouyang X, Ma X, Zheng S, Wei H. Transplantation of human gingiva-derived mesenchymal stem cells ameliorates neurotic erectile dysfunction in a Rat Model. Front Bioeng Biotechnol. 2021;9:630076. https://doi.org/10.3389/fbioe.2021.630076.
155. Wu JH, Wang DY, Sheng L, Qian WQ, Xia SJ, Jiang Q. Human umbilical cord Wharton's jelly-derived mesenchymal stem cell transplantation could improve diabetic intracavernosal pressure. Asian J Androl. 2022;24(2):171–5. https://doi.org/10.4103/aja.aja_33_21.
156. Xu Y, Zhang F, Li C, Hao H, Hao Y. Angiotensin-(1-7) improves diabetes mellitus-induced erectile dysfunction in rats by regulating nitric oxide synthase levels. Peptides. 2022;151:170765. https://doi.org/10.1016/j.peptides.2022.170765.
157. Xuan Z, Yu W, Dou Y, Wang T. Efficacy of platelet-rich plasma for low back pain: a systematic review and meta-analysis. J Neurol Surg A Cent Eur Neurosurg. 2020;81(6):529–34. https://doi.org/10.1055/s-0040-1709170.
158. Yang Q, Chen W, Zhang C, Xie Y, Gao Y, Deng C, Sun X, Liu G, Deng C. Combined transplantation of adipose tissue-derived stem cells and endothelial progenitor cells improve diabetic erectile dysfunction in a Rat Model. Stem Cells Int. 2020;2020:2154053. https://doi.org/10.1155/2020/2154053.
159. Yang Q, Chen X, Zheng T, Han D, Zhang H, Shi Y, Bian J, Sun X, Xia K, Liang X, Liu G, Zhang Y, Deng C. Transplantation of human urine-derived stem cells transfected with pigment epithelium-derived factor to protect erectile function in a rat model of cavernous nerve injury. Cell Transplant. 2016;25(11):1987–2001. https://doi.org/10.3727/096368916x691448.
160. Yang S, Zhang Y, Lyu X, Gu Y, Zhang G, Liu P, Zheng Y, Guo Z, Zhang Y, Hou H. The association between FGF21 and diabetic erectile dysfunction: evidence from clinical and animal studies. Front Endocrinol (Lausanne). 2022;13:874796. https://doi.org/10.3389/fendo.2022.874796.
161. Yao HX, Ma FZ, Tan YY, Liu LY. Endothelial nitric oxide synthase gene polymorphisms and risk of erectile dysfunction: an updated meta-analysis of genetic association studies. Int J Surg. 2018;54(Pt A):141–8. https://doi.org/10.1016/j.ijsu.2018.04.012.
162. Yin GN. Pericyte-derived heme-binding protein 1 promotes angiogenesis and improves erectile function in diabetic mice. Investig Clin Urol. 2022;63(4):464–74. https://doi.org/10.4111/icu.20220038.
163. Yin GN, Choi MJ, Kim WJ, Kwon MH, Song KM, Park JM, Das ND, Kwon KD, Batbold D, Oh GT, Koh GY, Kim KW, Ryu JK, Suh JK. Inhibition of Ninjurin 1 restores erectile function

through dual angiogenic and neurotrophic effects in the diabetic mouse. Proc Natl Acad Sci USA. 2014;111(26):E2731–40. https://doi.org/10.1073/pnas.1403471111.
164. Yin GN, Jin HR, Choi MJ, Limanjaya A, Ghatak K, Minh NN, Ock J, Kwon MH, Song KM, Park HJ, Kim HM, Kwon YG, Ryu JK, Suh JK. Pericyte-Derived Dickkopf2 regenerates damaged penile neurovasculature through an Angiopoietin-1-Tie2 pathway. Diabetes. 2018;67(6):1149–61. https://doi.org/10.2337/db17-0833.
165. Yin GN, Kim DK, Kang JI, Im Y, Lee DS, Han AR, Ock J, Choi MJ, Kwon MH, Limanjaya A, Jung SB, Yang J, Min KW, Yun J, Koh Y, Park JE, Hwang D, Suh JK, Ryu JK, Kim HM. Latrophilin-2 is a novel receptor of LRG1 that rescues vascular and neurological abnormalities and restores diabetic erectile function. Exp Mol Med. 2022;54(5):626–38. https://doi.org/10.1038/s12276-022-00773-5.
166. Yin GN, Kim WJ, Jin HR, Kwon MH, Song KM, Choi MJ, Park JM, Das ND, Kwon KD, Batbold D, Kim KW, Ryu JK, Suh JK. Nerve injury-induced protein 1 (Ninjurin-1) is a novel therapeutic target for cavernous nerve injury-induced erectile dysfunction in mice. J Sex Med. 2013;10(6):1488–501. https://doi.org/10.1111/jsm.12129.
167. Yin GN, Wu J, Cui Y, Lin C, Shi L, Gao ZL, Suh JK, Ryu JK, Jin HR. Transcriptional profiling of mouse cavernous pericytes under high-glucose conditions: implications for diabetic angiopathy. Investig Clin Urol. 2021;62(1):100–10. https://doi.org/10.4111/icu.20200272.
168. Yoshimura N, Kato R, Chancellor MB, Nelson JB, Glorioso JC. Gene therapy as future treatment of erectile dysfunction. Expert Opin Biol Ther. 2010;10(9):1305–14. https://doi.org/10.1517/14712598.2010.510510.
169. Zakrzewski W, Dobrzyński M, Szymonowicz M, Rybak Z. Stem cells: past, present, and future. Stem Cell Res Ther. 2019;10(1):68. https://doi.org/10.1186/s13287-019-1165-5.
170. Zaninovic N, Elemento O, Rosenwaks Z. Artificial intelligence: its applications in reproductive medicine and the assisted reproductive technologies. Fertil Steril. 2019;112(1):28–30. https://doi.org/10.1016/j.fertnstert.2019.05.019.
171. Zhang T, Li W, Qiu X, Liu B, Li G, Feng C, Liao J, Lin K. CRISPR/Cas9-mediated TEAD1 knockout induces phenotypic modulation of corpus cavernosum smooth muscle cells in diabetic rats with erectile dysfunction. Nan Fang Yi Ke Da Xue Xue Bao. 2021;41(4):567–73. https://doi.org/10.12122/j.issn.1673-4254.2021.04.13.
172. Zhang Z, Nie P, Yang W, Ma X, Chen Z, Wei H. Lipopolysaccharide-preconditioned allogeneic adipose-derived stem cells improve erectile function in a rat model of bilateral cavernous nerve injury. Basic Clin Androl. 2022;32(1):5. https://doi.org/10.1186/s12610-022-00156-w.
173. Zhu XB, Niu ZH, Fan WM, Sheng CS, Chen Q. Type 2 diabetes mellitus and the risk of male infertility: a Mendelian randomization study. Front Endocrinol (Lausanne). 2023;14:1279058. https://doi.org/10.3389/fendo.2023.1279058.
174. Zhuo C, Zhang J, Lee JH, Jiao J, Cheng D, Liu L, Kim HW, Tao Y, Li M. Spatiotemporal control of CRISPR/Cas9 gene editing. Signal Transduct Target Ther. 2021;6(1):238. https://doi.org/10.1038/s41392-021-00645-w.

Chapter 18
Erectile Function Preservation in Prostate Cancer Treatment: New Advances

Marlon Martinez, Dyandra Parikesit, Missy Savira, and David K. W. Leung

Epidemiology of Erectile Dysfunction Following Prostate Cancer Treatment

Prostate cancer (PCa) remains the second most commonly diagnosed cancer and the fifth leading cause of cancer-related death among men worldwide, with an estimated 1.5 million new cases and 397,000 deaths in 2022 [1]. Management of PCa is guided by tumor stage and risk profile, with available treatments including radical prostatectomy (RP), radiotherapy (RT), androgen deprivation therapy (ADT), and chemotherapy [2]. However, surgery and RT can disrupt cavernous nerve function and penile vascular integrity [3], leading to sexual dysfunction characterized by erectile dysfunction (ED), ejaculatory and orgasmic disturbances, and broader psychosexual effects such as reduced sexual confidence and libido [4]. Ultimately, ED

M. Martinez (✉)
Section of Urology, Department of Surgery, University of Santo Tomas Hospital, Manila, Philippines

D. Parikesit
Urology Medical Staff Group, Universitas Indonesia Hospital, Universitas Indonesia, Depok, West Java, Indonesia

M. Savira
Department of Urology, Faculty of Medicine, Universitas Indonesia, Dr. Cipto Mangunkusumo Hospital, Jakarta Pusat, DKI Jakarta, Indonesia

Global Andrology Forum, Moreland Hills, OH, USA

D. K. W. Leung
Department of Urology, Faculty of Medicine, Prince of Wales Hospital, The Chinese University of Hong Kong, Hong Kong, China
e-mail: davidleung@surgery.cuhk.edu.hk

E. Chung et al. (eds.), *Advances in Andrology*,
https://doi.org/10.1007/978-3-032-29112-7_18

continues to be the most prevalent sexual consequence, adversely affecting quality of life and the well-being of intimate partners [4, 5].

Estimating the true incidence of ED after PCa treatment is challenging because of heterogeneous diagnostic criteria and multiple patient- and treatment-related factors, including age, baseline EF, radicality of surgery with regards to nerve-sparing, follow-up duration, use of multimodal therapy, and penile rehabilitation [6, 7]. ED following PCa treatment is common, with reported incidence rates varying between 30% and 80%, depending on the specific treatment modality, patient characteristics, and pre-treatment erectile function (EF) [8]. In a cohort of men with localized PCa, ED occurred in 44.2% overall [9], with reported rates higher after RP (56.1–65.3%) than after RT (30.4%–33.8%) [9, 10]. Notably, these studies were based on clinical diagnosis of ED, while survey-based assessments of perceived EF have reported markedly higher prevalence, with rates up to 91% [5]. Additionally, the timing of assessment is important, as EF following RP has been shown to recover in a time-dependent manner, particularly within the first 2 years after surgery [11]. In contrast, ED after RT has been shown to increase over time, affecting roughly one-third of patients at 1 year and up to one half at 5 years [12]. In one study, RT was associated with a longer median time to ED diagnosis compared with RP (346 vs 133 days) [9]. Furthermore, RP was also associated with a higher likelihood of penile prosthesis implantation compared with RT (3.6% vs 1.4%) [9].

When stratified by surgical approach, robotic-assisted RP (RARP) demonstrates improved EF preservation relative to laparoscopic RP (LRP) and open techniques, whereas laparoscopic and open approaches showed comparable outcomes [13]. The use of nerve-sparing techniques is a major determinant of EF recovery after RP [14, 15], with non–nerve-sparing surgery associated with an approximately 70% lower likelihood of recovery compared with nerve-sparing procedures [16]. Conversely, reported rates of radiation-induced ED vary widely in the literature, ranging from 17% to 90% [11]. Interestingly, brachytherapy (BT) demonstrated superior erectile outcomes compared with external-beam radiotherapy (EBRT) or RP [12], with differences diminishing and outcomes becoming comparable at longer follow-up [17]. Another treatment-related factor influencing erectile outcomes is the use of ADT, with studies showing that patients receiving ADT have significantly poorer EF at follow-up compared with those not exposed to ADT [18].

Several patient-related factors have been shown to influence ED outcomes, including younger age, lower prostate-specific antigen (PSA) levels, and better pre-treatment sexual function scores [15]. Younger age has been associated with improved EF recovery following RP, with one study reporting a higher likelihood of return to baseline function among younger men, despite an overall recovery rate of only 23% [19]. Comorbid conditions such as diabetes have been associated with poorer erectile outcomes, including a reduced likelihood of EF recovery (OR 0.43) and an increased risk of severe ED (OR 1.85) [20]. The presence of vascular risk factors, including hypertension, cigarette smoking, and hypercholesterolemia, has been associated with poorer EF outcomes following RP [21].

Anatomy, Vascularization and Innervation of the Prostate and Penis

To understand how PCa treatments can lead to ED, it is important to first review the complex anatomy of the prostate and its relationship with the structures responsible for erection. The prostate gland is situated within the male pelvis and is commonly described as having an inverted conical shape. Its base lies adjacent to the bladder neck, while the apex is closely associated with the external urethral sphincter [22]. Improved understanding of prostate anatomy over recent decades has refined surgical techniques, with EF recovery closely linked to preservation of prostatic vascular supply and neurovascular bundles (NVBs) anatomy.

Vascularization of Prostate

The arterial supply to the prostate is variable, most commonly arising from the internal pudendal artery (35–56%), followed by the gluteal–pudendal trunk (15–28%), and less frequently from the obturator artery (10–12%). Typically, two bilateral arterial pedicles can be identified: a posterior branch that courses around the seminal vesicles and vas deferens toward the prostatic base, and an anterior branch that runs along the lateral surface of the prostate toward the apex [23]. Studies have suggested that the anterior arterial pedicle, which courses along the lateral aspect of the prostate toward the apex as an anterior capsular branch, may play a role in preserving postoperative erectile function and penile integrity, as preservation of these small branches has been associated with improved EF recovery [24].

Notably, substantial inter- and intraindividual variation exists in male pelvic vascular anatomy, including the presence of accessory or aberrant pudendal arteries (APAs), which have been reported in 4–75% of individuals [25]. These vessels generally originate from internal iliac, external iliac, or obturator arteries, coursing along the tendinous arch of the pelvis or the anterolateral aspect of the prostatic apex [26]. Transection of accessory pudendal arteries has not been shown to independently predict postoperative erectile dysfunction [27]. However, as these vessels may contribute to penile arterial inflow, their preservation during radical prostatectomy is generally advocated [27, 28].

Innervation of Prostate

The neural pathways governing erection, ejaculation, and urinary continence arise from the inferior hypogastric (pelvic) plexus, which is embedded within a sagittally oriented fibro-fatty plane between the bladder and rectum [29, 30]. The extent of pelvic lymph node dissection may expose this region to surgical manipulation, thereby increasing the risk of neural injury. Standard dissection, limited to the common iliac bifurcation or ureter, primarily endangers the pelvic plexus and erectile nerves near the internal iliac vessels, whereas extended dissection adds risk in the presacral region and medial to the common iliac arteries [31, 32].

NVBs consist of microscopic nerve fibers originating from the inferior hypogastric plexus and closely associated vascular structures, coursing along the lateral and anterolateral surfaces of the prostate [26, 33]. These fibers are predominantly concentrated posterolaterally, with a higher proportion located anterolaterally at the prostatic apex [34]. Overall, the NVBs are enclosed within a multilayered periprostatic fascia that variably adheres to or separates from the prostatic capsule and covers the outer surface of the prostate [26]. Multiple dissection planes can be identified within the periprostatic fascia, permitting varying degrees of nerve-sparing and forming the basis of the incremental nerve-sparing concept. Traditionally, three principal planes have been described: an intrafascial plane along the prostatic pseudocapsule that enables maximal preservation of the neurovascular bundles; an interfascial plane within the periprostatic fascia allowing partial or complete nerve sparing depending on anatomical variation; and an extrafascial plane lateral to the levator ani fascia, which results in complete excision of the neurovascular bundles [26]. With the introduction of robotic surgery and enhanced optical magnification, a four-grade nerve-sparing approach based on lateral prostatic venous landmarks has been proposed. In this system, grade 1 dissection follows the plane between the prostatic pseudocapsule and periprostatic veins and represents maximal nerve preservation, while progressively more lateral dissections toward the levator ani fascia (grades 2–4) correspond to decreasing degrees of nerve sparing, ultimately resulting in a non–nerve-sparing technique [35].

Physiology of Erection

Penile erection, also known as tumescence, refers to the physiological process during which the penis becomes engorged with blood, typically in response to sexual arousal but occasionally occurring spontaneously. A comprehensive understanding of penile anatomy, neurovasculature, and related hormonal and molecular factors is essential to understanding tumescence physiology. An understanding of the underlying physiology informs medical intervention, making it a fundamental aspect of ED management. The mechanism of penile erection is shown in Fig. 18.1.

The physiology underlying an erection can be delineated into processes of arterial dilation and venous occlusion. Typically, tumescence ensues following sexual stimulation. This sequence inhibits the sympathetic nervous system, activates the parasympathetic nervous system, and releases pro-erectogenic neurotransmitters from the cavernous nerves. Consequently, parasympathetic nerve activation results in a reduction of intracellular calcium levels, leading to relaxation of cavernosal and arterial smooth muscles. This relaxation effect significantly enhances blood flow,

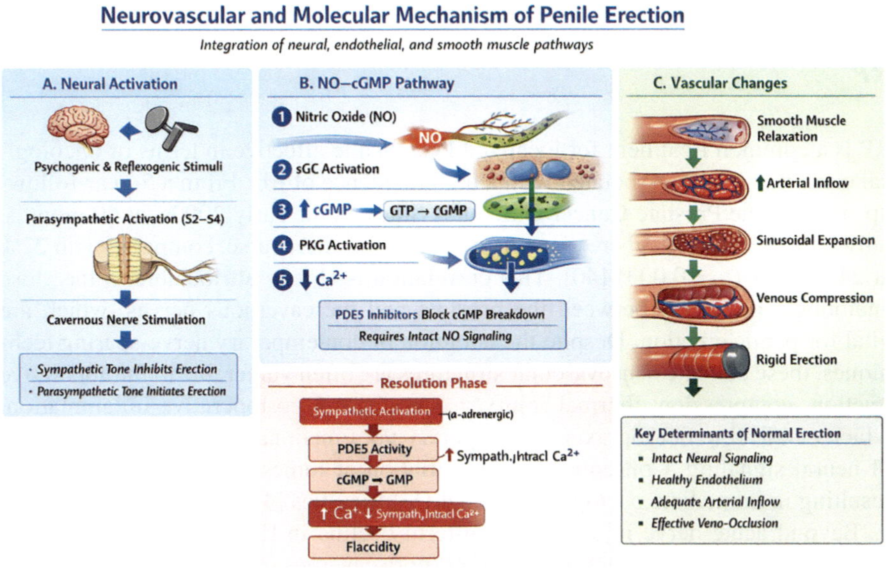

Fig. 18.1 Integrated neurovascular and molecular mechanisms of penile erection and detumescence

increasing it by approximately twenty to forty times within the expanding sinusoids of the corpora cavernosa. As these sinusoids expand, the peripheral regions of the corpora near the tunica albuginea commence venous occlusion. The emissary veins are compressed between the sinusoids and the inelastic tunica albuginea, thereby sustaining tumescence [36].

In most men, intracavernous pressure elevates to an average of approximately 100 mmHg. The pressure within the corpus spongiosum typically remains about one-third of that observed in the corpora cavernosa. This disparity is attributable to the weaker and more elastic tunica albuginea, which facilitates minimal venous occlusion. Contraction of the ischiocavernosus and bulbospongiosus muscles during the rigid erection phase elevates pressure within all three chambers and the glans penis. Sexual intercourse and repetitive penile stimulation induce robust contractions of these muscles, thereby forcing additional blood into all chambers and increasing rigidity. This stage is referred to as the rigid erection phase, during which intra-erectile pressures can attain several hundred millimeters of mercury [37, 38].

The intracorporeal pressure begins to decline only during the second phase of detumescence. The initial phase is characterized by a transient increase in pressure resulting from the contraction of trabecular smooth muscles within the sinusoids against an occluded venous system. During the subsequent phase of detumescence, expansion of the emissary veins facilitates drainage of the sinusoids, leading to a gradual decrease in intracorporeal pressure. The final phase of detumescence involves a rapid decline in pressure, coinciding with fully restored venous drainage and baseline arterial flow [39].

Treatment Effect Leading to ED

RP

RP is a common treatment for localized PCa. While effective in terms of oncological control, it is also associated with a high incidence of ED. From a 5-year-follow-up study of the Prostate Cancer Outcomes Study in the early 2000s, at 60 months, only 28% of the men had erections firm enough for intercourse, compared with 22% at 24 months ($p = 0.003$) [40]. This correlation is chiefly attributable to the close anatomical proximity between the prostate and the cavernous nerves, which are vital for penile erection. Despite the adoption of contemporary nerve-sparing techniques, these delicate neurovascular structures are often vulnerable to intraoperative traction, compression, thermal injury, ischemia, and postoperative inflammation, which can lead to neuropraxia—a temporary yet functionally impactful disruption of neural signaling. Consequently, the initiation of tumescence may be hindered, resulting in immediate postoperative erectile difficulties [41].

Beyond acute nerve injury, the long-term decline in EF after RP is caused by secondary structural changes within the corpora cavernosa. Extended penile flaccidity leads to chronic hypoxia, which encourages apoptosis, pyroptosis, and autophagy of cavernous smooth muscle cells, along with a phenotypic shift toward fibrosis (Fig. 18.2). This process results in cavernous fibrosis and veno-occlusive dysfunction, or "venous leak," making erections difficult or impossible to sustain. While recovery is possible, it is often slow. Nicolai et al. reported that 60–85% of men who undergo bilateral nerve-sparing RP eventually regain some EF, typically within 12–24 months [42].

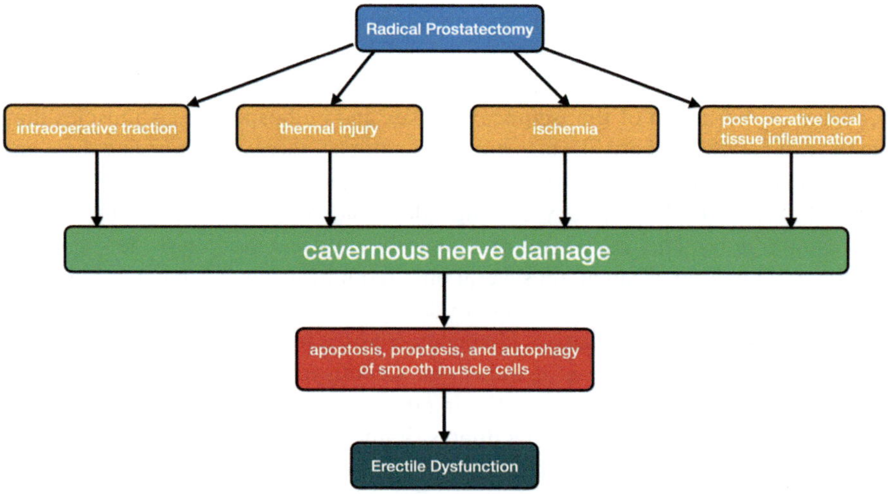

Fig. 18.2 Causes of erectile dysfunction following radical prostatectomy

Efforts to diminish the incidence of ED associated with RP have advanced over a period exceeding one hundred years. The initial description of the perineal approach to radical prostatectomy was provided by Young in 1905, subsequently followed by Millin's retropubic technique in 1945, which established the groundwork for contemporary radical retropubic prostatectomy (RRP). Early results were modest regarding sexual function, with nearly universal postoperative ED reported [43, 44]. A significant paradigm shift transpired in 1983 when Walsh delineated the posterolateral NBVs and subsequently pioneered the nerve-sparing RRP technique. Through meticulous dissection within the lateral pelvic fascia and the preservation of the NVBs, Walsh et al. demonstrated an early recovery of erectile function, with fifty percent of the patients attaining penetrative intercourse postoperatively [45, 46]. This innovation has considerably enhanced postoperative erectile outcomes and continues to serve as the fundamental element of contemporary RP.

Technological advances have further refined surgical precision, and the contemporary ED rates following RP were somewhat better. LRP emerged in the 1990s but was limited by its technical complexity. The widespread adoption of RARP followed the introduction of the da Vinci system in 2000. Menon et al. later optimized this approach through the Vattikuti Institute prostatectomy technique, which enhanced the preservation of the NVB and lateral prostatic fascia. As a result, RARP has become the leading surgical method for PCa in the United States [47–49]. According to a systematic review of 6 studies comparing RARP with RRP, and 4 studies comparing RARP with LRP, the 12- and 24-month potency rates ranged from 54% to 90% and from 63% to 94%, respectively. Higher 12-month potency rates after RARP were found, in comparison with RRP (odds ratio [OR]: 2.84; 95% confidence interval [CI]: 1.46–5.43; $p = 0.002$). There was no significant difference in potency rates between RARP and LRP [7]. Meta-analytic data exhibit enhanced recovery of EF following RALP in comparison to open and conventional laparoscopic techniques at both early and late postoperative intervals [41]. Recent innovations, such as transvesical RARP and Retzius-sparing or Hood techniques, seek to further preserve anatomical structures pertinent to erectile and urinary functions, although comprehensive outcome data from large-scale studies remain scarce [50, 51].

Intraoperative cavernous nerve monitoring has become an adjunctive strategy to minimize nerve injury. Electrical nerve stimulation systems, such as CaverMap, have been extensively researched; however, their application is constrained by low specificity and a high incidence of false-positive results [52, 53]. Advanced imaging technologies, including optical coherence tomography, provide real-time, high-resolution visualization of neural structures and are currently undergoing active investigation. Other modalities—such as optical nerve stimulation, fluorescence labeling, and multiphoton microscopy—continue to be experimental owing to practical and technical limitations [54–56].

Importantly, the psychosocial consequences of ED following RP are substantial, frequently contributing to depression, anxiety, and impaired quality of life [4]. As such, contemporary care increasingly integrates psychological counseling alongside medical therapy. Emerging regenerative approaches—including low-intensity shockwave therapy (LISWT) and stem cell-based interventions—aim to restore neurovascular integrity rather than merely manage symptoms, representing a promising future direction in post-RP sexual rehabilitation [57].

Overall, continued advancements in surgical technique, intraoperative nerve preservation, and structured postoperative rehabilitation remain essential to minimizing ED and improving long-term functional outcomes following RP.

EBRT

EBRT for pelvic malignancies is a well-recognized cause of radiation-induced ED (RiED), which typically manifests as a gradual and progressive decline in EF between 6 months and 3 years after treatment [58]. Contemporary studies indicate that approximately 30–50% of men encounter new-onset or deteriorating ED following EBRT, primarily attributable to cumulative radiation-induced damage to the penile vasculature and the progressive degeneration of the cavernous tissue nerves [59–61]. The peak incidence of ED generally occurs between 6 months and 2 years after RT [62, 63]. From a cohort of PCa patients who received EBRT without the use of antiandrogen, at 16 months post RT, only 60% (compared to 81% at baseline) could attain erection, and 27% (compared to 44% at baseline) could have erection that permitted intercourse [64].

RT-associated ED underscores the constraints of preceding methodologies and the biological susceptibility of erectile tissues to ionizing radiation. Initial two-dimensional radiotherapy and three-dimensional conformal RT (3DCRT) were characterized by imprecise target delineation, leading in overexposure of adjacent tissues to excessive radiation. Consequently, prospective investigations have documented a markedly heterogeneous range of ED incidences, spanning from 7% to 72% following 3DCRT [65–69]. The integration of computed tomography (CT) and magnetic resonance imaging (MRI) substantially enhanced target accuracy, with CT reducing target error by over 30% and MRI exhibiting superior soft-tissue resolution in comparison to CT alone [70–72].

These technological advancements in imaging facilitated the adoption of intensity-modulated radiation therapy (IMRT) during the 1990s, a technique that permits highly conformal dose delivery through computer-controlled beam modulation. IMRT diminishes radiation exposure to adjacent erectile structures while preserving oncologic efficacy. Nevertheless, ED persists as a prevalent issue; Brown et al. reported that 50% of patients treated with IMRT experienced severe ED (SHIM <10) at a median follow-up of 36.8 months [73]. Hypofractionated radiotherapy further enhances this approach by leveraging the differential DNA repair capacity between tumor and normal tissues. Stereotactic body radiotherapy (SBRT), an ultra-precise modality of hypofractionation, has demonstrated improved preservation of EF, with reported functional erection rates of 57% at 24 months and 45% at 60 months in patients with baseline intact erectile functionality [74].

More recently, image-guided radiation therapy (IGRT) has facilitated real-time visualization and adaptive treatment planning utilizing on-board CT or MRI. Data from the CHHiP trial IGRT substudy demonstrated a reduction in radiation dose to the penile bulb and a corresponding decrease in the risk of severe ED [75]. BT, which administers radiation directly to the prostate through implanted isotopes such as iodine-125 or palladium-103, has also been correlated with a reduced incidence of ED, with reported rates varying from 5% to 51% depending on the technique employed and its combination with EBRT [44]. Emerging particle therapies, such as proton and carbon-ion therapy, utilize the Bragg peak effect to optimize tumor dosing while minimizing damage to adjacent tissues. Extended follow-up of proton therapy indicates a reduction in EF from 90% at baseline to approximately 62–67% over a period of one to 5 years [76].

The pathophysiology of RiED is multifactorial and primarily vascular and neurogenic. Initial angiographic investigations revealed obstructive pathology in the internal pudendal arteries within irradiated pelvic regions [77]. In addition, Doppler ultrasound studies confirmed arterial insufficiency as a principal mechanism [78]. Preclinical data further indicate that radiation diminishes nerve fibers containing nitric oxide synthase within the corpora cavernosa, thereby impairing smooth muscle relaxation and penile hemodynamics [79]. Patient-related factors, including age, socioeconomic status, and access to specialized care, further influence the risk of ED subsequent to RT [80, 81].

Management of RiED emphasizes early intervention through structured penile rehabilitation, often initiated during or immediately after radiotherapy [42]. First-line therapy consists of PDE-5 inhibitors, followed by vacuum erection devices, intracavernosal alprostadil injections, or intraurethral therapy in nonresponders. LISWT has gained interest for its potential to promote neovascularization, while penile prosthesis implantation remains a definitive and highly effective option for refractory cases.

Ongoing technological refinements persist in their emphasis on reducing radiation exposure to vital sexual structures. Contemporary planning guidelines advocate for constraining the mean dose to the penile bulb to less than 50 Gy, with ultra-conformal techniques frequently aiming for doses below 20 Gy [82]. The utilization of hydrogel spacers, such as SpaceOAR, enhances the separation between the prostate and neighboring tissues and has been correlated with erectile preservation rates exceeding 60% [83]. Future advancements that incorporate molecular imaging, real-time adaptive IGRT, and more secure BT isotopes are anticipated to further diminish the incidence of ED caused by RT (Table 18.1).

Table 18.1 EBRT dose constraints and clinical protocol

Category	Component	Clinical recommendation
Dose constraints	Mean Penile Bulb Dose	Keep mean penile bulb dose below a specific threshold (e.g., <20–22 Gy) to significantly reduce severe ED risk [84]
	Max Penile Bulb Dose	Limit the near-maximum (D2%) to a specified maximum (e.g., <50–56 Gy) [85].
	Other Structures	Emerging protocols also limit mean dose to penile crura (e.g., <4.7 Gy) and internal pudendal arteries [86]
Clinical protocol	Targeting Method	Use IMRT or SBRT with daily IGRT to minimize margins [87]
	Protective Measures	Use of hydrogel spacers (e.g., SpaceOAR) to distance target volumes from healthy tissue [83]
Rehabilitation [42]	First-Line (Oral)	PDE5 inhibitors taken daily or on-demand, started during or shortly after treatment
	Mechanical Aids	Daily use of a VED to prevent penile shortening and tissue fibrosis
	Escalation	ICI or intraurethral alprostadil if oral medications are ineffective

ED Erectile dysfunction, *IMRT* Intensity-Modulated Radiotherapy, *SBRT* Stereotactic Body Radiotherapy, *IGRT* Image-Guided Radiation Therapy, *PDE-5* Phosphodiesterase-5, *VED* Vacuum Erection Device, *ICI* Intracavernosal injections

Systemic Therapies

Systemic therapies for PCa, particularly ADT and chemotherapy, can also impair EF. ADT works by reducing testosterone levels, which are critical for maintaining libido and EF. Testosterone plays a key role in the regulation of nitric oxide synthase, the enzyme responsible for producing nitric oxide in the corpora cavernosa, which is essential for initiating the erectile process [88]. By lowering testosterone levels, ADT diminishes sexual desire and reduces the ability of the penile arteries to dilate in response to sexual stimulation, leading to ED.

Although chemotherapy-induced ED has not been conclusively established in clinical studies, emerging evidence suggests an indirect association. In animal models, Kataoka et al. showed that docetaxel treatment led to reduced testosterone levels and a significant decrease in the intracavernosal pressure-to-mean arterial pressure (ICP/MAP) ratio, indicating impaired erectile hemodynamics [89]. Clinically, a multicenter study involving 428 PCa patients reported gonadal dysfunction in 48% of those receiving oral anticancer agents such as platinum compounds and paclitaxel, suggesting that chemotherapy may indirectly impair erectile function through endocrine disruption [90]. In addition, taxanes such as docetaxel are known to cause peripheral neuropathy, which may further compromise neural signaling involved in erection [91, 92]. Psychological sequelae of chemotherapy, including anxiety, depression, and fatigue, may further exacerbate ED by deteriorating overall physical and mental health. Nevertheless, direct clinical evidence linking chemotherapy to ED remains limited, highlighting the need for focused prospective studies.

In contrast, the mechanisms by which ADT induces ED are well characterized. Men undergoing long-term ADT often experience a profound loss of sexual interest and a marked decrease in the frequency of spontaneous erections. Testosterone plays a critical role in maintaining the structural and functional integrity of the corpora cavernosa [37, 41, 42, 90]. Androgen deprivation triggers smooth muscle atrophy and progressive replacement with collagen fibers, leading to corporal fibrosis and loss of elasticity [93]. This structural remodeling results in corporal veno-occlusive dysfunction, whereby venous outflow cannot be adequately restricted to sustain an erection. Simultaneously, diminished androgen levels lead to a decrease in the expression of nitric oxide synthase, resulting in reduced nitric oxide availability and compromised endothelial-dependent vasodilation. Consequently, this impairs erectile responses even during sexual stimulation, as demonstrated by Zhou et al. in an animal study [94]. From a retrospective review of a prospective RT cohort of PCa patients, the use of ADT was found to be associated with worse EF at 1 year regardless of the disease risk, and also at 3 years for the high-risk patients [95]. The efficacy of PDE-5 inhibitors in treating ED for men on ADT, however, was debatable. From a randomized double-blinded crossover trial among intermediate-risk PCa patients who received EBRT and ADT, sildenafil led to significant improvement in the probabilities of erectile response by approximately 20% for patients receiving ≤120 days of ADT. However, merely 21% of the patients had a treatment-specific response, that only lasted during the sildenafil phase, but not during the placebo phase [96]. While PDE-5 inhibitors improve ED related to ADT, at least in a subset of patients, the lack of testosterone might make it more challenging to achieve satisfactory erections, even with pharmacological assistance.

Despite advances in hormonal manipulation, most patients eventually progress to mCRPC, leading to the widespread adoption of androgen receptor pathway inhibitors. Abiraterone has demonstrated significant survival benefits in castration-resistant disease, with Ryan et al. reporting a median overall survival of 34.7 months in the abiraterone group compared with 30.3 months in the placebo group, along with marked improvements in radiographic progression-free survival [97]. Contemporary treatment strategies frequently combine ADT with androgen receptor antagonists to achieve maximal androgen blockade. Novel approaches, such as bipolar androgen therapy (BAT) and rapid androgen cycling (RAC), aim to exploit tumor vulnerability through abrupt hormonal fluctuations; however, clinical evidence remains limited. Notably, Teply et al. reported a ≥50% PSA reduction in 15 of 21 asymptomatic mCRPC patients treated with BAT after enzalutamide failure [98].

Regardless of therapeutic refinements, ED remains an almost inevitable consequence of ADT. A comprehensive review by Gryzinski et al. demonstrated a threefold increase in ED risk among patients receiving ADT [99]. This effect is primarily attributable to testosterone deficiency, which induces endothelial dysfunction, reduces penile blood flow, decreases nitric oxide bioavailability, and alters PDE-5 signaling, collectively impairing erection quality and durability [100]. While exogenous testosterone supplementation may improve EF, it is contraindicated during ADT due to the risk of stimulating tumor progression [101, 102]. Future ADT protocols may benefit from routine assessment of EF, enabling early identification and timely management of treatment-related ED.

Combination Treatment

Combination therapies, such as RP followed by RT or the combination of RT and ADT, are often used in patients with high-risk or locally advanced PCa. Unfortunately, these multimodal treatments are associated with a higher risk of ED compared to monotherapy. Although these multimodal strategies enhance oncologic outcomes, they significantly escalate the risk and severity of ED through cumulative and often synergistic mechanisms [103–105]. These cumulative effects of surgery, RT, and hormonal therapy increase the likelihood of damage to the neurovascular structures and penile vasculature that are critical for erections [106].

The combination of RP and RT exemplifies this additive injury. RP primarily impairs EF through cavernous nerve trauma and postoperative neuropraxia, while subsequent RT induces progressive vascular injury, smooth muscle loss, and corporal fibrosis [44, 107]. Together, these effects significantly diminish erectile recovery relative to either modality utilized independently, even amidst the era of nerve-sparing surgery and conformal RT planning [6]. Similarly, the combination of RT and ADT notably deteriorates erectile function outcomes. Neurovascular damage caused by radiation is exacerbated by hypogonadism associated with ADT, which suppresses libido, impairs endothelial function, and accelerates apoptosis of smooth muscle cells and collagen deposition within the corpora cavernosa [62, 78, 108]. When it comes to salvage RP following primary RT, the functional outcomes are notoriously adverse. According to a systematic review, the ED rates for salvage RP after RT could reach 80–100% [109]. These findings suggest that the detrimental effects of PCa treatments on erectile function can be cumulative in nature.

Clinical studies consistently demonstrate higher rates of persistent ED in patients receiving combined RT and ADT, particularly with prolonged androgen suppression [110]. In advanced PCa, combined systemic treatment modalities—such as ADT in conjunction with androgen receptor pathway inhibitors or chemotherapy—are commonly linked to nearly universal sexual dysfunction. The substantial and enduring suppression of androgen levels, coupled with the potential neurotoxic and vasculotoxic effects of systemic agents, results in irreversible structural and functional damage to erectile tissue [97, 111].

The increased risk of ED associated with combination therapy reflects the convergence of neurogenic injury, vascular compromise, hormonal depletion, and corporal remodeling [112]. Consequently, ED tends to be more severe, recovery becomes less predictable, and responsiveness to conventional treatments is diminished. Preservation strategies therefore prioritize prevention over restoration, including reducing the radiation dose to erectile structures, limiting

ADT duration when oncologically appropriate, and initiating early penile rehabilitation through the use of PDE-5 inhibitors, vacuum erection devices, or intracavernosal therapy [113, 114].

Emerging advances—such as ultra-conformal and image-guided RT, improved nerve-sparing and robotic surgical techniques, and regenerative approaches including LISWT—offer promise in mitigating the sexual morbidity of combination therapy [48, 115, 116]. Nonetheless, the preservation of EF in this context continues to be challenging, emphasizing the importance of individualized treatment planning, early intervention, and comprehensive patient counseling.

Predictors of Erectile Dysfunction Following Prostate Cancer Treatment

There are several variables influencing the EF outcomes after the treatment in men with PCa. Some of these disease-related factors are the PSA, Gleason score, and clinical or pathological cancer staging. These can indirectly predict the occurrence of ED following different treatment options as these factors can interact synergistically to influence EF.

PSA

PSA level itself does not directly lead to ED. Higher PSA levels per se or as one constituent of nomograms predict advanced disease and higher risk of extracapsular extension (ECE), which may indicate more extensive treatments such as non-nerve-sparing RP or high-dose RT [117]. These more aggressive treatments carry a higher risk of ED due to increased likelihood of damaging the neurovascular structures involved in EF [40, 117]. In a longitudinal study of 195 men with localized PCa, men with higher baseline PSA predicted a more rapidly declining sexual function over time [118].

Gleason Score

The Gleason score, which is used to grade the aggressiveness of PCa, also influences treatment decisions that impact EF. Patients with a high Gleason score are more likely to undergo radical treatments, including non-nerve-sparing surgery or high-dose RT [117]. These treatments are associated with a higher risk of ED compared to more conservative options, such as nerve-sparing surgery or active surveillance, which are often chosen for patients with lower Gleason scores [119]. In a retrospective review of 79 men who underwent bilateral nerve-sparing LRP, there was a significant association between ED and Gleason score [120]. A multivariate logistic regression identified Gleason score (OR 4.749) as independent predictor of ED. On the other hand, men with ED had a higher risk of high Gleason score. In a study of 1421 men, those in the low EF group were significantly associated with a higher Gleason score (OR 1.910) and large tumor volume (OR 1.390) [121]. Therefore, the Gleason score indirectly predicts the likelihood of post-treatment ED by guiding the selection of treatment modalities that have different risks for sexual dysfunction.

cT Staging

The clinical T stage of PCa is another important predictor of post-treatment ED. Men with organ-confined PCa have significantly better EF outcomes compared to those with locally advanced or metastatic diseases. EF in men with localized diseases is more often responsive to treatment strategies for ED. Patients with more advanced clinical stage (T3-T4) are more likely to require extensive surgical resection or higher doses of RT, both of which increase the likelihood of damaging the NVBs and penile blood vessels. Worse still, locally advanced diseases are more susceptible to the need for multimodal therapies [122]. In contrast, selected patients with early-stage disease (T1-T2) may be candidates for nerve-sparing surgery or even focal therapy which are associated with a lower risk of ED [64, 123].

Initial Erectile Function

One of the most reliable predictors of post-treatment EF is the patient's baseline EF prior to treatment. Patients who have good EF before treatment are more likely to retain some degree of EF after treatment, particularly if they undergo nerve-sparing surgery or are treated with lower doses of radiation. In contrast, patients who have pre-existing ED are at higher risk of experiencing further deterioration in their sexual function after treatment [107]. The presence of spontaneous erection before RT was found to positively predict the chance of attaining erection that allows intercourse post-treatment [123]. Pre-treatment documentation and counseling about EF preservation are therefore crucial, especially for men with pre-existing ED, who may be more motivated to choose treatments that maximize their chances of retaining sexual function.

Spontaneous Recovery of EF

While many men experience immediate or early ED following PCa treatment, some patients may experience spontaneous recovery of EF over time. This is particularly true for men who undergo nerve-sparing RP, as the cavernous nerves may gradually regenerate or recover from temporary injury caused by the surgical procedure. Studies have shown that EF can improve spontaneously within 24–48 months post-operatively, although the degree of recovery is variable and often incomplete [124]. Factors that may contribute to spontaneous recovery include the extent of nerve preservation, the patient's age, and their baseline EF [7].

Erectile Function Preservation in PCa Management

Oncological control remains the primary concern of PCa management. However, preservation of EF becomes equally important as this warrants active treatment in many men. Commencing sexual rehabilitation before the initiation of surgical treatment seems to ensure a better recovery of EF after the surgery [125]. This can be achieved through multimodal strategies. Emerging techniques in nerve-sparing refinement during RP, use of PDE5 inhibitors and regenerative therapies may preserve EF after PCa management.

Nerve Preservation

Nerve-sparing technique was introduced in the 1980s to decrease the adverse effects of RP particularly ED [44]. This approach comprises of meticulous dissection of the NBVs that are located within the posterolateral periprostatic fascial layers which are fundamental for penile erection. This can preserve erectile function without compromising oncologic control.

In a comparative study including 147 patients, the intrafascial nerve-sparing RP group was found to have a better potency rate and shorter time of return of continence, as compared to the interfascial nerve-sparing RP group. The benefit came with the cost of higher positive surgical margin rates in patients with pT3 disease in the intrafascial group [126]. Similarly, a relatively high positive surgical margin rate of 30.7% was found to be associated with the intrafascial approach, from another large cohort of LRP [127]. Ultimately, the success of nerve-sparing RP in preserving EF depends on several factors, including the surgeon's experience, the extent of the tumor, and the patient's preoperative sexual function. In a systematic review and meta-analysis of 124 studies comprising of 73,448 patients, the estimated absolute risk of ED was lowest in bilateral nerve-sparing surgery (30.6%) compared to unilateral-nerve-sparing (50.5%) and non-nerve-sparing surgery (72.1%) [128].

Several intraoperative strategies to enhance the preservation of EF have been investigated. For instance, some advocate the use of intraoperative nerve monitoring (IONM) to identify and protect the cavernous nerves during surgery. This technique involves the use of electrical stimulation to locate the nerves, allowing the surgeon to avoid damaging them during dissection [129]. However, from a recent randomized trial, the use of ProPep® Nerve Monitoring System did not result in better continence and erection outcomes following unilateral-nerve-sparing or non-nerve-sparing RARP [130]. Up to date, there has not been conclusive evidence to support the role of IONM in preserving erectile function after RP.

Minimal Invasive Versus Open Surgeries

RP has evolved from open surgery to include minimally invasive approaches such as laparoscopic and robot-assisted procedures. Open RRP is still considered as the gold standard for the surgical management of men with organ-confined PCa [131]. Sexual potency after bilateral nerve-sparing RP is 31–86% of sexually active men with non-metastatic disease [132]. Contemporary evidence showed that the incidence of ED after RP is more than half of cases despite the advances and innovation in surgical techniques [133]. After surgery, return to subjective baseline erection is rare [134].

In a comparative meta-analysis of 13 studies comprising of 6281 men, RARP was associated with significantly more effective in EF preservation at 3, 6, and 12 months after surgery compared to those who underwent LRP [135]. Similar results were demonstrated in another meta-analysis showing RARP provided not only superior oncological control but also better EF recovery compared to LRP as shown in the improvement of the IIEF-5 scores [136]. RARP has shown quicker potency recovery as compared to open RP [131]. Even in high-risk PCa, RARP is beneficial for the long-term EF recovery 12 months after the surgery [16]. Surgeon's expertise can be contributory to the recovery of EF after RP. Annual surgeon caseload of more than 25 RP cases per year or total cumulative experience of more than 1000 cases demonstrated superior erectile function outcomes after RP [137]. Younger men (<60 years old), preoperative potency and bilateral nerve-sparing surgery are positive predictors of EF following RARP [138]. Recovery in EF can occur after 12 months after surgery [139].

Despite the advantages of LRP and RARP, further prospective randomized studies are necessary to further determine the definitive role of these surgical techniques in the treatment of men with organ-confined PCa.

PDE-5 Inhibitors

PDE-5 inhibitors, which include sildenafil, tadalafil, avanafil, and vardenafil, are generally considered as the first line of treatment in properly selected men with PCa suffering with ED [140]. By enhancing blood flow, PDE-5 inhibitors can help improve erectile responses in men who have undergone PCa treatment [119].

The early use of PDE-5 inhibitors after RP—often referred to as "penile rehabilitation"—has been associated with better EF outcomes. A randomized study suggested that the early group (in which patients took sildenafil starting from their foley catheter removal) had better EF recovery than the delayed group (in which sildenafil was started 3 months after nerve-sparing RP) [141]. Likewise, the REACCT trial demonstrated the efficacy of daily 5 mg tadalafil in contributing to the recovery of EF after RP and the prevention of penile fibrosis. Nevertheless, the use of tadalafil failed to improve unassisted erection after cessation of active therapy for 9 months [113]. From a systematic review and network meta-analysis of penile rehabilitation strategy after nerve-sparing RP, only pelvic floor exercise and sildenafil used in regular high doses (100 mg daily) were associated with significantly higher likelihood of EF recovery. The on-demand use of PDE-5 inhibitors was no better than placebo [142].

However, care must be taken that the possible improvement in on-medication EF does not necessarily translate to improved spontaneous EF in the long-term. From a 2018 Cochrane review, scheduled PDE-5 inhibitors resulted in little to no difference in both short-term and long-term (greater than 12 months) self-reported potency (short-term: RR 0.97, 95% CI 0.62 to 1.53; long-term: RR 1.00, 95% CI 0.60 to 1.67; both very low quality evidence) [143]. There was a paucity of evidence to support the use of PDE-5 inhibitors in improving post-RP ED especially in the long-term [143].

Intracavernosal Injections

Intracavernosal injections (ICI) of alprostadil (prostaglandin E1) have been a widely utilized strategy to treat ED. Its vasodilatory effect encourages blood flow into the cavernosal bodies. In post-prostatectomy settings, ICI is commonly adopted in non-responders to PDE-5 inhibitors [107].

From a prospective cohort of 87 patients who received laparoscopic nerve-sparing RP, ICI was started 1 month after surgery; alprostadil ICI improved EF after 1 year in terms of the mean IIEF-15 score and erection hardness score (EHS), but remained below preoperative levels [144]. In that study, the adverse impact of pain on sexual rehabilitation was significant during the first 6 months and diminished over time [144]. ICI often causes penile pain, which may ultimately lead to a high treatment discontinuation rate [144, 145].

In a prospective non-randomized study, men with functional preoperative erections who underwent various forms of RP (bilateral-, unilateral-, or non-nerve-sparing RP) were treated with oral sildenafil postoperatively. Non-responders were switched to ICI using TriMix (papaverine, phentolamine, prostaglandin E1), starting on average 4 months post-surgery. At 18 months, none of the patients reported pain or prolonged erections, suggesting that non-alprostadil injectables may cause less pain. However, the authors urge caution due to unresolved issues regarding penile pain pathophysiology and the lack of comprehensive time-based assessments of ICI-related symptoms [146].

Mechanical Treatments

In addition to pharmacological interventions, mechanical devices such as vacuum erection devices (VEDs) and penile implants are used in the management of ED following PCa treatment. VEDs are external devices that create a vacuum around the penis, drawing blood into the corpora cavernosa and inducing an erection. VEDs have some initial promise as part of a penile rehabilitation program to increase blood flow to the penile tissues and prevent fibrosis [147].

Implantable penile prostheses (IPP), on the other hand, offer the last resort for men who fail to respond to other treatments. There are two main types of penile implants: inflatable and malleable. Inflatable implants consist of cylinders that are surgically placed inside the corpora cavernosa, a pump that is implanted in the scrotum, and a fluid reservoir that is placed in the abdomen. The patient can inflate the device manually to achieve an erection. Malleable implants consist of flexible rods that can be bent into an erect or flaccid position. For ED patients, penile implants are typically considered a last resort after other treatments have failed [148].

When it comes to treatment of post-prostatectomy ED, the role of early adoption of IPP has been investigated. From a study comparing tadalafil (20 mg three times/week) versus three-piece inflatable IPP among 174 patients who had ED 6 months following bilateral nerve-sparing RP, the IPP group not only had better improvement in IIEF scores from immediately after surgery to 2 years than the tadalafil group (20.4 1.3 vs 8.1 2.4, $P < 0.001$), but it also demonstrated better self-reported erection frequency, firmness, penetration ability, maintenance and erection confidence [149].

The choice of IPP after PCa treatment was also found to be related to the index PCa treatment. From a retrospective Surveillance, Epidemiology, and End Results (SEER) cohort, IPP implantation was more frequent for prostatectomy patients than for radiation patients (3.6% vs. 1.4%, $p < 0.001$) [9]. Technically, adhesions may develop in the retropubic space following RP, which increase the difficulty in dissection during placement of the fluid reservoir. The 3-year reoperation rates of IPP following RP and RT were reported to be 11.1% and 13.1%, respectively [150]. These risks and benefits of IPP should be balanced and discussed during preoperative counseling.

Regenerative Therapies

Emerging paradigms in regenerative medicine aim to preserve EF by repairing the nerves and vascular structures responsible for penile erection. Several regenerative therapies are classified into cellular-based biomaterials and device-related technology [151]. The main regenerative approaches include stem cell therapy (SCT), platelet-rich plasma (PRP) and LISWT.

SCT is a promising regenerative strategy by repairing damaged tissues through cellular proliferation and differentiation. Earlier study demonstrated injection of bone marrow mononucleated cells to manage ED after RP [152]. There were significant improvements of the intercourse satisfaction and EF in 12 men with localized PCa particularly those who received higher doses. In an open-label phase 1 clinical trial of men with ED after RP, 53% of continent men who received a single intracavernous injection of autologous adipose-derived regenerative cells (ADRC) reported EF sufficient for intercourse for 1 year [153]. SCT exhibited numerous concerns hindering it to be accepted as a standard of care in ED treatment in men with PCa. As of now, SCT is still in the experimental stages and not ready for routine clinical use due to the lack of high-level evidence.

Clinical application of PRP in the treatment of ED in men with PCa still lacks robust evidence and existing trials are not standardized. Proposed beneficial effects of PRP are the release of multiple growth factors and differentiation factors on platelet activation [154]. In a pilot study of 16 men with a median time since surgery of 24 months, use of PRP showed improvement of EF after bilateral nerve-sparing RP [155]. However, this did not proceed with unassisted erection enough for sexual intercourse.

The release of vascular endothelial growth factor and endothelial nitric oxide synthase is believed to be the main effect of LISWT [151]. This process is known to promote angiogenesis and neovascularization resulting to significant improvement in EF. Shockwave therapy for ED seems to have beneficial effects in the treatment of ED in men with PCa. LISWT showed significant increase in EF in men following bilateral nerve-sparing RP compared to those men with organic causes of ED [156]. Single treatment cycle which includes 4 sessions over 2 weeks and with application at least 6000 pulses in each session resulted in positive outcome. This is better achieved if the pulses are distributed throughout the crura and both corpora cavernous of the penis. A meta-analysis reviewed the outcomes of LISWT in men with ED post-RP, and found that in IIEF scores performed 3–4 months after LISWT, the group receiving LISWT showed statistically significantly better results than the control. Nevertheless, from the only two studies that measured the results after 9–12 months, there was no statistical difference between the two groups. However, the long-term efficacy and optimal treatment parameters, such as the intensity and duration of shockwave therapy, still warrant further investigations [157]. Up till now, there is no conclusive evidence that LISWT therapy confers clinically meaningful benefits to men suffering from ED after RP.

Despite the beneficial effects of these regenerative therapies, there are considerable concerns particularly the long-term efficacy and safety [158]. There is a scarcity of high-quality clinical trials that support these emerging treatments as a standard care. Further studies are warranted to define the role of these alternative treatment options in the management of men with PCa suffering from ED.

Conclusion

Preserving EF after PCa treatment remains a critical goal, but it depends on several factors including the type of treatment, the stage of cancer, and nerve-sparing techniques used during surgery. Advances in treatments, such as robotic-assisted surgeries, pharmacological and mechanical therapies, show promise in reducing the impact on sexual health. However, patient recovery varies, and long-term outcomes require individualized care plans and rehabilitation strategies. Ongoing research is essential to optimize post-treatment quality of life for PCa survivors.

References

1. Bray F, Laversanne M, Sung H, Ferlay J, Siegel RL, Soerjomataram I, et al. Global cancer statistics 2022: GLOBOCAN estimates of incidence and mortality worldwide for 36 cancers in 185 countries. CA Cancer J Clin. 2024;74(3):229–63.
2. Sekhoacha M, Riet K, Motloung P, Gumenku L, Adegoke A, Mashele S. Prostate cancer review: genetics, diagnosis, treatment options, and alternative approaches. Molecules. 2022;27(17):5730.
3. Hyun JS. Prostate cancer and sexual function. World J Mens Health. 2012;30(2):99–107.
4. Chambers SK, Chung E, Wittert G, Hyde MK. Erectile dysfunction, masculinity, and psychosocial outcomes: a review of the experiences of men after prostate cancer treatment. Transl Androl Urol. 2017;6(1):60–8.
5. Kinnaird W, Schartau P, Kirby M, Jenkins V, Allen S, Payne H. Sexual dysfunction in prostate cancer patients according to disease stage and treatment modality. Clin Oncol. 2025;41:103801.
6. Tal R, Alphs HH, Krebs P, Nelson CJ, Mulhall JP. Erectile function recovery rate after radical prostatectomy: a meta-analysis. J Sex Med. 2009;6(9):2538–46.
7. Ficarra V, Novara G, Ahlering TE, et al. Systematic review and meta-analysis of studies reporting potency rates after robot-assisted radical prostatectomy. Eur Urol. 2012;62(3):418–30.
8. van Tol-Geerdink JJ, Leer JW, van Oort IM, et al. Quality of life after prostate cancer treatments in patients comparable at baseline. Br J Cancer. 2013;108(9):1784–9.
9. Shen C, Jain K, Shah T, Schaefer E, Zhou S, Fried D, et al. Relationships between erectile dysfunction, prostate cancer treatment type and inflatable penile prosthesis implantation. Investig Clin Urol. 2022;63(3):316–24.
10. Muise A, Pan MM, Rose B, Buckley JC. Functional outcomes after prostate cancer treatment: a comparison between single and multiple modalities. Urol Oncol Semin Orig Investig. 2023;41(2):104.e1–9.
11. Nukala V, Incrocci L, Hunt AA, Ballas L, Koontz BF. Challenges in reporting the effect of radiotherapy on erectile function. J Sex Med. 2020;17(6):1053–9.

12. Putora PM, Engeler D, Haile SR, Graf N, Buchauer K, Schmid HP, et al. Erectile function following brachytherapy, external beam radiotherapy, or radical prostatectomy in prostate cancer patients. Strahlenther Onkol Organ Dtsch Rontgengesellschaft Al. 2016;192(3):182–9.
13. Kim DK, Moon YJ, Chung DY, Jung HD, Jeon SH, Kang SH, et al. Comparison of robot-assisted, laparoscopic, and open radical prostatectomy outcomes: a systematic review and network meta-analysis from KSER update series. Medicina (Mex). 2025;61(1):61.
14. Avulova S, Zhao Z, Lee D, Huang LC, Koyama T, Hoffman KE, et al. The effect of nerve sparing status on sexual and urinary function: 3-year results from the CEASAR study. J Urol. 2018;199(5):1202–9.
15. Alemozaffar M, Regan MM, Cooperberg MR, Wei JT, Michalski JM, Sandler HM, et al. Prediction of erectile function following treatment for prostate cancer. JAMA. 2011;306(11):1205.
16. Liu Y, Deng XZ, Qin J, Wen Z, Jiang Y, Huang J, et al. Erectile function, urinary continence and oncologic outcomes of neurovascular bundle sparing robot-assisted radical prostatectomy for high-risk prostate cancer: a systematic review and meta-analysis. Front Oncol. 2023;13:1161544.
17. Xie X, Zhang Y, Ge C, Liang P. Effect of brachytherapy vs. external beam radiotherapy on sexual function in patients with clinically localized prostate cancer: a meta-analysis. Front Cell Dev Biol. 2021;9:792597.
18. Donovan KA, Gonzalez BD, Nelson AM, Fishman MN, Zachariah B, Jacobsen PB. Effect of androgen deprivation therapy on sexual function and bother in men with prostate cancer: a controlled comparison. Psychooncology. 2018;27(1):316–24.
19. Nelson CJ, Scardino PT, Eastham JA, Mulhall JP. Back to baseline: erectile function recovery after radical prostatectomy from the patients' perspective. J Sex Med. 2013;10(6):1636–43.
20. Flores JM, Thorogood S, Jenkins LC, Miyagi H, Nelson CJ, Benfante N, et al. Does diabetes have a negative impact on erectile function recovery after radical prostatectomy? Urology. 2024;194:327–32.
21. Teloken PE, Nelson CJ, Karellas M, Stasi J, Eastham J, Scardino PT, et al. Defining the impact of vascular risk factors on erectile function recovery after radical prostatectomy. BJU Int. 2013;111(4):653–7.
22. McNeal JE. Anatomy of the prostate and morphogenesis of BPH. Prog Clin Biol Res. 1984;145:27–53.
23. Walz J, Epstein JI, Ganzer R, Graefen M, Guazzoni G, Kaouk J, et al. A critical analysis of the current knowledge of surgical anatomy of the prostate related to optimisation of cancer control and preservation of continence and erection in candidates for radical prostatectomy: an update. Eur Urol. 2016;70(2):301–11.
24. Patel VR, Schatloff O, Chauhan S, Sivaraman A, Valero R, Coelho RF, et al. The role of the prostatic vasculature as a landmark for nerve sparing during robot-assisted radical prostatectomy. Eur Urol. 2012;61(3):571–6.
25. Mulhall JP, Secin FP, Guillonneau B. Artery sparing radical prostatectomy—myth or reality? J Urol. 2008;179(3):827–31.
26. Walz J, Burnett AL, Costello AJ, Eastham JA, Graefen M, Guillonneau B, et al. A critical analysis of the current knowledge of surgical anatomy related to optimization of cancer control and preservation of continence and erection in candidates for radical prostatectomy. Eur Urol. 2010;57(2):179–92.
27. Williams SB, Morales BE, Huynh LM, Osann K, Skarecky DW, Ahlering TE. Analysis of accessory pudendal artery transection on erections during robot-assisted radical prostatectomy. J Endourol. 2017;31(11):1170–5.
28. Henry BM, Pękala PA, Vikse J, Sanna B, Skinningsrud B, Saganiak K, et al. Variations in the arterial blood supply to the penis and the accessory pudendal artery: a meta-analysis and review of implications in radical prostatectomy. J Urol. 2017;198(2):345–53.
29. Costello AJ, Brooks M, Cole OJ. Anatomical studies of the neurovascular bundle and cavernosal nerves. BJU Int. 2004;94(7):1071–6.

30. Drizenko A, Goullet E, Mauroy B, Demondion X, Bonnal JL, Biserte J, et al. The inferior hypogastric plexus (pelvic plexus): its importance in neural preservation techniques. Surg Radiol Anat. 2003;25(1):6–15.
31. Joniau S, Van Den Bergh L, Lerut E, Deroose CM, Haustermans K, Oyen R, et al. Mapping of pelvic lymph node metastases in prostate cancer. Eur Urol. 2013;63(3):450–8.
32. Yuh B, Artibani W, Heidenreich A, Kimm S, Menon M, Novara G, et al. The role of robot-assisted radical prostatectomy and pelvic lymph node dissection in the management of high-risk prostate cancer: a systematic review. Eur Urol. 2014;65(5):918–27.
33. Sievert KD, Hennenlotter J, Laible I, Amend B, Schilling D, Anastasiadis A, et al. The peri-prostatic autonomic nerves—bundle or layer? Eur Urol. 2008;54(5):1109–17.
34. Clarebrough EE, Challacombe BJ, Briggs C, Namdarian B, Weston R, Murphy DG, et al. Cadaveric analysis of periprostatic nerve distribution: an anatomical basis for high anterior release during radical prostatectomy? J Urol. 2011;185(4):1519–25.
35. Tewari AK, Srivastava A, Huang MW, Robinson BD, Shevchuk MM, Durand M, et al. Anatomical grades of nerve sparing: a risk-stratified approach to neural-hammock sparing during robot-assisted radical prostatectomy (RARP). BJU Int. 2011 Sept;108(6b):984–92.
36. Porst H, Burri A. Novel treatment for premature ejaculation in the light of currently used therapies: a review. Sex Med Rev. 2019;7(1):129–40.
37. Bhat GS, Shastry A. New tools to measure ejaculatory latency-arousal to ejaculation time interval and erection to ejaculation time interval: a pilot study. Urology. 2018;115:107–11.
38. Krassioukov A, Elliott S. Neural control and physiology of sexual function: effect of spinal cord injury. Top Spinal Cord Inj Rehabil. 2017;23(1):1–10.
39. Davoudzadeh EP, Davoudzadeh NP, Margolin E, Stahl PJ, Stember DS. Penile length: measurement technique and applications. Sex Med Rev. 2018;6(2):261–71.
40. Penson DF, McLerran D, Feng Z, et al. 5-year urinary and sexual outcomes after radical prostatectomy: results from the prostate cancer outcomes study. J Urol. 2005;173(5):1701–5.
41. Moretti TBC, Magna LA, Reis LO. Erectile dysfunction criteria of 131,350 patients after open, laparoscopic, and robotic radical prostatectomy. Andrology. 2024;12(8):1865–73.
42. Nicolai M, Urkmez A, Sarikaya S, Fode M, Falcone M, Albersen M. Penile rehabilitation and treatment options for erectile dysfunction following radical prostatectomy and radiotherapy. Syst Rev Front Surg. 2021;8:636974.
43. Young HH. The early diagnosis and radical cure of carcinoma of the prostate. Being a study of 40 cases and presentation of a radical operation which was carried out in four cases. J Urol 1905. 2002;168(3):914–21.
44. Walsh PC, Donker PJ. Impotence following radical prostatectomy: insight into etiology and prevention. J Urol. 1982;128(3):492–7.
45. Walsh PC, Lepor H, Eggleston JC. Radical prostatectomy with preservation of sexual function: anatomical and pathological considerations. Prostate. 1983;4(5):473–85.
46. Eggleston JC, Walsh PC. Radical prostatectomy with preservation of sexual function: pathological findings in the first 100 cases. J Urol. 1985;134(6):1146–8.
47. Binder J, Kramer W. Robotically-assisted laparoscopic radical prostatectomy. BJU Int. 2001;87(4):408–10.
48. Menon M, Tewari A, Peabody JO, Shrivastava A, Kaul S, Bhandari A. Vattikuti Institute prostatectomy, a technique of robotic radical prostatectomy for management of localized carcinoma of the prostate: experience of over 1100 cases. Urol Clin North Am. 2004;31(4):701–17.
49. Capogrosso P, Vertosick EA, Benfante NE, Eastham JA, Scardino PJ, Vickers AJ. Are we improving erectile function recovery after radical prostatectomy? Analysis of patients treated over the last decade. Eur Urol. 2019;75(2):221–8.
50. Yang Y, Wang J, Zhang D, Zhang Q. Efficacy of the transvesical approach for robotic-assisted radical prostatectomy via a bladder neck and prostate combined longitudinal incision for the treatment of localized prostate cancer. Front Surg. 2022;9:1053140.

51. Zhang H, Ning Z, Jia G, Zhang G, Wang J, Liu H. Modified hood technique for single-port robot-assisted radical prostatectomy contributes to early recovery of continence. Front Surg. 2023;10:1132303.
52. Kim HL, Stoffel DS, Mhoon DA, Brendler CB. A positive caver map response poorly predicts recovery of potency after radical prostatectomy. Urology. 2000;56(4):561–4.
53. Klotz L, Herschorn S. Early experience with intraoperative cavernous nerve stimulation with penile tumescence monitoring to improve nerve sparing during radical prostatectomy. Urology. 1998;52(4):537–42.
54. Aron M, Kaouk J, Hegarty N, Colombo JR Jr, Haber G, Chung B. Second prize: preliminary experience with the Niris optical coherence tomography system during laparoscopic and robotic prostatectomy. J Endourol. 2007;21(8):814–8.
55. Fried NM, Rais-Bahrami S, Lagoda GA, Chuang Y, Burnett AL, Su LM. Imaging the cavernous nerves in the rat prostate using optical coherence tomography. Lasers Surg Med. 2007;39(1):36–41.
56. Yadav R, Mukherjee S, Hermen M, Tan G, Maxfield FR, Webb WW. Multiphoton microscopy of prostate and periprostatic neural tissue: a promising imaging technique for improving nerve-sparing prostatectomy. J Endourol. 2009;23(5):861–7.
57. Asker H, Yilmaz-Oral D, Oztekin CV, Gur S. An update on the current status and future prospects of erectile dysfunction following radical prostatectomy. Prostate. 2022;82(12):1135–61.
58. Mahmood J, Shamah AA, Creed TM, Pavlovic R, Matsui H, Kimura M. Radiation-induced erectile dysfunction: recent advances and future directions. Adv Radiat Oncol. 2016;1(3):161–9.
59. Hunt AA, Choudhury KR, Nukala V, Nolan MW, Ahmad A, Ashcraft KA. Risk of erectile dysfunction after modern radiotherapy for intact prostate cancer. Prostate Cancer Prostatic Dis. 2021;24(1):128–34.
60. Takemura LS, Costa PHP, Claros OR, Tourinho-Barbosa RR, Teles SB, Sanchez-Salas R. Salvage local treatment for recurrent prostate cancer after focal therapy: a systematic review and meta-analysis. Urol Oncol. 2024;42(12):1–11.
61. Teunissen FR, Zyp JRN, Wortel RC. Advances in erectile function-preserving radiotherapy for prostate cancer. J Sex Med. 2023;20(2):121–3.
62. Incrocci L. Radiation therapy for prostate cancer and erectile (dys)function: the role of imaging. Acta Oncol. 2005;44(7):673–8.
63. Miller DC, Sanda MG, Dunn RL, Montie JE, Pimentel H, Sandler HM. Long-term outcomes among localized prostate cancer survivors: health-related quality-of-life changes after radical prostatectomy, external radiation, and brachytherapy. J Clin Oncol. 2005;23(12):2772–80.
64. Pinkawa M, Gagel B, Piroth MD, et al. Erectile dysfunction after external beam radiotherapy for prostate cancer. Eur Urol. 2009;55(1):227–34.
65. Beard CJ, Propert KJ, Rieker PP, Clark JA, Kaplan I, Kantoff PW. Complications after treatment with external-beam irradiation in early-stage prostate cancer patients: a prospective multiinstitutional outcomes study. J Clin Oncol. 1997;15(1):223–9.
66. Beckendorf V, Hay M, Rozan R, Lagrange JL, N'Guyen T, Giraud B. Changes in sexual function after radiotherapy treatment of prostate cancer. Br J Urol. 1996;77(1):118–23.
67. Borghede G, Hedelin H. Radiotherapy of localised prostate cancer. Analysis of late treatment complications. A prospective study. Radiother Oncol. 1997;43(2):139–46.
68. Tendulkar RD. Commentary RE: androgen deprivation with radiation therapy compared with radiation therapy alone for locally advanced prostatic carcinoma: a randomized comparative trial of the Radiation Therapy Oncology Group. Urology. 2020;145:312.
69. Turner SL, Adams K, Bull CA, Berry MP. Sexual dysfunction after radical radiation therapy for prostate cancer: a prospective evaluation. Urology. 1999;54(1):124–9.
70. Low NN, Vijayakumar S, Rosenberg I, Rubin S, Virudachalam R, Spelbring DR. Beam's eye view based prostate treatment planning: is it useful? Int J Radiat Oncol Biol Phys. 1990;19(3):759–68.

71. Chang JH, Lim Joon D, Nguyen BT, Hiew CY, Esler S, Angus D. MRI scans significantly change target coverage decisions in radical radiotherapy for prostate cancer. J Med Imaging Radiat Oncol. 2014;58(2):237–43.
72. Horsley PJ, Aherne NJ, Edwards GV, Benjamin LC, Wilcox SW, McLachlan CS. Planning magnetic resonance imaging for prostate cancer intensity-modulated radiation therapy: impact on target volumes, radiotherapy dose and androgen deprivation administration. Asia Pac J Clin Oncol. 2015;11(1):15–21.
73. Brown MW, Brooks JP, Albert PS, Poggi MM. An analysis of erectile function after intensity modulated radiation therapy for localized prostate carcinoma. Prostate Cancer Prostatic Dis. 2007;10(2):189–93.
74. Zelefsky MJ, Cowen D, Fuks Z, Shike M, Burman C, Jackson A. Long term tolerance of high dose three-dimensional conformal radiotherapy in patients with localized prostate carcinoma. Cancer. 1999;85(11):2460–8.
75. Murray J, Dean J, Mossop H, Griffin C, Hall E, Gulliford S. Effect of dose and Image Guided Radiation Therapy (IGRT) on patient-reported sexual function in prostate radiation therapy. Int J Radiat Oncol Biol Phys. 2016;96(2):E232.
76. Ho CK, Bryant CM, Mendenhall NP, Henderson RH, Mendenhall WM, Nichols RC. Long-term outcomes following proton therapy for prostate cancer in young men with a focus on sexual health. Acta Oncol. 2018;57(5):582–8.
77. Goldstein I, Feldman MI, Deckers PJ, Babayan RK, Krane RJ, Radiation-associated impotence. A clinical study of its mechanism. JAMA. 1984;251(7):903–10.
78. Zelefsky MJ, Eid JF. Elucidating the etiology of erectile dysfunction after definitive therapy for prostatic cancer. Int J Radiat Oncol Biol Phys. 1998;40(1):129–33.
79. Carrier S, Hricak H, Lee SS, Baba K, Morgan DM, Nunes L. Radiation-induced decrease in nitric oxide synthase–containing nerves in the rat penis. Radiology. 1995;195(1):95–9.
80. Goldstein I, Goren A, Li VW, Tang WY, Hassan TA. Epidemiology update of erectile dysfunction in eight countries with high burden. Sex Med Rev. 2020;8(1):48–58.
81. Pellegrino F, Sjoberg DD, Tin AL, Benfante NE, Briganti A, Montorsi F. Relationship between age, comorbidity, and the prevalence of erectile dysfunction. Eur Urol Focus. 2023;9(1):162–7.
82. Mangar SA, Sydes MR, Tucker HL, Coffey J, Sohaib SA, Gianolini S. Evaluating the relationship between erectile dysfunction and dose received by the penile bulb: using data from a randomised controlled trial of conformal radiotherapy in prostate cancer (MRC RT01, ISRCTN47772397). Radiother Oncol. 2006;80(3):355–62.
83. Guo X, Zhang J, Guan Y, Tian X, Gong Y, Xiao Y. Hydrogel technologies in andrology: advances in research and prospective applications. Front Pharmacol. 2025;16:1635007.
84. Murray J, Gulliford S, Griffin C, Wilkins A, Syndikus I, Staffurth J. Evaluation of erectile potency and radiation dose to the penile bulb using image guided radiotherapy in the CHHiP trial. Clin Transl Radiat Oncol. 2020;21:77–84.
85. Roach M, Nam J, Gagliardi G, El Naqa I, Deasy JO, Marks LB. Radiation dose–volume effects and the penile bulb. Int J Radiat Oncol. 2010;76(3):S130–4.
86. Achard V, Zilli T, Lamanna G, Jorcano S, Bral S, Rubio C. Urethra-sparing prostate cancer stereotactic body radiation therapy: sexual function and radiation dose to the Penile Bulb, the Crura, and the internal pudendal arteries from a randomized phase 2 trial. Int J Radiat Oncol Biol Phys. 2024;119(4):1137–46.
87. Gregoire V, Guckenberger M, Haustermans K, Lagendijk JJW, Menard C, Potter R. Image guidance in radiation therapy for better cure of cancer. Mol Oncol. 2020;14(7):1470–91.
88. Kaplan AL, Hu JC, Morgentaler A, Mulhall JP, Schulman CC, Montorsi F. Testosterone therapy in men with prostate cancer. Eur Urol. 2016;69(5):894–903.
89. Kataoka T, Sanagawa A, Suzuki J, Muto T, Hotta Y, Kawade Y. Influence of anticancer agents on sexual function: an in vivo study based on the US FDA Adverse Event Reporting System. Andrology. 2022;10(1):166–78.

90. Fleishman SB, Khan H, Homel P, Suhail MF, Strebel-Amrhein R, Mohammad F. Testosterone levels and quality of life in diverse male patients with cancers unrelated to androgens. J Clin Oncol. 2010;28(34):5054–60.
91. Cheng HL, Molassiotis A, Leung AKT, Wong KH. Docetaxel-induced peripheral neuropathy in breast cancer patients treated with adjuvant or neo-adjuvant chemotherapy. Breast Care Basel. 2021;16(3):269–75.
92. Micheli L, Collodel G, Moretti E, Noto D, Menchiari A, Cerretani D. Redox imbalance induced by docetaxel in the neuroblastoma SH-SY5Y cells: a study of docetaxel-induced neuronal damage. Redox Rep. 2021;26(1):18–28.
93. Zhang X, Pan J, Xu R, Fu Y, Lv B. Erectile dysfunction associated with prostate cancer treatment and therapeutic advances: a narrative review. Transl Androl Urol. 2024;13(11):2625–43.
94. Zhou W, Jiang J, Jiang R. A low androgenic state inhibits erectile function by suppressing endothelial glycosides in the penile cavernous tissue of rats. Sex Med. 2024;12(3):qfae039.
95. Joyce DD, Wallis CJD, Luckenbaugh AN, et al. Sexual function outcomes of radiation and androgen deprivation therapy for localized prostate cancer in men with good baseline function. Prostate Cancer Prostatic Dis. 2022;25(2):238–47.
96. Watkins Bruner D, James JL, Bryan CJ, et al. Randomized, double-blinded, placebo-controlled crossover trial of treating erectile dysfunction with sildenafil after radiotherapy and short-term androgen deprivation therapy: results of RTOG 0215. J Sex Med. 2011;8(4):1228–38.
97. Ryan CJ, Smith MR, Bono JS, Molina A, Logothetis CJ, Souza P. Abiraterone in metastatic prostate cancer without previous chemotherapy. N Engl J Med. 2013;368(2):138–48.
98. Teply BA, Wang H, Luber B, Sullivan R, Rifkind I, Bruns A. Bipolar androgen therapy in men with metastatic castration-resistant prostate cancer after progression on enzalutamide: an open-label, phase 2, multicohort study. Lancet Oncol. 2018;19(1):76–86.
99. Gryzinski GM, Fustok J, Raheem OA, Bernie HL. Sexual function in men undergoing androgen deprivation therapy. Androgens. 2022;3(1):233–41.
100. Castela A, Vendeira P, Costa C. Testosterone, endothelial health, and erectile function. ISRN Endocrinol. 2011;2011:839149.
101. Potosky AL, Knopf K, Clegg LX, Albertsen PC, Stanford JL, Hamilton AS. Quality-of-life outcomes after primary androgen deprivation therapy: results from the Prostate Cancer Outcomes Study. J Clin Oncol. 2001;19(17):3750–7.
102. Zhang XH, Morelli A, Luconi M, Vignozzi L, Filippi S, Marini M. Testosterone regulates PDE5 expression and in vivo responsiveness to tadalafil in rat corpus cavernosum. Eur Urol. 2005;47(3):409–16.
103. Resnick MJ, Koyama T, Fan KH, Albertsen PC, Goodman M, Hamilton AS. Long-term functional outcomes after treatment for localized prostate cancer. N Engl J Med. 2013;368(5):436–45.
104. Donovan JL, Hamdy FC, Lane JA, Mason M, Metcalfe C, Walsh E. Patient-reported outcomes after monitoring, surgery, or radiotherapy for prostate cancer. N Engl J Med. 2016;375(15):1425–37.
105. Potosky AL, Davis WW, Hoffman RM, Stanford JL, Stephenson RA, Penson DF. Five-year outcomes after prostatectomy or radiotherapy for prostate cancer: the prostate cancer outcomes study. J Natl Cancer Inst. 2004;96(18):1358–67.
106. Pisansky TM, Hunt D, Gomella LG, et al. Duration of androgen suppression before radiotherapy for localized prostate cancer: radiation therapy oncology group randomized clinical trial 9910. J Clin Oncol. 2015;33(4):332–9.
107. Mulhall JP, Bella AJ, Briganti A, McCullough A, Brock G. Erectile function rehabilitation in the radical prostatectomy patient. J Sex Med. 2010;7(4 Pt 2):1687–98.
108. Spratt DE, Pei X, Yamada J, Kollmeier MA, Cox B, Zelefsky MJ. Long-term survival and toxicity in patients treated with high-dose intensity modulated radiation therapy for localized prostate cancer. Int J Radiat Oncol Biol Phys. 2013;85(3):686–92.

109. Chade DC, Eastham J, Graefen M, et al. Cancer control and functional outcomes of salvage radical prostatectomy for radiation-recurrent prostate cancer: a systematic review of the literature. Eur Urol. 2012;61(5):961–71.
110. D'Amico AV, Chen MH, Renshaw AA, Loffredo M, Kantoff PW. Androgen suppression and radiation vs radiation alone for prostate cancer: a randomized trial. JAMA. 2008;299(3):289–95.
111. Beer TM, Armstrong AJ, Rathkopf DE, Loriot Y, Sternberg CN, Higano CS. Enzalutamide in metastatic prostate cancer before chemotherapy. N Engl J Med. 2014;371(5):424–33.
112. Burnett AL, Aus G, Canby-Hagino ED, Cookson MS, D'Amico AV, Dmochowski RR. Erectile function outcome reporting after clinically localized prostate cancer treatment. J Urol. 2007;178(2):597–601.
113. Montorsi F, Brock G, Stolzenburg JU, Mulhall J, Moncada I, Patel HR. Effects of tadalafil treatment on erectile function recovery following bilateral nerve-sparing radical prostatectomy: a randomised placebo-controlled study (REACTT). Eur Urol. 2014;65(3):587–96.
114. Raina R, Pahlajani G, Agarwal A, Jones S, Zippe C. Long-term potency after early use of a vacuum erection device following radical prostatectomy. BJU Int. 2010;106(11):1719–22.
115. Zelefsky MJ, Kollmeier M, Cox B, Fidaleo A, Sperling D, Pei X. Improved clinical outcomes with high-dose image guided radiotherapy compared with non-IGRT for the treatment of clinically localized prostate cancer. Int J Radiat Oncol Biol Phys. 2012;84(1):125–9.
116. Clavijo RI, Kohn TP, Kohn RJR. Effects of low-intensity extracorporeal shockwave therapy on erectile dysfunction: a systematic review and meta-analysis. J Sex Med. 2017;14(1):27–35.
117. Vis AN, van den Bergh RCN, van der Poel HG, et al. Selection of patients for nerve sparing surgery in robot-assisted radical prostatectomy. BJUI Compass. 2021;3(1):6–18.
118. Pearce SM, Wang CH, Victorson DE, Helfand BT, Novakovic KR, Brendler CB, et al. A longitudinal study of predictors of sexual dysfunction in men on active surveillance for prostate cancer. Sex Med. 2015;3(3):156–64.
119. Salonia A, Burnett AL, Graefen M, et al. Prevention and management of postprostatectomy sexual dysfunctions part 2: recovery and preservation of erectile function, sexual desire, and orgasmic function. Eur Urol. 2012;62(2):273–86.
120. Tekinaslan H, Köse O, Özcan S, Görgel SN, Akın Y. Clinical and surgical predictors of erectile dysfunction after bilateral nerve-sparing laparoscopic radical prostatectomy. Arch Esp Urol. 2025;78(6):671–6.
121. Jeong CW, Lee S, Jeong SJ, Hong SK, Byun SS, Lee SE. Preoperative erectile function and the pathologic features of prostate cancer. Int Braz J Urol. 2015;41(2):265–73.
122. Khauli R, Ferrigno R, Guimarães G, et al. Treatment of localized and locally advanced, high-risk prostate cancer: a report from the first prostate cancer consensus conference for developing countries. JCO Glob Oncol. 2021;7:530–7.
123. Budäus L, Bolla M, Bossi A, et al. Functional outcomes and complications following radiation therapy for prostate cancer: a critical analysis of the literature. Eur Urol. 2012;61(1):112–27.
124. Montorsi F, Guazzoni G, Strambi LF, et al. Recovery of spontaneous erectile function after nerve-sparing radical retropubic prostatectomy with and without early intracavernous injections of alprostadil: results of a prospective, randomized trial. J Urol. 1997;158(4):1408–10.
125. Schoentgen N, Califano G, Manfredi C, Romero-Otero J, Chun FKH, Ouzaid I, Hermieu JF, Xylinas E, Verze P. Is it worth starting sexual rehabilitation before radical prostatectomy? Results from a systematic review of the literature. Front Surg. 2021;8:648345.
126. Potdevin L, Ercolani M, Jeong J, Kim IY. Functional and oncologic outcomes comparing interfascial and intrafascial nerve sparing in robot-assisted laparoscopic radical prostatectomies. J Endourol. 2009;23(9):1479–84.
127. Curto F, Benijts J, Pansadoro A, et al. Nerve sparing laparoscopic radical prostatectomy: our technique. Eur Urol. 2006;49(2):344–52. https://doi.org/10.1016/j.eururo.2005.11.029.

128. Nguyen LN, Head L, Witiuk K, Punjani N, Mallick R, Cnossen S, et al. The risks and benefits of cavernous neurovascular bundle sparing during radical prostatectomy. Syst Rev Meta-Anal J Urol. 2017;198(4):760–9.
129. Song WH, Park JH, Tae BS, et al. Establishment of novel intraoperative monitoring and mapping method for the cavernous nerve during robot-assisted radical prostatectomy: results of the phase I/II, first-in-human, feasibility study. Eur Urol. 2020;78(2):221–8.
130. Nolsøe AB, Østergren PB, Jakobsen H, et al. Can nerve monitoring during radical prostatectomy improve functional outcomes? A randomised trial. BJU Int. 2024;133(6):742–51.
131. Pan XW, Cui XM, Teng JF, Zhang DX, Wang ZJ, Qu FJ, et al. Robot-assisted radical prostatectomy vs. open retropubic radical prostatectomy for prostate cancer: a systematic review and meta-analysis. Indian J Surg. 2015;77(Suppl 3):1326–33.
132. Dubbelman YD, Dohle GR, Schröder FH. Sexual function before and after radical retropubic prostatectomy: a systematic review of prognostic indicators for a successful outcome. Eur Urol. 2006;50(4):711–8:718–20.
133. Wallis CJD, Saskin R, Choo R, Herschorn S, Kodama RT, Satkunasivam R, et al. Surgery versus radiotherapy for clinically-localized prostate cancer: a systematic review and meta-analysis. Eur Urol. 2016;70(1):21–30.
134. Fode M, Frey A, Jakobsen H, Sønksen J. Erectile function after radical prostatectomy: do patients return to baseline? Scand J Urol. 2016;50(3):160–3.
135. Pina AJ, Melo VC, Carlos VW, Tristão LS, Santos CL, Bernardo WM, et al. Erectile function after laparoscopic versus robotic-assisted radical prostatectomy: a systematic review and meta-analysis. Asian J Urol. 2025;12(3):281–9.
136. Tian Z, Zhu Y, Sun X, Cui Q. Meta-analysis of radical prostatectomy outcomes: oncological control and functional recovery in prostate cancer patients. Med Baltim. 2025;104(32):e43444.
137. Ju IE, Trieu D, Chang SB, Mungovan SF, Patel MI. Surgeon experience and erectile function after radical prostatectomy: a systematic review. Sex Med Rev. 2021;9(4):650–8.
138. Woo SH, Kang DI, Ha YS, Salmasi AH, Kim JH, Lee DH, et al. Comprehensive analysis of sexual function outcome in prostate cancer patients after robot-assisted radical prostatectomy. J Endourol. 2014;28(2):172–7.
139. Jurys T, Burzynski B, Potyka A, Paradysz A. Post-radical prostatectomy erectile dysfunction assessed using the IIEF-5 questionnaire - a systematic literature review. Int J Sex Health. 2021;34(1):55–64.
140. Cui Y, Liu X, Shi L, Gao Z. Efficacy and safety of phosphodiesterase type 5 (PDE5) inhibitors in treating erectile dysfunction after bilateral nerve-sparing radical prostatectomy. Andrologia. 2016;48(1):20–8.
141. Jo JK, Jeong SJ, Oh JJ, et al. Effect of starting penile rehabilitation with sildenafil immediately after robot-assisted laparoscopic radical prostatectomy on erectile function recovery: a prospective randomized trial. J Urol. 2018;199(6):1600–6.
142. Sari Motlagh R, Abufaraj M, Yang L, et al. Penile rehabilitation strategy after nerve sparing radical prostatectomy: a systematic review and network meta-analysis of randomized trials. J Urol. 2021;205(4):1018–30.
143. Philippou YA, Jung JH, Steggall MJ, et al. Penile rehabilitation for postprostatectomy erectile dysfunction. Cochrane Database Syst Rev. 2018;10(10):CD012414.
144. Yiou R, Cunin P, de la Taille A, et al. Sexual rehabilitation and penile pain associated with intracavernous alprostadil after radical prostatectomy. J Sex Med. 2011;8(2):575–82.
145. Mulhall JP, Jahoda AE, Cairney M, et al. The causes of patient dropout from penile self-injection therapy for impotence. J Urol. 1999;162(4):1291–4.
146. Mulhall J, Land S, Parker M, Waters WB, Flanigan RC. The use of an erectogenic pharmacotherapy regimen following radical prostatectomy improves recovery of spontaneous erectile function. J Sex Med. 2005;2:532–40.
147. Köhler TS, Pedro R, Hendlin K, et al. A pilot study on the early use of the vacuum erection device after radical retropubic prostatectomy. BJU Int. 2007;100(4):858–62.

148. Wang J, Wu P, Liu Q, et al. Effect of a three-piece inflatable penile prosthesis combined with a phosphodiesterase-5 inhibitor on erectile dysfunction. J Int Med Res. 2021;49(4):300060520985365.
149. Megas G, Papadopoulos G, Stathouros G, Moschonas D, Gkialas I, Ntoumas K. Comparison of efficacy and satisfaction profile, between penile prosthesis implantation and oral PDE5 inhibitor tadalafil therapy, in men with nerve-sparing radical prostatectomy erectile dysfunction. BJU Int. 2013;112(2):E169–76.
150. Golan R, Patel NA, Sun T, Barbieri CE, Sedrakyan A, Kashanian JA. Impact of pelvic radiation therapy on inflatable penile prosthesis reoperation rates. J Sex Med. 2018;15(11):1653–8.
151. Chung E. Regenerative technology to restore and preserve erectile function in men following prostate cancer treatment: evidence for penile rehabilitation in the context of prostate cancer survivorship. Ther Adv Urol. 2021;13:17562872211026421.
152. Yiou R, Hamidou L, Birebent B, Bitari D, Lecorvoisier P, Contremoulins I, et al. Safety of intracavernous bone marrow-mononuclear cells for postradical prostatectomy erectile dysfunction: an open dose-escalation pilot study. Eur Urol. 2016;69(6):988–91.
153. Haahr MK, Harken Jensen C, Toyserkani NM, Andersen DC, Damkier P, Sørensen JA, et al. A 12-month follow-up after a single intracavernous injection of autologous adipose-derived regenerative cells in patients with erectile dysfunction following radical prostatectomy: an open-label phase I clinical trial. Urology. 2018;121:203.e6–203.e13.
154. Scott S, Roberts M, Chung E. Platelet-rich plasma and treatment of erectile dysfunction: critical review of literature and global trends in platelet-rich plasma clinics. Sex Med Rev. 2019;7(2):306–12.
155. Frey A, Sønksen J, Fode M. Low-intensity extracorporeal shockwave therapy in the treatment of postprostatectomy erectile dysfunction: a pilot study. Scand J Urol. 2016;50(2):123–7.
156. Juan-Casas C, Leirós-Rodríguez R, González-Castro A, Hernandez-Lucas P. Efficacy of extracorporeal shock waves therapy for erectile dysfunction treatment: a systematic review and meta-analysis. Basic Clin Androl. 2025;35(1):12.
157. Rho BY, Kim SH, Ryu JK, Kang DH, Kim JW, Chung DY. Efficacy of low-intensity extracorporeal shock wave treatment in erectile dysfunction following radical prostatectomy: a systematic review and meta-analysis. J Clin Med. 2022;11(10):2775.
158. Chung E, Lee J, Liu CC, Taniguchi H, Zhou HL, Park HJ. Clinical practice guideline recommendation on the use of low intensity extracorporeal shock wave therapy and low intensity pulsed ultrasound shock wave therapy to treat erectile dysfunction: the Asia-Pacific Society for Sexual Medicine Position Statement. World J Mens Health. 2021;39(1):1–8.

Chapter 19
Advances in Penile Implants and Mechanical Devices for Erectile Dysfunction

Eric Chung, Cesar Rojas-Cruz, and Rupin Shah

Introduction

Erectile dysfunction (ED) is a common male sexual dysfunction that adversely impacts beyond psychosexual domains to the general health problem, well-being, and other aspects of the patient's quality of life [41, 65]. Although it is estimated that ED affects 20% of men above 40 years of age, with the incidence increasing with the old age group and those with medical comorbidities such as diabetes mellitus and cardiovascular or neurological pathologies; younger men can develop ED secondary to recreational drug use and pornography addiction [41, 49, 65].

E. Chung (✉)
Department of Urology, Princess Alexandra Hospital, University of Queensland, Brisbane, QLD, Australia

AndroUrology Centre, Brisbane, QLD, Australia

C. Rojas-Cruz
Global Andrology Forum, Moreland, OH, USA

Urology Department University Hospital of Rostock, Rostock, Germany
e-mail: Cesar.RojasCruz@med.uni-rostock.de

R. Shah
Global Andrology Forum, Moreland, OH, USA

Division of Andrology, Department of Urology, Lilavati Hospital and Research Centre, Mumbai, India

E. Chung et al. (eds.), *Advances in Andrology*,
https://doi.org/10.1007/978-3-032-29112-7_19

The true dichotomy between psychogenic and organic causes of ED is likely not distinct in many cases, and most men often exhibit multifactorial causes that can contribute to ED [6, 18, 19, 51, 61]. It is thought that the basic pathophysiology of ED relates to underlying endothelial dysfunction in which the vasodilation of penile blood flow is not possible and/or coexisting veno-occlusive dysfunction. Because ED can pose as a silent marker and predictor of comorbidities, especially future cardiovascular disease, earlier diagnosis of ED and subsequent optimal management of ED may provide an opportunity to prevent future cardiovascular events. In men presenting with complaints of ED, screening for, monitoring, and appropriately treating diseases that are comorbid with ED is essential [6, 18, 19, 51, 61]. Screening for and appropriately treating ED is important for enhanced life quality and improved motivation in men with existing ED comorbidities or risk factors.

While conventional medical therapy such as phosphodiesterase type 5 inhibitors and intracavernosal injection of vasoactive agent(s) are effective, these medications are not without side effect profiles and their use negates sexual spontaneity [6, 18, 19, 51, 61]. Hence, mechanical therapy may offer a different approach to managing ED and circumvent some of the current limitations of medications. Mechanical devices for ED can largely be classified under 3 broad categories, namely (1) penile implants, (2) regenerative therapy (shockwave therapy and penile vibratory device), and (3) static (external) devices (such as penile vacuum erection pump, wearable sleeve, wearable dildos, and external penile exo-devices) [18, 19, 32, 33, 48, 68, 70]. The following book chapter provides a narrative overview of contemporary mechanical interventions for ED and examines the current understanding of the proposed mechanism(s) of action and scientific progress in this field.

Penile Prosthesis Implants

Types of Penile Implants

Penile prosthetic implants are broadly divided into two categories: inflatable and semi-rigid (or malleable) devices (see Fig. 19.1). The history of penile prostheses has been characterized by successive improvements in devices and techniques based on trial and error [50]. The non-inflatable (semi-rigid) penile prostheses maintain constant length, girth and axial rigidity but can be bent for concealment and straightened for intercourse [15]. Hydraulic implants rest in a state of soft flaccidity for easy concealment and can be inflated to a rigid state, with an increase in girth, length (some models) and rigidity, when intercourse is desired. These are the most frequently used types in Western developed countries [28] and are considered the (more) ideal implants since they mimic normal erections.

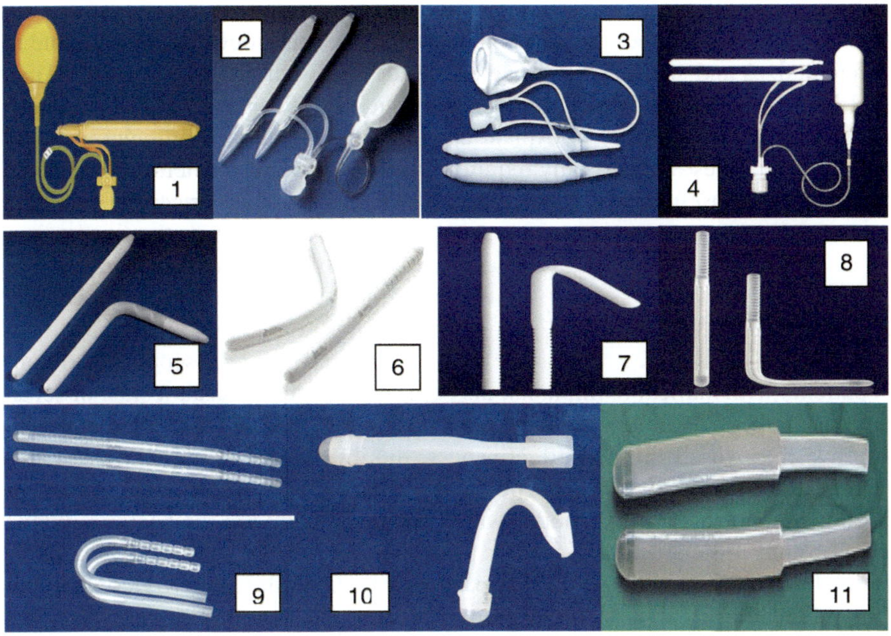

Fig. 19.1 Commercially available malleable and inflatable penile prosthesis devices. (Devices depicted are (1) Boston scientific AMS 700 IPP, (2) Coloplast Titan IPP, (3) Zephyr IPP and (4) Rigicon Infla10 IPP (5) Coloplast Genesis prosthesis; (5) Boston Scientific Tactra prosthesis; (7) Rigi10® prosthesis; (8) Promedon Tube malleable prosthesis; (9) Zephyr ZSI 100 (malleable) prosthesis; (10) Zephyr ZSI 100 FTM prosthesis; (11) Shah prosthesis. All images are obtained from online images and derived from the following scientific journals [15, 18, 19]. All images are open-access images and obtained directly from product websites

Inflatable Penile Implants

The most popular and common inflatable (hydraulic) penile implants have three-piece components: (1) a pair of cylinders to be placed inside the corpora cavernosa, (2) a reservoir that is placed either in the retropubic space or submuscular compartment, and (3) a pump that is located within the scrotum. The inflatable devices currently available are produced by four companies: Boston Scientific: AMS 700 Series™ (Marlborough, MA, USA), Coloplast: Titan™ (Humlebæk, Denmark), Zephyr ZSI™ (Switzerland) and Rigicon™ (Ronkonkoma, NY, USA) (Fig. 19.1). In contrast, the two-piece inflatable implants have a small hydraulic reservoir in the proximal part of the cylinders and a pump to move that liquid to the distal part of the corpora cavernosa. Currently, the only company that produces this type of implant is Boston Scientific under the name AMS Ambicor™ [18, 19]. The classic indication of considering them as an option for patients in whom it is desired to avoid reservoir implantation due to a surgical history is now obsolete given the currently described alternatives for ectopic location.

Various studies have evaluated overall satisfaction with these devices, observing high satisfaction rates between 76 and 98% [4, 28]. These devices are available in different sizes and smaller cylinder diameter devices such as AMS CXR™, Titan NB™, and Infla 10 NB™ are used in patients with significant corporal fibrosis such as in post-priapism, history of explant due to infection, and severe Peyronie's disease [18, 19]. These devices only require an intracorporeal diameter of 10 mm [60] and can also be useful in patients with sensory neurological lesions [5].

Malleable Penile Implants

In patients with malleable implants, the penis remains in a constant state of semirigidity. In recent decades, there have been technological and design advances to improve the overall clinical effectiveness, durability, and axial rigidity of this type of device (Fig. 19.1) [15]. The most recent addition to this market was the Boston Scientific Tactra™ model which includes a unique dual-layer silicone shell around a nickel-titanium alloy [54]. Among the malleable models, those with a hydrophilic coating are those produced by Coloplast and Rigicon companies. Shah hinged non-inflatable implant offers the benefits of very low cost (USD 300), two removable sleeves that allow the diameter of the implant to be changed from 15 to 13 to 11 mm (in the longer versions) or from 13 to 11 to 9 mm in the shorter versions, and can be cut or trimmed anywhere (since there is no metallic core) which allows it to be shortened or narrowed for a customized fit in cases of severe corporal fibrosis [15].

It is generally accepted that malleable implants have a lower risk of mechanical failure and revision surgeries than hydraulic implants [15]. Patients with malleable implants report a lower, although adequate, degree of satisfaction (66.1–88.7%) compared to inflatable devices [2]. None of the malleable implants available has been shown to be significantly superior in terms of satisfaction to others in its class.

Arguments for Opting for a Specific Type of Penile Prosthesis Implant

There are multiple factors to consider when deciding which implant should be chosen for each patient: indication for surgery, medical and surgical history, manual dexterity of the patient and availability of collaboration on the part of the couple to activate the device, costs, penile size, previous penile surgeries, experience, and training of the surgeon. In principle, the best devices available are hydraulic implants. However, in many countries, malleable implants are used more frequently due to their low cost (10–25% of the cost of hydraulic ones) or lack of reimbursement of hydraulic prostheses [28, 30].

Also, malleable implants are simpler devices, easier to implant and associated with fewer mechanical complications. These implants may be the best alternative for patients who do not have the dexterity or manual strength to manipulate the pump and who cannot count on the collaboration of their partner for this purpose [15]. The other clinical settings where malleable implants play an important role are as follows.

(a) Early implantation for patients with refractory ischaemic priapism [52]. Patients with priapism can develop severe ED and intracavernal fibrosis resulting in a marked decrease in penile size and making late implantation technically difficult. The experience of the acute or early use of malleable prosthesis implantation in these cases has been published with the idea of maintaining the dimensions of the corpora cavernosa as much as possible with a relatively easier and safer intervention than that of the implantation of a multi-component prosthesis. There is also the possibility of subsequently replacing it with a hydraulic prosthesis if the patient so wishes [76].
(b) Use of malleable implants during salvage procedures.

In cases where infection has occurred after penile prosthesis implantation and the implant is removed, there is a significant decrease in the size of the corpora cavernosa due to fibrosis. To avoid this complication, large-volume implanters recommend a salvage procedure where an extensive lavage is performed followed by immediate re-implantation of a new prosthesis. In these cases, advantages are attributed to the use of malleable implants: fewer components, faster intervention, lower potential for infection [29].

(c) It has classically been mentioned that patients with spinal cord injury are candidates for a malleable implant. However, the available data do not support the use of these devices given the higher rate of erosion due to continuous pressure on the especially labile tissues of these patients [77]. The lack of dexterity for patients with high lesions can be treated with the activation of a hydraulic implant by the partners. The mere presence of the hydraulic cylinders or their partial activation is sufficient support for those patients who use a condom catheter.

While malleable implants have been reported to have lower rates of revision, mechanical failure and overall satisfaction, published studies reported higher rates of erosion compared to hydraulic implants [10, 39, 47]. Inflatable implants have higher satisfaction rates and are the most frequently implanted, especially in Western developed countries and, in general, are the preferred devices [36].

Recent Advances in Penile Implants

In the last 50 years, penile prosthesis implants have gone through many modifications and technological advances. These have allowed the widespread use of implants for the definitive treatment of ED, and these advances have allowed the selection of the best materials, optimal designs, and robust components [58].

In the last three decades, there have been a series of very significant advances in these devices. One of them is specifically aimed at one of the most feared complications in the postoperative period: infection. The presence of infection leads to the need for device removal with subsequent shortening of the penis secondary to fibrosis. In 2000, AMS equipped its devices with "Inhibizone™" technology, which consists of a coating composed of rifampin and minocycline that has been shown to control the growth of the main bacteria that cause infection [9, 46]. Coloplast subsequently developed a hydrophilic coating (polyvinylpyrrolidone) that aims to reduce bacterial adhesion and can absorb any water-soluble antibiotics which allows the implant surgeon to select the antibiotics to be used as the coating [74]. The infection rates of implants with this type of coating are lower than those reported in series with implants without it [23].

One of the most frequent complaints of patients after the implant is the "loss" of penile length. Based on previous models (Ultrex™) and correcting the technical causes of the previously presented failures, AMS in 2006 introduced the LGX cylinders that allow controlled expansion in diameter and length [16]. These devices are preferably indicated in patients without fibrotic pathology. In terms of cylinder expansion, the Coloplast Titan provides a larger diameter when the cylinders are fully inflated compared to Rigicon Infla10 and AMS LGX devices [18, 19].

One of the drawbacks that previously occurred in hydraulic implants was spontaneous activation when liquid was transferred from the reservoir to the cylinders due to pressure changes (auto-inflation). To avoid this problem, Mentor™ developed a valve system (lock-out valve) [73]. This advance also created the opportunity to locate the reservoir in non-traditional "ectopic" locations outside of Retzius space. The device pump allows the liquid to be transferred from the reservoir to the cylinders and generate the necessary rigidity in them. This element of the implants has evolved to facilitate manipulation and make it more comfortable and easier to use [27]. AMS obtained authorization in 2004 for the "Tactile Pump™" which presents changes in the surface of the bulb to reduce the slippage of the pump during activation [22]. One of the most significant improvements in the deactivation system occurred 2 years later. The "momentary squeeze" system incorporates a one-touch deflate button that allows complete evacuation of the cylinders after a single compression of the button [37]. Until then, continuous pressure on the deflate button was required for deflation. In turn, the pumps of Coloplast devices have improved in different generations with One Touch Release™ (OTR) [66] and Titan Touch Pump. Zephyr Device Pump (ZSI 475 pump) is composed of a single open-close reinforced valve limiting the risk of mechanical failure and auto-inflation [21]. On Rigicon (Rapid Pump) models, the deactivation button is located on the side of the pump, potentially facilitating manipulation of the system [18, 19]. In November 2023, the FDA approved a new pump (Tenacio™) designed by Boston Scientific that requires fewer activation movements, has a greater distance between the activation bulb and the deactivation button and prominent grips for easier use.

Concerning the reservoir, relevant modifications have also been introduced in recent years. In 2000, Coloplast introduced changes in the layout of the implant neck that, associated with the described autoactivation system, allowed the development of implant techniques in cases where it is preferable not to use the Retzius space [56]. In 2010, Boston Scientific launched a flat profile reservoir called "Conceal™" that allows it to be implanted under the abdominal wall without producing the protrusion that the traditional spherical reservoir would generate [24]. For its part, Coloplast introduced the Cloverleaf reservoir, which also acquires a flattened configuration when full. These devices have allowed the expansion of the use of three-component hydraulic devices for patients who have undergone laparoscopic and Robot-assisted radical prostatectomy, by allowing ectopic implantation of that part of the system [34]. Rigicon markets the AdaptiveReservoir™ which is made of a material that assumes the shape of the site where it has been implanted. The Zephyr implant reservoir is cylindrical in shape and is pre-connected to the pump [21]. The recent rise of the infrapubic approach has meant that manufacturers produce three-element implants with adapted lengths of the connecting tubes between the cylinders and the pump according to the type of surgical approach chosen [3, 53]. Another technical advance is the subcoronal approach for 3-piece inflatable implants that allow unfettered access to the corpora in cases where simultaneous corporal reconstruction is needed [18, 19].

For FtoM transgender patients with neo-phallus, Zephyr has designed a specific model of hydraulic implant composed of a single cylinder with a glans-shaped distal tip and a 2.5-cm proximal plate for an anchorage that can be fixed to the pubic periosteum to give implant stability [57].

Current Limitations of These Devices

Despite the enormous advances in this area of medical devices and surgical techniques, challenges remain to be overcome. The fact of placing a foreign body in a closed cavity with a vascularization system that favours venous stasis, such as the corpora cavernosa, makes the natural defence mechanisms insufficient to prevent associated infections. The implications that the development of an infection in their genitals has on the patient with the physical and psychological impacts and subsequent consequences make it necessary to further develop techniques to prevent infections associated with implants. There is currently no medical device that is free of associated infections when implanted, but in penile prosthesis implants, prevention, and strategies to reduce associated complications become more relevant. The progressive increase in the resistance of microorganisms against antibiotics and antifungals puts pressure on the implants of the future to evolve to the use of new technologies that do not depend on the use of antibiotics susceptible to generating resistance [60].

The available implants still have a considerable number of failures associated with mechanical problems due to material wear or failure of the pump or its deflation mechanism.

The use of systems that use liquid to generate the rigidity of the cylinders has been the essential concept of implants that resemble the physiological conditions of the penis. The advantages have been evident in these decades, but the fact of depending on the use of this principle implies a system of multiple components subject to failure due to loss of liquid from the system in its elements or failure of the systems to move it. The development of new materials/systems could simplify the mechanism for obtaining rigidity in the shaft of the penis. An example of these investigations was presented with a prototype of an implant composed of a nickel-titanium alloy with changes in structure generated by temperature [40].

A considerable percentage of patients present significant postoperative difficulties in activating and deactivating hydraulic implants. In some cases where dexterity limitations are not evident in the pre-implant evaluation, serious difficulties arise for the patient to properly manipulate the pump. Studies are in development where the hydraulic system uses a piezoelectric pump activated wirelessly [54]. Another proposed version of electronic IPP resides in a wirelessly controlled external module and an implantable module in which the external control module may transmit wireless power and control signals to be received by circuitry on a flexible printed circuit board in the implantable module to cause a motor and pump combination to transfer fluid from a reservoir in the implantable device [71]. The flexible printed circuit board, motor, and pump may be placed within the fluid reservoir, which provides a heat sink that prevents overheating of the implant.

The shape of the implant cylinders is standard and this fact has been questioned recently. When obtaining three-dimensional models of normal cavernous bodies and comparing them with those of cylinders, significant discrepancies in size and shape are observed, especially at the distal tips. Currently, when performing the implant surgery, we adapt the albuginea of the corpus cavernosum around the device, and in some patients, especially in cases of Peyronie's or fibrosis, this can pose a challenge. In the future, it would be desirable to have the possibility of modelling the design of the implants according to the anatomy of the corpus cavernosum of the patients, especially in those with a significant corporal fibrosis [31].

The information related to the implant life, mechanical failures, percentage of infection and satisfaction with the implants is still quite limited [18, 19]. There are no prospective comparative studies of the clinical course of patients with different types and brands of implants. A common multicentre international research effort in collaboration with manufacturers would shed more light on being able to offer the best alternative available according to the characteristics of each patient and allow better decision-making in a consensual manner that reduces the associated anxiety on the part of both patients and infrequent implanters.

One of the main limitations to access to this excellent therapeutic option for patients with erectile dysfunction is the cost of the implants and the coverage of the procedure and devices by the different health systems. The consequent advances undoubtedly imply an increase in the cost of the devices, which will impose greater access restrictions on many patients within the already tight global health payment system [38]. Additionally, the awareness about penile prosthesis among the general medical community and even among urologists who are not dedicated to sexual medicine is low and, consequently, the general population has a very limited idea of this treatment option and its benefits. The open dissemination of this therapeutic option is faced with barriers associated with the taboo on topics related to sexuality and must be overcome according to an approach adapted to different cultures.

Without a doubt, penile prosthesis implants are the best therapeutic alternative for patients with refractory ED. Despite this fact, it is estimated that only 5% of potential candidates in industrialized countries receive an implant as a treatment solution. This figure is likely significantly lower in countries with fewer health resources. There are economic barriers, training of the medical team, and information on the availability of the treatment as well as the implant that must be overcome. Likewise, the implants of the future must be simpler devices that come closer to physiological flaccidity and erection (increase in diameter, length, and size) and not just intracavernosal rigidity.

Mechanical Devices

Regenerative Therapy (Shockwave Therapy and Penile Vibratory Device)

Contemporary treatment for ED improves the penile rigidity without altering the underlying pathogenesis of ED which often relates to endothelial dysfunction. Hence, there is a strong interest in regenerative therapy that improves endothelial dysfunction to increase penile blood flow, regenerate cavernous nerve, and reverse trophic changes within the cavernosal smooth muscle [7, 12].

Since its initial introduction in the early 2010s, low-intensity extracorporeal shockwave therapy (LIESWT) has gained popularity as a treatment for ED. It is postulated that LIESWT causes repetitive shear stress (microtrauma) to target tissue stimulating vascular regeneration (neovascularization) through the release of various angiogenic growth factors and cytokines and recruitment of stem cells responsible for endothelial remodelling and tissue regeneration [13, 14, 67]. Published systematic reviews and meta-analyses reported good clinical efficacy and safety profile [20, 25, 43, 45, 78], while published guidelines advocate the use of LiESWT as treatment in younger "healthy" men with vasculogenic ED [8, 17, 42].

While literature supports the benefits of LIESWT with improved erectile function in the short-term, longer-term outcomes in terms of clinical durability and physiological changes to the corporal tissue remain uncertain [17]. The patient selection appears paramount to treatment success and patients with mild-moderate ED, younger age group, those with minimal cardiovascular comorbidities, and the absence of diabetes or cavernous nerve injury are likely going to report higher EF recovery and spontaneous erection. To date, there is no widely adopted treatment template and treatment protocols are often based on manufacturer's guidelines and it remains unknown if one machine is superior to another [14]. At this stage, long-term multi-institutional randomized placebo-controlled studies with dose-finding studies are required to compare various treatment protocols and shock wave machines, and the potential synergistic role of concurrent use of adjunctive measures such as PDE5i. Future research should incorporate a cost-effective analysis model, how to miniaturize shock wave technology with better energy delivery for use at home, and the role of concurrent administration of similar regenerative technology to treat men with ED.

Like LIESWT for ED, impulse magnetic-field therapy has gained interest in the field of sexual medicine. Magnetic pulse fields induce an alternating current within the body's electrolytes to increase oxygen uptake by the cell, enhance blood circulation, and reverse functional impairment. Older literature showed that impulse magnetic stimulation can improve erectile function in men with ED [55, 64], although there have not been any recent studies since the delivery of this treatment modality can be cumbersome, not readily available, and expensive when compared to the more "mobile" and simpler LiESWT.

Penile vibratory stimulation (PVS) has been marketed as a safe and effective mechanical device to aid erection. The proposed mechanism of action is thought to occur through vibratory stimulation to cavernosal nerve fibres to induce NO release and reflex parasympathetic erection [63]. To date, 2 PVS devices have been commercialized namely Viberect (Reflexonic, Chambersburg, Pennsylvania, USA) and Ferti Care (Multicept, Albertslund, Denmark), although the latter is designed more towards patients with ejaculatory dysfunction [11, 59].

Another proposed option for using the device is for penile rehabilitation after nerve-sparing radical prostatectomy [1, 26]. Nonetheless, it is important to note that PVS alone is unlikely to be "more" effective than the current standard of therapy such as PDE5i or ICI therapy. Furthermore, vibrator use can cause bothersome physical side effects when used improperly. At present, no good data is supporting or refuting the idea that vibrator use habituates individuals to certain ways of sexual stimulation even in patients with orgasmic disorder.

Static (External) Devices (Penile Pump, Wearable Sleeve, Wearable Dildos, External Penile Exo-devices)

In contrast to mechanical devices that regenerate tissue and promote neovascularization, these mechanical devices provide an external "exo-skeleton" to improve penile rigidity [48, 68]. The static (external) device offers a less invasive alternative to penile prosthesis implantation since patients do not need to undergo surgery, can use these devices anytime and it is essentially "reversible" in nature.

The vacuum erection device (VED) has been around since the 1980s as an easy, readily available, and simple device for ED, consisting of a cylinder and a pump which can be powered manually or by battery. It employs negative pressure to dilate the cavernous venous sinuses, increase the perfusion of the cavernous artery and venous blood, and ultimately achieve the goal of producing penile erection. An external constriction ring is placed at the base of the penis to prevent blood flow during intercourse to maintain an erection. This device can bypass the limitations of PDE5i and ICI therapy to directly achieve an (artificial) erection. In recent years, VED has regained popularity as a form of penile rehabilitation by preserving erectile function through anti-hypoxic, antiapoptotic, and anti-fibrotic mechanisms by improving the arterial blood flow into the penis [72, 75].

The use of VED may complement a PDE5i, especially in diabetic men with severe ED who have only a partial response to a PDE5i. One study reported that the combined use of sildenafil and a VED significantly enhanced erectile function and improved the outcome [69]. Interestingly, more recent studies have highlighted that frequent VED use could promote the recovery of penis function and size through the release of certain growth factors and cytokines to improve corporal oxygenation [35, 62]. However, the optimal duration of VED use remains unknown based on cavernosal oxygenation profile, and there is no clarity on which device is best since there is no regulatory governance in the production of VED. Compared to contemporary penile rehabilitation strategies, VED therapy has the advantages of being non-invasive and having fewer systemic side effects. Nonetheless, common adverse effects include penile bruising if used excessively (especially in patients on anticoagulants), and penile sensory changes such as numbness, coldness and/or pain.

Over the years, several wearable penile external devices have allowed men with ED to be able to achieve sexual penetration and have been developed to assist patients with medical-refractory ED who are not suitable for or cannot afford penile prosthesis implants [48, 68, 70]. The 'Erektor' or "Elator" (San Diego, California, USA) external penile support device is composed of a rigid rod with two rings at either end with the base rings available in different sizes. The device frame is adapted to be fitted to the penis with the two rings encircling the penis and is individually customized to the patient's phallic length. This device has been shown to enhance the penile length, provide support along the ventral aspect of the penis, and strengthen penile rigidity during sexual intercourse [44]. Similarly, another penile support device consists of a penile cast that can also be worn externally during intercourse akin to a "dildo" but has a window available in the distal part of the cast as the corona and glans opening to allow for glans sensation during intercourse (Takehisa Iwai T. Iwai, personal communication). This penile cast is available in 3 sizes based on the user's penile size. There have been no published trials to establish the efficacy of the device currently. Other silicone-made sexual aids such as penile sleeves which function like a hollow, strap-on dildo are designed to fit the outer surface of the penile shaft and can provide sexual penetration and improve sexual pleasure. It is important to acknowledge that while commercially available products from reputable companies such as Tenga (Tokyo, Japan) and Doc Johnson (North Hollywood, California, USA) have assisted men with ED to have satisfactory sexual lives and alleviate the psychosexual distress, there have been no independent trials or research done to validate the devices' intended functions and the specific circumstances for use [48, 68, 70].

The medical literature concerning the use of sex aids is very limited and consists predominantly of observational studies. Although sex aids can often be used in a non-discriminatory fashion, their clinical effectiveness and safety risks in real-life scenarios are poorly discussed in the scientific literature. To date, none of the major international organizations have provided formal recommendations. Nonetheless, these devices can be integrated into existing sexual practice and may provide adjunctive assistance to the individual or couple might have some physical and/or psychological consequences. Hence, clinicians need to familiarize themselves with the range of sex aids aimed at augmenting sexual function and sexual satisfaction in men with sexual dysfunction.

Future Directions

While contemporary and standardized treatment for ED predominantly alleviates the symptom of ED rather than underlying endothelial dysfunction, scientific advances in regenerative technology such as LIESWT offer these patients the opportunity to regain erection with or without medications. Given that ED affects men beyond psychosexual impairment, it is important to address other non-sexual issues including concomitant medical comorbidities since the presence of ED is often a precursor of underlying cardiovascular health risk. Innovations in surgical techniques and device technology have resulted in better design, more robust devices and greater clinical outcomes, especially patient satisfaction rates following penile prosthesis implantation. Sexual aids such as external mechanical penile devices have clinical and research relevance and their utility invariably increases in the future through the incorporation of state-of-the-art technology such as the sex-bots (humanoid sexual robots), integration of virtual reality and remotely accessed devices. Nonetheless, in these evolving sexual treatment options, governmental regulations and higher-level clinical evidence are necessary for these advances in penile prosthesis implants and mechanical devices for ED to continue to provide effective and safe treatments for this group of vulnerable patients.

References

1. Abdel Raheem A, Ralph D. Penile vibratory stimulation: a novel approach for penile rehabilitation after nerve-sparing radical prostatectomy. BJU Int. 2014;114(1):2–3.
2. Akakpo W, Pineda MA, Burnett AL. Critical analysis of satisfaction assessment after penile prosthesis surgery. Sex Med Rev. 2017;5(2):244–51.
3. Antonini G, Busetto GM, De Berardinis E, Giovannone R, Vicini P, Del Giudice F, Conti SL, Gentile V, Perito PE. Minimally invasive infrapubic inflatable penile prosthesis implant for erectile dysfunction: evaluation of efficacy, satisfaction profile and complications. Int J Impot Res. 2016;28(1):4–8.

4. Bernal RM, Henry GD. Contemporary patient satisfaction rates for three-piece inflatable penile prostheses. Adv Urol. 2012;2012:707321.
5. Bertero EB, Antunes DL. Surgical treatment of erectile dysfunction. Sex Med Rev. 2015;3(4):316–27.
6. Burnett AL, Nehra A, Breau RH, et al. Erectile dysfunction: AUA guideline. J Urol. 2018;200(3):633–41.
7. Campbell JD, Milenkovic U, Usta MF, Albersen M, Bivalacqua TJ. The good, bad, and the ugly of regenerative therapies for erectile dysfunction. Transl Androl Urol. 2020;9(Suppl 2):S252–61.
8. Capogrosso P, Frey A, Jensen CFS, et al. Low-intensity shock wave therapy in sexual medicine- clinical recommendations from the European Society of Sexual Medicine (ESSM). J Sex Med. 2019;16(10):1490–505.
9. Carson CC 3rd, Mulcahy JJ, Harsch MR. Long-term infection outcomes after original antibiotic impregnated inflatable penile prosthesis implants: up to 7.7 years of followup. J Urol. 2011;185(2):614–8.
10. Casabe AR, Sarotto N, Gutierrez C, Bechara AJ. Satisfaction assessment with malleable prosthetic implant of spectra (AMS) and genesis (Coloplast) models. Int J Impot Res. 2016;28(6):228–33.
11. Chong W, Ibrahim E, Aballa TC, Lynne CM, Brackett NL. Comparison of three methods of penile vibratory stimulation for semen retrieval in men with spinal cord injury. Spinal Cord. 2017;55(10):921–5.
12. Chung E. A review of regenerative therapies as penile rehabilitation in men following primary prostate cancer treatment: evidence for erectile restoration and cavernous nerve regeneration. Asian J Urol. 2022;9(3):287–93.
13. Chung E, Cartmill R. Evaluation of long-term clinical outcomes and patient satisfaction rate following low-intensity shock wave therapy in men with erectile dysfunction: a minimum 5-year follow-up on a prospective open-label single-arm clinical study. Sex Med. 2021;9(4):100384.
14. Chung E, Wang J. A state-of-art review of low intensity extracorporeal shock wave therapy and lithotripter machines for the treatment of erectile dysfunction. Expert Rev Med Devices. 2017;14(12):929–34.
15. Chung E, Wang J. State-of-art review of current malleable penile prosthesis devices in the commercial market. Ther Adv Urol. 2023;15:17562872231179008.
16. Chung PH, Siegel JA, Tausch TJ, Klein AK, Scott JM, Morey AF. Inflatable penile prosthesis as tissue expander: what is the evidence? Int Braz J Urol. 2017;43(5):911–6.
17. Chung E, Lee J, Liu CC, et al. Clinical practice guideline recommendation on the use of Low Intensity Extracorporeal Shock Wave Therapy (LIESWT) and Low Intensity Pulsed Ultrasound Shockwave (LIPUS) therapy to treat erectile dysfunction: an Asia-Pacific position statement. World J Mens Health. 2021;39(1):1–8.
18. Chung E, Bettocchi C, Egydio P, Love C, Osmonov D, Park S, et al. The international penile prosthesis implant consensus forum: clinical recommendations and surgical principles on the inflatable 3-piece penile prosthesis implant. Nat Rev Urol. 2022a;19(9):534–46.
19. Chung E, Lowy M, Gillman M, Love C, Katz D, Neilson G. Urological Society of Australia and New Zealand (USANZ) and the Australasian Chapter of Sexual Health Medicine (AChSHM) for the Royal Australasian College of Physicians (RACP) clinical guidelines on the management of erectile dysfunction. Med J Aust. 2022b;217(6):318–32.
20. Clavijo RI, Kohn TP, Kohn JR, Ramasamy R. Effects of low-intensity extracorporeal shockwave therapy on erectile dysfunction: a systematic review and meta-analysis. J Sex Med. 2017;14:27–35.
21. Colombo F, Gentile G, Vagnoni V, Fiorillo A, Piazza P, Sartorio F, Franceschelli A. Initial experience of a single center with the use of ZSI 475 penile prosthesis. Asian J Urol. 2021;8(2):176–82.
22. Delk J, Knoll LD, McMurray J, Shore N, Wilson S. Early experience with the American Medical Systems new tactile pump: results of a multicenter study. J Sex Med. 2005;2(2):266–71.

23. Dhabuwala C, Sheth S, Zamzow B. Infection rates of rifampin/gentamicin-coated titan Coloplast penile implants. Comparison with Inhibizone-impregnated AMS penile implants. J Sex Med. 2001;8(1):315–20.
24. Dinerman BF, Telis L, Eid JF. New advancements in inflatable penile prosthesis. Sex Med Rev. 2021;9(3):507–14.
25. Dong L, Chang D, Zhang X, et al. Effect of low-intensity extracorporeal shock wave on the treatment of erectile dysfunction: a systematic review and meta-analysis. Am J Mens Health. 2019;13(2):1557988319846749.
26. Fode M, Borre M, Ohl DA, Lichbach K, Sønksen J. Penile vibratory stimulation in the recovery of urinary continence and erectile function after nerve-sparing radical prostatectomy: a randomized, controlled trial. BJU Int. 2014;114(1):111–7.
27. Giordano A, Smarrazzo F, Cilio S, Califano G, Colla Ruvolo C, Verze P. History of penile implants: from implants made of bone to modern inflatable penile implants. Int J Impot Res. 2023;35(7):601–8.
28. Goodstein T, Jenkins LC. A narrative review on malleable and inflatable penile implants: choosing the right implant for the right patient. Int J Impot Res. 2023;35(7):623–8.
29. Gross MS, Phillips EA, Balen A, Eid JF, Yang C, Simon R, Martinez D, et al. The malleable implant salvage technique: infection outcomes after Mulcahy salvage procedure and replacement of infected inflatable penile prosthesis with malleable prosthesis. J Urol. 2016;195(3):694–7.
30. Habous M, Tealab A, Farag M, Soliman T, Williamson B, Mahmoud S, Elserafy A, et al. Malleable penile implant is an effective therapeutic option in men with Peyronie's disease and erectile dysfunction. Sex Med. 2018;6(1):24–9.
31. Hakky TS, Ferguson D, Spiess PE, Bradley P, Lue TF, Carrion RE. Three-dimensional mapping and comparative analysis of the distal human corpus cavernosum and the inflatable penile prosthesis. Asian J Androl. 2013;5(4):567–70.
32. Hellstrom WJG, Montague DK, Moncada I, Carson C, Minhas S, Faria G, Krishnamurti S. Implants, mechanical devices, and vascular surgery for erectile dysfunction. J Sex Med. 2010;7(1 Pt 2):501–23.
33. Ismail EA, El-Sakka AI. Innovative trends and perspectives for erectile dysfunction treatment: a systematic review. Arab J Urol. 2016;14(2):84–93.
34. Karpman E, Sadeghi-Nejad H, Henry G, Khera M, Morey AF. Current opinions on alternative reservoir placement for inflatable penile prosthesis among members of the Sexual Medicine Society of North America. J Sex Med. 2013;10(8):2115–20.
35. Katz PG, Haden HT, Mulligan T, Zasler ND. The effect of vacuum devices on penile hemodynamics. J Urol. 1990;143(1):55–6.
36. Khera M, Mulcahy J, Wen L, Wilson SK. Is there still a place for malleable penile implants in the United States? Wilson's workshop #18. Int J Impot Res. 2023;35(2):82–9.
37. Knoll LD, Henry G, Culkin D, Ohl DA, Otheguy J, Shabsigh R, et al. Physician and patient satisfaction with the new AMS 700 momentary squeeze inflatable penile prosthesis. J Sex Med. 2009;6(6):1773–8.
38. Kohler TS. The future of penile implants IJIR special edition: 50(th) year anniversary on penile implants. Int J Impot Res. 2023;35(7):593–5.
39. Lacy JM, Walker J, Gupta S, Davenport DL, Preston DM. Risk factors for removal or revision of penile prostheses in the veteran population. Urology. 2016;98:189–94.
40. Le B, McVary K, McKenna K, Colombo A. A novel thermal-activated shape memory penile prosthesis: comparative mechanical testing. Urology. 2017;99:136–41.
41. Lewis RW, Fugl-Meyer KS, Bosch R, et al. Epidemiology/risk factors of sexual dysfunction. J Sex Med. 2004;1:35–9.
42. Liu JL, Chu KY, Gabrielson AT, Wang R, Trost L, Broderick G, Davies K, Brock G, Mulhall J, Ramasamy R, Bivalacqua TJ. Restorative therapies for erectile dysfunction: position statement from the Sexual Medicine Society of North America (SMSNA). Sex Med. 2021 Jun;9(3):100343.

43. Lu Z, Lin G, Reed-Maldonado A, Wang C, Lee YC, Lue TF. Low-intensity extracorporeal shock wave treatment improves erectile function: a systematic review and Metaanalysis. Eur Urol. 2017;71:223–33.
44. Mainwaring JM, Wibowo E, Wassersug RJ, Jagervall CD. Assessment of the Elator penile support device for patients with prostate cancer and their partners affected by severe erectile dysfunction. Urol Nurs. 2022;42(4):189–97.
45. Man L, Li G. Low-intensity extracorporeal shock wave therapy for erectile dysfunction: systematic review and meta-analysis. Urology. 2018;119:97–103.
46. McKim SE, Carson CC 3rd. AMS 700 inflatable penile prosthesis with InhibiZone. Expert Rev Med Devices. 2010;7(3):311–7.
47. Minervini A, Ralph DJ, Pryor JP. Outcome of penile prosthesis implantation for treating erectile dysfunction: experience with 504 procedures. BJU Int. 2006;97(1):129–33.
48. Miranda EP, Taniguchi H, Cao DL, et al. Application of sex aids in men with sexual dysfunction: a review. J Sex Med. 2019;16(6):767–80.
49. Montorsi F, Adaikan G, Becher E, et al. Summary of the recommendations on sexual dysfunctions in men. J Sex Med. 2010;7:3572–88.
50. Mulcahy JJ. The development of modern penile implants. Sex Med Rev. 2016;4(2):177–89.
51. Mulhall JP, Giraldi A, Hackett G, et al. The 2018 revision to the process of care model for evaluation of erectile dysfunction. J Sex Med. 2018;15:1280–92.
52. Muneer A, Ralph DJ. Immediate placement of a penile prosthesis as first-line treatment for the Management of Ischaemic Priapism. Eur Urol Focus. 2019;5(4):529–30.
53. Otero JR, Manfredi C, Wilson SK. The good, the bad, and the ugly about surgical approaches for inflatable penile prosthesis implantation. Int J Impot Res. 2022;34(2):128–37.
54. Patel J, Zakkar B, Polchert M, Tannenbaum J, Dick B, Raheem O. Recent technological development of penile prosthesis: a literature review. Transl Androl Urol. 2024;13(1):165–84.
55. Pelka R, Jaenicke C, Gruenwald J. Impulse magnetic-field therapy for erectile dysfunction: a double-blind, placebo-controlled study. Adv Ther. 2002;19:53–60.
56. Perito PE, Wilson SK. Traditional (retroperitoneal) and abdominal wall (ectopic) reservoir placement. J Sex Med. 2011;8(3):656–9.
57. Preto M, Blecher G, Timpano M, Gontero P, Falcone M. The frontier of penile implants in Phalloplasty: is the ZSI 475 FTM what we have been waiting for? Int J Impot Res. 2020;33(7):779–83.
58. Quesada-Olarte J, Nelwan D, Donato U, Fernandez-Crespo R, Parker J, Carrion RE. Penile implant instrument innovations. Curr Urol Rep. 2023;24(2):59–67.
59. Reece M, Herbenick D, Sanders SA, Dodge B, Ghassemi A, Fortenberry JD. Prevalence and characteristics of vibrator use by men in the United States. J Sex Med. 2009;6(7):1867–74.
60. Rodriguez KM, Kohn TP, Davis AB, Hakky TS. Penile implants: a look into the future. Transl Androl Urol. 2017;6(Suppl 5):S860–6.
61. Salonia A, Bettochi C, Boeri L, et al. European Association of Urology guidelines on sexual and reproductive health-2021 update: male sexual dysfunction. Eur Urol. 2021;80(3):333–57.
62. Salvatore FT, Sharman GM, Hellstrom WJ. Vacuum constriction devices and the clinical urologist: an informed selection. Urology. 1991;38(4):323–7.
63. Segal RL, Tajkarimi K, Burnett AL. Viberect penile vibratory stimulation system: evaluation of its erectogenic efficacy. Can J Urol. 2013;20(4):6844–7.
64. Shafik A, El-Sibai O, Shafik A. Magnetic stimulation of the cavernous nerve for the treatment of erectile dysfunction in humans. Int J Impot Res. 2000;12:137–41.
65. Shamloul R, Ghanem H. Erectile dysfunction. Lancet. 2013;381(9861):153–65.
66. Shaw T, Garber BB. Coloplast titan inflatable penile prosthesis with one-touch release pump: review of 100 cases and comparison with genesis pump. J Sex Med. 2011;8(1):310–4.
67. Sokolakis I, Dimitriadis F, Teo P, Hatzichristodoulou G, Hatzichristou D, Giuliano F. The basic science behind low-intensity extracorporeal shockwave therapy for erectile dysfunction: a systematic scoping review of pre-clinical studies. J Sex Med. 2019;16(2):168–94.
68. Stein MJ, Lin H, Wang R. New advances in erectile technology. Ther Adv Urol. 2014;6(1):15–24.

69. Sun L, Peng FL, Yu ZL, Liu CL, Chen J. Combined sildenafil with vacuum erection device therapy in the management of diabetic men with erectile dysfunction after failure of first-line sildenafil monotherapy. Int J Urol. 2014;21(12):1263–7.
70. Trost LW, Munarriz R, Wang R, Morey A, Levine L. External mechanical devices and vascular surgery for erectile dysfunction. J Sex Med. 2016;13(11):1579–617.
71. US patent US20170079760A1. https://patents.google.com/patent/US20170079760A1/en. 2021. last Accessed 1 May 2024.
72. Wang R. Vacuum erectile device for rehabilitation after radical prostatectomy. J Sex Med. 2017;14(2):184–6.
73. Wilson SK, Henry GD, Delk JR Jr, Cleves MA. The mentor alpha 1 penile prosthesis with reservoir lock-out valve: effective prevention of auto-inflation with improved capability for ectopic reservoir placement. J Urol. 2002;168(4 Pt 1):1475–8.
74. Wilson SK, Salem EA, Costerton W. Anti-infection dip suggestions for the Coloplast titan inflatable penile prosthesis in the era of the infection retardant coated implant. J Sex Med. 2011;8(9):2647–54.
75. Yuan J, Lin H, Li P, Zhang R, Luo A, Berardinelli F, et al. Molecular mechanisms of vacuum therapy in penile rehabilitation: a novel animal study. Eur Urol. 2010;58(5):773–80.
76. Zacharakis E, De Luca F, Raheem AA, Garaffa G, Christopher N, Muneer A, Ralph DJ. Early insertion of a malleable penile prosthesis in ischaemic priapism allows later upsizing of the cylinders. Scand J Urol. 2015;49(6):468–71.
77. Zermann DH, Kutzenberger J, Sauerwein D, Schubert J, Loeffler U. Penile prosthetic surgery in neurologically impaired patients: long-term followup. J Urol. 2006;175(3 Pt 1):1041–4. discussion 1044
78. Zou ZJ, Tang LY, Liu ZH, Liang JY, Zhang RC, Wang YJ, et al. Short-term efficacy and safety of low-intensity extracorporeal shock wave therapy in erectile dysfunction: a systematic review and meta-analysis. Int Braz J Urol. 2017;43:805–21.

Chapter 20
Pharmacological Formulation for ED Management: ODF and ODT

Maged Ragab, Muhammed Arif Ibis, and Kaan Aydos

Medical Treatment of ED

Erectile dysfunction (ED) is a common sexual disorder in men that significantly impacts quality of life. Although the true global burden continues to evolve, it was previously estimated that approximately 322 million men would be affected by ED worldwide by 2025 [21]. Among men diagnosed with ED, 68% present with comorbid conditions such as hypertension, dyslipidemia, diabetes mellitus (DM), and depression [29]. ED is also a common complication among men with cancer. A systematic review and meta-analysis estimated an overall prevalence of 40.7% with approximately 42.7% of cases occuring after cancer treatment [27].

Accordingly, the initial approach to ED management should include lifestyle modifications and the treatment of underlying chronic conditions. Subsequent therapeutic strategies may involve oral phosphodiesterase type 5 inhibitors (PDE5i), intracavernosal injections, topical or intraurethral alprostadil, vacuum erection devices, and penile prothesis implantation [14], in line with the guidelines of the American Urological Association (AUA) and the European Association of Urology (EAU). Moreover, several novel agents are being explored as potential advancements in ED therapy. These include low intensity shock wave therapy (LISWT) stem cell therapy, platelet-rich plasma (PRP) injections, gene therapy, amniotic fluid matrices, Rho-kinase inhibitors, melanocortin receptor antagonists, maxi-K channel activators, soluble guanylate cyclase stimulators, and nitric oxide donors [20].

M. Ragab (✉)
Department of Urology, Tanta University, Tanta, Egypt

M. A. Ibis · K. Aydos
Department of Urology, Ankara University School of Medicine, Ankara, Turkey

Center for Research on Human Reproduction, Ankara University School of Medicine, Ankara, Turkey

E. Chung et al. (eds.), *Advances in Andrology*,
https://doi.org/10.1007/978-3-032-29112-7_20

Classification of Drugs for the Treatment of ED

The therapeutic approaches for ED can be broadly categorized into two main groups based on their route of administration: local treatments, including intracavernosal, topical, and intraurethral agents and systemic treatments, such as oral and sublingual formulations.

Intracavernous, Topical, and Intraurethral Agents

Alprostadil is the primary agent administered via intracavernosal injection for the treatment of ED. It may also be used in combination with papaverine and phentolamine. In 1996, prostaglandin E1 (PGE-1) became the first and only penile injectable approved by the U.S. Food and Drug Administration (FDA) for ED treatment. Papaverine, an opium alkaloid originally derived from Papaver somniferum, was identified as a potential intracavernosal agent by the French surgeon Ronald Virág in Paris in 1982. Phentolamine, introduced in 1978, is a non-selective alpha-adrenergic antagonist that inhibits smooth muscle contraction. Although it exhibits limited efficacy as monotherapy, phentolamine remains effective in combination regimens. Prostaglandins E1 and E2 are also utilized in intraurethral therapies for ED.

More recently, transdermal delivery systems have emerged as safe and convenient alternatives to oral administration by bypassing hepatic metabolism. Studies involving sildenafil citrate-loaded nanostructured lipid carriers and solid lipid nanoparticles have demonstrated effective local release through penile skin [31]. Similarly, tadalafil—owing to its low aqueous solubility—benefits from transdermal administration via nanostructured lipid carriers [3]. Avanafil, which is practically water-insoluble, has been formulated using solid lipid nanoparticles embedded in hydrogel films to enhance skin penetration and improve bioavailability [19]. In addition to PDE5 inhibitors, compounds such as alprostadil, papaverine, testosterone, and minoxidil are being explored in various topical and transdermal formulations. For example, alprostadil creams containing penetration enhancers have demonstrated promising efficacy in clinical studies.

Oral and Sublingual Agents

A variety of PDE5i are available for the treatment of ED. U.S. FDA-approved agents include sildenafil, vardenafil, tadalafil, and avanafil. In addition to these, other commercially available PDE5is—such as lodenafil, udenafil, and mirodenafil—are marketed in certain countries, although they have not received FDA approval.

Overview of Oral PDE5i

History of the Development of PDE5 Inhibitors

The observation of penile erection as a side effect during Phase I clinical trials of sildenafil—originally developed for the treatment of angina—led to the hypothesis that PDE5i could be effective in managing ED [6]. Following a series of clinical trials, sildenafil became the first PDE5 inhibitor approved by the U.S. FDA for the treatment of ED in 1998.

Sildenafil has since become a widely used and transformative therapy for millions of patients, generating substantial market demand and spurring the development of several additional PDE5 inhibitors, including tadalafil, vardenafil, avanafil, udenafil, and mirodenafil. Vardenafil, the second PDE5 inhibitor to be introduced, received FDA approval in August 2003. Later that year, tadalafil was also approved. Avanafil became the most recent addition, obtaining FDA approval in 2012.

A comparative overview of the approved PDE5 inhibitors with respect to their pharmacokinetic parameters, duration of action, food interactions, enzyme selectivity, and adverse event profiles is presented in Table 20.1.

Table 20.1 Comparison of Pharmacokinetics, Pharmacodynamics, and Side Effect Profiles of Approved PDE5i

Parameter	Sildenafil	Tadalafil	Vardenafil	Avanafil
Onset of action	30–60 min	30 min	30–60 min	15–30 min
Tmax	~0.8 h	~2 h	~0.7–0.9 h	~0.6–0.75 h
T½	2.6–3.7 h	17.5 h	3.9 h	6–17 h
Duration of effect	Up to 12 h	Up to 36 h	4–6 h	6–8 h
Food effect	Delayed by high-fat meal	No significant effect	Delayed by high-fat meal	Minimal effect
Selectivity (PDE5)	Moderate	High	High	Very high
PDE6 inhibition (visual SE)	Yes (blue vision)	Minimal	Moderate	Minimal
PDE11 inhibition (myalgia)	No	Yes	Minimal	No
Common adverse effects	Headache, flushing, visual changes	Myalgia, back pain	Headache, nasal congestion	Headache, flushing
FDA approval year	1998	2003	2003	2012

PDE5i Phosphodiesterase type 5 inhibitors, *Tmax* Time to maximum plasma concentration, *T½* Elimination half-life, *PDE5* Phosphodiesterase type 5, *PDE6* Phosphodiesterase type 6, *SE* Side effect, *PDE11* Phosphodiesterase type 11, *FDA* U.S. Food and Drug Administration

Phosphodiesterase Selectivity

Sildenafil, vardenafil, and tadalafil are all selective inhibitors of phosphodiesterase type 5 (PDE5), with vardenafil demonstrating the highest in vitro potency against PDE5 and minimal cross-reactivity with other phosphodiesterase isoforms. Tadalafil is also highly selective for PDE5 but exhibits strong inhibitory activity against PDE11, which is believed to contribute to the back and muscle pain (myalgia) reported by some men during treatment. This is likely due to the abundant expression of PDE11 in skeletal muscle cells.

PDE1, expressed in the brain, myocardium, and vascular smooth muscle, may also be affected by non-selective inhibition, potentially resulting in vasodilation and tachycardia. Among the three agents, tadalafil exhibits the highest selectivity for PDE5 over PDE1, followed by vardenafil and sildenafil.

Inhibition of PDE6 which is exclusively expressed in the retina and plays a key role in visual signal transduction—may lead to transient visual disturbances. Inhibition of PDE6, particularly by sildenafil and to a lesser degree by vardenafil, may cause transient visual disturbances, whereas tadalafil has minimal effect on this enzyme [4].

Dosing and Absorption

Sildenafil is available in 25 mg, 50 mg, and 100 mg tablet formulations. Vardenafil is typically initiated at a dose of 10 mg, which may be titrated to 5 mg or 20 mg based on individual efficacy and tolerability. Tadalafil is commonly prescribed at an initial on-demand dose of 10 mg, while daily dosing regimens include 2.5 mg and 5 mg preparations. Avanafil is usually started at 100 mg, with alternative doses of 50 mg or 200 mg employed depending on clinical response.

The absorption and bioavailability of sildenafil and vardenafil are known to be delayed and reduced when taken with a high-fat meal. In contrast, the pharmacokinetics of tadalafil are not significantly affected by dietary fat intake [9].

Udenafil is initiated at a dose of 100 mg, with the option to increase to 200 mg if necessary; daily dosing of 25 mg, 50 mg, or 75 mg is also used in clinical practice [16]. Lodenafil is available in 20 mg, 40 mg, and 80 mg doses, while mirodenafil is marketed in 100 mg tablet formulations.

Duration of Action

Sildenafil reaches a maximum plasma concentration (Tmax) at approximately 0.81-1 h and has a terminal half-life T½ of 2.6–3.7 h. Its onset of action occurs within 30 to 60 min after administration, with effects lasting up to 12 h. However, its efficacy is reduced when taken with a high-fat meal. Vardenafil has a Tmax of 0.7–0.9 h and a T½ of 3.9 h, with an onset of action similarly observed at 30 to

60 min post-administration. Tadalafil, in contrast, demonstrates a longer pharmacokinetic profile, with a Tmax of approximately 2 h and a T½ of 17.5 h. Its effects begin within 30 min, reaching peak efficacy around 2 h after ingestion, and may persist for up to 36 h.

Metabolism and Excretion

Each PDE5i is primarily metabolized by the hepatic cytochrome P450 (CYP) isoenzyme system, particularly CYP3A4. Additional minor metabolic pathways include CYP2C9 for sildenafil, CYP3A5 and CYP2C for vardenafil, and CYP2C for avanafil.

Sildenafil undergoes biotransformation to produce an active metabolite that retains approximately 50% of the parent compound's potency and contributes to around 20% of its total pharmacological activity. Similarly, vardenafil and avanafil also form active metabolites that enhance their overall pharmacodynamic effects [13]. PDE5 inhibitors are predominantly excreted as metabolites via feces, with a smaller proportion eliminated through the urine [13].

Adverse Events

PDE5i differ in their side effect profiles. Common adverse events associated with these agents include headache, facial flushing, nasal congestion, nasopharyngitis, and dyspepsia. Although rare, serious complications such as prolonged erections lasting more than 4 h and priapism have been reported. In addition, cases of non-arteritic anterior ischemic optic neuropathy (NAION) have been documented following PDE5i use.

Tadalafil is uniquely associated with back pain and myalgia. These symptoms are typically mild to moderate in severity, appear 12–24 h post-administration, and generally resolve within 48 h without the need for medical intervention. Visual disturbances—most notably a bluish tint to vision—have been observed with sildenafil and are attributed to its inhibitory action on the PDE6 isoenzyme in the retina. Compared to sildenafil and vardenafil, tadalafil exhibits significantly lower inhibitory activity against PDE6 [37].

Safety and Drug Interactions

For patients with mild to moderate renal impairment, dose adjustments are generally not required for sildenafil, vardenafil, or avanafil. However, in individuals with severe renal dysfunction, sildenafil should be initiated at a reduced dose of 25 mg. In those with moderate renal impairment (creatinine clearance [CrCl] 30–50 mL/

min), tadalafil should be initiated at 5 mg, with a maximum cumulative dose of 10 mg within a 48-h period, and should not be administered more than once daily.

In cases of mild to moderate hepatic impairment, the recommended starting dose is 25 mg for sildenafil and 5 mg for vardenafil, with a maximum daily dose of 10 mg. Tadalafil should not be used at doses exceeding 10 mg in this population, while no dosage adjustment is necessary for avanafil. In the presence of severe hepatic impairment, the use of any of the four agents is not recommended.

The co-administration of moderate to strong CYP3A4 inhibitors (e.g., erythromycin, ketoconazole, itraconazole, ritonavir) or CYP3A4 inducers (e.g., rifampin, phenytoin) can significantly affect the plasma concentrations of PDE5is, potentially altering their efficacy and safety profiles.

Nitroglycerin and other organic nitrates increase the synthesis of cyclic guanosine monophosphate (cGMP), while PDE5i inhibit the enzymatic degradation of cGMP. The concomitant use of these agents can result in excessive accumulation of intracellular cGMP, leading to a synergistic and potentially dangerous drop in blood pressure. Therefore, the combined use of PDE5İs and any form of organic nitrate is contraindicated.

If nitrate administration becomes necessary, appropriate time intervals must be observed based on the specific PDE5 inhibitor used. At least 24 h should elapse after the last dose of sildenafil or vardenafil, 12 h for avanafil, and 48 h for tadalafil. Nitrates should only be administered under strict medical supervision following these intervals. In emergency situations where patients experience chest pain after recent PDE5i use, alternative non-nitrate anti-anginal agents—such as calcium channel blockers or beta-blockers—may be considered when clinically appropriate [28].

Efficacy

PDE5i are widely regarded as the first-line pharmacological treatment for ED. Clinical studies have demonstrated that PDE5 inhibitors are both effective and well tolerated, with efficacy reported in over 80% of patients compared to placebo [11]. Despite their overall success, discontinuation rates remain high, ranging from 30% to 70%. These dropouts are primarily attributed to suboptimal therapeutic response, lack of satisfaction, and adverse events [7, 35].

Recent Technological Advances in Oral Drug Delivery

ODx Types

Orally disintegrating tablets (ODTs) and oral disintegrating films (ODFs), collectively referred to as orodispersible dosage forms (ODx), are fast-dissolving drug delivery systems designed to disintegrate rapidly upon contact with approximately 2 mL of saliva in the oral cavity. This rapid disintegration enables direct drug absorption through the buccal mucosa, allowing the active compound to bypass

Table 20.2 Comparison between Orodispersible Tablets (ODT) and Orodispersible Films (ODF)

Feature	ODT	ODF
Form	Solid tablet	Thin, flexible polymeric film
Disintegration time	Rapid (<60 seconds), but may depend on pressure/position on tongue	Typically faster disintegration than ODT
Need for water	No	No
Ease of swallowing	Easier than tablets, but may still pose difficulty for some	Excellent option for patients with dysphagia
Taste masking	Generally more challenging	Easier to incorporate sweeteners/flavors via film coating
Stability	Sensitive to humidity and heat	Generally more sensitive than ODT
Manufacturing complexity	Moderate	High (requires film casting and precise drying conditions)
Patient compliance (elderly/children)	High	Very high

ODT: Orodispersible Tablets, *ODF*: Orodispersible Films

first-pass hepatic metabolism and enter systemic circulation efficiently. By improving bioavailability and reducing the frequency of dosing, ODx formulations aim to enhance patient compliance and minimize systemic side effects.

Orally Disintegrating Tablets (ODTs) These solid dosage forms disintegrate quickly on the tongue, releasing the drug for absorption through the buccal mucosa. Examples include Adcirca® ODT and Cialis® Rapid-Dissolve.

Orodispersible Films (ODFs) These thin, flexible polymer-based films adhere to the tongue and dissolve rapidly, providing a discreet and convenient alternative. An example is Tadanerfi®.

The key differences between ODTs and ODFs—including disintegration time, manufacturing complexity, stability, and patient compliance—are summarized in Table 20.2.

ODx Formulations

One of the major challenges in pharmaceutical development is the poor aqueous solubility of many active pharmaceutical ingredients (API). Several strategies have been employed to enhance solubility, including nanoparticle systems, lipid-based formulations, solid dispersions (SDs), particle size reduction, salt formation, and prodrug synthesis [34]. Among these, solid dispersion (SD)—a homogeneous mixture of one or more APIs dispersed in an inert polymeric carrier—is considered a particularly promising approach for improving both solubility and oral bioavailability.

The most effective form of SD is molecular dispersion, in which the API is uniformly distributed at the molecular level within the polymer matrix. Various manufacturing techniques can be used to produce amorphous SDs, including solvent evaporation, melting, spray drying, freeze-drying, hot-melt extrusion, and milling [32]. Solid dispersions offer several advantages, such as particle size reduction to the molecular level, decreased crystallinity, and enhanced wettability and porosity. Upon contact with aqueous media, the polymer carrier dissolves, releasing the API as fine colloidal particles. This increased surface area facilitates faster dissolution and improved bioavailability [36].

Orodispersible films (ODFs) are a relatively novel dosage form consisting of thin polymeric strips—approximately the size of a postage stamp—that rapidly dissolve or disintegrate upon contact with the tongue, typically within 1 min, without the need for water or swallowing. Compared to conventional oral dosage forms such as tablets or capsules, ODFs have been shown to improve drug delivery and enhance clinical outcomes [8, 12]. Their ease of administration, reduced risk of choking, precise dosing, and suitability for patients with dysphagia make them particularly beneficial for elderly and pediatric populations. Furthermore, advancements in manufacturing technologies have made ODFs increasingly cost-effective alternatives to traditional dosage forms [12].

In the context of ED, tadalafil (TAD), a long-acting PDE5i, has significantly transformed treatment paradigms due to its favorable safety profile, prolonged duration of action, and high permeability. Since its market introduction in 2003, tadalafil has been commercially available in yellow, film-coated tablets (FCTs) for oral administration [26]. However, its clinical performance is limited by poor aqueous solubility and a slow dissolution rate, which contribute to inconsistent absorption, fluctuating plasma drug levels, and variable therapeutic responses [5]. Additionally, some patients experience difficulties with conventional tablets due to swallowing challenges or psychological discomfort.

Pharmaceutical researchers have created tadalafil ODx in response to these worries, providing a practical and possibly more approachable method of treating ED.

In response to these limitations, pharmaceutical research has focused on developing alternative formulations of tadalafil that improve patient adherence and pharmacokinetic reliability. ODx, including ODFs and solid dispersion-based systems, have emerged as promising solutions. Strategies include the use of solid dispersions (SDs) to enhance solubility and dissolution [30], and the development of tadalafil ODFs to offer faster onset of action and improved convenience.

Metabolism and Excretion

ODx, including ODTs and ODFs, are designed to dissolve rapidly in the oral cavity. These formulations may allow partial absorption of the drug through the oral mucosa before it reaches the gastrointestinal tract. As a result they achieve a faster onset of action compared with conventional oral tablets offer several pharmacokinetic advantages over conventional oral formulations. One notable benefit is their ability to bypass enzymatic degradation in the gastrointestinal (GI) tract and avoid first-pass metabolism in the liver. As a result, ODx formulations can potentially enhance drug bioavailability by facilitating direct absorption through the oral mucosa.

However, current evidence indicates that the metabolic profiles of ODTs and ODFs do not significantly differ from their conventional counterparts at later pharmacokinetic stages.

Park et al., compared tadalafil pharmacokinetics after administration of a new ODF vs a film-coated tablet and found that the T_{max}, time to maximum plasma concentration; C_{max}, maximum plasma concentration were comparable between the two forms and concluded that the ODF formulation of tadalafil exhibited comparable pharmacokinetic, safety, and tolerability profiles to the film-coated tablet (FCT) formulation [26].

Following the success of orodispersible tadalafil formulations, recent developments have focused on similarly creating sildenafil products that dissolve rapidly in the mouth. Novel sublingual films containing sildenafil citrate have shown very fast disintegration times—under 30 s—and bioavailability similar to standard oral tablets. Importantly, these films can reach peak plasma concentrations (Tmax) up to 20 min faster in healthy volunteers. Early Phase I trials indicate that therapeutic blood levels (Cmax and Cmin) remain within the effective range, without requiring increased doses. Additionally, incorporating cyclodextrin complexes has effectively masked the drug's characteristic bitterness, which improves patient adherence and allows discreet administration without water [15].

Benefits of ODx

- *Improved medication adherence:* Rapid disintegration and ease of administration facilitate consistent drug intake, particularly among patients with dysphagia or pill aversion.
- *Faster onset of action:* Buccal and sublingual absorption routes may enable quicker systemic absorption compared to traditional oral tablets, potentially shortening the time to achieve an erection.
- *Enhanced patient satisfaction and confidence:* The convenience and potentially quicker efficacy of ODx formulations may positively influence patient perception and satisfaction with ED therapy.
- *Greater compliance for mobile or busy individuals:* The ability to administer the medication without water makes ODx formulations suitable for individuals who travel frequently or have limited access to water during daily activities.
- *Discreet administration:* Particularly relevant for orodispersible films, the unobtrusive mode of use can reduce psychological barriers and self-consciousness often associated with ED treatment [26].

Challenges and Considerations

- *Stability concerns:* Compared to conventional tablets, ODTs and ODFs are generally more sensitive to moisture and temperature variations, requiring stringent formulation and protective packaging measures to maintain stability.
- *Taste-masking requirements:* Tadalafil possesses an inherently bitter taste, which may reduce patient acceptability. Effective taste-masking strategies, such as the incorporation of sweeteners, flavoring agents, or polymeric coatings, are essential to ensure compliance.
- *Potential need for dosage adjustments:* Although buccal and sublingual absorption can accelerate drug onset, overall systemic bioavailability may be lower than with traditional oral routes, necessitating dose modifications in some cases.
- *Higher production costs:* The development and manufacturing of ODx formulations involve specialized technologies and materials, which may lead to increased production costs compared to conventional tablets [10].

Optimizing the ODx Experience: Novel Excipients, Nanotechnology, and Taste Masking

While current tadalafil ODx offer significant advantages over conventional tablets, there's always room for improvement. This section explores promising optimization strategies focusing on novel excipients, nanotechnology, and taste-masking approaches.

(i) *Novel Excipients*

- *Advanced superdisintegrants:* Novel agents such as sodium starch glycolate and croscarmellose sodium can accelerate disintegration times and facilitate rapid drug release, thereby improving onset of action.
- *Bioadhesive polymers*: Incorporating bioadhesive excipients—such as hyaluronic acid and chitosan—can improve buccal mucosal adhesion, potentially enhancing local residence time and systemic absorption, which may lead to improved bioavailability.
- *Taste-masking polymers*: To address the inherent bitterness of tadalafil, polymers such as cyclodextrins and cellulose derivatives have been employed for taste masking. These materials not only improve palatability but also support effective drug release and patient adherence [2].

(ii) *Nanotechnology*

- *Nano-carrier systems:* Encapsulation of tadalafil in nanocarriers such as liposomes or micelles may enhance its aqueous solubility, facilitate improved absorption through the buccal mucosa, and enable more targeted interaction with specific receptors. These systems hold promise for increasing both therapeutic efficiency and selectivity [22].

- *Tadalafil-loaded nanofilms*: The incorporation of tadalafil into nanostructured orodispersible films may enable even faster dissolution upon contact with the tongue. This rapid disintegration can lead to a quicker onset of action and potentially improve patient adherence due to ease of use and enhanced convenience [22].

(iii) *Taste-Masking Polymers*

- *Sweeteners and flavoring agents*: The use of sweeteners such as sucralose, combined with pleasant flavoring agents like citrus or mint, can substantially improve the palatability of tadalafil orodispersible formulations, which is essential for ensuring patient acceptability and compliance.
- *Microencapsulation techniques:* Tadalafil particles can be coated with taste-masking polymers using microencapsulation methods to prevent their direct interaction with oral taste receptors. This approach offers a more pleasant mouthfeel while maintaining rapid drug release.
- *Liposomal formulations*: In addition to enhancing absorption, liposomal encapsulation of tadalafil also provides effective taste masking by enveloping the drug within phospholipid bilayers, minimizing its exposure to taste buds during buccal administration [17].

Charting the Future: Research and Development Directions for ODx

While current orally disintegrating tadalafil formulations represent a significant advancement in the management of ED, substantial opportunities remain for further innovation and refinement. Future research is anticipated to focus on both enhanced drug delivery mechanisms and personalized treatment strategies.

(i) *Enhanced Drug Delivery Technologies*

- *Mucoadhesive systems:* The use of novel mucoadhesive polymers or nanoparticles may prolong buccal residence time, facilitating sustained drug release and potentially extending therapeutic efficacy [33].
- *Triggered-release systems:* Incorporating pH-sensitive or enzyme-responsive polymers into ODx formulations can enable site-specific drug release within the oral cavity, thereby maximizing local absorption and minimizing systemic variability [1].

(ii) *Personalized Medicine Approaches*

- *Pharmacogenomics-based formulation design:* Understanding how genetic polymorphisms affect tadalafil metabolism and absorption may guide the creation of individualized ODTs tailored to patient-specific metabolic profiles [23].

- *Genetic markers:* The identification of genetic markers linked to a person's reaction to tadalafil may allow for the modification of ODT dosages to maximize effectiveness and reduce side effects [23].

(iii) *Combination Therapies*

- *Combination with PDE5 inhibitors:* Combining tadalafil and other PDE5 inhibitors together may have synergistic effects, decrease dosage requirements and minimize side effects [25].

(iv) *Innovative Manufacturing Methods*

- *3D printing*: Additive manufacturing technologies such as 3D printing enable the production of personalized ODTs with precise drug dosages, customizable drug combinations, and rapid disintegration profiles tailored to individual patient needs [24].
- *Microfluidic chip technologies*: Microfluidic platforms offer highly controlled environments for ODT fabrication, enabling uniform dispersion of active pharmaceutical ingredients and consistent drug release characteristics across batches [10].

(v) *Patient-Centric Design Features*

- *Enhanced palatability:* Improving taste and mouthfeel remains a critical factor in increasing patient acceptability and adherence, particularly for populations with heightened taste sensitivity.
- *Dispenser innovations*: User-friendly, portable, and protective dispensing devices—especially for orodispersible films—can improve ease of administration, dose accuracy, and product stability during storage and transport.
- *Integration with telemedicine platforms*: Incorporating ODT-based ED therapies into digital health ecosystems may enhance accessibility for patients in remote or underserved areas, especially those with limited mobility or reluctance to seek in-person care [18].

References

1. Liu L, Yao W, Rao Y, Lu X, Gao J. pH-Responsive carriers for oral drug delivery: challenges and opportunities of current platforms. Drug Deliv. 2017;24(1):569–81.
2. Ali HS, Ahmed SA, Alqurshi AA, Alalawi AM, Shehata AM, Alahmadi YM. Boosting tadalafil bioavailability via sono-assisted nano-emulsion-based oral jellies: box–behnken optimization and assessment. Pharmaceutics. 2022;14(12):2592.
3. Baek J-S, Pham CV, Myung C-S, Cho C-W. Tadalafil-loaded nanostructured lipid carriers using permeation enhancers. Int J Pharm. 2015;495(2):701–9.
4. Bischoff E. Potency, selectivity, and consequences of nonselectivity of PDE inhibition. Int J Impot Res. 2004;16(1):S11–4.
5. Choi J-S, Lee S-E, Jang WS, Byeon JC, Park J-S. Tadalafil solid dispersion formulations based on PVP/VA S-630: improving oral bioavailability in rats. Eur J Pharm Sci. 2017;106:152–8.

6. Corona G, Mondaini N, Ungar A, Razzoli E, Rossi A, Fusco F. Phosphodiesterase type 5 (PDE5) inhibitors in erectile dysfunction: the proper drug for the proper patient. J Sex Med. 2011;8(12):3418–32.
7. Corona G, Rastrelli G, Burri A, Serra E, Gianfrilli D, Mannucci E, et al. First-generation phosphodiesterase type 5 inhibitors dropout: a comprehensive review and meta-analysis. Andrology. 2016;4(6):1002–9.
8. Dixit R, Puthli S. Oral strip technology: overview and future potential. J Control Release. 2009;139(2):94–107.
9. Forgue ST, Patterson BE, Bedding AW, Payne CD, Phillips DL, Wrishko RE, Mitchell MI. Tadalafil pharmacokinetics in healthy subjects. Br J Clin Pharmacol. 2006;61(3):280–8.
10. Ghourichay MP, Kiaie SH, Nokhodchi A, Javadzadeh Y. Formulation and quality control of orally disintegrating tablets (ODTs): recent advances and perspectives. Biomed Res Int. 2021;2021:1–12.
11. Hatzimouratidis K, Salonia A, Adaikan G, Buvat J, Carrier S, El-Meliegy A, et al. Pharmacotherapy for erectile dysfunction: recommendations from the Fourth International Consultation for Sexual Medicine (ICSM 2015). J Sex Med. 2016;13(4):465–88.
12. Hoffmann EM, Breitenbach A, Breitkreutz J. Advances in orodispersible films for drug delivery. Expert Opin Drug Deliv. 2011;8(3):299–316.
13. Huang SA, Lie JD. Phosphodiesterase-5 (PDE5) inhibitors in the management of erectile dysfunction. Pharm Ther. 2013;38(7):407.
14. İbis MA, Ozkaya F, Tokatli Z, Akpinar C, Yaman O. Efficacy of low-intensity shockwave therapy with different tadalafil regimens in patients with PDE5 inhibitor-resistant erectile dysfunction: a retrospective cohort study. Int Urol Nephrol. 2024;56(2):407–13.
15. Jannini EA, Vignesh SO, Hassan T. Next-generation pharmaceuticals: the rise of sildenafil citrate ODF for the treatment of men with erectile dysfunction. Ther Deliv. 2025;16:365–78.
16. Kang SG, Kim JJ. Udenafil: efficacy and tolerability in the management of erectile dysfunction. Ther Adv Urol. 2013;5(2):101–10.
17. Sanjay L, Ashokbhai M, Ghatole S, Roy S, Kashinath K, Kaity S: Strategies for beating the bitter taste of pharmaceutical formulations towards better therapeutic outcomes. RSC Pharm., 2025;2:59.
18. Pallavi PA, Yashpal MM, Vinay RK, Pradnya DL: Review on Orodispersible Tablet. Res. J. Pharma. Dosage Forms and Tech.2024;16(1):55–9.
19. Kurakula M, Ahmed OA, Fahmy UA, Ahmed TA. Solid lipid nanoparticles for transdermal delivery of avanafil: optimization, formulation, in-vitro and ex-vivo studies. J Liposome Res. 2016;26(4):288–96.
20. Langarizadeh MA, Salary A, Tavakoli MR, Nejad BG, Fadaei S, Jahani Z, Forootanfar H. An overview of the history, current strategies, and potential future treatment approaches in erectile dysfunction: a comprehensive review. Sex Med Rev. 2023;11(3):253–67.
21. MIMaiorinoGBellastellaKEsposito2015Lifestyle modifications and erectile dysfunction: what can be expected?Asian J Androl171510Maiorino MI, Bellastella G, Esposito K. Lifestyle modifications and erectile dysfunction: what can be expected? Asian J Androl. 2015;17(1):5–10.
22. Mikušová V, Mikuš P. Advances in chitosan-based nanoparticles for drug delivery. Int J Mol Sci. 2021;22(17):9652.
23. Mini E, Nobili S. Pharmacogenetics: implementing personalized medicine. Clin Cases Miner Bone Metab. 2009;6(1):17.
24. Mohammed AA, Algahtani MS, Ahmad MZ, Ahmad J, Kotta S. 3D printing in medicine: technology overview and drug delivery applications. Ann 3D Print Med. 2021;4:100037.
25. Mykoniatis I, Pyrgidis N, Sokolakis I, Ouranidis A, Sountoulides P, Haidich A-B, et al. Assessment of combination therapies vs monotherapy for erectile dysfunction: a systematic review and meta-analysis. JAMA Netw Open. 2021;4(2):e2036337.
26. Park SI, Heo SH, Kim G, Chang S, Song KH, Kim MG, et al. Comparison of tadalafil pharmacokinetics after administration of a new orodispersible film versus a film-coated tablet. Drug Des Devel Ther. 2018; 12:935–942.

27. Pizzol D, Xiao T, Smith L, Sánchez GFL, Garolla A, Parris C, et al. Prevalence of erectile dysfunction in male survivors of cancer: a systematic review and meta-analysis of cross-sectional studies. Br J Gen Pract. 2021;71(706):e372–80.
28. Rosen RC, Jackson G, Kostis JB. Erectile dysfunction and cardiac disease: recommendations of the Second Princeton Conference. Curr Urol Rep. 2006;7(6):490–6.
29. Seftel AD, Sun P, Swindle R. The prevalence of hypertension, hyperlipidemia, diabetes mellitus and depression in men with erectile dysfunction. J Urol. 2004;171(6 Part 1):2341–5.
30. Sharma PK, Sharma PK, Darwhekar GN, Birendra S. Formulation and evaluation of solid dispersion of tadalafil. Int J Drug Regulat Affairs (IJDRA). 2018;6(1):26–34.
31. Shitole M, Dugam S, Tade R, Desai N, Nangare S. Progress in erectile dysfunction therapy through drug delivery system. Thai J Pharm Sci. 2020;44(2):73–81.
32. Slamova M, Školáková T, Školáková A, Patera J, Zámostný P. Preparation of solid dispersions with respect to the dissolution rate of active substance. J Drug Delivery Sci Technol. 2020;56:101518.
33. Subramanian P. Mucoadhesive delivery system: a smart way to improve bioavailability of nutraceuticals. Foods. 2021;10(6):1362.
34. Vasconcelos T, Marques S, das Neves J, Sarmento B. Amorphous solid dispersions: rational selection of a manufacturing process. Adv Drug Deliv Rev. 2016;100:85–101.
35. Verze P, Cai T, Palmieri A, Mirone V. 17 years of clinical experience with phosphodiesterase type 5 inhibitors: what do we have yet to learn? Eur Urol. 2015;4(68):681–2.
36. Vo CL-N, Park C, Lee B-J. Current trends and future perspectives of solid dispersions containing poorly water-soluble drugs. Eur J Pharm Biopharm. 2013;85(3):799–813.
37. Yuan J, Zhang R, Yang Z, Lee J, Liu Y, Tian J, et al. Comparative effectiveness and safety of oral phosphodiesterase type 5 inhibitors for erectile dysfunction: a systematic review and network meta-analysis. Eur Urol. 2013;63(5):902–12.

Chapter 21
LUTS, ED and PE: Common Pathogenic Pathways and New Treatment Options

Widi Atmoko, Eric Chung, and Nguyen Quang

Introduction

Male lower urinary tract symptoms (LUTS) and benign prostatic hyperplasia (BPH) are common conditions that are closely associated with sexual dysfunction. Although initially considered as normal consequences of ageing, growing evidence shows that these conditions are closely related [1]. With the development of new medical and minimally invasive treatment options, major professional organizations such as the EAU and AUA have adapted treatment considerations, particularly in patients with coexisting sexual dysfunction [2, 3]. This chapter will discuss the relationship between LUTS/BPH and male sexual dysfunction in detail.

W. Atmoko (✉)
Department of Urology, Dr Cipto Mangunkusumo Hospital, Faculty of Medicine, Universitas Indonesia, Jakarta, Indonesia

E. Chung
Department of Urology, Princess Alexandra Hospital, University of Queensland, Brisbane, QLD, Australia

AndroUrology Centre, Brisbane, QLD, Australia

N. Quang
Center for Andrology and Sexual Medicine, VietDuc University Hospital, Hanoi, Vietnam

Department of Urology, Andrology and Sexual Medicine, University of Medicine and Pharmacy, Vietnam National University, Hanoi, Vietnam

E. Chung et al. (eds.), *Advances in Andrology*,
https://doi.org/10.1007/978-3-032-29112-7_21

Epidemiology of LUTS and Sexual Dysfunction

Epidemiology of LUTS

Male LUTS are divided into three groups: storage (or irritative) symptoms, voiding (or obstructive) symptoms and post micturition complaints [2, 4]. These symptoms were majorly linked to bladder outlet obstruction (BOO) that develops as benign prostatic hyperplasia (BPH). Although it is majorly correlated to BPH (28%–33% in men over 70 years), a growing of research shows that LUTS also frequently arise from causes other than the prostate [2]. Bladder disorders such as detrusor overactivity (overactive bladder), detrusor underactivity (underactive bladder), bladder stones or malignancy can also be the cause of male LUTS [4, 5]. Another cause of LUTS came from neurological aspect such as multiple sclerosis, Parkinson disease, stroke, spinal cord injury. Notably, there are some neurological conditions where LUTS can be an early symptom in the presentation of the neurological disease [5]. Metabolic syndrome such as obesity, hyperinsulinaemia and inflammation causing LUTS through endocrine and vascular mechanism [6]. Other less common contributors such as urinary tract infection; urethral strictures; drug-induced urinary dysfunction (e.g. anticholinergics, opioid analgesics, antidepressants, first-generation antipsychotics and certain cardiovascular agents like β-blockers, thiazide and potassium-sparing diuretics) can all produce urinary retention or incontinence [7, 8].

Globally, approximately 63% of adult men experience LUTS. When symptom severity is considered, about 31% are affected by moderate-to-severe LUTS. The prevalence of moderate-to-severe LUTS has increased over the past three decades, rising from 27.4% in 1990–1999 to 31.9% in 2000–2009, and reaching 36.2% in 2010–2019 [9]. Age is one of the key epidemiologic determinant of LUTS. Approximately 25% of men aged 40–49 years experienced LUTS, while more than 80% of men aged 70–79 years reported symptoms, often with histologic evidence of benign prostatic hyperplasia [10, 11]. Studies conducted across five European countries and Canada highlight regional differences in LUTS type and frequency. In the European Prospective Investigation into Cancer (EPIC), 26% of men reported obstructive LUTS, while 51% reported irritative LUTS [12]. In contrast, a Malaysian community survey found that 16.3% of men aged 40 years and older had clinically significant LUTS, defined as an International Prostate Symptom Score (IPSS) of ≥8 [13]. LUTS tend to worsen over time, with a U.S. cohort of men aged 40–75 years showing progression rates of 18.5 per 1000 person-years from mild to moderate–severe LUTS and 44.9 per 1000 person-years from moderate-to-severe LUTS. Over 3 years, symptoms worsened in 54.8% of men, while 27.1% improved [11].

Epidemiology of Sexual Dysfunction

Reported prevalence rates of erectile dysfunction (ED) vary considerably across studies. Globally, estimates range from 13% to 71%, whereas in the United States, figures fall between 18% and 69%. It is projected that by 2025, the total number of men affected by ED will exceed 322 million worldwide [14]. The prevalence of ED increases substantially with advancing age [15]. Among adults younger than 40 years, approximately 1% to 10% are affected. For men aged 60 to 69 years, prevalence increases to 20% to 40%. In men aged 70 years and older, prevalence rates rise to between 50% and 100% [14]. Severity, as measured by the five-item International Index of Erectile Function (IIEF-5), also correlates with age. In a large community-based sample: Among young adults aged 18–34 years, 6.5% exhibited severe ED, defined as an IIEF-5 score of 0– 7. Among men aged 50 to 64 years, 13.7% were classified as having severe ED. Among elderly individuals aged 65 years and older, 24.9% were classified as having severe ED [15].

On the other hand, the prevalence of premature ejaculation in adult males ranges from 6–40% worldwide [16]. There are several premature ejaculation definitions published from 1970 to 2021 [17]. The reported incidence of premature ejaculation is primarily a function of how the condition is defined, and psychological factors are the most common underlying cause. The prevalence rate of premature ejaculation mean-weighted is 14.19%. But in comparison, a psychogenic ejaculatory complaint shows dominate over somatogenic impaired ejaculatory control (18.22% vs 9.97%) [18].

Epidemiologic Association of LUTS and Sexual Dysfunction

A meta-analysis indicated that individuals with more severe LUTS had 3.31 times higher odds of experiencing sexual dysfunction [19]. Erectile dysfunction and ejaculatory dysfunction are highly prevalent among men with LUTS, with both conditions demonstrating strong associations with advancing age and increased LUTS severity. A European clinical characteristics study reported erectile dysfunction in 40% of men younger than 60 years and in 80% of those aged 70 years or older. Additionally, a significant correlation exists between age and LUTS severity, with 55% of cases classified as mild and 70% as severe [20]. The prevalence of PE among men with LUTS ranges from 12% to 77%, with most studies demonstrating significant associations between LUTS and PE [21]. Multiple studies have demonstrated that greater LUTS severity correlates with increased risk and severity of PE [19, 20]. In the EpiLUTS study, the overall prevalence of PE was 16%. Additional findings indicate that men with multiple LUTS experienced more frequent PE, and specific symptoms such as terminal dribble, incomplete emptying and split stream were significantly associated with PE [22]. Furthermore, a study in Korea reported that

Surgical Alternatives to TURP for LUTS/BPH

In recent years, there has been an increased emphasis and renewed interest in the role of minimally invasive surgical therapy (MIST) for male LUTS/BPH [69, 131]. These new technologies for BPH surgical interventions have been designed to target rapid recovery and symptom relief with relatively low complication rates compared to TURP [132]. These MISTs aim to preserve various male sexual function domains such as erectile and ejaculatory functions with an improvement in urinary function for sexually active men who are contemplating BPH surgery [133]. While conventional TURP resects prostate tissue to open the prostatic urethra and bladder outlet, these novel minimally invasive surgical interventions either expand the prostatic tissue or cause delayed prostatic tissue cavitation. Current commercially available MISTs for male LUTS/BPE can be largely divided into 2 categories, namely endourological and endovascular. Endourological interventions can be either prostatic ablative or non-ablative technology, with the Rezum water vapour thermal therapy (Boston Scientific, MA, USA) in the former group while Prostatic Urethral Lift (also known as Urolift) (Teleflex Inc., Pleasanton, CA, USA), Temporary implantable nitinol device (TIND) (Medi-Tate Ltd., Hadera, Israel), and Optilume BPH catheter system (Urotronic, Inc. MN, USA) in the latter group. Prostatic artery embolization constitutes the main endovascular approach in the treatment of male LUTS/BPE.

It is difficult to directly compare these MISTs since there are limited direct comparative clinical trials with available studies reporting short-term outcomes, and there was considerable heterogeneity in the patient demographics and study methodology. Nonetheless, a network meta-analysis tried to compare monopolar TURP, bipolar TURP (bTURP), PVP, holmium laser enucleation of the prostate (HoLEP), diode LEP, thulium LEP (ThuLEP), bipolar enucleation of the prostate, open prostatectomy, laparoscopic simple prostatectomy, prostatic urethral lift (PUL), prostatic arterial embolisation (PAE), Aquablation and sham. PUL showed higher mean difference in IIEF-5 score in the first month up to 60 months post-intervention. However, the data of PUL is limited on prostate volume under 60 mL. Moreover, open prostatectomy was found to have significantly lower IIEF-5 score compared to HoLEP, but no other comparison reached statistical significance [134]. Another network meta-analysis comparing different MiSTs concluded an uncertain result on its effect towards sexual function, both erectile function and ejaculatory function, compared to TURP. The study noted many major concerns towards the available studies, including inconsistency, within-study bias and imprecision [135]. Moreover, a meta-analysis study of 10 articles comparing endoscopic enucleation of the prostate (EEP) and TURP found that EEP has a slightly better benefit on erectile function in the long term (mean difference 1.00, 95% CI: 0.95–1.05 at 48 months and mean difference 1.08, 95% CI: 1.03–1.13 at 60 months for IIEF-5 score) [136]. In studies with longer follow-up (>5 years), similar preservation of sexual outcomes has been reported for PUL, Rezum and Aquablation [137–139]. Data has shown that most BPH surgeries have comparable adverse effect on erectile function. Similar evidence from other published systematic reviews and network meta-analyses [82, 140–143] support these MISTs as effective treatments with considerable improvements in various urinary parameters with the preservation of various male sexual domains postoperatively especially erectile function and, to a larger extent, ejaculatory function too, in men with male LUTS/BPH compared to TURP.

Several alternatives are available to make ejaculatory function better after prostate surgery, including urethral-sparing robotic-assisted prostatectomy, ejaculatory-preserving TURP and MiSTs [100, 144, 145]. Ejaculatory dysfunction was reported as low as 3.2%–10.8% for Rezum, 7%–15% for Aquablation, and 13.3%–56% for embolization. Meanwhile, PUL, iTIND and the optilume BPH catheter system were found to have the superiority in preserving ejaculatory function compared to other conventional treatments [145].

Despite the attractiveness of these MISTs, there remains a concern about whether longer-term preservation of ejaculation is possible if prostate volume involutes over time, and the indirect injury of erectile (cavernous) nerves from the transmission of energy by prostatic ablative MIST could potentially lead to ED and indirectly EjD with longer follow-up [146]. The concept of sexual rehabilitation with specialized pelvic floor exercises and the use of PDE5i in the early postoperative period in men following BPH surgery is intriguing and requires formal evaluation given the positive outcomes observed in the penile rehabilitation cohort following radical prostatectomy [147].

Future Directions

Increased awareness of the association between male sexual function and LUTS/BPH coupled with greater public demands for more effective but safer treatments have resulted in clinical challenges and new priorities reshaping consumer needs and clinician decision-making. In the search for the optimal BPH therapy, it has become clear that sexually active men are keen to maintain, if not improve their sexual function with BPH treatment. BPH medical therapy that targets bladder neck and prostate volume invariably causes unwanted ED and EjD, and newer drug designs would need to offset these structural alterations while improving penile blood flow and safeguarding the ejaculatory apparatus. Drugs targeting oxidative stress (chronic inflammatory process) and NO-cGMP pathways will likely offer the best of both worlds in terms of clinical improvements in urinary and sexual functions.

Numerous innovative MISTs are in various research, development and clinical testing stages to enhance surgical outcomes with excellent safety records and importantly, minimal to no adverse impact on various male sexual domains. The difficulty in surgical intervention resides in successfully 'un-obstructing' the bladder outlet while preserving key structures responsible for erection and ejaculatory functions. Mechanical devices that open the prostatic urethra with minimal prostatic apoptosis would maintain the prostatic contribution to seminal fluid and should preserve the ejaculatory function. Further validation with validated objective assessments and direct comparative large well-designed and multi-centre studies are desired to examine the actual role of MIST in clinical practice and whether MIST can replace TURP as the new standard of surgical care in male LUTS/BPH.

References

1. Rosen RC, Giuliano F, Carson CC. Sexual dysfunction and lower urinary tract symptoms (luts) associated with benign prostatic hyperplasia (bph). Eur Urol. 2005;47(6):824–37.
2. Cornu JN, Gacci M, Hashim H, Herrmann TRW, Malde S, Netsch C, et al. EAU guidelines on non-neurogenic male lower urinary tract symptoms (luts). In: EAU Guidel Off. EAU; 2025.
3. Sandhu JS, Bixler BR, Dahm P, Goueli R, Kirkby E, Stoffel JT, et al. Management of lower urinary tract symptoms attributed to benign prostatic hyperplasia (bph): aua guideline amendment 2023. J Urol. 2024;211(1):11–9.
4. Wei JT, Dauw CA, Brodsky CN. Lower urinary tract symptoms in men: a review. JAMA. 2025;334(9):809–21.
5. Panicker JN, Fowler CJ, Kessler TM. Lower urinary tract dysfunction in the neurological patient: clinical assessment and management. Lancet Neurol. 2015;14(7):720–32.
6. Oztekin CV, Kaya-Sezginer E, Yilmaz-Oral D, Gur S. Male urogenital disorders and metabolic syndrome: possible links, characteristics and potential treatment strategies. Curr Pharm Des. 2018;24(9):1019–33.
7. Wessells H, Morey A, Souter L, Rahimi L, Vanni A. Urethral stricture disease guideline amendment (2023). J Urol. 2023;210(1):64–71.
8. Dobrek L. Lower urinary tract disorders as adverse drug reactions—a literature review. Pharmaceuticals. 2023;16(7):1031.
9. Huang J, Chan CK, Yee S, Deng Y, Bai Y, Chan SC, et al. Global burden and temporal trends of lower urinary tract symptoms: a systematic review and meta-analysis. Prostate Cancer Prostatic Dis. 2023;26(2):421–8.
10. Maharajh S, Abdel Goad EH, Ramklass SS, Conradie MC. Lower urinary tract symptoms (luts) in males: a review of pathophysiology. S Afr Fam Pract. 2015;57(2):88–92.
11. McNicholas T, Kirby R. Benign prostatic hyperplasia and male lower urinary tract symptoms (luts). BMJ Clin Evid. 2011;2011:1801.
12. Irwin DE, Milsom I, Hunskaar S, Reilly K, Kopp Z, Herschorn S, et al. Population-based survey of urinary incontinence, overactive bladder, and other lower urinary tract symptoms in five countries: results of the epic study. Eur Urol. 2006;50(6):1306–15.
13. Mohamad Anuar MF, Solihin Rezali M, Mohamed Daud MA, Ismail SB. A community-based study on lower urinary tract symptoms in malaysian males aged 40 years and above. Sci Rep. 2022;12(1):2345.
14. Shamloul R, Ghanem H. Erectile dysfunction. Lancet Lond Engl. 2013;381(9861):153–65.
15. Amand C, Tong S, Tardy AL, McGraw T, Stewart A, Cruz-Rivera M. A population-based survey of self-reported and iief-defined erectile dysfunction among adult men in the United States in 2021. BMC Public Health. 2025;25(1):4172.
16. Sihotang RC, Alvonico T, Taher A, Birowo P, Rasyid N, Atmoko W. Premature ejaculation in patients with lower urinary tract symptoms: a systematic review. Int J Impot Res. 2021;33(5):516–24.
17. Althof SE, McMahon CG, Rowland DL. Advances and missteps in diagnosing premature ejaculation: analysis and future directions. J Sex Med. 2022;19(1):64–73.
18. Opolony M, Rettenberger M, Briken P, Turner D. Examining the prevalence of premature ejaculation as a three-dimensional construct of sexual dysfunction-a systematic review. J Sex Med. 2025;22(10):1718–36.

19. Song G, Wang M, Chen B, Long G, Li H, Li R, et al. Lower urinary tract symptoms and sexual dysfunction in male: a systematic review and meta-analysis. Front Med. 2021;8:653510.
20. Vallancien G, Emberton M, Harving N, van Moorselaar RJA, Alf-One Study Group. Sexual dysfunction in 1,274 european men suffering from lower urinary tract symptoms. J Urol. 2003;169(6):2257–61.
21. Lee JH. Associations between premature ejaculation, lower urinary tract symptoms, and erectile dysfunction in middle-aged korean policemen. J Sex Med. 2014;11(6):1512–8.
22. Coyne KS, Sexton CC, Thompson CL, Milsom I, Irwin D, Kopp ZS, et al. The prevalence of lower urinary tract symptoms (luts) in the USA, the UK and Sweden: results from the epidemiology of luts (epiluts) study. BJU Int. 2009;104(3):352–60.
23. Wein AJ, Coyne KS, Tubaro A, Sexton CC, Kopp ZS, Aiyer LP. The impact of lower urinary tract symptoms on male sexual health: epiluts. BJU Int. 2009;103(Suppl 3):33–41.
24. Gacci M, Eardley I, Giuliano F, Hatzichristou D, Kaplan SA, Maggi M, et al. Critical analysis of the relationship between sexual dysfunctions and lower urinary tract symptoms due to benign prostatic hyperplasia. Eur Urol. 2011;60(4):809–25.
25. McVary KT, McKenna KE. The relationship between erectile dysfunction and lower urinary tract symptoms: epidemiological, clinical, and basic science evidence. Curr Urol Rep. 2004;5(4):251–7.
26. Ückert S, Richter K, Fischer K, Tsikas D, Kuczyk MA. Re-evaluation of the immunohistochemical distribution of isoforms of nitric oxide synthase in the human prostate: a light and electron microscopical study. Andrologia. 2021;53(7) Available from: https://onlinelibrary.wiley.com/doi/10.1111/and.14098.
27. Andersson KE. Erectile physiological and pathophysiological pathways involved in erectile dysfunction. J Urol. 2003;170(2S) Available from: http://www.jurology.com/doi/10.1097/01.ju.0000075362.08363.a4.
28. Kedia GT, Ückert S, Jonas U, Kuczyk MA, Burchardt M. The nitric oxide pathway in the human prostate: clinical implications in men with lower urinary tract symptoms. World J Urol. 2008;26(6):603–9.
29. McVARY K. Lower urinary tract symptoms and sexual dysfunction: epidemiology and pathophysiology. BJU Int. 2006;97(s2):23–8.
30. Gradini R, Realacci M, Ginepri A, Naso G, Santangelo C, Cela O, et al. Nitric oxide synthases in normal and benign hyperplastic human prostate: immunohistochemistry and molecular biology. J Pathol. 1999;189(2):224–9.
31. Hedlund P, Ekström P, Larsson B, Alm P, Andersson KE. Heme oxygenase and no-synthase in the human prostate—relation to adrenergic, cholinergic and peptide-containing nerves. J Auton Nerv Syst. 1997;63(3):115–26.
32. Bloch W, Klotz T, Loch C, Schmidt G, Engelmann U, Addicks K. Distribution of nitric oxide synthase implies a regulation of circulation, smooth muscle tone, and secretory function in the human prostate by nitric oxide. Prostate. 1997;33(1):1–8.
33. Burnett AL, Maguire MP, Chamness SL, Ricker DD, Takeda M, Lepor H, et al. Characterization and localization of nitric oxide synthase in the human prostate. Urology. 1995;45(3):435–9.
34. Ückert S, Küthe A, Jonas U, Stief CG. Characterization and functional relevance of cyclic nucleotide phosphodiesterase isoenzymes of the human prostate. J Urol. 2001;166(6):2484–90.
35. Takeda M, Tang R, Shapiro E, Burnett AL, Lepor H. Effects of nitric oxide on human and canine prostates. Urology. 1995;45(3):440–6.
36. Klotz T, Bloch W, Loch C, Engelmann U, Addicks K. Distribution of the constitutive no-synthase isoforms (bnos and ecnos) in the normal and hyperplastic human prostate. The Urologist. 1997;36(4):318–22.
37. Luo J, Dunn T, Ewing C, Sauvageot J, Chen Y, Trent J, et al. Gene expression signature of benign prostatic hyperplasia revealed by cdna microarray analysis. Prostate. 2002;51(3):189–200.
38. Haynes JM, Cook AM. Protein kinase g-induced activation of k_{ATP} channels reduces contractility of human prostate tissue. Prostate. 2006;66(4):377–85.

39. Waldkirch ES, Ückert S, Langnäse K, Richter K, Jonas U, Wolf G, et al. Immunohistochemical distribution of cyclic gmp-dependent protein kinase-1 in human prostate tissue. Eur Urol. 2007;52(2):495–502.
40. Yu Q, Li T, Li J, Zhong L, Mao X. Nitric oxide synthase in male urological and andrologic functions. In: Saravi SSS, editor. Nitric oxide synthase–simple enzyme-complex roles. InTech; 2017. Available from: http://www.intechopen.com/books/nitric-oxide-synthase-simple-enzyme-complex-roles/nitric-oxide-synthase-in-male-urological-and-andrologic-functions.
41. Chitaley K, Wingard CJ, Clinton Webb R, Branam H, Stopper VS, Lewis RW, et al. Antagonism of rho-kinase stimulates rat penile erection via a nitric oxide-independent pathway. Nat Med. 2001;7(1):119–22.
42. Wang H, Eto M, Steers WD, Somlyo AP, Somlyo AV. RhoA-mediated ca2+ sensitization in erectile function. J Biol Chem. 2002;277(34):30614–21.
43. Christ GJ, Andersson KE. Rho-kinase and effects of rho-kinase inhibition on the lower urinary tract. Neurourol Urodyn. 2007;26(S6):948–54.
44. Kimura K, Ito M, Amano M, Chihara K, Fukata Y, Nakafuku M, et al. Regulation of myosin phosphatase by rho and rho-associated kinase (rho-kinase). Science. 1996;273(5272):245–8.
45. Sopko NA, Hannan JL, Bivalacqua TJ. Understanding and targeting the rho kinase pathway in erectile dysfunction. Nat Rev Urol. 2014;11(11):622–8.
46. Peters SLM, Schmidt M, Michel MC. Rho kinase: a target for treating urinary bladder dysfunction? Trends Pharmacol Sci. 2006;27(9):492–7.
47. Schneider T, Fetscher C, Krege S, Michel MC. Signal transduction underlying carbachol-induced contraction of human urinary bladder. J Pharmacol Exp Ther. 2004;309(3):1148–53.
48. Durlu-Kandilci NT, Brading AF. Involvement of rho kinase and protein kinase c in carbachol-induced calcium sensitization in beta-escin skinned rat and Guinea-pig bladders. Br J Pharmacol. 2006;148(3):376–84.
49. Takahashi R, Nishimura J, Hirano K, Seki N, Naito S, Kanaide H. Ca2+ sensitization in contraction of human bladder smooth muscle. J Urol. 2004;172(2):748–52.
50. Rees RW, Foxwell NA, Ralph DJ, Kell PD, Moncada S, Cellek S. Y-27632, a rho-kinase inhibitor, inhibits proliferation and adrenergic contraction of prostatic smooth muscle cells. J Urol. 2003;170(6 Pt 1):2517–22.
51. Takahashi R, Nishimura J, Seki N, Yunoki T, Tomoda T, Kanaide H, et al. RhoA/rho kinase-mediated Ca2+ sensitization in the contraction of human prostate. Neurourol Urodyn. 2007;26(4):547–51.
52. Schwinn DA, Roehrborn CG. α_1 -adrenoceptor subtypes and lower urinary tract symptoms. Int J Urol. 2008;15(3):193–9.
53. Dean RC, Lue TF. Physiology of penile erection and pathophysiology of erectile dysfunction. Urol Clin North Am. 2005;32(4):379–95.
54. Golomb E, Rosenzweig N, Eilam R, Abramovici A. Spontaneous hyperplasia of the ventral lobe of the prostate in aging genetically hypertensive rats. J Androl. 2000;21(1):58–64.
55. Persson K, Pandita RK, Spitsbergen JM, Steers WD, Tuttle JB, Andersson KE. Spinal and peripheral mechanisms contributing to hyperactive voiding in spontaneously hypertensive rats. Am J Phys. 1998;275(4):R1366–73.
56. Behr-Roussel D, Chamiot-Clerc P, Bernabe J, Mevel K, Alexandre L, Safar ME, et al. Erectile dysfunction in spontaneously hypertensive rats: pathophysiological mechanisms. Am J Physiol Regul Integr Comp Physiol. 2003;284(3):R682–8.
57. Kim IH, Choi JB, Kim SJ, Kim YS, Kim JC, Lee JG. Relationship between autonomic nervous system activity and lower urinary tract symptoms: an analysis of heart rate variability in men with lower urinary tract symptoms. LUTS Low Urin Tract Symptoms. 2009;1(1):25–8.
58. Choi JB, Lee JG, Kim YS. Characteristics of autonomic nervous system activity in men with lower urinary tract symptoms (luts): analysis of heart rate variability in men with luts. Urology. 2010;75(1):138–42.

59. Juszczak K, Mazur M, Wyczokowski M, Filipek M, Thor PJ. Autonomic nervous system activity in patients with lower urinary tract symptoms secondary to benign prostatic hyperplasia estimated by heart rate variability. Open Urol Nephrol J. 2008;1(1):44–9.
60. Shim KH, Kim TW, Chung BH, Lee SW, Park JK, Park K, et al. Changes in autonomic nervous system activity after treatment with alpha-blocker in men with lower urinary tract symptoms. Investig Clin Urol. 2018;59(1):49–54.
61. Azadzoi KM, Tarcan T, Siroky MB, Krane RJ. Atherosclerosis-induced chronic ischemia causes bladder fibrosis and non-compliance in the rabbit. J Urol. 1999;161(5):1626–35.
62. Azadzoi KM, Babayan RK, Kozlowski R, Siroky MB. Chronic ischemia increases prostatic smooth muscle contraction in the rabbit. J Urol. 2003;170(2 Pt 1):659–63.
63. Kozlowski R, Kershen RT, Siroky MB, Krane RJ, Azadzoi KM. Chronic ischemia alters prostate structure and reactivity in rabbits. J Urol. 2001;165(3):1019–26.
64. Papaefstathiou E, Gatsos S, Tigkiropoulos K, Apostolidis I, Koukourikis P, Lazaridis I, et al. Role of pelvic ischemia in human lower urinary tract symptoms and sexual function among patients with common iliac artery obstruction undergoing revascularization surgery. Int Neurourol J. 2023;27(2):129–38.
65. Antunes-Lopes T, Vasconcelos A, Costa D, Charrua A, Neves J, Silva J, et al. The impact of chronic pelvic ischemia on luts and urinary levels of neuroinflammatory, inflammatory, and oxidative stress markers in elderly men: a case-control study. Urology. 2019;123:230–4.
66. De Nunzio C, Cindolo L, Gacci M, Pellegrini F, Carini M, Lombardo R, et al. Metabolic syndrome and lower urinary tract symptoms in patients with benign prostatic enlargement: a possible link to storage symptoms. Urology. 2014;84(5):1181–7.
67. De Nunzio C, Aronson W, Freedland SJ, Giovannucci E, Parsons JK. The correlation between metabolic syndrome and prostatic diseases. Eur Urol. 2012;61(3):560–70.
68. Hammarsten J, Högstedt B. Hyperinsulinaemia as a risk factor for developing benign prostatic hyperplasia. Eur Urol. 2001;39(2):151–8.
69. De Nunzio C, Roehrborn CG, Andersson KE, McVary KT. Erectile dysfunction and lower urinary tract symptoms. Eur Urol Focus. 2017;3(4–5):352–63.
70. Martin SA, Tully PJ, Kahokehr AA, Jay A, Wittert GA. The bidirectional association between depression and lower urinary tract symptoms (luts) in men: a systematic review and meta-analysis of observational studies. Neurourol Urodyn. 2022;41(2):552–61.
71. Martin S, Vincent A, Taylor AW, Atlantis E, Jenkins A, Januszewski A, et al. Lower urinary tract symptoms, depression, anxiety and systemic inflammatory factors in men: a population-based cohort study. Seedat S, editor. PLoS One. 2015;10(10):e0137903.
72. Liu Q, Zhang Y, Wang J, Li S, Cheng Y, Guo J, et al. Erectile dysfunction and depression: a systematic review and meta-analysis. J Sex Med. 2018;15(8):1073–82.
73. Velurajah R, Brunckhorst O, Waqar M, McMullen I, Ahmed K. Erectile dysfunction in patients with anxiety disorders: a systematic review. Int J Impot Res. 2022;34(2):177–86.
74. Pacák K. Stressor-specific activation of the hypothalamic-pituitary-adrenocortical axis. Physiol Res. 2000;49(Suppl 1):S11–7.
75. Herman J, Flak J, Jankord R. Chronic stress plasticity in the hypothalamic paraventricular nucleus. In: Progress in brain research. Elsevier; 2008. p. 353–64. Available from: https://linkinghub.elsevier.com/retrieve/pii/S0079612308004299.
76. Kalantaridou SN, Zoumakis E, Makrigiannakis A, Lavasidis LG, Vrekoussis T, Chrousos GP. Corticotropin-releasing hormone, stress and human reproduction: an update. J Reprod Immunol. 2010;85(1):33–9.
77. Wang Z, Chang HH, Gao Y, Zhang R, Guo Y, Holschneider DP, et al. Effects of water avoidance stress on peripheral and central responses during bladder filling in the rat: a multidisciplinary approach to the study of urologic chronic pelvic pain syndrome (mapp) research network study. PLoS One. 2017;12(9):e0182976.
78. Matos R, Serrão P, Rodriguez L, Birder LA, Cruz F, Charrua A. The water avoidance stress induces bladder pain due to a prolonged alpha1a adrenoceptor stimulation. Naunyn Schmiedeberg's Arch Pharmacol. 2017;390(8):839–44.

79. Kullmann FA, McDonnell BM, Wolf-Johnston AS, Kanai AJ, Shiva S, Chelimsky T, et al. Stress-induced autonomic dysregulation of mitochondrial function in the rat urothelium. Neurourol Urodyn. 2019;38(2):572–81.
80. Coyne KS, Wein AJ, Tubaro A, Sexton CC, Thompson CL, Kopp ZS, et al. The burden of lower urinary tract symptoms: evaluating the effect of luts on health-related quality of life, anxiety and depression: epiluts. BJU Int. 2009;103(s3):4–11.
81. Manfredi C, García-Gómez B, Arcaniolo D, García-Rojo E, Crocerossa F, Autorino R, et al. Impact of surgery for benign prostatic hyperplasia on sexual function: a systematic review and meta-analysis of erectile function and ejaculatory function. Eur Urol Focus. 2022;8(6):1711–32.
82. Franco JVA, Jung JH, Imamura M, Borofsky M, Omar MI, Escobar Liquitay CM, et al. Minimally invasive treatments for benign prostatic hyperplasia: a cochrane network meta-analysis. BJU Int. 2022;130(2):142–56.
83. La Torre A, Palleria C, Tamanini I, Scardigli A, Cai T, Colosimo M, et al. Sexual dysfunctions related to drugs used in the management of lower urinary tract symptoms due to benign prostatic hyperplasia: a narrative review on α-blockers and 5-alpha reductase inhibitors. Uro. 2021;1(3):82–98.
84. La Vignera S, Aversa A, Cannarella R, Condorelli RA, Duca Y, Russo GI, et al. Pharmacological treatment of lower urinary tract symptoms in benign prostatic hyperplasia: consequences on sexual function and possible endocrine effects. Expert Opin Pharmacother. 2021;22(2):179–89.
85. Singh D, Nguyen T, Burnam P, Greenberg J, Raheem O, Hellstrom W. Benign prostatic hyperplasia and sexual dysfunction: review of the impact of new medical and surgical therapies on sexual health. Curr Urol Rep. 2025;26(1):49.
86. Cornu JN, Baboudjian M, Netsch C, Hashim H, Creta M, Pyrgidis N, et al. Management of non-neurogenic male lower urinary tract symptoms: better holistic than sequential. Eur Urol. 2025;88(3):223–7.
87. Kaplan SA. Side effects of alpha-blocker use: retrograde ejaculation. Rev Urol. 2009;11(Suppl 1):S14–8.
88. Bapir R, Bhatti KH, Eliwa A, García-Perdomo HA, Gherabi N, Hennessey D, et al. Effect of alpha-adrenoceptor antagonists on sexual function. A systematic review and meta-analysis. Arch Ital Urol E Androl. 2022;94(2):252–63.
89. Giuliano F. Impact of medical treatments for benign prostatic hyperplasia on sexual function. BJU Int. 2006;97(s2):34–8.
90. McVary KT. Sexual function and alpha-blockers. Rev Urol. 2005;7(Suppl 8):S3–11.
91. Gur S, Kadowitz PJ, Hellstrom WJ. Effects of 5-alpha reductase inhibitors on erectile function, sexual desire and ejaculation. Expert Opin Drug Saf. 2013;12(1):81–90.
92. Zhang JJ, Shi X, Wu T, Zhang MD, Tang J, Yin GM, et al. Sexual, physical, and overall adverse effects in patients treated with 5α-reductase inhibitors: a systematic review and meta-analysis. Asian J Androl. 2022;24(4):390–7.
93. Liu L, Zhao S, Li F, Li E, Kang R, Luo L, et al. Effect of 5α-reductase inhibitors on sexual function: a meta-analysis and systematic review of randomized controlled trials. J Sex Med. 2016;13(9):1297–310.
94. Diviccaro S, Herian M, Cioffi L, Audano M, Mitro N, Caruso D, et al. Exploring rat corpus cavernosum alterations induced by finasteride treatment and withdrawal. Andrology. 2024;12(3):674–81.
95. Gacci M, Ficarra V, Sebastianelli A, Corona G, Serni S, Shariat SF, et al. Impact of medical treatments for male lower urinary tract symptoms due to benign prostatic hyperplasia on ejaculatory function: a systematic review and meta-analysis. J Sex Med. 2014;11(6):1554–66.
96. Corona G, Tirabassi G, Santi D, Maseroli E, Gacci M, Dicuio M, et al. Sexual dysfunction in subjects treated with inhibitors of 5α-reductase for benign prostatic hyperplasia: a comprehensive review and meta-analysis. Andrology. 2017;5(4):671–8.
97. Traish AM. Post-finasteride syndrome: a surmountable challenge for clinicians. Fertil Steril. 2020;113(1):21–50.

98. Leong JY, Patel AS, Ramasamy R. Minimizing sexual dysfunction in bph surgery. Curr Sex Health Rep. 2019;11(3):190–200.
99. Rassweiler J, Teber D, Kuntz R, Hofmann R. Complications of transurethral resection of the prostate (turp)—incidence, management, and prevention. Eur Urol. 2006;50(5):969–79. discussion 980
100. Tawfeek AM, Radwan A, Esmat M, Ismail AM, ElSaeed KO, Higazy A. Ejaculation-preserving transurethral resection of the prostate: a randomized controlled trial. J Endourol. 2025;39(2):166–71.
101. Muntener M, Aellig S, Kuettel R, Gehrlach C, Sulser T, Strebel RT. Sexual function after transurethral resection of the prostate (turp): results of an independent prospective multicentre assessment of outcome. Eur Urol. 2007;52(2):510–6.
102. Alwaal A, Breyer BN, Lue TF. Normal male sexual function: emphasis on orgasm and ejaculation. Fertil Steril. 2015;104(5):1051–60.
103. Kennedy WP. The nocebo reaction. Med World. 1961;95:203–5.
104. Wartolowska K, Colloca L, Amanzio M. Editorial: the nocebo effect and its consequences for clinical trials and clinical practice. Front Psychol. 2023;13:1111324.
105. Fertig R, Shapiro J, Bergfeld W, Tosti A. Investigation of the plausibility of 5-alpha-reductase inhibitor syndrome. Skin Appendage Disord. 2016;2(3–4):120–9.
106. Mondaini N, Gontero P, Giubilei G, Lombardi G, Cai T, Gavazzi A, et al. Finasteride 5 mg and sexual side effects: how many of these are related to a nocebo phenomenon? J Sex Med. 2007;4(6):1708–12.
107. Sertkaya Z, Ozkaya F. Silodosin has nocebo effect on sexual adverse effects: a randomized controlled trial. Eurasian J Med. 2019;51(3):277–9.
108. Mónica FZ, De Nucci G. Tadalafil for the treatment of benign prostatic hyperplasia. Expert Opin Pharmacother. 2019;20(8):929–37.
109. Gonzalez RR, Kaplan SA. Tadalafil for the treatment of lower urinary tract symptoms in men with benign prostatic hyperplasia. Expert Opin Drug Metab Toxicol. 2006;2(4):609–17.
110. Kallidonis P, Adamou C, Kotsiris D, Ntasiotis P, Verze P, Athanasopoulos A, et al. Combination therapy with alpha-blocker and phosphodiesterase-5 inhibitor for improving lower urinary tract symptoms and erectile dysfunction in comparison with monotherapy: a systematic review and meta-analysis. Eur Urol Focus. 2020;6(3):537–58.
111. Zhou Z, Zheng X, Wu J, Gao Z, Xu Z, Cui Y. Meta-analysis of efficacy and safety of tadalafil plus tamsulosin compared with tadalafil alone in treating men with benign prostatic hyperplasia and erectile dysfunction. Am J Mens Health. 2019;13(5):1557988319882597.
112. Sebastianelli A, Spatafora P, Morselli S, Vignozzi L, Serni S, McVary KT, et al. Tadalafil alone or in combination with tamsulosin for the management for luts/bph and ed. Curr Urol Rep. 2020;21(12):56.
113. Wang Y, Bao Y, Liu J, Duan L, Cui Y. Tadalafil 5 mg once daily improves lower urinary tract symptoms and erectile dysfunction: a systematic review and meta-analysis. Low Urin Tract Symptoms. 2018;10(1):84–92.
114. Liu J, Zhou W, Zhang P, Zhang W, Chang C, Fu G. Comparison of monotherapies and combination therapy of tamsulosin and tadalafil for treating lower urinary tract symptoms caused by benign prostatic hyperplasia with or without erectile dysfunction: a meta-analysis. Urol Int. 2024;108(2):89–99.
115. Elkelany OO, Owen RC, Kim ED. Combination of tadalafil and finasteride for improving the symptoms of benign prostatic hyperplasia: critical appraisal and patient focus. Ther Clin Risk Manag. 2015;11:507–13.
116. Olesovsky C, Kapoor A. Evidence for the efficacy and safety of tadalafil and finasteride in combination for the treatment of lower urinary tract symptoms and erectile dysfunction in men with benign prostatic hyperplasia. Ther Adv Urol. 2016;8(4):257–71.
117. Ma C, Zhang J, Cai Z, Li H. To evaluate the efficacy and safety of different kinds of pde5-is with tamsulosin as a medical therapy for luts secondary to benign prostatic hyperplasia: a protocol for systematic review and meta analysis. Medicine (Baltimore). 2020;99(3):e18712.

118. Kang TW, Kim SJ, Kim MH, Jung JH. Beta 3 adrenoreceptor agonist for the management of lower urinary tract symptoms in men with benign prostatic hyperplasia: a systematic review. Int Neurourol J. 2021;25(3):182–91.
119. Dahm P, Brasure M, MacDonald R, Olson CM, Nelson VA, Fink HA, et al. Comparative effectiveness of newer medications for lower urinary tract symptoms attributed to benign prostatic hyperplasia: a systematic review and meta-analysis. Eur Urol. 2017;71(4):570–81.
120. Mitidieri E, Tramontano T, Gurgone D, Imbimbo C, Mirone V, Fusco F, et al. B3 adrenergic receptor activation relaxes human corpus cavernosum and penile artery through a hydrogen sulfide/cgmp-dependent mechanism. Pharmacol Res. 2017;124:100–4.
121. Cirino G, Sorrentino R, di Villa BR, d'Emmanuele PA, Palmieri A, Imbimbo C, et al. Involvement of beta 3-adrenergic receptor activation via cyclic gmp- but not no-dependent mechanisms in human corpus cavernosum function. Proc Natl Acad Sci USA. 2003;100(9):5531–6.
122. Ückert S, Kedia GT, Tsikas D, Simon A, Bannowsky A, Kuczyk MA. Emerging drugs to target lower urinary tract symptomatology (luts)/benign prostatic hyperplasia (bph): focus on the prostate. World J Urol. 2020;38(6):1423–35.
123. Cao D, Sun R, Peng L, Li J, Huang Y, Chen Z, et al. Immune cell proinflammatory microenvironment and androgen-related metabolic regulation during benign prostatic hyperplasia in aging. Front Immunol. 2022;13:842008.
124. Tong Y, Zhou RY. Review of the roles and interaction of androgen and inflammation in benign prostatic hyperplasia. Mediat Inflamm. 2020;2020:7958316.
125. Choi JH, Hwa JS, Kam SC, Jeh SU, Hyun JS. Effects of tamsulosin on premature ejaculation in men with benign prostatic hyperplasia. World J Mens Health. 2014;32(2):99–104.
126. Modi NB, Kell S, Aquilina J, Rivas D. Effect of dapoxetine on the pharmacokinetics and hemodynamic effects of tamsulosin in men on a stable dose of tamsulosin. J Clin Pharmacol. 2008;48(12):1438–50.
127. Rieken M, Antunes-Lopes T, Geavlete B, Marcelissen T. EAU young academic urologists functional urology and BPH group. What is new with sexual side effects after transurethral male lower urinary tract symptom surgery? Eur Urol Focus. 2018;4(1):43–5.
128. Calik G, Laguna MP, Gravas S, Albayrak S, de la Rosette J. Preservation of antegrade ejaculation after surgical relief of benign prostatic obstruction is a valid endpoint. World J Urol. 2021;39(7):2277–89.
129. Chung E, Brock G. Sexual rehabilitation and cancer survivorship: a state of art review of current literature and management strategies in male sexual dysfunction among prostate cancer survivors. J Sex Med. 2013;10(Suppl 1):102–11.
130. Otani T. Clinical review of ejaculatory dysfunction. Reprod Med Biol. 2019;18(4):331–43.
131. Zhao H, Kim HH. The complex relationship between lower urinary tract symptoms and sexual health. Curr Urol Rep. 2019;20(10):58.
132. Elterman D, Gao B, Lu S, Bhojani N, Zorn KC, Chughtai B. New technologies for treatment of benign prostatic hyperplasia. Urol Clin North Am. 2022;49(1):11–22.
133. Ng BHS, Chung E. A state-of-art review on the preservation of sexual function among various minimally invasive surgical treatments for benign prostatic hyperplasia: impact on erectile and ejaculatory domains. Investig Clin Urol. 2021;62(2):148–58.
134. Light A, Jabarkhyl D, Gilling P, George G, Van Hemelrijck M, Challacombe B, et al. Erectile function following surgery for benign prostatic obstruction: a systematic review and network meta-analysis of randomised controlled trials. Eur Urol. 2021;80(2):174–87.
135. Franco JV, Jung JH, Imamura M, Borofsky M, Omar MI, Escobar Liquitay CM, et al. Minimally invasive treatments for lower urinary tract symptoms in men with benign prostatic hyperplasia: a network meta-analysis. Cochrane Database Syst Rev. 2021;2021(12) Available from: http://doi.wiley.com/10.1002/14651858.CD013656.pub2.
136. Liu Y, Cheng Y, Zhuo L, Liu K, Xiao C, Zhao R, et al. Impact on sexual function of endoscopic enucleation *vs* transurethral resection of the prostate for lower urinary tract symptoms due to benign prostatic hyperplasia: a systematic review and meta-analysis. J Endourol. 2020;34(10):1064–74.

137. McVary KT, El-Arabi A, Roehrborn C. Preservation of sexual function 5 years after water vapor thermal therapy for benign prostatic hyperplasia. Sex Med. 2021;9(6):100454.
138. Roehrborn CG, Barkin J, Gange SN, Shore ND, Giddens JL, Bolton DM, et al. Five year results of the prospective randomized controlled prostatic urethral l.i.f.t. study. Can J Urol. 2017;24(3):8802–13.
139. Gilling PJ, Barber N, Bidair M, Anderson P, Sutton M, Aho T, et al. Five-year outcomes for aquablation therapy compared to turp: results from a double-blind, randomized trial in men with luts due to bph. Can J Urol. 2022;29(1):10960–8.
140. Checcucci E, Veccia A, De Cillis S, Piramide F, Volpi G, Amparore D, et al. New ultra-minimally invasive surgical treatment for benign prostatic hyperplasia: a systematic review and analysis of comparative outcomes. Eur Urol Open Sci. 2021;33:28–41.
141. Cantiello F, Fimognari D, Di Mauro M, Crocerossa F, Carbonara U, Ferro M, et al. Mechanical and ablative minimally invasive techniques for male luts due to benign prostatic obstruction: a systematic review according to bph-6 evaluation. Urol Int. 2021;105(9–10):858–68.
142. Shin BNH, Qu L, Rhee H, Chung E. Systematic review and network meta-analysis of re-intervention rates of new surgical interventions for benign prostatic hyperplasia. BJU Int. 2024;134(2):155–65.
143. Tanneru K, Jazayeri SB, Alam MU, Kumar J, Bazargani S, Kuntz G, et al. An indirect comparison of newer minimally invasive treatments for benign prostatic hyperplasia: a network meta-analysis model. J Endourol. 2021;35(4):409–16.
144. Ying J, Zhou C, Jin Y. Efficacy and safety of urethral sparing versus other robot-assisted simple prostatectomy for large volume benign prostatic hyperplasia: a systematic review and meta-analysis. BMC Urol. 2025;25(1):251.
145. Akgul B, Aydin A, Cakir OO, Tozsin A, Noel O, Balasar M, et al. Impact of minimally invasive surgical therapies on sexual function in benign prostatic hyperplasia: a systematic review. Minerva Urol Nephrol. 2025;77(4) Available from: https://www.minervamedica.it/index2.php?show=R19Y2025N04A0459.
146. Mykoniatis I, Renterghem KV, Sokolakis I. How can we preserve sexual function after ablative surgery for benign prostatic hyperplasia? Curr Drug Targets. 2021;22(1):4–13.
147. Chung E, Gillman M. Prostate cancer survivorship: a review of erectile dysfunction and penile rehabilitation after prostate cancer therapy. Med J Aust. 2014;200(10):582–5.

Chapter 22
Simultaneous Surgery for Erectile Dysfunction and Stress Urinary Incontinence

Charalampos Thomas, Aykut Baser, and Ponco Birowo

Introduction

Despite significant advancements in the technological landscape for the treatment of major pelvic surgeries such as urological surgeries for prostate cancer, invasive bladder cancer, and colorectal surgeries, a considerable number of patients continue to grapple with the dual challenges of erectile dysfunction (ED) and stress urinary incontinence (SUI) following their initial treatments. Pelvic trauma can also lead to both ED and SUI as well. Additionally, climacturia, described as urinary leakage during sexual intercourse, can also occur. These complications significantly impact the quality of life and overall well-being of affected individuals, underscoring the importance of elucidating the frequency, etiology, and optimal management strategies for these concurrent conditions.

Studies have reported varying incidences of both ED and SUI, both separately and in combination, among patients undergoing treatment for prostate cancer and invasive bladder cancer. The incidence rates for these two complications have been reported to range between 6% and 94% for ED and between 3% and 74% for SUI [1–5]. Climacturia can occur in up to 68% of men following prostatectomy [6]. While the prevalence of ED following prostate cancer treatment has been extensively documented, relatively fewer studies have focused on the incidence of SUI in

C. Thomas (✉)
Department of Urology, General Hospital of Corinth, Corinth, Greece

A. Baser
Department of Urology, Bandirma Onyedi Eylul University, Faculty of Medicine, Surgical Medical Sciences, Balikesir, Turkey

P. Birowo
Department of Urology, Faculty of Medicine, Universitas Indonesia, Cipto Mangunkusumo Hospital, Jakarta, Indonesia

E. Chung et al. (eds.), *Advances in Andrology*,
https://doi.org/10.1007/978-3-032-29112-7_22

this population. The reported impairment in quality of life for SUI and ED is 13% and 46%, respectively [7]. Despite the identification of quality-of-life impairment, the combined prevalence of ED and SUI has not been adequately defined, necessitating further research to better understand the epidemiological landscape of these conditions in the context of cancer treatment. Blunt pelvic trauma account for almost 10% of all traumatic injuries in U.S.A [8]. and 2% of them will have urethral disruption [9]. Pelvic fracture after blunt pelvic trauma is associated with post-injury ED. Its true incidence is hard to estimate, due to many factors, such as the time from injury till data collection and biased subjective reports of patients. Taken these under account, the estimated incidence of ED after pelvic fracture is approximately 5% to 20% which in cases of pelvic fracture urethral injuries (PFUI) rises up to 42–62% [10, 11]. Pelvic trauma in men can also cause SUI, in cases of blunt or penetrating lacerations at the bladder neck and prostatic urethra which eventually compromise the internal sphincter mechanism [12], but data are very limited since this particular population is poorly evaluated in the literature [13], therefore its true incidence cannot be estimated. Radiation therapy can also cause both ED and SUI with different mechanisms. ED is a common side effect of both external beam radiation therapy (EBRT) and brachytherapy due to neuronal, vascular and muscular damage. Radiation may also affect the bladder wall by causing a rare condition called radiation cystitis, which includes hematuria, urge incontinence and decreased bladder capacity but even rarer may weaken the pelvic floor muscles thus leading to SUI in the long term.

The initial step in the treatment of both ED and SUI typically involves conservative management strategies, including lifestyle modifications, pharmacotherapy, and pelvic floor exercises. While these interventions may yield positive outcomes for some patients, a subset may experience persistent or resistant symptoms, necessitating surgical intervention.

The decision to pursue surgical intervention for ED and SUI requires a comprehensive assessment of patient-specific factors, including the severity of symptoms, underlying etiology, and patient preferences. Various surgical options are available for the treatment of ED and SUI, ranging from minimally invasive procedures to more extensive surgical interventions. However, the optimal surgical approach will vary based on individual patient characteristics and treatment goals. Regardless of the approaches, the surgical treatment of ED is primarily focused on penile prosthesis implantation. On the other hand, artificial urinary sphincter (AUS) is highlighted for SUI, while male sling surgeries are prominent for mild to moderate cases. Additionally, treatments such as Mini-Jupette suspension may be recommended for climacturia [6]. Patients may be considered for surgical treatment in the first year after conservative and medical treatments have been attempted and failed to alleviate their symptoms.

Available Surgical Methods for ED and SUI

ED:

Modern penile implants replaced the use of rudimentary penile stiffeners more than 50 years ago, when Scott et al. in 1972 [14] and Small in 1978 [15] introduced the use of the three-piece inflatable implant and the semirigid (malleable) rod prosthesis, respectively. Even now, despite the major advances in pharmacotherapy, such as the discovery of PDE5 inhibitors and intracavernosal injections of vasoactive agents, they still are men's suffering from ED last resort, either when they are not suitable for any pharmacotherapy or when they do not respond to them.

Since the beginning, there were two types of penile implants: the Scott inflatable and the Small-Carrion semirigid rod. Through the years many improvements have been made, regarding the material, coating, etc., but these two categories stand still, the hydraulic and the semirigid. The hydraulic group includes the two-piece and the three-piece inflatable devices, which give the patient the element of spontaneity and can be inflated at any given time. It can be coated with antibiotic or not. The two-piece devices are mostly preserved for patients at higher risk of complications with the site of reservoir placement, especially in patients who have had a previous abdominal operation. The most popular three-piece devices are the AMS 700CX/CXR (Boston Scientific, Minnetonka, USA) and the Titan (Coloplast, Minneapolis, USA). On the other hand, the semirigid devices are easier to implant, easier to manage and of course cheaper, but they have the disadvantage of having the patient in a permanent erection status, which may cause discomfort. Regarding the efficacy, all types are efficacious but in terms of patient's satisfaction there aren't any prospective RCTs comparing the different types.

SUI:

Persistent post-prostatectomy incontinence is one of the most severe adverse effects with a tremendous impact on patient's quality of life. After conservative treatment's (lifestyle interventions, weight loss, physical activity, and pelvic floor muscle training-PFMT) and medical (duloxetine, anticholinergic, or b3 agonist) failure, surgical treatment is a one-way solution. In order to achieve continence, urethral resistance must be restored, either passively or actively. Depending on the severity of SUI, various techniques and devices have been developed.

Bulking Agents

Urethral bulking agents consist a minimal invasive treatment for men with mild to moderate SUI or those who are unfit for a more aggressive approach. When injected in the urethral wall, at the level of external sphincter, they add bulk, thus increasing the passive urethral resistance. In terms of efficacy, there is only one RCT which fulfilled the inclusion criteria for a Cochrane review, which compared the Macroplastique injection versus the implantation of an artificial urethral sphincter (AUS). The study reported a significant improvement for both procedures in men with mild SUI, and a significant supremacy of AUS in cases of severe SUI [16].

There is very limited evidence that bulking agents are effective for the treatment of PPI. The data for their long-term efficacy, even for cases of mild SUI are discouraging, since the long-term cure rate is about 10.3% [17]. Although the complications are mild and rare, the low cure rates make them an option only for men with mild SUI or for those who cannot undergo a more invasive operation, hence the weak strength of recommendation by the EAU 2023 guidelines [18].

Male Slings

Various kinds of male slings have been proposed for mild and moderate PPI, including non-adjustable and adjustable sling, autologous or synthetic, while their fixation can be achieved either via a transobturator or a retropubic approach. They restore continence by compressing directly the bulbar urethra resulting in coaptation of the urethral lumen and/or by repositioning it [19, 20]. Autologous slings are practically abandoned, except in some neurogenic cases and bone anchored also, due to their high complication rates.

(a) Non-adjustable Slings

Non-adjustable male slings are placed under the urethra and after any adjustments made during the operation no further can be performed postoperatively. Currently, there are 4 slings commercially available: AdVance (Boston Scientific, Minnetonka, USA), Virtue (Coloplast, Minneapolis, USA), Surgimesh M-SLING (Aspide Medical, France) and I-STOP TOMS (CL Medical, France).

(b) Adjustable Slings

Adjustable male slings offer tension adjustment at the level of compression of the urethra postoperatively. Three main systems are commercially available at this moment, the Argus, Argus classic and Argus T (Promedon, Cordova, Argentina [21] the ATOMS (A.M.I., Feldkirch, Austria) [22], and the Remeex [23].

Compression Devices

(a) Artificial Urinary Sphincter

Artificial Urethral Sphincter (AUS) is one of the oldest surgical treatments for SUI and till now the standard treatment for moderate to severe male SUI. AUS restores continence by applying circumferential compression to the urethra via its cuff which is placed around and is filled with liquid. The cuff can be inflated and deflated, just like an IPP, allowing the patient voluntary control over micturition.

The AMS 800 (Boston Scientific, Marlborough, MA, USA) is a three-component device, consisting of an inflatable cuff, a control pump and pressure regulating balloon and is still the reference system worldwide, [24] although other systems have been developed, such as the two-component ZSI 375 [25] or Br-SL-AS 904 [26], the Victo and Victo+ (Promedon, Cordoba, Argentina), and the Rigicon Conticlassic and Contireflex devices, with little so far data regarding their efficacy and safety.

(b) Periurethral Balloons

The ProAct (Uromedica, Inc., Plymouth, MN, USA) system is actually a set of 2 balloons which are implanted via a perineal incision laterally under the bladder neck. Each balloon has 2 lumen and a volume-adjustment-port. Once the device is placed, the surgeon can adjust the volume of the balloon postoperatively, thus achieving the optimal peri-urethral compression. The device should be avoided in men who have had pelvic radiotherapy, but it can be used as a salvage therapy, after a failed male sling implantation [27].

Simultaneous Operation for ED and SUI

Simultaneous surgeries for ED and SUI represent a complex but increasingly recognized approach in the treatment of patients with concurrent urological conditions. The feasibility of performing both surgeries simultaneously has been a highly intriguing topic.

Historically, the concept of simultaneous surgery for ED and SUI dates back several decades, alongside early pioneers in the field investigating the feasibility and safety of such interventions. In 1987, Scott et al. shared their initial experiences in the literature with the application of IPP and AUS in 72 patients without a control group between 1973 and 1986 [28]. Subsequently, numerous studies have continued to emphasize the feasibility and potential benefits of this groundbreaking approach. Evaluating the advantages and disadvantages of this simultaneous surgical approach in terms of success (efficacy and satisfaction), complications (perioperative, postoperative), cost, and surgical duration would be more appropriate, akin to conducting a SWOT (strength, weakness, opportunity, and threat) analysis.

Parulkar et al. [29] conducted a study in which they applied combined implants for both ED and urinary incontinence and followed up with 60 patients grouped according to different sphincter implantations. In the study, it was reported that in two patients, all components of the sphincter had to be removed due to infection. Additionally, in the same study, it was noted that penile prostheses were removed in two patients due to infection limited to the penile prosthesis components, and in three patients, both the sphincter and penile implants had to be removed due to infection. Therefore, as a significant disadvantage of simultaneous surgical intervention, they highlighted the difficulty in preventing the spread of infection to other components when an infection occurs in any component [9]. In 2005, Rhee [30] reported a series where penile prosthesis (PP) + male sling was applied to four patients without a control group, achieving a 100% success rate and observing no complications.

In the same year, Sellers et al. [31] compared inflatable penile prosthesis (IPP) + artificial urinary sphincter (AUS), AUS only, and IPP only groups. They reported that dual implantation in a single-stage procedure reduced the operation time by 24.7%, and there were no infections or erosions in the prostheses. Additionally, they provided the initial cost and cost-benefit analysis of dual implantation compared to single implantation [31]. Simultaneous implantation also provided approximately $7000 in cost savings [31]. In the same study, they highlighted the delayed widespread adoption of dual prosthesis implantation due to perceived increased infection rates. On contrary, dual implantation theoretically reduces the risk of infection compared to staged procedures [31]. In 2006, Kendirci et al. [32] reported the outcomes of a study involving 22 patients who underwent IPP + AUS application. They noted complications including urethral erosion in 2 patients (9%) and reservoir migration in 2 patients (9%). They also stated that no prosthetic infections occurred postoperatively, and the overall revision rate was 14%. The reasons for revision included urethral erosion associated with AUS device in 2 patients and reservoir migration in 1 patient. They determined that urethral erosions occurred in patients who had received radiotherapy [32].

In 2008, Mancini et al. [33] conducted a study involving a total of 95 patients comparing PP + AUS vs. PP vs. AUS, where all surgical procedures were performed by two staff surgeons. They reported that there was no difference in satisfaction between the combined surgical with prosthesis group and the prosthesis-only group for penile prosthesis outcomes. They also noted that although there was no statistically significant difference in revision rates, three out of 33 patients (9.1%) in the combined surgery group underwent revision surgery, while one out of 31 patients (3.3%) in the prosthesis-only group underwent revision surgery [33]. In the same study, similar results were also expressed for AUS outcomes. Regarding AUS revision, 6 patients (18.2%) in the combined surgery group and 4 patients (12.6%) in the AUS-only surgery group required revision, with 1 patient in each group requiring prosthesis removal. As a result, Mancini et al. stated that with careful preoperative evaluation of patients and in indicated cases, synchronized implantation could be offered initially, potentially preventing additional time, pain, cost, and risk associated with secondary procedures [33].

In their study comparing PP + sling with PP and sling groups, Gorbatiy et al. [34] analyzed the surgical duration, length of hospital stay, bleeding, and cost outcomes. They found no significant differences between groups in terms of surgical duration (98 ± 24 min for PP; 86 ± 24 min for sling; 177 ± 17 min for dual implant), estimated blood loss (57 ± 30 mL for IPP; 48 ± 59 mL for sling; 49 ± 5 mL for dual implant), and postoperative hospital stay (1.2 ± 0.45 days for IPP, 0.7 ± 0.48 days for sling, and 1.1 ± 0.50 days for dual implant). Interestingly, they found that dual implantation with approximately $9000 in cost savings when compared to the aggregated cost of individual procedures, similar to that reported by Sellers eta al

[31, 34]. Rolle et al. [35] retrospectively compared PP + AUS with asynchronous PP + AUS applications. They found similar success rates between PP + AUS (87%) and asynchronous PP + AUS (86%) groups, with only one case of infection requiring reoperation observed in the PP + AUS group. They stated that synchronous surgery was more advantageous in terms of surgical duration and noted the absence of any major complications in surgery [35]. In their study, Segal et al. [36] compared PP + AUS with asynchronous PP + AUS and PP vs. AUS in a larger patient cohort, published one year after the aforementioned study. Segal and colleagues reported that insertion of IPP was halted in one case due to intraoperatively detected distal urethral injury. They indicated no difference in terms of infection, erosion, and mechanical failure between combined procedures with both IPP and AUS and other groups. Furthermore, in the same study, consistent with previous research, they confirmed that combined procedures had longer implantation times compared to single prosthesis placement, with combined procedures taking longer (218.1 min) and individual procedures being shorter in total (145.9 min for IPP only and 114.7 min for AUS only), consistent with previous studies [16]. In a study with the same study groups designed, Patel et al. [37] conducted a much larger study in 2019, indicating a different situation regarding reoperation. When compared with men who underwent only penile prosthesis implantation, they found that those with both penile prosthesis and artificial urinary sphincter had a higher likelihood of undergoing revision surgery for inflatable penile prosthesis at 1 year (OR 2.08, 95% CI 1.32–3.27, $p < 0.01$) and 3 years (OR 2.60, 95% CI 1.69–3.99, $p < 0.01$). In the same study, when compared with those with only an artificial urinary sphincter, they showed that patients with both inflatable penile prosthesis and artificial urinary sphincter did not have a higher likelihood of undergoing artificial urinary sphincter revision surgery at 1 year ($p = 0.76$) or 3 years ($p = 0.73$) [37]. In the studies conducted by Bolat et al. with 11 cases and Martinez-Salamanca et al. with 32 cases, where AUS + IPP was applied and there was no control group; Bolat et al. [38] reported a success rate of 89%, with one case experiencing urinary infection and one case requiring reoperation due to infection. Martinez-Salamanca et al. [39], on the other hand, reported a success rate of over 96% and performed reoperation in a total of 4 cases, with 2 cases of urethral erosion, and 1 case each of reservoir migration and corporal extrusion. Martinez-Salamanca et al. [39] highlighted that three additional patients planned for device removal had a history of prior adjuvant/salvage radiotherapy. In this study, they presented a short surgical duration for PPI + AUS application with a median (range) of 57 [42–84] minutes, contributing to the literature.

In recent years, studies without control groups have drawn attention to the simultaneous application of IPP with mini-Jupette, modified mini-Jupette, and ProACT incontinence surgeries. The information about the surgical methods has been highlighted here only by their names, as further details regarding the procedures will be discussed in subsequent sections. Andrianne R [40]. reported an average surgical duration of 72 min (SD = 19.8) in a series of 15 patients who underwent mini-Jupette Sling + IPP application. Surgically, they observed a 93% improvement in incontinence and an 80% improvement in climacturia by the end of the sixth month.

They noted no postoperative immediate or delayed complications related to IPP or “Mini-Jupette” procedures, except for one case of urinary retention and two cases of postoperative dysuria (20%) [40]. Valenzuela et al. [41], who employed a similar method, reported a 93% improvement in climacturia and an 85% improvement in subjective SUI. They noted one case requiring reoperation for mesh removal due to urethral erosion, while the prosthesis was preserved. Yiou & Binhas [42] reported the surgical duration in patients undergoing PP + ProACT and asynchronous PP + ProACT applications. The average operation time was 133.4 ± 14 minutes in cases of combined implantation, while it was reported as 33.8 ± 4.8 minutes for ProACT device and penile prosthesis asynchronous implantation, and 78.8 ± 8.5 minutes, respectively. They noted satisfaction among patients in both scenarios and observed no reoperations. However, Yafi et al. [43], who applied a similar method, reported complications in 5 out of 38 patients (13.2%) who underwent Mini-Jupette placement, with 4 patients requiring device removal. They noted that the overall complication rates were similar to those reported with male suburethral slings. Regarding success rates, they reported a subjective improvement of 89.3% in incontinence and 92.8% in climacturia.

The results of the most recent study conducted by Van Huele & Van Renterghem [44] in 2023, where they applied simultaneous three-piece IPP implantation with AUS, found a median (IQR) surgical duration of 45 (41.25–58) minutes, a social continence rate of 96%, and a patient satisfaction rate of 88%. No complications related to infection were noted. With a revision rate reported as 16% (4 patients), they mentioned that revision was necessary in two cases (8%) due to sphincter prosthesis leakage, in one case (4%) due to glans erosion, and in another case due to urethral atrophy requiring cuff downsizing [44].

It is important to note that comparing simultaneous operations with two-stage synchronous operations involves various challenges. Firstly, the differences among operating surgeons and the surgical techniques applied are the most significant parameters affecting reoperation, infection, and success outcomes. Additionally, the variations in healthcare reimbursement systems across countries and the differences in prosthetic and sphincter brands also pose challenges in cost assessment. Regarding the treatment of ED, surgical penile prosthesis implantation is performed, and within this practice, there are variations such as penoscrotal and suprapubic applications, as well as options for malleable and inflatable penile prosthesis applications. For SUI, the choice of treatment depends on the severity of symptoms, discomfort level, and history of radiotherapy. Options may include AUS procedures, male sling surgeries (such as AdVance or InVance), or methods like ProACT [42], Mini-Jupette [43], and modified Mini-Jupette [41]. All these factors make it challenging to conduct a homogeneous evaluation.

Pyrgidis et al. [45] provided a comprehensive review of the current literature, stating that simultaneous surgical procedures for ED and SUI reduce costs and rehabilitation duration, and are safe and effective. In our clinical experience, with appropriate patient education, simultaneous surgery offers various potential advantages, including reducing the overall treatment burden for patients, shortening recovery times, and potentially lowering healthcare expenditure. Additionally, simultaneous surgery reduces the need for repeated hospitalizations and exposure to anesthesia, thereby minimizing associated risks and optimizing patient comfort. While we may not have experienced a significant difference in mechanical failure and infection rates, it is evident that the surgical complexity associated with perioperative complications in simultaneous operations would affect both surgeries.

However, skepticism regarding simultaneous surgery persists within the medical community, primarily driven by concerns surrounding perioperative complications, surgical complexity, and the potential for compromised outcomes. Critics caution that simultaneous surgery may increase the risk of intraoperative and postoperative complications, such as infection, bleeding, and device malfunction. Furthermore, the technical intricacies of performing two distinct procedures concurrently may necessitate a higher level of surgical expertise and precision, posing challenges for some urological surgeons.

To facilitate a comprehensive understanding of the advantages and disadvantages of simultaneous surgery versus two-stage sequential operations, a comparative analysis can be conducted, summarizing key considerations in a structured format. A table outlining the benefits and drawbacks of each approach, including factors such as perioperative risks, recovery times, functional outcomes, and patient satisfaction, can serve as a valuable tool for clinicians and patients alike in making informed treatment decisions.

Advantages and disadvantages of simultaneous surgery for erectile dysfunction (ED) and stress urinary incontinence (SUI) represent crucial considerations in the decision-making process for clinicians and patients. A comprehensive understanding of the potential benefits and drawbacks associated with this approach is essential for informed treatment decisions.

Advantages of Simultaneous Surgery

- Comprehensive management: Simultaneous surgery offers the opportunity for comprehensive management of both ED and SUI in a single operative session, addressing multiple urological concerns simultaneously.
- Reduced treatment burden: By combining procedures into a single operative session, patients may experience reduced treatment burden, including fewer hospital visits, decreased recovery time, and potentially lower overall healthcare costs.
- Improved patient convenience: Simultaneous surgery may enhance patient convenience by minimizing the need for multiple surgical interventions and associated recovery periods, allowing for a more streamlined treatment experience.
- Potential synergistic effects: Some studies suggest that simultaneous surgery for ED and SUI may yield synergistic effects, with improvements in one condition potentially enhancing outcomes in the other.

Disadvantages of Simultaneous Surgery

- Increased perioperative risks: Performing two distinct procedures concurrently may increase the overall perioperative risks, including complications such as infection, bleeding, and anesthesia-related adverse events.

- Technical complexity: Simultaneous surgery requires a higher level of technical expertise and precision due to the complexity of performing two distinct procedures concurrently, posing challenges for some urological surgeons.
- Potential for compromised outcomes: Critics of simultaneous surgery raise concerns regarding the potential for compromised outcomes, including suboptimal functional outcomes, device malfunction, and the need for revision surgery.

Patient selection challenges: Identifying suitable candidates for simultaneous surgery requires careful patient selection and consideration of individual factors such as overall health status, comorbidities, and surgical risk profile.

In conclusion, while simultaneous surgery for ED and SUI offers several potential advantages, including comprehensive management and reduced treatment burden, it is not without its challenges and limitations. Careful patient selection, meticulous surgical planning, and ongoing research are essential to optimize outcomes and ensure patient safety in the context of simultaneous surgery for ED and SUI.

Selection of the Appropriate Combined Method of Synchronous Management. Patients' Assessment

The choice of an appropriate combined treatment strategy for patients with concomitant ED and SUI is a critical aspect of urological practice. Central to this decision-making process is the evaluation of the severity of SUI, given that the placement of a penile prosthesis often emerges as the sole viable option for ED treatment in the context of combined pathology.

Assessing the severity of SUI involves a comprehensive evaluation of urinary symptoms and functional impairment. Various clinical tools and diagnostic modalities can be employed to gauge the severity of SUI and inform treatment decisions. Video urodynamics, a dynamic imaging study that combines conventional urodynamic testing with fluoroscopy or ultrasound, offers valuable insights into bladder and urethral function during voiding, providing detailed information about bladder capacity, detrusor pressure, and urinary flow rates. Additionally, pad usage quantification, wherein patients record the frequency and volume of urinary leakage using absorbent pads, serves as a practical and cost-effective method for assessing the severity of SUI and monitoring treatment outcomes over time.

Once the severity of SUI has been established, a range of treatment options may be considered based on individual patient characteristics, treatment goals, and preferences. Non-invasive interventions, such as lifestyle modifications, pelvic floor muscle exercises, and pharmacotherapy, may be recommended as initial management strategies for mild to moderate SUI. For patients with persistent or refractory symptoms, minimally invasive procedures, such as urethral bulking agents or mid-urethral slings, may be considered to provide additional support to the urethra and improve continence.

In cases where conservative and minimally invasive interventions fail to adequately address the severity of SUI, surgical intervention may be warranted. The placement of an artificial urinary sphincter (AUS) represents a gold standard surgical treatment for severe SUI, offering reliable and durable control of urinary leakage. Additionally, the combined placement of an AUS and a penile prosthesis during a single surgical procedure, known as synchronous surgery, offers several potential advantages, including reduced overall treatment burden, streamlined recovery periods, and improved patient satisfaction.

Since individuals tend to experience more complaints related to SUI on a daily basis compared to those related to ED (such as the expectation of a higher frequency of urination per day than the need for daily sexual intercourse), prioritizing SUI has emerged as the forefront. However, it should be evaluated in conjunction with the algorithm presented below.

The algorithm for AUS implantation and PP for both ED and SUI is displayed in Table 22.1:

Table 22.1 AUS implantation algorithm

Patient evaluation
Obtaining a detailed medical history, assessing symptoms and complaints. Measurement of symptoms of erectile dysfunction and urinary incontinence using validated questionnaires such as the international index of erectile function (IIEF) and the international consultation on incontinence questionnaire (ICIQ)
Physical examination
Conducting a general physical examination and pelvic examination. Evaluation of specific findings, such as penile deformities or urethral stricture
Laboratory tests
Measurement of serum hormone levels, especially testosterone levels. Performing other laboratory tests as necessary
Psychosocial assessment
Identification of psychosocial factors such as anxiety, depression, or relationship problems Measurement of psychological effects using validated questionnaires (e.g., Beck depression inventory)
Imaging and other tests
Performing imaging tests such as ultrasonography, radiography, or other imaging modalities as necessary Conducting urodynamic tests, especially for evaluating stress urinary incontinence
Evaluation of treatment options
Considering various treatment options including medication, surgery, or other interventions Conducting a benefit-risk analysis of treatment options
Involvement of the patient in the decision-making process
Providing information about treatment options to the patient and considering their preferences. (if the patient does not prefer simultaneous surgery, prioritization between ED and SUI surgeries should be determined. For this purpose, each condition should be evaluated separately in a joint assessment, and discussed with the patient regarding treatment options.) Offering patient education and support services
Follow-up and monitoring
Regularly assessing the effectiveness of treatment and revising the treatment plan as needed Monitoring treatment outcomes using validated questionnaires such as the IIEF and ICIQ

In summary, the selection of the appropriate combined method of synchronous management for patients with ED and SUI requires a comprehensive assessment of SUI severity and consideration of individual patient factors. By employing a multimodal approach to SUI evaluation and treatment, clinicians can optimize outcomes and improve quality of life for affected individuals.

Combination Therapy

PP + AUS

It was Wilson et al. [46] who realized that the traditional implantation of an AUS which required 2 incision, one perineal for the cuff and one suprapubic for the balloon and pump, was time and effort consuming, therefore, a single penoscrotal incision was proposed, which allows the simultaneous implantation of a penile prothesis along with an artificial sphincter.

Just a few centimeters below the penoscrotal junction, a single incision is made, which provides an excellent exposure to both the corpora and the proximal bulbar urethra. The advantage of performing an upper transverse scrotal incision is that the bulbocavernous muscle is left intact, thus allowing the AUS cuff to be placed at the bulb, if it is retracted ventrally. After a circumferential dissection of the urethra, adequate space is made for the cuff to be placed properly.

Next step is PP implantation. Vertical corporotomies are performed, followed by dilation and accurate measurement to input the cylinders. Once the cylinders are in place, the corporotomies are water-tight closed. The reservoirs for both IPP and AUS are placed prevesically, within the retropubic space, through the transversalis fascia, or alternatively in the epigastric are, superior to the transversalis fascia, while the pumps are placed into the scrotum, underneath the scrotal skin and the dartos, leaving the tunica vaginalis intact [32, 46, 47].

PP + Male Sling

Rhee et al. [30] were the first to describe a technique for the concomitant implantation of inflatable and malleable penile prostheses along with a synthetic (silicone coated polypropylene) male sling. The procedure was performed by the same surgeon. A total of 4 patients suffering from post-prostatectomy ED and urinary incontinence underwent the implantation of an InVance (AMS) male sling using 6 bone screws drilled into the descending pelvic rami bilaterally via a 2 cm perineal raphe incision. One end of the silicone coated propylene synthetic mesh was tied down with the preloaded sutures attached to the bone screws. The penile prosthesis (inflatable or semirigid) was placed via a penoscrotal incision, with extra care taken when the drilling was performed, in order to avoid extreme bleeding in case of corpora violation.

Gorbatiy and his associates, 5 years later, described a new technique where a single incision was required to achieve a simultaneous placement of both a bulbo-urethral male sling and a penile prothesis [34]. A 4 cm midline perineal incision is performed, providing access to the inferior pubic rami for the placement of the AdVance sling. Bone drill is used to insert 3 screws on each side of it. When placing the sling, the bulbospongiosus muscle is dissected for a triangle to be created, with corpus spongiosum being the medial portions and the ischiocavernosus the hypotenuse. The central tendon is dissected off the bulbous urethra. The transobturator fossa is accessed with the helical trocars exiting at the apex of the dissection between urethra and the pubic rami. After that, dissection of the perineal-scrotal fat takes place, until both corpora cavernosa are visible. The Buck's fascia is uncovered and a vertical corporotomy is made bilaterally, followed by dilation of the corpora thus making proper space for cylinders implantation. The placement of the reservoir is facilitated through the same perineal incision, sometimes with an extension of it superiorly, for the surgeon to safely reach the inguinal ring. Tubes are connected and then the pump is left to rest in the dependent dartos pouch of the scrotum, which lies right above the primal incision, providing an easy access to it.

PP + "Adrianne Mini-Jupette"

It was Robert Adrianne in 2005 who described a new surgical technique which allowed the placement of a graft across the male urethra while implanting a penile prothesis, having two birds killed with one stone, meaning dealing with both ED along with climacturia and/or mild SUI, after a radical prostatectomy. The graft was sutured to medial aspect of each corporotomy, lying there just like a miniskirt, hence the name "Mini-Jupette" in French.

The success of this technique is based on the hypothesis that as the cylinders of the penile prothesis are expanding, the graft itself would apply tension on the urethra, thus reducing climacturia, perhaps and a mild SUI, via a passive and an active compression of the urethra. He never formally published his results, but he inspired many to pursuit this approach.

The perfect candidate for this procedure is a patient suffering from ED and climacturia with/or mild SUI (the patient is using no more than 2 pads per day), after a radical prostatectomy. After placing the patient in a supine position with a slight Trendelenburg position a 4 cm transverse incision is made 2–3 cm below the penoscrotal junction, or a sub-coronal one, providing an excellent exposure of proximal crural corpora cavernosa and bulbar urethra. Two bilateral symmetrical corporotomies are made as any standard IPP implantation and the distance between the medial aspects of them is carefully measured. Afterward, a mini-jupette graft is fashioned based on these measurements. Its dimensions are the size of the corporotomy which represents the length, and the medial inter-corporal distance which represents the width of the graft. After the size of the graft is determined it is sewn in place to the medial corporotomies, in such a way to avoid urethral injury. After the sling installment, the IPP is implanted, and the device is activated to achieve sling's optimal compression on the urethra [43]. There is an ongoing debate regarding the material of which the graft is made of. It is up to the surgeon, but many believe that a synthetic one is better than cadaver fascia.

Recently a new, modified approach was proposed by Valenzuela et al. [41]. It is a modified approach of standard mini-jupette where a male urethral minimal sling (MUMS), in particular a Virtue (Coloplast Corporation, Humlebaeke, Denmark) monofilament polypropylene mesh sling is placed more proximally along the bulbar urethra (proximal to the corporotomy) and sutured to the lateral corpora. This approach requires a smaller corporotomy and minimizes the risk of suture injury of the prothesis during closure.

PP + ProACT

The ProAct (Uromedica, Plymouth, MN, USA) device was designed to fill the gap between the artificial sphincter, which attempts to replace the physiological function of the external sphincter, and male slings, which restore continence by compressing the urethra more proximally, most of the times at the level of bulbar urethra. The rationale behind this device is that the underlying detrusor function is most likely to change as the patient grows older, therefore the need for adjusting the outlet resistance in order to achieve continence.

The device was introduced by Hubner and Schlarp in 2005 [48] and is made from silicon elastomer, a material very similar to the one used for AUS. It consists of an expandable silicon balloon attached to a re-injectable titanium port and the kit includes two of them, each one to be placed to either side of the bladder neck, at the vesicourethral anastomosis, above the pelvic diaphragm.

Under general anesthesia, patient is placed in lithotomy position. A rigid cystoscope is used to inject contrast medium to identify the bladder neck. A horizontal perineum incision of 1.5 cm is made to expose the urethra and the descending pubic ramus under fluoroscopic control. A sharp tipped, reusable trocar combined with a "U-shaped" canula is used to insert the balloons bilaterally, with the fixed cystoscope acting as a guide for proper implantation of them. Each balloon has two lumens, the first one contains a push wire while the second one serves as a conduit for inflation with a maximum capacity of 8 ml.

At the beginning, the implantation was performed under endoscopical and fluoroscopical guidance [48–50], but Gregori et al. [51] proposed the use of transrectal ultrasound guidance for the implantation, to avoid unnecessary radiation exposure for both the patient and the surgical team.

Having the device placed, the physician can easily adjust the volume of the balloons, thus achieving the optimal urethral resistance, without the need of another surgical operation.

Yiou and Binhas in 2015 [42] were the first to propose the implantation of an IPP and ProAct for ED and SUI. Ten patients with severe ED and moderate SUI, after radical prostatectomy were enrolled in this study, where 6 of them underwent a synchronous implantation of IPP and the ProAct device (with the prothesis implanted first) while the other four had an asynchronous placement of the devices. At all patients, a transverse scrotal incision was performed to gain access for the IPP placement and the ProAct device was inserted under endoscopic and fluoroscopic control as described above.

PP + Bulking Agents

There aren't any data in the literature regarding PP implantation after bulking agents for SUI, or bulking agents after PP, let alone supporting simultaneous placement of penile protheses and bulking agents. It would be interesting to design a study focused on sequential implantation of PP and bulking agents, but it would be prudent to first inject the agent, in order to avoid any instrumentation damage, once the PP is in place.

Complications, Prevention, and Treatment

Performing a sole implantation of a PP, an AUS or any other device includes the risk of complications, let alone performing two at the same time. It is more than reasonable that one can assume that the rate of complications should be at least the sum of those expected when performing each one. Unfortunately, in this case, the level of difficulty increases, even in the most skillful hands. Therefore, surgeons need to understand and recognize the risks to eliminate or at least minimize complications. There are few studies comparing head-to-head the rate of complications when performing a two-stage or one-stage surgery for both ED and SUI after radical prostatectomy [35, 36], not to mention studies comparing head-to-head different combinations of implants, which surprisingly both are in favor of synchronous and in fact Rolle et al. [15] reported that patients who underwent a two-staged operation would have chosen the one-stage if they have been asked in the first place, while Segal et al. [36] reported that those who experienced a complication with one device didn't have one with the other one.

Complications can be categorized in intraoperatively or postoperatively, they can be infectious or non-infectious, and they can be device or tissue related.

Infection

The greatest fear of a surgeon performing implantation of any kind is the colonization of a graft or a prothesis, during or after the operation. Infection rates vary depending on the combination of implants. Wilson et al. reported an overall infection rate of 9% at synchronous implantation of IPP and AUS (Wilson) while Parulkar and Barrett had an overall infection rate of 11% [29]. On the other hand, Martinez-Salamanca et al. reported zero prosthetic infections in a series of 32 participants who underwent synchronous dual implantation [39]. When it comes to IPP plus male sling the incidence of infection is practically zero [30, 34], but the number of participants were small. As for IPP plus mini-Jupette, Yafi et al. reported only one incident of infection out of 38 participants in their study [43].

The procedure begins when the patient is placed on the operating table and not when the first cut is being made. Infection generally occurs at the time of surgery or due to early postoperative bacteremia and can be surgical site infections (SSI) or infections of the device itself. SSIs develop right after surgery with only skin involvement and can be treated relatively easy as any other SSI by administrating antibiotics. On the other hand, device infections can be acute or chronic. Acute infections usually occur within 6 weeks of implantation and involve Gram-negative rod bacteria while chronic infections occur after 6 weeks and most of the times are subclinical, due to common skin flora, such as S. aureus. The underlying mechanism is biofilm formation due to bacterial contamination at the time of implantation [52]. Shaving must be performed in the operating theater with clippers. Surgeons must meticulously wash their hands for at least 5 to 10 min. Proper sterilization of the area with chlorhexidine-alcohol solution [53, 54], as it has shown to be superior to a standard povidone-iodine solution and prophylactic chemoprophylaxis with antibiotics covering Gram-positive and Gram-negative bacteria complete the list of minimum measures that should be taken to avoid infections. AUA guidelines insist on avoiding such an operation in presence of systematic, cutaneous, or urinary tract infection [55]. Unfortunately, there is no consensus regarding which kind of antibiotic regimens one should use as prophylaxis. AUA guidelines till 2012 edition recommended the use of aminoglycoside plus vancomycin or a first- or second-generation cephalosporin one hour before surgery [56], but Gross et al. demonstrated that microorganisms isolated from infected protheses were not covered by the antibiotics recommended in both EUA and AUA guidelines at the time [57], therefore none of them proposes a specific combination. In order to further minimize the risk of infections, advances in device engineering have been made. AMS developed an antibiotic-impregnated prosthesis with rifampin and minocycline, the AMS Inhibizone in 2001 [58] to be later followed in 2002 by Coloplast (former Mentor Corporation) with the addition of a hydrophilic-coating to their successful Alpha-1 model, which can uptake antibiotics when immersed in solution [59]. The coating is up to surgeon's discretion. There is no consensus upon the best choice for antimicrobial solution, but a large cohort, multicenter, retrospective analysis by Towe et al. in men with diabetes who underwent a Coloplast Titan implant, highlighted that combination of vancomycin with gentamicin was the most efficacious for preventing postoperative infections [60]. All these break-throughs reduced the overall rate of infection to 1–2% [61–66].

In order to further minimize the risk of infection during the operation, the "no-touch" technique was introduced in 2011 by Eid et al. [67]. The concept is really simple, after initial dissection down to Buck's fascia, all the instruments and gloves must be replaced, along with all the covers of the surgical field, since they are considered contaminated. A new drape is placed, and a small window is created above the original incision. This manipulation ensures minimal contact with patient's skin, surgeon's hands, instruments involved and above all the prosthesis itself. Authors have reported a remarkably decreased infection rate to 0.46%.

The duration of postoperative prophylaxis is also debatable. Dropkin et al. demonstrated that patients who undergo IPP insertion most likely will not benefit from routine administration of any antibiotic regimen after they have been discharged [68] but many experts believe that a 5 to 14 days administration of a combination of oral agents including quinolones, penicillin and cephalosporins, with use of trimethoprime or doxycycline in areas with high prevalence of MRSA is in order [65].

The majority of postoperative infections occur within 3 months period of time. In the unfortunate event of prosthetic infection, removal of the prosthesis is mandatory, with antibiotic administration. Mulcahy was the first to describe a "salvage" technique [69] which includes replacement of the infected device and wash-out protocol with an infection-free rate of 82%. Since then, significant improvements have been made [70–72] but this isn't the rule. Any attempt should be avoided in case of sepsis, unregulated diabetes urethral erosion or tissue necrosis. The patient should be fully informed about the pros and cons of such an approach.

Finally, one can argue that performing a two-staged operation can lead to increased rates of infection, due to longer operative time, but in experienced centers, the total operative time needed for synchronous procedures is slightly longer, therefore, it is in safe range.

Urethral Injury

A rare but serious and significant complication of placing a PP is urethral injury. The true incidence is unknown, but many studies estimate it from 0.1% to 3% [73–76]. Urethral injuries occur either during the operation as a direct injury, while the surgeon is performing dilation of the corpora (mostly in cases of excessive fibrosis such as concomitant Peyronie's disease and previous use of intracavernous injections) [75], or after the surgery, due to erosion by the implanted cylinders. Depending on the site of injury, its extent, and surgeon's experience, it could lead to operation termination and late implantation; therefore, one should be able of preventing and dealing with such a complication.

Regarding the sequence of a dual PP and AUS implantation, most surgeons prefer to perform the AUS procedure first. Such a thing requires the circumferential mobilization of the bulbar urethra, along with corpora dissection, which is a prerequisite for the AUS cuff implantation, so if a urethral injury occur, there will be no reason for discarding any of the prosthesis in case of procedure cancelation [77].

A total of 71% of urethral injuries involve distal urethra and occur during distal corpus cavernosum dilation [78]. In the same study, the majority of urologists performing implantations would abort the procedure (55%) and revisit after a minimum of 6-month delay, while only a few (10.7%) would continue, repairing the urethral defect, before placing the cylinders, thus increasing the chance of infections. If someone chooses to repair the injury, then the defect should be closed in 2 layers.

Mid-urethral injuries are very rare. Most of the times they occur during the initial corporotomy or at distal corpora dilation. If the defect is easily accessible, then the closure will be performed in 2 layers, if not, then a penis degloving is mandatory for proper exposure and repairment.

Proximal urethral injuries comprise only 12.5% of urethral injuries and they occur during the initial dissection and exposure of the corpora. Because of their location they can be easily recognized during the operation, therefore late presentations of such injuries are very rare [76, 78]. Since they can easily be detected, a primary two-layer repair is the treatment of choice. When the defect is small, urethral catheterization only and healing on second degree is also an alternative. Proximal urethral injuries occur before the dilation of corpora; therefore, the next logical step for a surgeon is to abort the procedure [79–81], but Anele et al. demonstrated that synchronous urethroplasty during the time of implantation is feasible [75]. Interestingly, in Sexton's survey 20.6% of surgeons answered that they would proceed to such an approach, with this percentage rising with surgeon's self-confidence and experience (surgeons performing more than 50 procedures per year) [78].

Although urethral injury during penile prosthesis is relatively rare, 73% of respondents in Sexton's survey reported at least one career injury [78]. Managing urethral injuries depends on location and surgeon's experience. Although most of the times abortion seems to be a one-way street, in selected cases and experienced hands, synchronous urethral repair, and prosthesis placement could be a safe alternative.

Erosion

Erosion of IPP cylinders can occur into the urethra, the glans, or the distal corpora, and the overall rate is 1–6% [82]. Risk factors include diabetes mellitus, spinal cord injury, and patients with vascular disease [83, 84]. Urethral erosion after AUS implantation can occur in about 8.5% of the cases [85] and is mostly associated with previous radiotherapy and penoscrotal approach [86]. Parulkar and Barrett [29] were the first to report a combined rate of 11% for infection/erosion after dual implantation of IPP and AUS with no comparative data though, between synchronous and asynchronous dual implantation. Erosion is also one of the most common complications in adjustable male slings with an estimated rate of around 10% [87]. As for mini-slings, Valenzuela et al. reported only one incidence out of 27 participants in their dual implantation of IPP and a MUMS [41].

Urethral Atrophy

Urethral atrophy can occur in 7.9% of AUS implantation [85] and it is mostly associated with previous radiation therapy, older age and delay in placing an AUS after prostate cancer treatment [88].

Dual implantation of AUS and IPP has been criticized in the past for harnessing an increased risk of urethral atrophy, since the original approach did not offer as proximal as needed urethral cuff placement, but this hazard has been minimized since Wilson introduced his modified approach in 2010 which allows a more proximal cuff placement [89].

Glans Hypermobility

Floppy glans is a common complication with a reported incidence up to 5% [82] after penile prosthesis implantation, and it can be associated with some anatomic variation, where the corpora do not extend the full distance into the glans and there is a lack of underlying support from the corpora-glans ligament [90], or it can be the result of inserting an undersized cylinder.

Often it is "self-corrected," as part of normal healing and capsule formation, otherwise surgical intervention is needed, which includes a hemi-circumcisional incision at the opposite side of the defect and anchoring of the of the glans to the adjacent tunica albuginea [91].

Decreased Glans Sensation

Glans numbness is a very rare condition, and it can theoretically occur after an infrapubic approach or after a surgical intervention for restoring glans hypermobility [92].

Glans Ischemia and Necrosis

Glandular ischemia is a rare postoperative complication, after IPP surgery, with only a few cases reported in the literature [93–95] with the largest series being those of Wilson et al., including 21 patients [96]. The underlying mechanism seems to be disruption of glanural blood supply which is facilitated by the dorsal penile arteries and corpus spongiosum muscle. The risk can be minimized by avoiding sub-coronal incisions or penile degloving in high-risk patients such as diabetics, smokers, and patients who had undergone radiotherapy. Salvage techniques can be applied [88] but usually immediate removal of the device should be performed to avoid glans necrosis [87].

Hematoma

Scrotal hematoma is a dreadful complication and its incidence ranges from 0.2 to 22.2% [97]. Prevention measures include running corporotomy closures, meticulous bleeding restriction and rarely use of suction draining, which if necessary, can be placed at the lowest point of the scrotal dissection [98, 99]. "Mummy wrap" technique was described by Gerard Henry in 2009 [100] which decreases hematoma formation.

Mechanical Failure

All implants are prone to failure over time. The current IPP and AUS devices have gone through multiple revisions to minimize device malfunction and mechanical failure [101]. Cylinder, tubing or reservoir leaks, cylinder aneurysms, and connector disruption are the most common incidents for penile protheses [102], while pressure-regulation balloon is the main cause of AUS failure, followed by cuff or pump malfunction [103]. The true incidence is difficult to be estimated since data are conflicting. Parulkar and Barrett [29] reported an overall rate of 48% mechanical failure for AUS, with a proportional high rate when older versions of AUS were implanted. Kendirci et al. [32] reported 2 incidents of reservoir migrations out of 22 patients (9%). Recent data estimate the risk for AUS alone at 2.2–2.5% [25]. The rate for IPP alone is less than 5% after 5 years of follow-up [61, 106, 107] and for the Remeex system is 21% [108].

Little can be done to avoid a mechanical failure besides the obvious: meticulous implantation, proper measurement of cylinders [52], and AUS cuff [109].

Other complications, less specific, are postoperative pain and edema which can easily be addressed with anti-inflammatory agents and cold dressings. Bladder perforation is a rare but severe complication. It can be easily confirmed by cystoscopy. If it is minor, then placing a simple urethral catheter for a few days can solve the day, but when it is major, then an open bladder repair should be performed to restore the damage. The easiest way to avoid such a complication is of course having the bladder emptied prior the operation.

A comparative list of complications type and rates, regarding synchronous dual implantation for ED and SUI can be found in Table 22.2, while tips and tricks can be found summarized in Table 22.3.

Patients considered for a synchronous implantation should be carefully evaluated as mentioned before, and wisely selected. One must offer tailor-made solutions for every patient, meaning that the surgeon must consider the severity of each condition alone. PP implantation is a one-way street, in cases of severe ED, which do not respond to any conservative treatments, but the choice of AUS over a male sling depends on the severity of SUI. In cases of severe SUI, implantation of AUS seems the only solution, but for mild to moderate degree of SUI a male sling is a considerable option, even though there are data supporting that AUS can be significantly better than fixed sling for moderate post-prostatectomy SUI [109] but we have to take into account also the combined cost. The ideal candidate for male sling is someone with an estimated 24-h pad weight of less than 500 g at least 6 months following radical prostatectomy (although pad test isn't always accurate regarding SUI severity) with some residual urinary sphincteric function and adequate detrusor contraction for overcoming the artificial resistance of the sling [20, 77, 108, 110].

Patient's or partner's dexterity is a prerequisite, in order to have a happy ending for both of them. Comorbidities such as diabetes mellitus or immunosuppression may increase the risk of complications. Evidence about diabetes is conflicting. There is a large review by Christodoulidoy and Pearce in 2016, which did not demonstrate any statistically significant increased infection rate [111], while Gon et al. highlighted that there is an increased risk of PP prosthesis infection with an odds ratio of 1.53 [112]. Most surgeons believe that diabetes is an independent risk factor for infection after PP implantation, but unfortunately, there isn't a safe threshold of preoperative HbA1c levels that would predict a positive outcome of the surgery [113] although a study by Habous et al. determined that the statistically ideal is 8.5% even though the optimal one is 7.5% [114].

Table 22.2 Complication types and rates

Author	Reference number	Year	Type of Implants	Number of patients	mean age	Complications	Number of explanations	Mean follow-up (months)
Parulkar and Barrett	[29]	1989	PP (various) + AUS (AMS 792/800)	40	55.1		3 explantations due to infection (IPP or AUS)	35.7
Wilson et al	[46]	2003	PP (N/A) + AMS 800 AUS	14	N/A		1 IPP explantation due to infection, AUS was salvaged	12
Sellers	[31]	2005	IPP + AUS	15	N/A	0	0	N/A
Rhee	[30]	2005	Semirigid AMS 650 + InVAnce ($N = 1$)	4	70.5	0	0	14.75
			Inflatable 700CX + InVAnce ($N = 3$)					17
Kendirci et al	[32]	2005	AMS 700 CX+ AMS 800 AUS	22	64	Urethral erosion $n = 2$ (9%)		
						Reservoir migration $n = 2$ (9%)		
						Revision 14%		
Gorbatiy et al	[34]	2010	IPP AMS 700 CX + InVance/advance	8	N/A	0		
Segal et al	[36]	2013	IPP + AUS	55	65.3	IPP erosion $N = 2$ (3.6%)		
						Infection $N = 0$		
						Mechanical failure $N = 3$ (5.5%)		
						AUS erosion $N = 3$ (5.5%)		
						Infection $N = 2$ ((3.6%)		
						Mechanical failure $N = 9$ (16.4%)		

Yiou and Binhas	[42]	2015	Coloplast titan + ProAct	6	66.8	0	0	22.7
Salamanka et al	[39]	2015	N/A	32	66		1 IPP explantation	12
							2 Aus explantation	
Yafi et al	[43]	2018	IPP + mini-Jupette	38	65.3	Significant postoperative pain $n = 1$	$n = 4$	5.1
			Coloplast titan 31			Hematoma formation $n = 1$		
			AMS 700 LGX 4			Urethro-corporal fistula $n = 1$		
			AMS 700 CX 3			Death due to pulmonary embolism $n = 1$		
Valenzuela et al	[41]	2019	IPP (various) + MUMS	36	67.7	Transient urinary retention $n = 2$, (6%)	1 explantation	5.9
						Prolonged urinary retention $n = 1$, (3%)		
						Mesh erosion $n = 1$, (3%)		
						Persistent scrotal pain (5 months) $n = 1$, (3%)		
Andrianne	[40]	2019	PP (various) + mini Jupette	15	65.9	1 urinary retention		107

Table 22.3 Tips and tricks

Preoperative measures	1. Advise the patient to quit smoking 2. Advise the patient to be euglycemic 3. Be aware of any skin infections 4. Must have a negative urine culture
Peri/intraoperative measures	1. Meticulous hand-washing, some surgeons advocate in favor of at least 10 min 2. Proper antimicrobial prophylaxis 3. Highly trained and experienced personnel 4. Safety checklist implementation 5. Appropriate instruments 6. Proper sterilization of the area with chlorhexidine-alcohol solution 7. Change gloves frequently in critical steps 8. Place a urethral catheter in order to avoid bladder injury 9. No-touch technique minimizes infection rates 10. Standardized technique minimizes complications 11. Usage of antibiotic coated implants 12. Wilsons'modified approach allows a more proximal cuff placement 13. In cases of PP + AUS implant the AUS first, so if a urethral injury occur, there will be no reason for discarding any of the prosthesis in case of procedure cancellation
Postoperative measures	1. "Mummy wrap" technique 2. Drain placement to reduce the formation of hematoma

Conclusions

Simultaneous prosthetic implantation surgery for both ED and SUI after radical prostatectomy promises to kill two birds with one stone. In terms of efficacy and safety, the results are comparable to two-stage procedures. In terms of cost, it saves money and time (lesser days and cost of hospitalization, lesser anesthesia time, lesser cost of operations, lesser days of absence form work). Patients considered for a dual implantation should be thoroughly evaluated prior the procedure. They should be informed about the pros and cons of such an operation. Last but not least, the patient's and his partner's needs and expectations should be totally taken into account; after all, a well-informed patient is a happy and satisfied patient.

Despite the promising data, we still need more prospective studies, with more participants to evaluate and standardize the techniques. It is crucial also that such procedures be performed by experienced surgeons in specialized centers with large numbers of operations to provide the patients with the best of care.

References

1. Ficarra V, Novara G, Ahlering TE, Costello A, Eastham JA, Graefen M, et al. Systematic review and meta-analysis of studies reporting potency rates after robot-assisted radical prostatectomy. Eur Urol. 2012;62:418–30.
2. Ficarra V, Novara G, Rosen RC, Artibani W, Carroll PR, Costello A, et al. Systematic review and meta-analysis of studies reporting urinary continence recovery after robot-assisted radical prostatectomy. Eur Urol. 2012;62:405–17.
3. Dubbelman YD, Dohle GR, Schröder FH. Sexual function before and after radical retropubic prostatectomy: a systematic review of prognostic indicators for a successful outcome. Eur Urol. 2006;50(4):711–20. https://doi.org/10.1016/j.eururo.2006.06.009.
4. Lee D, Romero C, Alba F, Westney OL, Wang R. Simultaneous penile prosthesis and male sling/artificial urinary sphincter. Asian J Androl. 2013;15(1):10–5. https://doi.org/10.1038/aja.2012.115. Epub 2012 Dec 3. PMID: 23202702; PMCID: PMC3739112.
5. Stanford JL, Feng Z, Hamilton AS, Gilliland FD, Stephenson RA, et al. Urinary and sexual function after radical prostatectomy for clinically localized prostate cancer: the prostate cancer outcomes study. JAMA. 2000;283:354–60.
6. Lee J, Hersey K, Lee CT, Fleshner N. Climacturia following radical prostatectomy: prevalence and risk factors. J Urol 2006;176(6 Pt 1):2562–5; discussion 2565. https://doi.org/10.1016/j.juro.2006.07.158. PMID: 17085160.
7. Penson DF, McLerran D, Feng Z, Li L, Albertsen PC, Gilliland FD, Hamilton A, Hoffman RM, Stephenson RA, Potosky AL, Stanford JL. 5-year urinary and sexual outcomes after radical prostatectomy: results from the prostate cancer outcomes study. J Urol. 2005;173(5):1701–5. https://doi.org/10.1097/01.ju.0000154637.38262.3a. PMID: 15821561
8. Inaba K, Sharkey PW, Stephen DJ, Redelmeier DA, Brenneman FD. The increasing incidence of severe pelvic injury in motor vehicle collisions. Injury. 2004;35(8):759–65. https://doi.org/10.1016/S0020-1383(03)00308-5. PMID: 15246798
9. Demetriades D, Karaiskakis M, Toutouzas K, Alo K, Velmahos G, Chan L. Pelvic fractures: epidemiology and predictors of associated abdominal injuries and outcomes. J Am Coll Surg. 2002;195(1):1–10. https://doi.org/10.1016/s1072-7515(02)01197-3. PMID: 12113532
10. Johnsen NV, Kaufman MR, Dmochowski RR, Milam DF. Erectile dysfunction following pelvic fracture urethral injury. Sex Med Rev. 2018;6(1):114–123. https://doi.org/10.1016/j.sxmr.2017.06.004. Epub 2017 Jul 27. PMID: 28757357.
11. Blaschko SD, Sanford MT, Schlomer BJ, Alwaal A, Yang G, Villalta JD, Wessells H, McAninch JW, Breyer BN. The incidence of erectile dysfunction after pelvic fracture urethral injury: A systematic review and meta-analysis. Arab J Urol. 2015;13(1):68–74. https://doi.org/10.1016/j.aju.2014.09.004. Epub 2014 Oct 16. PMID: 26019983; PMCID: PMC4435659.
12. Mundy AR, Andrich DE. Pelvic fracture-related injuries of the bladder neck and prostate: their nature, cause and management. BJU Int 2010;105(9):1302–1308. https://doi.org/10.1111/j.1464-410X.2009.08970.x. Epub 2009 Oct 28. PMID: 19874306.
13. Johnsen NV, Dmochowski RR, Young JB, Guillamondegui OD. Epidemiology of blunt lower urinary tract trauma with and without pelvic fracture. Urology 2017;102:234–239. https://doi.org/10.1016/j.urology.2016.11.015. Epub 2016 Dec 30. PMID: 28043650.
14. Scott FB, Bradley WE, Timm GW. Management of erectile impotence. Use of implantable inflatable prosthesis Urology. 1973;2(1):80–2. https://doi.org/10.1016/0090-4295(73)90224-0. PMID: 4766860
15. Small MP. Small-Carrion penile prosthesis: a report on 160 cases and review of the literature. J Urol. 1978;119(3):365–8. https://doi.org/10.1016/s0022-5347(17)57492-3. PMID: 642091
16. Silva LA, Andriolo RB, Atallah AN, da Silva EM. Surgery for stress urinary incontinence due to presumed sphincter deficiency after prostate surgery. Cochrane Database Syst Rev. 2011;(4):CD008306. https://doi.org/10.1002/14651858.CD008306.pub2. Update in: Cochrane Database Syst Rev. 2014;9:CD008306. PMID: 21491408.

17. Choinière R, Violette PD, Morin M, Tu LM, Guyatt GH, Reed C, Philie CA, Legault B, Beaudry MM, Ahmed MM, Richard PO. Evaluation of benefits and harms of surgical treatments for post-radical prostatectomy urinary incontinence: a systematic review and meta-analysis. Eur Urol Focus 2022;8(4):1042–1052. https://doi.org/10.1016/j.euf.2021.09.007. Epub 2021 Sep 22. PMID: 34563480.
18. EAU Guidelines. Edn. presented at the EAU Annual Congress Milan March 2023. ISBN 978-94-92671-19-6.
19. Zeif H-J, Almallah Z. The male sling for post-radical prostatectomy urinary incontinence: urethral compression versus urethral relocation or what is next? Brit J Med Surgic Urol. 2010;3(4):134–43. https://doi.org/10.1016/j.bjmsu.2010.01.006.
20. Bole R, Hebert KJ, Gottlich HC, Bearrick E, Kohler TS, Viers BR. Narrative review of male urethral sling for post-prostatectomy stress incontinence: sling type, patient selection, and clinical applications. Transl Androl Urol 2021;10(6):2682–2694. https://doi.org/10.21037/tau-20-1459. PMID: 34295753; PMCID: PMC8261433.
21. Shamout S, Huang YQ, Kabbara H, Corcos J, Campeau L. Short-term evaluation of the adjustable bulbourethral male sling for post-prostatectomy urinary incontinence. Low Urin Tract Symptoms 2019;11(2):O111–O116. https://doi.org/10.1111/luts.12227. Epub 2018 Jun 4. PMID: 29869450.
22. Esquinas C, Angulo JC. Effectiveness of Adjustable Transobturator Male System (ATOMS) to treat male stress incontinence: a systematic review and meta-analysis. Adv Ther. 2019;36(2):426–441. https://doi.org/10.1007/s12325-018-0852-4. Epub 2018 Dec 17. PMID: 30560525; PMCID: PMC6824356.
23. Navalón-Monllor V, Ordoño-Domínguez F, Pallás-Costa Y, Vilar-Castro LA, Monllor-Peidro ME, Juan-Escudero J, Navalón-Verdejo P. Long-term follow-up for the treatment of male urinary incontinence with the Remeex system. Actas Urol Esp. 2016 40(9):585–591. English, Spanish. https://doi.org/10.1016/j.acuro.2016.03.009. Epub 2016 May 26. PMID: 27237411.
24. Kretschmer A, Nitti V. Surgical treatment of male postprostatectomy incontinence: current concepts. Eur Urol Focus 2017 3(4–5):364–376. https://doi.org/10.1016/j.euf.2017.11.007. Epub 2017 Nov 23. PMID: 29174616.
25. Ostrowski I, Golabek T, Ciechan J, Śledź E, Przydacz M, Dyś W, Blewniewski M, von Heyden B, Pottek T, Neugart F, Carrieri G, Selvaggio O, Iori F, Arjona MF, Foley S, Yang B, Llorens C, Różanski W, Chłosta PL. Preliminary outcomes of the European multicentre experience with the ZSI 375 artificial urinary sphincter for treatment of stress urinary incontinence in men. Cent European J Urol. 2019;72(3):263–269. https://doi.org/10.5173/ceju.2019.1920. Epub 2019 Jul 12. PMID: 31720028; PMCID: PMC6830485.
26. Lima SVC, de Barros EGC, Vilar FO, Pinto FCM, Barros TDP, Truzzi JC, de Toledo LGM, Kanasiro F, Amaro JL. Artificial sphincter "BR–SL–AS 904" in the treatment of urinary incontinence after radical prostatectomy: efficacy, practicality and safety in a prospective and multicenter study. Int Braz J Urol 2018;44(6):1215–1223. https://doi.org/10.1590/S1677-5538.IBJU.2018.0128. PMID: 30325613; PMCID: PMC6442165.
27. Cornu JN, Sèbe P, Ciofu C, Peyrat L, Cussenot O, Haab F. Mid-term evaluation of the transobturator male sling for post-prostatectomy incontinence: focus on prognostic factors. BJU Int 2011;108(2):236–240. https://doi.org/10.1111/j.1464-410X.2010.09765.x. Epub 2010 Oct 18. PMID: 20955265.
28. Scott FB, Fishman IJ, Shotland Y. Experience with simultaneous implantation of inflatable penile prosthesis and artificial urinary sphincter in 72 patients. J Urol. 1987;137:374A.
29. Parulkar BG, Barrett DM. Combined implantation of artificial sphincter and penile prosthesis. J Urol. 1989;142(3):732–5. https://doi.org/10.1016/s0022-5347(17)38870-5. PMID: 2769850
30. Rhee EY. Technique for concomitant implantation of the penile prosthesis with the male sling. J Urol. 2005;173(3):925–7. https://doi.org/10.1097/01.ju.0000154023.93188.9c. PMID: 15711332

31. Sellers CL, Morey AF, Jones LA. Cost and time benefits of dual implantation of inflatable penile and artificial urinary sphincter prosthetics by single incision. Urology. 2005;65(5):852–3. https://doi.org/10.1016/j.urology.2004.11.017. PMID: 15882709
32. Kendirci M, Gupta S, Shaw K, Morey A, Jones L, Hakim L, Hellstrom WJ. Synchronous prosthetic implantation through a transscrotal incision: an outcome analysis. J Urol. 2006;175(6):2218–22. https://doi.org/10.1016/S0022-5347(06)00345-4. PMID: 16697843
33. Mancini JG, Kizer WS, Jones LA, Mora RV, Morey AF. Patient satisfaction after dual implantation of inflatable penile and artificial urinary sphincter prostheses. Urology 2008;71(5):893–896. https://doi.org/10.1016/j.urology.2007.10.018. Epub 2008 Mar 28. PMID: 18374398.
34. Gorbatiy V, Westney OL, Romero C, Wang R. Outcomes of simultaneous placement of an inflatable penile prosthesis and a male urethral sling through a single perineal incision. J Sex Med 2010;7(2 Pt 1):832–838. https://doi.org/10.1111/j.1743-6109.2009.01506.x. Epub 2009 Sep 29. PMID: 19796057.
35. Rolle L, Ceruti C, Sedigh O, Timpano M, Destefanis P, Lillaz B, Galletto E, De Maria C, Falcone M, Dalmasso E, Fontana D. Surgical implantation of artificial urinary device and penile prosthesis through trans-scrotal incision for postprostatectomy urinary incontinence and erectile dysfunction: synchronous or delayed procedure? Urology 2012 Nov;80(5):1046–1050. https://doi.org/10.1016/j.urology.2012.08.003. Epub 2012 Sep 19. PMID: 22999451.
36. Segal RL, Cabrini MR, Harris ED, Mostwin JL, Bivalacqua TJ, Burnett AL. Combined inflatable penile prosthesis-artificial urinary sphincter implantation: no increased risk of adverse events compared to single or staged device implantation. J Urol 2013 Dec;190(6):2183–2188. https://doi.org/10.1016/j.juro.2013.06.084. Epub 2013 Jul 2. PMID: 23831315.
37. Patel N, Golan R, Halpern JA, Sun T, Asafu-Adjei AD, Chughtai B, Stahl P, Sedrakyan A, Kashanian JA. A contemporary analysis of dual inflatable penile prosthesis and artificial urinary sphincter outcomes. J Urol. 2019;201(1):141–6. https://doi.org/10.1016/j.juro.2018.07.046. PMID: 30059687
38. Bolat D, Kozacioglu Z, Polat S, Koras O, Arslan M, Minareci S. Synchronous penoscrotal implantation of penile prosthesis and artificial urinary sphincter after radical prostatectomy. Arch Esp Urol 2017;70(3):367–372. English. PMID: 28422042.
39. Martínez-Salamanca JI, Espinós EL, Moncada I, Portillo LD, Carballido J. Management of end-stage erectile dysfunction and stress urinary incontinence after radical prostatectomy by simultaneous dual implantation using a single trans-scrotal incision: surgical technique and outcomes. Asian J Androl 2015 Sep-Oct;17(5):792–6. https://doi.org/10.4103/1008-682X.143757. PMID: 25657083; PMCID: PMC4577592.
40. Andrianne R. The "mini-Jupette" sling at the time of inflatable penile prosthesis implantation: adequate treatment for erectile dysfunction with mild incontinence and/or climacturia after radical prostatectomy. Prog Urol 2019;29(8–9):456–463. https://doi.org/10.1016/j.purol.2019.05.003. Epub 2019 Jul 9. PMID: 31300267.
41. Valenzuela RJ, Ziegelmann MJ, Hillelsohn JH, Farrell MR, Kent MA, Levine LA. Preliminary outcomes of the male urethral "mini-sling": a modified approach to the Andrianne Mini-Jupette procedure with penile prosthesis placement for Climacturia and mild stress urinary incontinence. J Sex Med 2019 Aug;16(8):1310–1317. https://doi.org/10.1016/j.jsxm.2019.04.009. Epub 2019 May 17. PMID: 31109775.
42. Yiou R, Binhas M. Combined implantation of a penile prosthesis and adjustable continence therapy ProACT in patients with erectile dysfunction and urinary incontinence after radical prostatectomy: results of a prospective pilot study. J Sex Med 2015(12):2481–2484. https://doi.org/10.1111/jsm.13059. Epub 2015 Nov 27. PMID: 26611356.
43. Yafi FA, Andrianne R, Alzweri L, Brady J, Butcher M, Chevalier D, DeLay KJ, Faix A, Hatzichristodoulou G, Hellstrom WJG, Jenkins L, Kohler TS, Osmonov D, Park SH, Schwabb MD, Valenzuela R, van Renterghem K, Wilson SK. Andrianne Mini-Jupette graft at the time of inflatable penile prosthesis placement for the management of post-prostatectomy

Climacturia and minimal urinary incontinence. J Sex Med 2018 May;15(5):789–796. https://doi.org/10.1016/j.jsxm.2018.01.015. Epub 2018 Mar 6. PMID: 29523479.
44. Van Huele A, Van Renterghem K. Simultaneous implant of inflatable penile prosthesis and artificial urinary sphincter: a single high-volume center experience. Int J Impot Res. 2023;15 https://doi.org/10.1038/s41443-023-00718-0. Epub ahead of print. PMID: 37188772
45. Pyrgidis N, Barham DW, Hammad M, Sokolakis I, Hatzichristodoulou G, Lentz AC, Simhan J, Yafi FA, Gross MS. Synchronous surgical Management of Erectile Dysfunction and Stress Urinary Incontinence: a systematic review and meta-analysis of reoperation rates. Sex Med Rev. 2022;10(4):782–90. https://doi.org/10.1016/j.sxmr.2022.08.003. PMID: 37051965
46. Wilson S, Delk J II, Henry GD, Siegel AL. New surgical technique for sphincter urinary control system using upper transverse scrotal incision. J Urol. 2003;169(1):261–4. https://doi.org/10.1016/S0022-5347(05)64082-7. PMID: 12478150
47. Zafirakis H, Wang R, Westney OL. Combination therapy for male erectile dysfunction and urinary incontinence. Asian J Androl. 2008;10(1):149–54. https://doi.org/10.1111/j.1745-7262.2008.00364.x. PMID: 18087654
48. Hübner WA, Schlarp OM. Treatment of incontinence after prostatectomy using a new minimally invasive device: adjustable continence therapy. BJU Int. 2005;96:587–94.
49. Lebret T, Cour F, Benchetrit J, Grise P, Bernstein J, Delaporte V, Chartier-Kastler E, Botto H, Costa P. Treatment of postprostatectomy stress urinary incontinence using a minimally invasive adjustable continence balloon device, ProACT: results of a preliminary, multicenter, pilot study. Urology. 2008;71(2):256–60. https://doi.org/10.1016/j.urology.2007.08.062. PMID: 18308096
50. Trigo-Rocha F, Gomes CM, Pompeo ACL, Lucon AM, Arap S. Prospective study evaluating efficacy and safety of Adjustable Continence Therapy (ProACT) for post radical prostatectomy.
51. Gregori A, Simonato A, Lissiani A, Scieri F, Rossi R, Gaboardi F. Transrectal ultrasound guided implantation of the ProACT adjustable continence therapy system in patients with post-radical prostatectomy stress urinary incontinence: a pilot study. J Urol. 2006;176:2109–13.
52. Krzastek SC, Smith R. An update on the best approaches to prevent complications in penile prosthesis recipients. Ther Adv Urol 2019 8;11:1756287218818076. https://doi.org/10.1177/1756287218818076. PMID: 30671142; PMCID: PMC6329024.
53. Pineda M, Burnett AL. Penile prosthesis infections—a review of risk factors, prevention, and treatment. Sex Med Rev. 2016 4(4):389–398. https://doi.org/10.1016/j.sxmr.2016.03.003. Epub 2016 May 13. PMID: 27872031.
54. Dropkin BM, Kaufman MR. Antibiotics and inflatable penile prosthesis insertion: a literature review. Sex Med Rev. 2021 9(1):174–180. https://doi.org/10.1016/j.sxmr.2020.04.005. Epub 2020 Jul 3. PMID: 32631811.
55. Burnett AL, Nehra A, Breau RH, Culkin DJ, Faraday MM, Hakim LS, Heidelbaugh J, Khera M, McVary KT, Miner MM, Nelson CJ, Sadeghi-Nejad H, Seftel AD, Shindel AW. Erectile Dysfunction: AUA Guideline. J Urol. 2018 Sep;200(3):633–641. https://doi.org/10.1016/j.juro.2018.05.004. Epub 2018 May 7. Erratum in: J Urol. 2022 Mar;207(3):743. PMID: 29746858.
56. Wolf JS Jr, Bennett CJ, Dmochowski RR, Hollenbeck BK, Pearle MS, Schaeffer AJ; Urologic surgery antimicrobial prophylaxis best practice policy panel. Best practice policy statement on urologic surgery antimicrobial prophylaxis. J Urol. 2008 Apr;179(4):1379–90. https://doi.org/10.1016/j.juro.2008.01.068. Epub 2008 Feb 20. Erratum in: J Urol 2008;180(5):2262–2263. PMID: 18280509.
57. Gross MS, Phillips EA, Carrasquillo RJ, et al. Multicenter investigation of the microorganisms involved in penile prosthesis infection: an analysis of the efficacy of the AUA and EAU guidelines for penile prosthesis prophylaxis. J Sex Med. 2017;14:455–63.
58. Carson CC 3rd. Efficacy of antibiotic impregnation of inflatable penile prostheses in decreasing infection in original implants. J Urol. 2004 Apr;171(4):1611–4. https://doi.

org/10.1097/01.ju.0000118245.66976.e1. Erratum in: J Urol 2004 Aug;172(2):781. PMID: 15017233.

59. Wolter CE, Hellstrom WJ. The hydrophilic-coated inflatable penile prosthesis: 1-year experience. J Sex Med. 2004;1(2):221–4. https://doi.org/10.1111/j.1743-6109.2004.04032.x. PMID: 16429621
60. Towe M, Huynh LM, Osman MM, El-Khatib FM, Andrianne R, Barton G, Broderick G, Burnett AL, Campbell JD, Clavell-Hernandez J, Connor J, Gross M, Guillum R, Guise AI, Hatzichristodoulou G, Henry GD, Hsieh TC, Jenkins LC, Koprowski C, Lee KB, Lentz A, Munarriz RM, Osmonov D, Pan S, Parikh K, Park SH, Patel AS, Perito P, Sadeghi-Nejad H, Sempels M, Simhan J, Wang R, Yafi FA. Impact of antimicrobial dipping solutions on postoperative infection rates in patients with diabetes undergoing primary insertion of a Coloplast titan inflatable penile prosthesis. J Sex Med 2020 17(10):2077–2083. https://doi.org/10.1016/j.jsxm.2020.07.009. Epub 2020 Aug 15. PMID: 32807707.
61. Hellstrom WJ, Montague DK, Moncada I, Carson C, Minhas S, Faria G, Krishnamurti S. Implants, mechanical devices, and vascular surgery for erectile dysfunction. J Sex Med. 2010;7(1 Pt 2):501–23. https://doi.org/10.1111/j.1743-6109.2009.01626.x. PMID: 20092450
62. Carson CC 3rd, Mulcahy JJ, Harsch MR. Long-term infection outcomes after original antibiotic impregnated inflatable penile prosthesis implants: up to 7.7 years of followup. J Urol 2011;185(2):614–618. https://doi.org/10.1016/j.juro.2010.09.094. Epub 2010 Dec 18. PMID: 21168870.
63. Mandava SH, Serefoglu EC, Freier MT, Wilson SK, Hellstrom WJ. Infection retardant coated inflatable penile prostheses decrease the incidence of infection: a systematic review and meta-analysis. J Urol 2012 Nov;188(5):1855–1860. https://doi.org/10.1016/j.juro.2012.07.022. Epub 2012 Sep 19. PMID: 22999690.
64. Serefoglu EC, Mandava SH, Gokce A, Chouhan JD, Wilson SK, Hellstrom WJ. Long-term revision rate due to infection in hydrophilic-coated inflatable penile prostheses: 11-year follow-up. J Sex Med 2012 9(8):2182–2186. https://doi.org/10.1111/j.1743-6109.2012.02830.x. Epub 2012 Jul 3. PMID: 22759917.
65. Darouiche RO, Bella AJ, Boone TB, Brock G, Broderick GA, Burnett AL, Carrion R, Carson C 3rd, Christine B, Dhabuwala CB, Hakim LS, Henry G, Jones LA, Khera M, Montague DK, Nehra A. North American consensus document on infection of penile prostheses. Urology 2013 Oct;82(4):937–942. https://doi.org/10.1016/j.urology.2013.05.048. Epub 2013 Aug 16. PMID: 23958508.
66. Zargaroff S, Sharma V, Berhanu D, Pearl JA, Meeks JJ, Dupree JM, Le BV, Cashy J, McVary KT. National trends in the treatment of penile prosthesis infections by explantation alone vs. immediate salvage and reimplantation. J Sex Med 2014;11(4):1078–1085. https://doi.org/10.1111/jsm.12446. Epub 2014 Mar 13. PMID: 24628707.
67. Eid JF, Wilson SK, Cleves M, Salem EA. Coated implants and "no touch" surgical technique decreases risk of infection in inflatable penile prosthesis implantation to 0.46%. Urology. 2012;79(6):1310–5. https://doi.org/10.1016/j.urology.2011.11.076. Epub 2012 Apr 21. PMID: 22521187
68. Dropkin BM, Chisholm LP, Dallmer JD, Johnsen NV, Dmochowski RR, Milam DF, Kaufman MR. Penile prosthesis insertion in the era of antibiotic stewardship-are postoperative antibiotics necessary? J Urol. 2020;203(3):611–4. https://doi.org/10.1097/JU.0000000000000578. Epub 2019 Oct 3. PMID: 31580192
69. Mulcahy JJ. Long-term experience with salvage of infected penile implants. J Urol. 2000;163(2):481–2. PMID: 10647660
70. Henry GD, Donatucci CF, Conners W, Greenfield JM, Carson CC, Wilson SK, Delk J, Lentz AC, Cleves MA, Jennermann CJ, Kramer AC. An outcomes analysis of over 200 revision surgeries for penile prosthesis implantation: a multicenter study. J Sex Med. 2012;9(1):309–15. https://doi.org/10.1111/j.1743-6109.2011.02524.x. Epub 2011 Nov 14. PMID: 22082149

71. Trost LW, McCaslin R, Linder B, Hellstrom WJ. Long-term outcomes of penile prostheses for the treatment of erectile dysfunction. Expert Rev Med Devices. 2013;10(3):353–66. https://doi.org/10.1586/erd.12.92. PMID: 23668707
72. Gross MS, Phillips EA, Balen A, Eid JF, Yang C, Simon R, Martinez D, Carrion R, Perito P, Levine L, Greenfield J, Munarriz R. The malleable implant salvage technique: infection outcomes after Mulcahy salvage procedure and replacement of infected inflatable penile prosthesis with malleable prosthesis. J Urol. 2016;195(3):694–7. https://doi.org/10.1016/j.juro.2015.08.091. Epub 2015 Sep 3. PMID: 26343986
73. Minervini A, Ralph DJ, Pryor JP. Outcome of penile prosthesis implantation for treating erectile dysfunction: experience with 504 procedures. BJU Int. 2006;97(1):129–33. https://doi.org/10.1111/j.1464-410X.2005.05907.x. PMID: 16336342
74. Chung E, Van CT, Wilson I, Cartmill RA. Penile prosthesis implantation for the treatment for male erectile dysfunction: clinical outcomes and lessons learnt after 955 procedures. World J Urol 2013 Jun;31(3):591–595. https://doi.org/10.1007/s00345-012-0859-4. Epub 2012 Mar 29. PMID: 22457032.
75. Anele UA, Le BV, Burnett AL. Suprapubic cystostomy for the management of urethral injuries during penile prosthesis implantation. Sex Med 2014 2(4):178–181. https://doi.org/10.1002/sm2.44. PMID: 25548649; PMCID: PMC4272249.
76. Qi RB, Grimberg DC, Lentz AC. Management of urethral injury during penile prosthesis surgery. Curr Sex Health Rep. 2020;12:62–7. https://doi.org/10.1007/s11930-020-00259-3.
77. Kumar R, Nehra A. Dual implantation of penile and sphincter implants in the post-prostatectomy patient. Curr Urol Rep. 2007;8(6):477–81. https://doi.org/10.1007/s11934-007-0052-2. PMID: 18042328
78. Sexton SJ, Granieri MA, Lentz AC. Survey on the contemporary management of intraoperative urethral injuries during penile prosthesis implantation. J Sex Med 2018 15(4):576–581. https://doi.org/10.1016/j.jsxm.2018.01.026. Epub 2018 Mar 6. PMID: 29523475.
79. Mulcahy JJ. The prevention and management of noninfectious complications of penile implants. Sex Med Rev. 2015 3(3):203–213. https://doi.org/10.1002/smrj.41. Epub 2015 Oct 8. PMID: 27784610.
80. Minhas S. Urethral perforation during penile implant surgery: what to do? J Sex Med. 2017;14(7):867–9. https://doi.org/10.1016/j.jsxm.2017.05.003. PMID: 28673431
81. Carlos EC, Sexton SJ, Lentz AC. Urethral injury and the penile prosthesis. Sex Med Rev. 2019 7(2):360–368. https://doi.org/10.1016/j.sxmr.2018.06.003. Epub 2018 Aug 2. PMID: 30078620.
82. Scherzer ND, Dick B, Gabrielson AT, Alzweri LM, Hellstrom WJG. Penile prosthesis complications: planning, prevention, and decision making. Sex Med Rev 2019 7(2):349–359. https://doi.org/10.1016/j.sxmr.2018.04.002. Epub 2018 Jul 19. PMID: 30033128.
83. Carson CC, Noh CH. Distal penile prosthesis extrusion: treatment with distal corporoplasty or Gortex windsock reinforcement. Int J Impot Res. 2002;14(2):81–4. https://doi.org/10.1038/sj.ijir.3900829. PMID: 11979321
84. Botkin H, Barnes B, Pearlman A. Bulbar urethrocavernous fistula in setting of inflatable penile prosthesis: a case report. BMC Urol 2021 21(1):25. https://doi.org/10.1186/s12894-021-00793-9. PMID: 33581719; PMCID: PMC7881336.
85. Van der Aa F, Drake MJ, Kasyan GR, Petrolekas A, Cornu JN; Young academic urologists functional urology group. The artificial urinary sphincter after a quarter of a century: a critical systematic review of its use in male non-neurogenic incontinence. Eur Urol 2013;63(4):681–689. https://doi.org/10.1016/j.eururo.2012.11.034. Epub 2012 Nov 23. PMID: 23219375.
86. Queissert F, Huesch T, Kretschmer A, Anding R, Kurosch M, Kirschner-Hermanns R, Pottek T, Olianas R, Friedl A, Pfitzenmaier J, Naumann CM, Wotzka C, Nyarangi-Dix J, Hoffmann T, Herrmann E, Obaje A, Rose A, Homberg R, Abdunnur R, Loertzer H, Bauer RM, Haferkamp A, Schrader AJ. Artificial Urinary Sphincter Cuff Size Predicts Outcome in Male Patients Treated for Stress Incontinence: Results of a Large Central European Multicenter Cohort

Study. Int Neurourol J. 2019 Sep;23(3):219–225. https://doi.org/10.5213/inj.1938032.016. Epub 2019 Sep 30. PMID: 31607101; PMCID: PMC6790824.
87. Silva LAD, Simonetti R, Silva EMKD. Adjustable sling for the treatment of post-prostatectomy urinary incontinence: systematic review and meta-analysis. Einstein (Sao Paulo) 2019 Sep 23;17(4):eRW4508. https://doi.org/10.31744/einstein_journal/2019RW4508. PMID: 31553360; PMCID: PMC6748345.
88. Viers BR, Linder BJ, Rivera ME, Rangel LJ, Ziegelmann MJ, Elliott DS. Long-term quality of life and functional outcomes among primary and secondary artificial urinary sphincter implantations in men with stress urinary incontinence. J Urol 2016 Sep;196(3):838–843. https://doi.org/10.1016/j.juro.2016.03.076. Epub 2016 Mar 17. PMID: 26997310.
89. Wilson SK, Aliotta PJ, Salem EA, Mulcahy JJ. New enhancements of the scrotal one-incision technique for placement of artificial urinary sphincter allow proximal cuff placement. J Sex Med. 2010;7(10):3510–5. https://doi.org/10.1111/j.1743-6109.2010.01933.x. PMID: 20584110
90. O'Rourke TK, Erbella A, Zhang Y, et al. Prevention, identification, and management of post-operative penile implant complications of infection, hematoma, and device malfunction. Transl Androl Urol. 2017;5:832–48.
91. Gurtner K, Saltzman A, Hebert K, Laborde E. Erectile Dysfunction: A Review of Historical Treatments With a Focus on the Development of the Inflatable Penile Prosthesis. Am J Mens Health. 2017;11(3):479–486. https://doi.org/10.1177/1557988315596566. Epub 2015 Jul 23. PMID: 26206161; PMCID: PMC5675239.
92. Palmisano F, Boeri L, Cristini C, Antonini G, Spinelli MG, Franco G, Longo F, Gadda F, Colombo F, Montanari E. Comparison of Infrapubic vs Penoscrotal approaches for 3-piece inflatable penile prosthesis placement: do we have a winner? Sex Med Rev. 2018;6(4):631–639. https://doi.org/10.1016/j.sxmr.2018.03.007. Epub 2018 May 2. PMID: 29730314.
93. García Gómez B, Romero Otero J, Díez Sicilia L, Jiménez Alcaide E, García-Cruz E, Rodríguez Antolín A. Ischemic Gangrene of the Glans following Penile Prosthesis Implantation. Case Rep Urol. 2013;2013:323574. https://doi.org/10.1155/2013/323574. Epub 2013 Jul 11. PMID: 23956919; PMCID: PMC3728554.
94. Hebert KJ, Kohler TS. Glans ischemia following inflatable penile prosthesis surgery. Transl Androl Urol 2020;9(2):824–827. https://doi.org/10.21037/tau.2020.01.04. PMID: 32420191; PMCID: PMC7215035.
95. Garrido-Abad P, Estéve-Sánchez DA, Fernández-Arjona M. Superficial glans ischemia after penile prosthesis successfully treated by conservative treatment. Rev Int Androl 2021;19(4):281–284. https://doi.org/10.1016/j.androl.2020.04.001. Epub 2020 Jul 11. PMID: 32660866.
96. Wilson SK, Mora-Estaves C, Egydio P, Ralph D, Habous M, Love C, Shamsodini A, Valenzuela R, Yafi FA. Glans necrosis following penile prosthesis implantation: prevention and treatment suggestions. Urology 2017 107:144–148. https://doi.org/10.1016/j.urology.2017.06.020. Epub 2017 Jun 23. PMID: 28648967.
97. Braun AE, Swerdloff D, Sudhakar A, Patel RD, Gross MS, Simhan J. Defining the incidence and management of postoperative scrotal hematoma after primary and complex three-piece inflatable penile prosthesis surgery. Int J Impot Res 2023 8:1–5. https://doi.org/10.1038/s41443-023-00697-2. Epub ahead of print. PMID: 37156930; PMCID: PMC10166027.
98. Al-Shaiji TF. Dual implantation of artificial urinary sphincter and inflatable penile prostheses for concurrent male urinary incontinence and erectile dysfunction. Adv Urol. 2011;2011:178312. https://doi.org/10.1155/2011/178312. Epub 2011 Nov 17. PMID: 22162678; PMCID: PMC3226319.
99. Mykoniatis I, Albersen M, Andrianne R, Sokolakis I, Hatzichristodoulou G, Sempels M, van Renterghem K. Synchronous surgery for the combined treatment of post-radical prostatectomy erectile dysfunction and stress urinary incontinence: a lucrative evolution or an unnecessary complexity? Int J Impot Res 2021 33(1):6–15. https://doi.org/10.1038/s41443-020-0253-5. Epub 2020 Mar 17. PMID: 32203423.

100. Henry GD. The Henry mummy wrap and the Henry finger sweep surgical techniques. J Sex Med 2009 6(3):619–622. https://doi.org/10.1111/j.1743-6109.2008.01200.x. PMID: 19284470
101. Sadeghi-Nejad H. Penile prosthesis surgery: a review of prosthetic devices and associated complications. J Sex Med. 2007 Mar;4(2):296–309. https://doi.org/10.1111/j.1743-6109.2007.00434.x. Erratum in: J Sex Med 2007 Sep;4(5):1520. PMID: 17367425.
102. Smelser AM, VanDyke ME, Nealon SW, Badkhshan S, Langford BT, Peedikayil J, El-Eishy AF, Monaghan TF, Sanders SC, Franzen BP, Morey AF. Mechanical indications for inflatable penile prosthesis revision: analysis and implications for revision surgery. J Sex Med. 2023;20(7):1044–51. https://doi.org/10.1093/jsxmed/qdad064. PMID: 37189017
103. Srivastava A, Joice GA, Patel HD, Manka MG, Sopko NA, Wright EJ. Causes of artificial urinary sphincter failure and strategies for surgical revision: implications of device component survival. Eur Urol Focus 2019 5(5):887–893. https://doi.org/10.1016/j.euf.2018.02.014. Epub 2018 Mar 12. PMID: 29545058.
104. Carson CC, Mulcahy JJ, Govier FE. Efficacy, safety and patient satisfaction outcomes of the AMS 700CX inflatable penile prosthesis: results of a long-term multicenter study. AMS 700CX Study Group. J Urol. 2000;164(2):376–80. PMID: 10893589
105. Wilson SK, Cleves MA, Delk JR 2nd. Comparison of mechanical reliability of original and enhanced Mentor alpha I penile prosthesis. J Urol. 1999;162(3 Pt 1):715–8. https://doi.org/10.1097/00005392-199909010-00022. PMID: 10458350
106. Kim J. Long term follow-up of readjustable urethral sling procedure (Remeex system) for male stress urinary incontinence. Neurourol Urodyn. 2011;30:209.
107. Eswara JR, Chan R, Vetter JM, Lai HH, Boone TB, Brandes SB. Revision techniques after artificial urinary sphincter failure in men: results from a multicenter study. Urology. 2015;86(1):176–80. https://doi.org/10.1016/j.urology.2015.04.023. PMID: 26142602
108. Sandhu JS, Breyer B, Comiter C, Eastham JA, Gomez C, Kirages DJ, Kittle C, Lucioni A, Nitti VW, Stoffel JT, Westney OL, Murad MH, McCammon K. Incontinence after prostate treatment: AUA/SUFU guideline. J Urol 2019 202(2):369–378. https://doi.org/10.1097/JU.0000000000000314. Epub 2019 Jul 8. PMID: 31059663.
109. Sacco E, Gandi C, Marino F, Totaro A, Di Gianfrancesco L, Palermo G, Pierconti F, Racioppi M, Bassi P. Artificial urinary sphincter significantly better than fixed sling for moderate post-prostatectomy stress urinary incontinence: a propensity score-matched study. BJU Int 2021 127(2):229–237. https://doi.org/10.1111/bju.15197. Epub 2020 Aug 26. PMID: 32744793.
110. Meisterhofer K, Herzog S, Strini KA, Sebastianelli L, Bauer R, Dalpiaz O. Male slings for Postprostatectomy incontinence: a systematic review and meta-analysis. Eur Urol Focus 2020 6(3):575–592. https://doi.org/10.1016/j.euf.2019.01.008. Epub 2019 Feb 2. PMID: 30718160.
111. Christodoulidou M, Pearce I. Infection of penile prostheses in patients with diabetes mellitus. Surg Infect 2016 17(1):2–8. https://doi.org/10.1089/sur.2015.164. Epub 2015 Oct 1. PMID: 26426099.
112. Gon LM, de Campos CCC, Voris BRI, Passeri LA, Fregonesi A, Riccetto CLZ. A systematic review of penile prosthesis infection and meta-analysis of diabetes mellitus role. BMC Urol 2021 21(1):35. https://doi.org/10.1186/s12894-020-00730-2. PMID: 33691670; PMCID: PMC7945372.
113. Bettocchi C, Ditonno P, Palumbo F, Lucarelli G, Garaffa G, Giammusso B, Battaglia M. Penile prosthesis: what should we do about complications? Adv Urol. 2008;2008:573560. https://doi.org/10.1155/2008/573560. Epub 2008 Nov 4. PMID: 19009029; PMCID: PMC2581729
114. Habous M, Tal R, Tealab A, et al. Defining a glycated haemoglobin (HbA1c) level that predicts increased risk of penile implant infection. BJU Int. 2018;121:293–300.

Chapter 23
Advances in the Management of Peyronie's Disease

Hyun Jun Park, Hussain Alnajjar, and Eric Chung

Introduction

Peyronie's disease (PD) is characterized by the development of fibrous plaque within the tunica albuginea, which prevents the tunica albuginea from expanding during an erection, resulting in a characteristic penile curvature. Clinically, this penile curvature is most problematic as it often leads to sexual difficulties. In severe cases, it can also result in a penis deformity such as a collar or hour-glass penis during erection, which can add to the patient's psychological distress.

The disease primarily affects middle-aged men and is increasing in prevalence, with a prevalence of 0.4–20% of adult men [1–3]. The prevalence is estimated to be much higher if asymptomatic patients are included. Recently published studies often report higher prevalence rates than in the past, likely due to the underestimation of past prevalence rates and increased awareness and interest in Peyronie's disease in recent years.

Currently, the most widely accepted and used guidelines for PD are the guidelines published by the European Association of Urology (EAU), the American Urological Association (AUA), and International Consultation on Sexual Medicine (ICSM), respectively [4–6]. The definition of PD in each guideline is listed in Table 23.1.

H. J. Park (✉)
Department of Urology, Pusan National University School of Medicine, Pusan National University Hospital, Busan, South Korea

H. Alnajjar
University College London Hospitals, London, UK

E. Chung
Department of Urology, Princess Alexandra Hospital, University of Queensland, Brisbane, QLD, Australia

AndroUrology Centre, Brisbane, QLD, Australia

E. Chung et al. (eds.), *Advances in Andrology*,
https://doi.org/10.1007/978-3-032-29112-7_23

Table 23.1 Definitions of Peyronie's disease

EAU [4]	A connective tissue disorder, characterized by the formation of a fibrotic lesion or plaque in the tunica albuginea, which leads to penile deformity
AUA [5]	An acquired penile abnormality characterized by fibrosis of the tunica albuginea, which may be accompanied by pain, deformity, erectile dysfunction (ED), and/or distress
ICSM [6]	Psychosexual condition characterized by the presence of penile pain, curvature and/or deformity, with a potential palpable plaque and concomitant sexual dysfunction

Pathophysiology and Etiology

The exact pathogenesis of PD is unclear, but it can be described as the result of chronic microtrauma to the penis resulting in improper wound healing. When microscopic damage is caused by ongoing behaviors such as sexual activity, blood leaks from the microvessels of the corpora cavernosa tissue and pools in the subtunical layer of the tunica albuginea. Here, fibrin deposits, macrophages, neutrophils, etc., gather, causing an inflammatory response. These cells secrete cytokines and vasoactive factors that accelerate the fibrosis process, most notably transforming growth factor-β1 (TGF-β1), which increases the synthesis of collagen. Over time, defects in tissue recombination, i.e., dysregulation of collagen synthesis and inadequate dissolution of nodules, develop [7, 8]. In addition to trauma, genetic predisposition such as HLA-B27 and autoimmune abnormalities are also involved in the pathogenesis of Peyronie's disease [9].

Commonly reported risk factors or comorbidities include hypertension, diabetes, dyslipidemia, ischemic heart disease, autoimmune disease, erectile dysfunction, smoking, alcohol consumption, low testosterone levels, and a history of pelvic surgery [10–12].

Symptom and Clinical Manifestation

The clinical course can be divided into active and stable phases, and treatment is differentiated accordingly [13].

Active Disease

This phase is characterized by rapidly changing symptoms, and pain in the penis or glans during erection or flaccid state is common. The onset of these symptoms may coincide with an injury to the penis during sexual activity, although in vast majority of cases there is no etiological history of penile injury. At this stage, a tender fibrous plaque may be palpable with a concomitant de novo penile curvature. During this period, the symptoms are dynamic and largely progressive. This results in increased anxiety and mental distress. Erectile function may be normal or decrease as the disease progresses.

Stable Disease

This is when clinical symptoms are no longer changing and are stable, usually 12–18 months after the first symptoms. Characteristically, the penile pain tends to subside. Penile curvature is common, which is independent of the size or extent of the fibrous plaque. Penile deformity is common in the ventral, dorso-lateral, and dorsal regions (e.g., wasting, S shape, hour-glass).

Penis curvature resolves spontaneously in 3–13% of cases, becomes fixed in 36–67% of cases, and continues to progress in 21–48% of cases. Erectile pain is present in 20–70% of patients and gradually decreases, disappearing in 90% of patients after 12 months [1–3].

Erectile dysfunction is present in as many as half of cases (8–52%), and Dupuytren's contracture is reported in 4–26% [14, 15].

Diagnostics

A diagnosis of PD can often be made based on medical history and physical examination alone. It is important to determine whether the disease is progressive or stable, which is essential in determining when and how to treat it. In addition, a history of penile surgery, mechanical manipulation of the urethra, penile injury, medications, Dupuytren's contracture/plantar fascial contracture, family history of fibrotic disease, smoking, dyslipidemia, hypertension, diabetes, and cardiovascular disease are all risk factors for erectile dysfunction. Abnormalities of the penis during erection, such as pain, fibrous plaque, hour glass deformity, penis shortening, distal flaccidity, hinge effect, direction and degree of penile curvature, and the degree of erectile dysfunction should be evaluated. When assessing the penis, the size, location, intensity and number of the fibrous plaques should be noted. The patient may take a picture of their erect penis from 2 angles at home to document the distorted erection. Additionally, an erection may be induced in the clinic, using intracavernosal injection, to assess the curvature in the erect state and to judge whether there is significant ED. In some cases, an artificially induced erection and a penile duplex ultrasonography [16] is necessary; this can help delineate calcified plaques and their nature. Doppler ultrasound is helpful in assessing erectile function and haemodynamics of the penis. MRI of the penis can occasionally be requested to assess a detailed anatomy of the erect penis.

Treatment

In the early stages of PD, or the active phase, penile pain is common, especially during erections, and treatment with non-steroidal anti-inflammatory drugs is recommended. Psychological distress is common during this active phase due to the pain, development of penile plaque, and rapid progression of penile deformity, so psychological counseling or therapy is also recommended to alleviate this distress.

Once the pain has subsided and the penile plaque or deformity is no longer problematic, a variety of treatment options are available, depending on the severity of the symptoms and the patient's wishes. Over time, it is not uncommon for multiple penile deformities or side effects to develop. The active and stable phases can exist on a continuum, and the disease can at times revert from one phase to the other. Pain can be an issue in the stable phase due to the torque of the penis during sexual intercourse. In general, treatment is usually started when penile pain appears or penile curvature becomes problematic. Specific treatments include oral medications that act systemically or locally, injectable drugs that are injected directly into the lesion, and surgical treatments. The current recommendations from the European Association of Urology (EAU) [4], American Urological Association (AUA) [6], and International Consultation on Sexual Medicine (ICSM) [5] guidelines are summarized in Table 23.2.

Table 23.2 Treatment recommendations for Peyronie's disease

Treatment methods	EAU	AUA	ICSM
Oral non-steroidal anti-inflammatory medications	N.A.	O	N.A
Oral phosphodiesterase type 5 inhibitors	X	N.A	O
Oral potassium para-aminobenzoate	O	X	O
Oral vitamin E, tamoxifen	X	X	X
Oral acetyl esters of carnitine, pentoxifylline, colchicine	X	X	X
Intralesional treatment with steroids	O	O	O
Intralesional interferon	O	O	O
Intralesional verapamil	O	O	O
Topical verapamil	O	O	X
Electromotive therapy with verapamil	O	X	X
Penile traction devices, vacuum devices	O	O	O
Extracorporeal shockwave for curvature and plaque	X	X	X
Extracorporeal shockwave for pain	O	O	O
Intralesional collagenase clostridium histolyticum	O	O	O
Tunical shortening procedures	O	O	O
Grafting techniques	O	O	O
Penile prosthesis implantation	O	O	O
Radiotherapy	N.A.	X	N.A

N.A no comments in the guidelines, *O* recommended or possible, *X* not recommended, *EAU* European Association of Urology, *AUA* American Urological Association, *ICSM* International Consultation on Sexual Medicine

Nonsurgical Treatment

Conservative or nonsurgical treatment of Peyronie's disease is an adjunctive, supportive treatment that is usually performed to relieve symptoms and control disease progression in patients in the early stages of the disease [17, 18].

Intralesional Therapy

This method is an attractive treatment alternative as it increases the drug concentration locally in the area of constriction of the lesion and avoids systemic side effects [19]. The main indications for this treatment are when the penile curvature is not severe ($\leq$ 30), the size of the penile fibrous plaque is small and it is not calcified, the deformity of the penis is minimal, and especially when the patient wants to avoid surgical treatment.

In the past, several non-specific therapeutic drugs had been used, but their efficacy has been unclear. Recently, collagenase clostridium histolyticum (Xiaflex®, Auxilium Pharmaceuticals, Inc.) has been developed as an injectable therapy to reduce curvature without the need for surgery.

Collagenase Clostridium Histolyticum

Collagenase clostridium histolyticum (CCH) (Xiaflex®) is an injectable drug that contains a mixture of two enzymes, class I and class II collagenase, which cleaves collagen at different sites, making it easier to break down fibrous plaques [20].

With the recent demonstration of the drug's intralesional efficacy in Dupuytren's contracture, its efficacy in Peyronie's disease has also been demonstrated, making it the only FDA-approved treatment for Peyronie's disease. Its primary effect is to reduce penile curvature in Peyronie's disease at rest.

The use of CCH is contraindicated in hour-glass deformity, ventral curvature, calcified fibrous plaques, and fibrous plaques at the base of the penis.

The treatment regimen consists of two Xiaflex® injections administered into the peyronie's plaque, 3 days apart with gentle penile stretching and modeling to help break the collagen. The process is repeated at 6 weeks, up to a maximum of 4 treatment cycles. The price for a treatment cycle can range between $ 8000–$12,000 in the USA. Each vial of Xiaflex® costs around $ 4000–$ 5000. Xiaflex® was fully withdrawn from the European market in March 2020, due to commercial reasons.

Ecchymosis of the penis, penile swelling, and penile pain occurred in almost all patients, but most resolved spontaneously. Rupture of the body of the penis is rare, but intercourse should be avoided for 4 weeks after injection to prevent this. Based on the results of previous studies, [21–23] improvement in penis curvature is consistent, with 31.4–42.9% of patients showing improvement, with an average improvement of 17° and 50–60% of cases reported improved ability to have intercourse. However, there was no improvement in pain, nodule size, or ED. [24]

Interferon

Theoretically, it may improve penis curvature by decreasing fibroblast production of collagen and increasing collagenase production [25]. In clinical studies, it has been shown to help relieve penile pain and improve penile blood flow [26, 27]. Side effects such as sinusitis, penis swelling, and flu-like symptoms occurred in 40–100% of patients, but were usually mild and rarely required further treatment. Currently, this treatment modality is not widely utilized due to its poor efficacy, practical drawbacks, and side effects.

Verapamil

It is a typical calcium channel blocker that controls fibroblast function, fibrous tissue production, and inhibits inflammatory responses, and has been used as a typical intralesional treatment for Peyronie's disease in the past. However, in recent years, it has been reported that the improvement in penile curvature is not as pronounced as in the early clinical results. Therefore, verapamil 10 mg injected into the plaques every 2–4 weeks may be used to reduce the size and intensity of penile fibrous plaque. It has no significant side effects and is inexpensive to utilize, so it may still play a role in the treatment of this condition [28].

Oral Medications

The effectiveness of oral therapy in treating Peyronie's disease remains largely uncertain, with existing studies showing only minimal impact on reducing penile deformity. This is likely due to variations in the studies, such as small sample sizes, different stages of the disease, and limited measurable outcomes [5, 6]. Although vitamin E, tamoxifen, carnitine, colchicine, L-arginine, and pentoxifylline have been tried in the past for their antioxidant, anti-inflammatory, and anti-fibrotic properties, none have successfully corrected penile curvature. While randomized trials have found that oral treatments like vitamin E, colchicine, carnitine, potassium aminobenzoate, and tamoxifen are mostly ineffective, more recent research suggests that pentoxifylline and low-dose tadalafil may offer some benefits in managing Peyronie's disease [29–31]. Oral therapy might be especially useful in the early stages of the disease, particularly for men experiencing unstable or worsening penile curvature and painful erections, or for those who are not ready or willing to pursue surgical options.

Other Therapies

Penile Traction Therapy and Vacuum Erection Device (VED)

It involves wearing a device that physically elongates the penis for a certain number of hours per day to stretch the penis to provide additional length, reduce curvature, or shorten it. It can be applied during both the active and stable phases of the disease, and is particularly effective when combined with intralesional drug injection therapy, or as an adjunctive procedure before or after radical penile surgery. However, traction of the penis for a prolonged period of time can be uncomfortable for the patient and should be performed selectively [32]. Martinez-Salamanca et al. showed in 55 men with acute-phase Peyronie's disease using PTT for 6 months improved their curvature from 33° to 15° at 6 months and 13° at 9 months when compared to 41 untreated controls [33]. Macdonald et al. reviewed 20 men with Peyronie's using VED 10 min twice daily with mean curvature improvement of 23° with mean follow-up period of 14 months [34].

Extracorporeal Shock Wave Therapy

In theory, it is thought to disrupt fibrous plaque and induce its dissolution and resorption [33, 34]. Taken together, clinical studies have shown that it is helpful in relieving pain during erection, but not in reducing the size or curvature of penile fibrous plaque [35, 36]. It may be considered as a treatment for pain in Peyronie's disease, but the benefit-cost ratio should be considered [37].

Surgical Treatments

In patients with Peyronie's disease, the goal of surgery is to correct the penile curvature to the point where sexual activity is not impaired and erectile function is maintained at preoperative levels. In general, the younger the patient, the more likely it is that the penile curvature will cause mental distress in addition to physical disability. In addition, if there is a ventral curvature, vaginal penetration is more difficult. Therefore, the following cases of Peyronie's disease, i.e., [1] severe penile curvature, [2] deformity such as hour-glass or wasting, which causes difficulty in sexual penetration, [3] severe penis shortening, [4] erectile dysfunction, and [5] a combination of the above factors, are indications for surgery. On the other hand, patients who have unrealistically high expectations or those with early-stage Peyronie's disease are not suitable candidates for surgical treatment. It is also important to determine the timing of surgery, which should only be performed when the disease is stable, usually around 12 months after the first symptoms. A detailed examination for penile vascular disorders or sexual dysfunction should be performed prior to surgery, and the appropriate surgical procedure should be selected after evaluation of all factors. Peyronie's disease corrective surgery can be categorized into three types: penile tunical shortening procedure, penile tunical lengthening procedure, and insertion of penile prosthesis. Penile tunical shortening and penile tunical lengthening procedures are recommended for patients who have normal erections or for whom oral pharmacotherapy is effective. Penile implants are a good option for patients with severe erectile dysfunction who have failed medications [38, 39]. The treatment algorithm is summarized in Fig. 23.1.

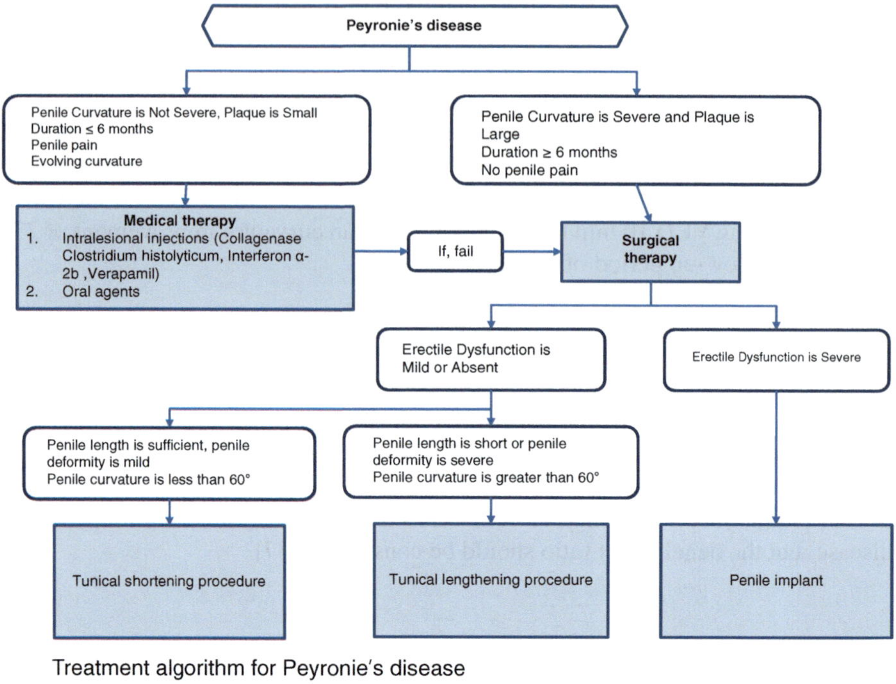

Fig. 23.1 Algorithm for surgical treatment of Peyronie's disease

Preoperative Preparation

The basic principle when considering surgery is that it should be performed when Peyronie's disease is in a stable phase. Surgery is usually considered at least 6–12 months after onset, when there is no change in fibrous plaque or curvature for 3–6 months, or when there is severe deformity that interferes with or makes intercourse difficult [40]. Surgery may also be considered when conservative treatment fails, when penile fibrous plaque is extensive to begin with, or when the patient wants quick results. It is also possible to skip nonsurgical treatment and proceed directly to surgery, but patients should be fully informed of the potential side effects of surgery and give informed consent [29, 41].

It is of utmost importance that patients considering surgery are fully counseled and informed of realistic expectations for the outcome of surgery. Patients often have unrealistic expectations, which can lead to post-operative difficulties for both patients and healthcare providers.

Components of informed consent should include a discussion of possible treatment options and their advantages and disadvantages, and an explanation of how they apply to the patient's current state of Peyronie's disease. Realistic expectations and potential complications of the proposed surgery should be fully explained and agreed upon [40, 42].

Tunical Shortening Procedure

The tunica albuginea shortening procedure is a surgical technique to straighten the penis by shortening the long and convex part of the penis to equalize with the opposite side. In patients with good erectile function, moderate penile length, without complicated deformities such as hour-glass deformity or hinge effect, and/or severe curvature (e.g., > 60°), the tunica albuginea shortening procedure may be an appropriate surgical option. Although various methods and variations have been described, no one method is superior to the others, and each should be tailored to the individual patient.

The *Nesbit procedure* involves removing a portion of the tunica albuginea opposite the point of curvature and suturing it [43, 44]. The traditional Nesbit procedure with excision of an ellipse of tunica may rarely increase the risk of ED secondary to postoperative veno-occlusive dysfunction [45]. However, several modifications of the Nesbit procedure have been published recently, which are considered the safer option and preferred method nowadays since they do not cause veno-occlusive ED. The *Yachia technique,* instead of removing a portion of the tunica albuginea, involves making a longitudinal incision and suturing it in a transverse direction. The *penile plication technique* involves shortening the tunica albuginea by passing sutures through an appropriate range of the tunica albuginea and tying them in a knot, rather than resection or incision of the tunica albuginea [46–48].

In general, tunical shortening procedures are successful in correcting the curvature in more than 85% of patients. Recurrence of curvature and penis hypoesthesia are uncommon (~10%) and the risk of postoperative ED is low. Disadvantages include penis shortening, and it does not resolve hinge or hour-glass deformity and may even worsen it. Other complications may include persistent penile pain, persistence or recurrence of penile curvature (>30°, 8–11%), penile hematoma (0–9%), requirement for circumcision, palpable suture knots, and decreased penile sensation. These are rarely the cause of postoperative sexual dysfunction, but patients may perceive penis shortening to be greater than it actually is. Therefore, measuring and recording stretched penile length intra-operatively before and after surgery, regardless of the technique used, is paramount for both patient information and medico-legal cases [49–52, 53].

Tunical Lengthening Procedure

The tunica albuginea lengthening procedure is a surgical method that involves incision or partial excision of the fibrous plaque or concavity of the penis, followed by the use of a graft to cover the defect. In patients with good erectile function, the tunica albuginea lengthening procedure may be an appropriate option if there is severe penis shortening, complex curvature, simple curvature greater than 60°, large fibrous plaque, or complex deformity such as hour-glass or hinge effect.

The ideal graft should be traction-resistant, easy to suture and manipulate, flexible, readily available, cost-effective, and minimize infection, especially when using

Table 23.3 Summary of grafts used in plaque incision and grafting and their advantages versus disadvantages

Graft	Type	Advantages	Disadvantages
Saphenous vein	Autologous	Easily available, good handling characteristics	Additional operative time, donor site morbidity
Buccal mucosa	Autologous	Easily available, excellent take	Donor site morbidity, limited size for larger defects
Tunica vaginalis	Autologous	Thin and pliable, single operative field	Limited structural strength, limited surface area
Dermal grafts	Autologous	Pliable and readily available	Donor site scar, variable thickness, quality, lack of anchorage
Cadaveric human pericardium	Allograft	Readily available off the shelf, good handling	High cost, risk of contracture, risk of disease transmission
Fascia lata	Allograft	Strong, durable	Limited availability, cost
Small intestinal submucosa (SIS	Xenograft	Excellent remodelling properties	Potential for calcification, cost
Bovine/porcine pericardium	Xenograft	Good strength and tensile properties	Contraction and possible immune reaction
Synthetic	PTFE/ Dacron	Unlimited supply, consistent	Higher infection risk, poor long-term outcomes

autografts (Table 23.3). However, no graft meets all of these requirements. In the case of the tunica albuginea lengthening procedure, structures within the deep penile fascia, such as the neurovascular bundle, are mobilized and temporarily retracted; hence, there is a risk of temporary neuropraxia or even permanent numbness. Although damage to the cavernosal artery is rare, the likelihood of postoperative erectile dysfunction is reported to be higher (10–50%) than in the tunica albuginea shortening procedure for a variety of reasons. The presence of preoperative erectile dysfunction, the use of larger grafts, age over 60 years, and dorsal curvature are considered poor prognostic factors for surgical outcome [54].

There are four main types of grafts: autograft, allograft, xenograft, and synthetic graft, each with its own advantages and disadvantages, and there is no consistent evidence that any one graft is superior to the others [55].

For autografts, venous grafts, mainly saphenous vein, are commonly used, and recently buccal mucosal grafts have also been used. Dermal grafts are rarely used due to their lack of anchorage and potential for venogenic erectile dysfunction [56, 57]. Tunica albuginea grafts are the most histologically suitable, but caution should be exercised due to the limited size that can be obtained and the possibility of weakening penile support [58, 59].

For allografts, cadaveric pericardium is commonly used. Cadaveric dura mater is no longer used due to concerns about possible infection [60].

For xenografts, type I collagen-based xenografts such as small intestinal submucosa or bovine pericardium are commonly used. Recently, grafting with collagen fleece (TachoSil©) has been increasingly used due to several key advantages, such as shorter surgical time, ease of application, and hemostatic effect [61].

For synthetic grafts, polyester (Dacron®) and polytetrafluoroethylene (Gore-Tex®) have been introduced, but are not recommended due to the potential for infection, inflammation, allergic reactions, and significant fibrosis [62–64].

The tunica albuginea lengthening procedure does not actually lengthen the penis, but rather extends the fibrous plaque to the length of the original tunica albuginea. Nevertheless, postoperative penile shortening has been reported, with rates ranging from around 30% for saphenous vein grafts, 23% to 30% for allografts, and 13% to 20% for xenografts, depending on the type of graft used to cover the fibrous plaque [4]. The exact cause of penile shortening after tunica albuginea lengthening procedures has not been reported.

In tunica albuginea lengthening procedures, the risk of erectile dysfunction is greater than in tunica albuginea shortening procedures, with rates of up to 50% reported.

Recurrence of curvature occurs due to failure to wait for the disease to stabilize, reactivation of the condition after stable disease has occurred, or use of absorbable sutures which lose their hold before healing is complete. Therefore, it is recommended that non-absorbable sutures or slowly resorbing absorbable sutures (e.g., polydioxanone) be used. If non-absorbable sutures are used, the knots should be buried to avoid irritation of the penile skin, but the use of slow resorbable sutures (e.g., polydioxanone) may reduce the likelihood of this occurring [65]. Changes in penile sensation are associated with damage to the neurovascular bundle, the degree of dissection required to remove fibrous plaque, and postoperative inflammation and fibrosis at the graft site. Reduction in penile sensation has been reported in rates up to 25%, but most studies report 5% or less [55].

Penile Prosthesis Implantation with Penile Reconstruction

For men with ED who want to preserve penile size, penile prosthesis implantation is advised [54]. The inflatable penile prosthesis generally provides higher functional outcomes and greater patient satisfaction compared to malleable implants [5, 6]. Although penile prosthesis implantation alone is usually adequate to correct minor penile curvature, patients with a residual curvature greater than 30° may require additional procedures such as repeated manual modeling, penile plication, or plaque incision with grafting during surgery [4–6]. However, using graft material is linked to an increased risk of prosthetic infection [5]. New surgical methods aimed at enhancing penile length and girth during prosthesis implantation, utilizing various modified sliding techniques, [38] have shown high rates of patient satisfaction but carry serious risks, including glans necrosis and penile gangrene [66].

Novel Pharmacological Treatments

Recent advancements in the treatment of Peyronie's disease have introduced novel therapeutic options that show promise in improving patient outcomes. Among these, stem cell therapy and platelet-rich plasma (PRP) injections are gaining attention for their potential to promote tissue repair and reduce fibrosis [67]. Stem cells, particularly mesenchymal stem cells, have demonstrated anti-fibrotic and regenerative properties in early studies, suggesting their potential to reverse the effects of Peyronie's disease [68]. PRP therapy, which utilizes a concentration of the patient's own platelets, is believed to release growth factors that can facilitate tissue healing and decrease plaque formation. In addition to these injectable therapies, H100 topical gel has emerged as a non-invasive treatment option [69]. This gel contains a combination of verapamil, a calcium channel blocker with anti-fibrotic effects, along with other active ingredients that aim to soften the plaques and improve penile curvature. Preliminary studies on H100 gel have shown promising results in reducing penile curvature and improving patient-reported outcomes. These novel therapies, though still under investigation, offer exciting new avenues for the management of Peyronie's disease, potentially improving efficacy while minimizing invasiveness compared to traditional surgical approaches.

Conclusion

Peyronie's disease is one of the most difficult conditions to treat in the field of andrology. Patients vary in the nature and severity of their symptoms, their level of psychological distress, and their desires and expectations for treatment. Treatment for this condition must take these variables into account. In general, in the acute phase of the disease, oral pharmacotherapy, such as anti-inflammatory medications, is indicated, along with psychological counseling. In the stable phase of the disease, a variety of treatment options are available to relieve the patient's sexual dysfunction. Various surgical treatments have been developed to correct penile curvature and have become the mainstay of treatment. However, each of these surgical procedures has its own disadvantages and should be used judiciously in properly selected patients. The recent development of collagenase clostridium histolyticum as an intralesional injection has opened up a new therapeutic option for nonsurgical treatment to reduce penile curvature, but cost is a concern. Advances in intralesional injections and newer drugs may alter the treatment in the future and lead to optimal management of the disease.

References

1. Mulhall JP, Schiff J, Guhring P. An analysis of the natural history of Peyronie's disease. J Urol. 2006;175(6):2115–8. discussion 2118
2. Grasso M, Lania C, Blanco S, Limonta G. The natural history of Peyronie's disease. Arch Esp Urol. 2007;60(3):326–31.
3. Berookhim BM, Choi J, Alex B, Mulhall JP. Deformity stabilization and improvement in men with untreated Peyronie's disease. BJU Int. 2014;113(1):133–6.
4. Hatzimouratidis K, Eardley I, Giuliano F, Hatzichristou D, Moncada I, Salonia A, et al. EAU guidelines on penile curvature. Eur Urol. 2012;62(3):543–52.
5. Chung E, Ralph D, Kagioglu A, Garaffa G, Shamsodini A, Bivalacqua T, et al. Evidence-based management guidelines on Peyronie's disease. J Sex Med. 2016;13(6):905–23.
6. Nehra A, Alterowitz R, Culkin DJ, Faraday MM, Hakim LS, Heidelbaugh JJ, et al. Peyronie's disease: AUA guideline. J Urol. 2015;194(3):745–53.
7. Somers KD, Dawson DM. Fibrin deposition in Peyronie's disease plaque. J Urol. 1997;157(1):311–5.
8. Mulhall JP. Expanding the paradigm for plaque development in Peyronie's disease. Int J Impot Res. 2003;15(Suppl 5):S93–102.
9. Mitsui Y, Yamabe F, Hori S, Uetani M, Kobayashi H, Nagao K, et al. Molecular mechanisms and risk factors related to the pathogenesis of Peyronie's disease. Int J Mol Sci. 2023;24(12):9583.
10. Sommer F, Schwarzer U, Wassmer G, Bloch W, Braun M, Klotz T, et al. Epidemiology of Peyronie's disease. Int J Impot Res. 2002;14(5):379–83.
11. Rhoden EL, Riedner CE, Fuchs SC, Ribeiro EP, Halmenschlager G. A cross-sectional study for the analysis of clinical, sexual and laboratory conditions associated with Peyronie's disease. J Sex Med. 2010;7(4 Pt 1):1529–37.
12. Mitsui Y, Kobayashi H, Yamabe F, Nakajima K, Nagao K. ABO blood type and risk of Peyronie's disease in Japanese males. World J Mens Health. 2022;40(3):509–16.
13. Di Maida F, Cito G, Lambertini L, Valastro F, Morelli G, Mari A, et al. The natural history of Peyronie's disease. World J Mens Health. 2021;39(3):399–405.
14. Arafa M, Eid H, El-Badry A, Ezz-Eldine K, Shamloul R. The prevalence of Peyronie's disease in diabetic patients with erectile dysfunction. Int J Impot Res. 2007;19(2):213–7.
15. Shindel AW, Sweet G, Thieu W, Durbin-Johnson B, Rothschild J, Szabo R. Prevalence of Peyronie's disease-like symptoms in men presenting with Dupuytren contractures. Sex Med. 2017;5(3):e135–41.
16. McCauley JF, Dean RC. Diagnostic utility of penile ultrasound in Peyronie's disease. World J Urol. 2020;38(2):263–8.
17. Lee HY, Pyun JH, Shim SR, Kim JH. Medical treatment for Peyronie's disease: systematic review and network Bayesian meta-analysis. World J Mens Health. 2024;42(1):133–47.
18. Joice GA, Burnett AL. Nonsurgical interventions for Peyronie's disease: update as of 2016. World J Mens Health. 2016;34(2):65–72.
19. Cai T, Tiscione D, Favilla V, Puglisi M, Palumbo F, Zucchi A, et al. Oral administration and intralesional injection of hyaluronic acid versus intralesional injection alone in Peyronie's disease: results from a phase III study. World J Mens Health. 2021;39(3):526–32.
20. Cocci A, Di Maida F, Russo GI, Di Mauro M, Cito G, Falcone M, et al. How atypical penile curvature influences clinical outcomes in patients with Peyronie's disease receiving collagenase clostridium histolyticum therapy. World J Mens Health. 2020;38(1):78–84.
21. Gelbard M, Lipshultz LI, Tursi J, Smith T, Kaufman G, Levine LA. Phase 2b study of the clinical efficacy and safety of collagenase clostridium histolyticum in patients with Peyronie's disease. J Urol. 2012;187(6):2268–74.
22. Gelbard M, Hellstrom WJ, McMahon CG, Levine LA, Smith T, Tursi J, et al. Baseline characteristics from an ongoing phase 3 study of collagenase Clostridium histolyticum in patients with Peyronie's disease. J Sex Med. 2013;10(11):2822–31.

23. Zhang F, Xiong Y, Wang W, Wu C, Qin F, Yuan J. The efficacy and safety of intralesional injection of collagenase Clostridium histolyticum for Peyronie's disease: a meta-analysis of published prospective studies. Front Pharmacol. 2022;13:973394.
24. Sun AJ, Li S, Eisenberg ML. The impact of Clostridium histolyticum collagenase on the prevalence and management of Peyronie's disease in the United States. World J Mens Health. 2019;37(2):234–9.
25. Duncan MR, Berman B, Nseyo UO. Regulation of the proliferation and biosynthetic activities of cultured human Peyronie's disease fibroblasts by interferons-alpha, -beta and -gamma. Scand J Urol Nephrol. 1991;25(2):89–94.
26. Kendirci M, Usta MF, Matern RV, Nowfar S, Sikka SC, Hellstrom WJ. The impact of intralesional interferon alpha-2b injection therapy on penile hemodynamics in men with Peyronie's disease. J Sex Med. 2005;2(5):709–15.
27. Hellstrom WJ, Kendirci M, Matern R, Cockerham Y, Myers L, Sikka SC, et al. Single-blind, multicenter, placebo controlled, parallel study to assess the safety and efficacy of intralesional interferon alpha-2B for minimally invasive treatment for Peyronie's disease. J Urol. 2006;176(1):394–8.
28. Cocci A, Di Maida F, Cito G, Verrienti P, Laruccia N, Campi R, et al. Comparison of intralesional hyaluronic acid vs. verapamil for the treatment of acute phase Peyronie's disease: a prospective, open-label non-randomized clinical study. World J Mens. Health. 2021;39(2):352–7.
29. Smith JF, Walsh TJ, Lue TF. Peyronie's disease: a critical appraisal of current diagnosis and treatment. Int J Impot Res. 2008;20(5):445–59.
30. Brant WO, Dean RC, Lue TF. Treatment of Peyronie's disease with oral pentoxifylline. Nat Clin Pract Urol. 2006;3(2):111–5. quiz 6
31. Chung E, Deyoung L, Brock GB. The role of PDE5 inhibitors in penile septal scar remodeling: assessment of clinical and radiological outcomes. J Sex Med. 2011;8(5):1472–7.
32. Chung E, Gillman M, Tuckey J, La Bianca S, Love C. A clinical pathway for the management of Peyronie's disease: integrating clinical guidelines from the International Society of Sexual Medicine, American urological association and European Urological Association. BJU Int. 2020;126(Suppl 1):12–7.
33. Martínez-Salamanca JI, Egui A, Moncada I, Minaya J, Ballesteros CM, Del Portillo L, et al. Acute phase Peyronie's disease management with traction device: a nonrandomized prospective controlled trial with ultrasound correlation. J Sex Med. 2014;11(2):506–15.
34. MacDonald LP, Armstrong ML, Lehmann KJ, Acker MR, Langille GM. Outcome analysis of patients with Peyronie's disease who elect for vacuum erection device therapy. Can Urol Assoc J. 2020;14(9):E428–31.
35. Husain J, Lynn NN, Jones DK, Collins GN, O'Reilly PH. Extracorporeal shock wave therapy in the management of Peyronie's disease: initial experience. BJU Int. 2000;86(4):466–8.
36. Kim KS, Choi YS, Bae WJ, Cho HJ, Ha US, Hong SH, et al. Efficacy of low-intensity extracorporeal shock wave therapy for the treatment of chronic pelvic pain syndrome IIIb: a prospective-randomized, double-blind, placebo-controlled study. World J Mens Health. 2022;40(3):473–80.
37. Chitale S, Morsey M, Swift L, Sethia K. Limited shock wave therapy vs sham treatment in men with Peyronie's disease: results of a prospective randomized controlled double-blind trial. BJU Int. 2010;106(9):1352–6.
38. Hatzichristodoulou G, Meisner C, Gschwend JE, Stenzl A, Lahme S. Extracorporeal shock wave therapy in Peyronie's disease: results of a placebo-controlled, prospective, randomized, single-blind study. J Sex Med. 2013;10(11):2815–21.
39. Di Mauro M, Russo GI, Della Camera PA, Di Maida F, Cito G, Mondaini N, et al. Extracorporeal shock wave therapy in Peyronie's disease: clinical efficacy and safety from a single-arm observational study. World J Mens Health. 2019;37(3):339–46.
40. Chung E. Penile reconstructive surgery in Peyronie disease: challenges in restoring normal penis size, shape, and function. World J Mens Health. 2020;38(1):1–8.

41. Segal RL, Burnett AL. Surgical management for Peyronie's disease. World J Mens Health. 2013;31(1):1–11.
42. Matsushita K, Stember DS, Nelson CJ, Mulhall JP. Concordance between patient and physician assessment of the magnitude of Peyronie's disease curvature. J Sex Med. 2014;11(1):205–10.
43. Kadioglu A, Kucukdurmaz F, Sanli O. Current status of the surgical management of Peyronie's disease. Nat Rev Urol. 2011;8(2):95–106.
44. Taylor FL, Levine LA. Surgical correction of Peyronie's disease via tunica albuginea plication or partial plaque excision with pericardial graft: long-term follow up. J Sex Med. 2008;5(9):2221–8. discussion 9–30
45. Nesbit RM. Congenital curvature of the phallus: report of three cases with description of corrective operation. J Urol. 1965;93:230–2.
46. Sokolakis I, Schonbauer P, Mykoniatis I, Kubler H, Gschwend J, Lahme S, et al. Long-term results after surgical treatment of congenital penile curvature using a modified Nesbit technique. World J Mens Health. 2020;38(4):564–72.
47. Carson CC, Levine LA. Outcomes of surgical treatment of Peyronie's disease. BJU Int. 2014;113(5):704–13.
48. Sassine AM, Wespes E, Schulman CC. Modified corporoplasty for penile curvature: 10 years' experience. Urology. 1994;44(3):419–21.
49. Licht MR, Lewis RW. Modified Nesbit procedure for the treatment of Peyronie's disease: a comparative outcome analysis. J Urol. 1997;158(2):460–3.
50. Yachia D. Modified corporoplasty for the treatment of penile curvature. J Urol. 1990;143(1):80–2.
51. Nooter RI, Bosch JL, Schroder FH. Peyronie's disease and congenital penile curvature: long-term results of operative treatment with the plication procedure. Br J Urol. 1994;74(4):497–500.
52. Klevmark B, Andersen M, Schultz A, Talseth T. Congenital and acquired curvature of the penis treated surgically by plication of the tunica albuginea. Br J Urol. 1994;74(4):501–6.
53. Thiounn N, Missirliu A, Zerbib M, Larrouy M, Dje K, Flam T, et al. Corporeal plication for surgical correction of penile curvature. Experience with 60 patients. Eur Urol. 1998;33(4):401–4.
54. Chahal R, Gogoi NK, Sundaram SK, Weston PM. Corporal plication for penile curvature caused by Peyronie's disease: the patients' perspective. BJU Int. 2001;87(4):352–6.
55. Geertsen UA, Brok KE, Andersen B, Nielsen HV. Peyronie curvature treated by plication of the penile fasciae. Br J Urol. 1996;77(5):733–5.
56. Mulhall J, Anderson M, Parker M. A surgical algorithm for men with combined Peyronie's disease and erectile dysfunction: functional and satisfaction outcomes. J Sex Med. 2005;2(1):132–8.
57. Langston JP, Carson CC 3rd. Peyronie disease: plication or grafting. Urol Clin North Am. 2011;38(2):207–16.
58. Devine CJ Jr, Horton CE. Surgical treatment of Peyronie's disease with a dermal graft. J Urol. 1974;111(1):44–9.
59. Garcia-Gomez B, Ralph D, Levine L, Moncada-Iribarren I, Djinovic R, Albersen M, et al. Grafts for Peyronie's disease: a comprehensive review. Andrology. 2018;6(1):117–26.
60. Teloken C, Grazziotin T, Rhoden E, Da Ros C, Fornari A, Soares FC, et al. Penile straightening with crural graft of the corpus cavernosum. J Urol. 2000;164(1):107–8.
61. Da Ros CT, Graziottin TM, Ribeiro E, Averbeck MA. Long-term follow-up of penile curvature correction utilizing autologous albugineal crural graft. Int Braz J Urol. 2012;38(2):242–7. discussion 8–9
62. Collins JP. Experience with lyophilized human dura for treatment of Peyronie disease. Urology. 1988;31(5):379–81.
63. Lahme S, Gotz T, Bichler KH. Collagen fleece for defect coverage following plaque excision in patients with Peyronie's disease. Eur Urol. 2002;41(4):401–5.
64. Schiffman ZJ, Gursel EO, Laor E. Use of Dacron patch graft in Peyronie disease. Urology. 1985;25(1):38–40.

65. Faerber GJ, Konnak JW. Results of combined Nesbit penile plication with plaque incision and placement of Dacron patch in patients with severe Peyronie's disease. J Urol. 1993;149(5 Pt 2):1319–20.
66. Ganabathi K, Dmochowski R, Zimmern PE, Leach GE. Peyronie's disease: surgical treatment based on penile rigidity. J Urol. 1995;153(3 Pt 1):662–6.
67. Asmundo MG, Durukan E, von Rohden E, Thy SA, Jensen CFS, Fode M. Platelet-rich plasma therapy in erectile dysfunction and Peyronie's disease: a systematic review of the literature. World J Urol. 2024;42(1):359.
68. Israeli JM, Lokeshwar SD, Efimenko IV, Masterson TA, Ramasamy R. The potential of platelet-rich plasma injections and stem cell therapy for penile rejuvenation. Int J Impot Res. 2022;34(4):375–82.
69. Twidwell J, Mahon J, Tortorelis D, Levine L. Transdermal application of H100 gel to the penile shaft in patients with Peyronie's disease infiltrates the tunica albuginea. Int J Impot Res. 2024;36(2):107–9.

Chapter 24
Diagnosis and Management of Ejaculatory Dysfunction

Eric Chung, Balantine Eze, and Selahittin Çayan

Introduction

Ejaculation and orgasm can be distinct yet synchronized events that occur at the peak of sexual arousal culminating in overall sexual satisfaction. The interplay between the 'objective' (i.e. ejaculation) and 'subjective' (i.e. orgasmic) elements of male sexual climax are complex and remain incompletely understood. While most men have some control over the timing of ejaculation during a sexual encounter, men who ejaculate before or shortly after penetration, without a sense of control, or unable to ejaculate after prolonged sexual intimacy, will experience psychosexual distress related to ejaculatory dysfunction (EjD). The spectrum of EjD extends from premature ejaculation (PE) and retrograde ejaculation (RE) to delayed ejaculation (DE) and anejaculation (AE) [7, 21, 24, 50, 58]. The specific diagnosis is determined by whether ejaculation occurs early, late or not at all.

E. Chung (✉)
Department of Urology, Princess Alexandra Hospital, University of Queensland, Brisbane, QLD, Australia

AndroUrology Centre, Brisbane, QLD, Australia

B. Eze
Global Andrology Forum, Moreland Hills, OH, USA

Urology Division, Department of Surgery, Enugu State University of Science and Technology Teaching Hospital, Enugu, Nigeria
e-mail: balantine.eze@esut.edu.ng

S. Çayan
Global Andrology Forum, Moreland Hills, OH, USA

Faculty of Medicine, Department of Urology, Mersin University, Mersin, Turkey

E. Chung et al. (eds.), *Advances in Andrology*,
https://doi.org/10.1007/978-3-032-29112-7_24

While PE and RE are well-defined with set criteria, DE, AE and anorgasmia are among the least common and least understood domains of male sexual health dysfunction [39, 45, 58]. Current treatment strategies for EjD involve psychosexual counselling, behavioural modifications, topical and mechanical devices, as well as pharmaceutical and surgical interventions. It is important to understand the complex nature of the human mind and the interactions between various neurobiology and pelvic structures responsible for male ejaculation [45, 50, 58]. Hence, no one treatment likely solves EjD but rather a holistic, multifaceted approach that is personalized to one's needs and preferences to the maximum clinical efficacy and least side effect profile.

The following book chapter provides a narrative review of the various definitions and underlying pathophysiological mechanisms responsible for PE, RE, DE and AE. This review provides a targeted clinical assessment and an overview of the treatment strategies will be covered although it is impossible to provide a full comprehensive review on this very broad topic of EjD.

Definitions

Major scientific organisations have carefully defined PE based on two key factors namely the lack of control with a short time to ejaculation during coitus and the ensuing psychosexual distress experienced by the patient. The International Society of Sexual Medicine (ISSM) and subsequently the International Consultation on Sexual Medicine (ICSM) defined PE as 'a male sexual dysfunction characterized by ejaculation which always or nearly always occurs prior to or within about one minute of vaginal penetration (lifelong PE), or, a clinically significant and bothersome reduction in latency time, often to about 3 min or less (acquired PE), with associated negative personal consequences, such as distress, bother, frustration, and/or the avoidance of sexual intimacy' [39, 47, 52].

On the other hand, the American Psychiatric Association's Diagnostic and Statistical Manual of Mental Disorders 5th edition (DSM-V) defines PE as 'a persistent or recurrent pattern of ejaculation occurring during partnered sexual activity within approximately 1 minute following vaginal penetration and before the individual wishes it' with this disorder must be present in 75% or more of sexual encounters and persistent over at least the last 6 months and the man must experience personal distress related to the dysfunction, and the condition cannot be better explained by a comorbid or concomitant diagnosis [8]. The DSM-V definition permits the categorization of PE into lifelong versus acquired and generalized versus situational sub-types. Similarly, the World Health Organization's International Classification of Diseases 11th edition (ICD-11) mirrors that of DSM-V to define PE as 'ejaculation that occurs prior to or within a very short duration of the initiation of vaginal penetration or other relevant sexual stimulation, with no or little perceived control over ejaculation' and 'the pattern of early ejaculation has occurred episodically or persistently over a period of at least several months and is associated with clinically significant distress' [26].

In contrast to the specific end-point criteria to define PE, the exact definition of DE appears more ambiguous and not time-defined [46]. Patients with DE experience difficulty achieving sexual climax, sometimes to the point that they are unable to climax during sexual activity. The ISSM and ICSM defined DE as the persistent or recurrent difficulty, delay in, or absence of attaining orgasm after sufficient sexual stimulation, which causes personal distress, and that DE is further subclassified as lifelong and acquired (secondary) DE [39]. Lifelong, alternatively classified as primary, delayed ejaculation was defined as a lifelong experience or inability to ejaculate in almost all (75–100%) occasions of coital activity, associated with distress. Voluntary cessation of coital activity may subsequently occur after a variable time to avoid frustration, physical exhaustion or genital irritation of self or partner. Men with lifelong DE might or might not be able to achieve ejaculation by subsequent non-coital activity, including masturbation. The DSM-V also defines DE as the condition in which a man experiences 'a marked delay in ejaculation' or 'marked infrequency or absence of ejaculation' and the disorder must be present in 75% or more of partnered sexual encounters and persistent over at least the last 6 months, with the patient must not desire delay of ejaculation and he must experience personal distress [8].

On the other hand, RE is a unique form of EjD that refers to the condition in which semen is not ejected antegrade but rather flows into the bladder during climax [26]. Interestingly, it does not specify whether there is an early ejaculatory component although to qualify for the strict definition of RE, a post-orgasmic urine sample should be collected to confirm the presence of spermatozoa.

AE refers specifically to the absence of seminal ejaculation with sexual climax and may be subclassified as (1) emission less; when the patient is unable to discharge semen into the posterior urethra, and (2) expulsion less; when the patient is unable to vigorously discharge semen from the external urethral meatus [27, 39, 58]. Anorgasmia may be conceptualized as an extreme variant of DE or AE in which orgasm cannot be achieved. The ICD-11 defines anorgasmia as 'the absence or marked infrequency of the orgasm experience or markedly diminished intensity of orgasmic sensations. The pattern of absence, delay or diminished frequency or intensity of orgasm occurs despite adequate sexual stimulation, including the desire for sexual activity and orgasm, has occurred episodically or persistently over a period of at least several months, and is associated with clinically significant distress' [26].

Ejaculatory dysfunction has a wide range of severity as symptomatology varies based on subjective interpretation by the patient. Moreover, there is no standard characterization of symptom bother as an unbearable change in sexual function to one man who may be of little bother to another. The term dysfunction is thus reserved for ejaculatory issues that cause significant distress to the patient.

Pathophysiology and Neurobiology of Various Forms of EjD

The male sexual response cycle is thought to occur in four stages sexual excitement and fulfilment, starting with sexual desire and followed by arousal, then climax and finally resolution. The sexual climax consists of orgasm, a sensation of intense pleasure, relaxation or intimacy that accompanies peak sexual arousal, followed by ejaculation with antegrade expulsion of semen from the penis [4]. While these events occur typically simultaneously, these are distinct physiological processes that may occur, or not occur, independently.

The process of ejaculation is highly coordinated and modulated through a network of spinal centres (see Fig. 24.1). The ejaculatory reflex comprises sensory receptors and areas, afferent pathways, cerebral sensory areas, cerebral motor centres, spinal motor centres and efferent pathways. Ejaculation is triggered by the integration of tactile (e.g. sensation from genital or other peripheral nerves) and non-tactile (e.g. sexually arousing audio and visual inputs) stimuli in the brain. Although ejaculation occurs in the pelvis, central nervous system (CNS) involvement plays a critical role, and various aspects of the brain such as the amygdala, hypothalamus, and cerebellum are connected through a complex ejaculatory network to the spinal 'ejaculatory' centres [22]. Neurotransmitters involved include dopamine, norepinephrine, serotonin, acetylcholine, oxytocin, gamma-aminobutyric acid and nitric oxide although it emerged that the balance between dopamine and serotonin is critical to normal ejaculation. In general, dopaminergic and oxytocinergic activation stimulates ejaculation and orgasm whereas serotonergic and GABA-ergic activation opposes ejaculation and orgasm.

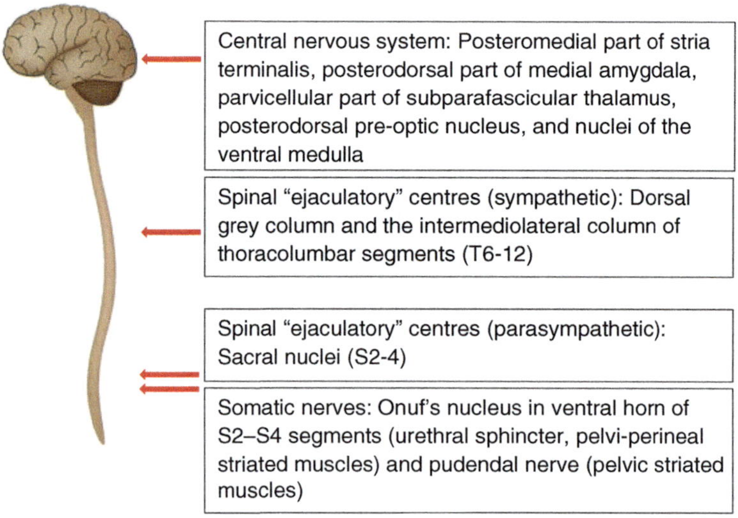

Fig. 24.1 Ejaculatory reflex is highly coordinated and modulated through a network of sensory receptors and areas, afferent pathways, cerebral sensory areas, cerebral motor centres, spinal motor centres and efferent pathways

Within the spinal centre, the dorsal grey column and the intermediolateral column of thoracolumbar segments provide sympathetic outflow while the sacral parasympathetic nuclei are responsible for parasympathetic outflow. Somatic fibres innervating the urethral sphincter and pelvi-perineal striated muscles are located in Onuf's nucleus, in the ventral horn of S2–S4 segments. It is thought that the sympathetic effect is dominant during ejaculation, responsible for controlling the contractile activity of the seminal tract smooth muscle. The role of the parasympathetic nervous system in ejaculation remains somewhat unclear, and is thought to play a role in preventing the reflux of seminal fluid through the ejaculatory duct, as well as the secretion of seminal fluid. Finally, somatic fibres carried by the pudendal nerve are thought to play a role in ejaculation through control of pelvic striated muscles [4, 16]. The penis is innervated by a complex system of somatic and autonomic nerve fibres that mediate sexual response. The dorsal nerve branches from the pudendal nerve provides somatic innervation to the penis and mediates contraction of the pelvic floor muscles to achieve rigidity and plays a role in discharging ejaculatory fluid.

Ejaculation consists of two distinct phases namely emission and expulsion of seminal fluid. Emission is a centrally mediated action characterized by the secretion of seminal fluid (from seminal vesicles, prostate and bulbourethral glands) into the proximal urethra, closure of the bladder neck, and contraction of smooth muscles throughout the seminal tract (mediated by the sympathetic nervous system). The expulsion of seminal fluid, a reflex driven by the somatic nervous system (pudendal nerve) with nominal input elicited through an involuntary sympathetic spinal cord reflex, consists of rhythmic contractions of the bulbospongiosus and ischiocavernous muscles leading to forceful expulsion of seminal fluid from the urethral meatus and penis. Normal antegrade ejaculation relies heavily on the normal function of the prostate and bladder neck.

Orgasm is the cerebral processing of sensory stimuli from the pudendal nerve related to the pleasurable sensation associated with the contraction of the relevant pelvic muscles and presents a transient neurological state characterized by intense feelings of pleasure, relaxation and intimacy [4, 16, 22]. Orgasm is typically experienced at peak sexual arousal and is followed in men by a refractory period during which arousal and sexual climax are not possible.

Diagnostic Evaluation

The key to identifying the various forms of EjD resides in the accurate diagnosis of the sexual complaint. It is important to distinguish whether the patient has EjD or other forms of male sexual dysfunction such as low sexual desire, erectile dysfunction or orgasmic, disorders. In many instances, it is not uncommon for these sexual complaints to coexist together since the underlying pathophysiology and contributing causes could be similar [36, 39, 45, 50, 58]. The history should establish the time of onset of EjD, whether ejaculation occurs on every/almost every attempt and with every partner, latency time to ejaculation and the presence or absence of other sexual dysfunction/s such as erection or orgasm. Questionnaires such as the Premature Ejaculatory Diagnostic Toll (PEDT), Premature Ejaculation Profile (PEP), and the Male Sexual Health Questionnaire (MSHQ) have been validated for use to provide a clearer diagnosis [39, 50, 58]. The time between penetration and ejaculation, the patient's ability to control or delay ejaculation, and the presence and extent of negative psychological consequences such as bother, distress and/or the avoidance of sexual activity are keys to the diagnosis of EjD. The interpersonal dynamics, relationship stress. Presence of dyspareunia, genital pain disorder, history of STI, a sexual aversion disorder and/or any other sexual dysfunction in the patient and his partner should be established. The identification of other relevant factors such as medical comorbidities (such as mental well-being, cardiovascular disease, diabetes mellitus, thyroid disorders, neurological conditions or pelvic dysfunction) and certain medications (such as antidepressants, antipsychotics, opioids, benzodiazepines or recreational drugs) can play a critical role in the development and/or progression of EjD [36, 45, 50, 58].

A focused physical examination is useful to assess for risk factors and exclude causal diseases such as testicular mass, prostate abnormality, penile deformity or signs of neurological disorders. Various standardized questionnaires have been developed to aid the diagnosis of specific male sexual dysfunction and these include validated instruments such as the Male Sexual Health Questionnaire, Male Sexual Quotient, Index of Premature Ejaculation, Premature Ejaculation Profile or the Premature Ejaculation Diagnostic Tool. Laboratory or imaging studies are rarely required although serum testosterone should be pursued as indicated and PSA for suspected prostatitis [36, 45, 50, 58]. Urine culture and STI screen may be conducted in the setting of patients with a history of urethral discharge, hematuria or STI. It is also important to establish whether ejaculation is absent or (actually) retrograde by examining the presence of spermatozoa in post-ejaculation first void urine. Highly specialized investigations such as nerve conduction studies and functional brain imaging tests are usually conducted by specialists following appropriate consultation and only in carefully selected patients with EjD. Cystoscopy can be both diagnostic and therapeutic in the settings of urethral stricture or ejaculatory duct obstruction.

Clinical Management for PE, DE and AE

Clinical management for PE, DE and AE in terms of providing a holistic and multidisciplinary approach with the incorporation of the following treatments.

1. Psychosexual and behavioural modifications
2. Pharmacological agents—established and novel drugs
3. Surgical interventions

Psychosexual and Behavioural Modifications

The major aim of psychosexual and behavioural modification therapy in the management of ejaculatory dysfunction is to identify psychological issues such as performance anxiety, strains in interpersonal relationships and loss of self-confidence occasioned by a history of non-satisfactory sexual performances that may have contributed to the development of ejaculatory dysfunction. To address those issues psychosexual and behavioural modification therapy plays a key role [5].

Psychotherapy is usually given by psychologists or sex therapists who are specially trained and dedicated to administering this type of therapy. Therapy sessions could be held for individuals, couples or as a group therapy. Psychosocial variables are always important to consider in the setting of delayed ejaculation (DE). The fact that approximately 75% of males with DE can achieve ejaculation through solitary masturbation, infers that a large proportion of DE is influenced by psychological or environmental factors and can be ameliorated by psychosexual and behavioural therapy [40].

Behavioural modification therapy works by helping men recognize mid-level ranges of excitement before the point where ejaculation becomes inevitable and helping them delay ejaculation by decreasing stimulation. This can be achieved by the man contracting the pelvic muscles and or his partner firmly squeezing the glans penis between the thumb ventrally and the index/middle fingers dorsally (squeeze technique); or temporal withdrawal or/and change of position or a pause in thrusting movement (start/stop technique). Behavioural modification therapy techniques commonly supplement psychotherapeutic modalities [38]. These behavioural modification techniques function by gradually increasing IELT, sexual confidence and self-esteem [38]. For delayed ejaculation, behavioural modification therapy involves asking individuals and couples to experiment with various forms of sexual stimulation, such as manual stimulation of the penis or perineum, oral sex, use of lubricants or vibrators, or change in position, as this additional stimulation may trigger orgasm [40].

Usually, psychological therapy, behavioural therapy and pharmacotherapy are combined to harness the synergistic power of these therapies to provide patients with ejaculatory dysfunction rapid symptom improvement. This is important because of the multifaceted domains of sex and ejaculation which are often affected by the complex interplay of psychological, religious, social and biological factors.

Established Pharmacotherapy

Some medications have been tested over time and proven to be effective in the management of ejaculatory dysfunction (see Table 24.1). Most of the medications are prescribed off-label without the approval of governmental regulatory

Table 24.1 Established drugs for ejaculatory dysfunction

Drugs	Mechanism of action	Ejaculatory dysfunction
Selective serotonin reuptake inhibitors	Increases the concentration of serotonin in the synaptic junction by inhibiting the post-synaptic reuptake	Premature ejaculation
Tricyclic antidepressants	Inhibiting serotonin and norepinephrine reuptake within the presynaptic terminals	Premature ejaculation
Opioids	Acts on opioid mu-receptor agonist and weak serotonin-norepinephrine receptor inhibitor activities	Premature ejaculation
PDE5 inhibitors	Inhibits the breakdown of cyclic guanosine monophosphate	Premature ejaculation
Topical anaesthetics	Reduces glans sensitivity	Premature ejaculation
Cabergoline	Dopamine D2 receptor agonist that increases dopamine neurotransmission and reduces the level of prolactin	Delayed ejaculation or anejaculation
Bupropion	Inhibits the reuptake of dopamine and norepinephrine	Delayed ejaculation or anejaculation
Flibanserin	Serotonin 1A agonist and a serotonin 2A antagonist	Delayed ejaculation or anejaculation
Pseudoephedrine or phenylephrine, and midodrine	Alpha-adrenergic agonist	Retrograde ejaculation

agencies except paroxetine which has received approval for the management of PE in more than 50 countries [32]. These medications include the following classes of drugs.

Selective Serotonin Reuptake Inhibitors (SSRI)

The use of SSRIs has revolutionized and has become the bedrock of the pharmacological management of premature ejaculation. Drugs in this class have become first-line drugs and work by increasing the concentration of serotonin in the synaptic junction by inhibiting the post-synaptic reuptake of serotonin and exploiting the inhibitory effect of serotonin on ejaculation to increase the intravaginal ejaculatory latency time [6]. SSRIs can be administered on demand (4–6 h before intercourse) or daily. Daily treatment is preferable for people with lifelong premature ejaculation but is less effective in ejaculation delay [41, 61].

Unwanted side effects may occur at the onset of treatment but usually resolve within 2–3 weeks of initiation of therapy with SSRI. These include fatigue, nausea, diarrhoea, increased perspiration, reduced sexual desire and erectile dysfunction [20, 32]. SSRI should be avoided in men less than 18 years of age (because of increased risk of suicidal ideation/suicide) and in men with a history of bipolar disorder (because of increased rate of agitation and hypomania) [35].

SSRIs usually used in the treatment of PE include paroxetine (10–40 mg/day), sertraline (50–200 mg/day), fluoxetine (20–40 mg/day) and citalopram (20–40 mg/day). They are safe, well-tolerated and effective. Paroxetine has been shown to be the most efficacious in increasing IELT over baseline [32, 65]. Since patients can experience SSRI withdrawal symptoms (dizziness, headache, nausea, vomiting, diarrhoea and irritation), sudden cessation of therapy with SSRI or rapid dose reduction is not advised.

Dapoxetine is the first to receive approval specifically as a drug for the treatment of PE. As a short-acting SSRI with a half-life of about 1.4 h [34], it is suitable for on-demand use (1–2 h) before intercourse) and has been found to increase IELT in a dose-dependent fashion [12]. It is rapidly absorbed and eliminated, with minimal accumulation and no withdrawal symptoms after abrupt discontinuation and reduction of dosage. In men with PE and erectile dysfunction, it is effective and well-tolerated in combination with phosphodiesterase-5 inhibitors (PDE5i) [63]. Treatment-related ASEs were uncommon, dose-dependent and largely mild to moderate in severity. The most common adverse events are headache (5.6–8.8%), dizziness (5.9–10.9%) and nausea (11.0–22.2%) Severe or serious side effects occurred infrequently in less than 5% of patients and included syncope [63]. The usual daily dose is 30–60 mg.

Tricyclic Antidepressants (TCA)

The only tricyclic antidepressant that has been in use for premature ejaculation is clomipramine. It also has a serotonin-norepinephrine reuptake inhibitor effect. It is used as a second line to SSRI because it has more adverse effects. Adverse effects are common and occur in more than 50% of patients [18] taking these medications and are attributable to their antimuscarinic effects; they include dry mouth, constipation, loss of appetite, sleepiness, weight gain, sexual dysfunction and obstructive lower urinary tract symptoms [31]. It can be used on demand (2–6 h before intercourse) or daily at a dose of 12.5–50 mg/day. Sudden cessation of medications and dose reduction can cause withdrawal symptoms (dizziness, headache, sweating).

Opioids

Opioids have been used off-label for the treatment of PE. Tramadol is a centrally acting opioid mu-receptor agonist but its efficacy in treating PE is due to its SSRI and weak serotonin-norepinephrine receptor inhibitor (SNRI) activities [12]. Tramadol at a dose of 25–100 mg are safe and effective and can be used on a daily dosing regimen or on demand [30]. Tramadol is often not used as first-line therapy for PE as it is associated with more adverse side effects (terminal dribble, ED, somnolence, headache, dizziness, constipation, nausea, vomiting, dry mouth, dizziness, pruritus and vomiting) than paroxetine [37]. There is also a potential for addiction since it is an opioid.

PDE5 Inhibitors

PDE5 inhibitors as monotherapy for the treatment of PE have yielded mixed results. It is usually used in combination with SSRI. Even though PDE5i's are significantly more effective than placebo at increasing IELT [10], therapy for isolated PE or PE associated with ED with SSRIs plus PDE-5 inhibitors is associated with a significantly greater increase in mean IELT compared with SSRI or PDE-5 inhibitor alone [11].

Topical Anaesthetics

Topical/ local therapy for PE is appealing as an effective topical therapy that will circumvent the systemic effects of oral therapy. Topical anaesthetics work under the assumption that PE may result from increased/abnormally high glans sensitivity and that topical anaesthetics can reduce glans sensitivity and thereby delay ejaculation. Common topical local anaesthetics available as a cream, gel or spray for the management of PE include EMLA (a cream consisting of 2.5 g prilocaine eutectic and 2.5 lidocaine), Severance Secret (SS) cream (a mixture of *Bufonis veneum* extract, *Asiasari radix* extract, *Caryophylli flos* extract, *Cinnamomicortex* extract, and Ginseng Radix Alba fructose), topical eutectic mixture for premature ejaculation (TEMPE) or PSD502 (a combination of 7.5 mg prilocaine eutectic mixture and 22.5 mg lidocaine), and lidocaine spray 5% [11]. Though topical anaesthetics have been found to increase IELT in men with premature ejaculation more effectively than placebo, sildenafil, tadalafil, paroxetine and dapoxetine, they have unique adverse effects which include reduced sensation in the penile shaft, loss of erection, localized irritations and (when not used with a condom) numbing of the partner's vagina and female anorgasmia [53].

Dopamine Receptor Agonist/Dopamine Reuptake Inhibitors

Cabergoline is a potent dopamine receptor agonist and acts at D2 receptors. By increasing dopamine neurotransmission and reducing the level of prolactin, it is thought to promote ejaculation. Cabergoline is usually administered at a dose of 0.5 mg twice/week. Bupropion is an atypical antidepressant that inhibits the reuptake of dopamine and norepinephrine. Compared to other antidepressants, bupropion has been shown to have lower rates of adverse sexual side effects and may even enhance sexual function in some patients; it is commonly used as an agent in depressed men when SSRIs cause delayed or anejaculation at a daily dose of 150–300 mg [20].

Hormonal Treatment

Hormonal regulation plays a critical role in the physiology of orgasm and ejaculation. Correction of identified endocrinopathies has a crucial place in the treatment of DE. Testosterone replacement has been evaluated as a potential treatment for DE. Corona et al. [17] compared T levels among 2437 men with PE or DE versus those without ejaculatory dysfunction and demonstrated lower total and free T levels among patients with DE; patients with DE also had a higher prevalence of testosterone deficiency than patients with PE. In men with DE with proven testosterone deficiency, a trial of testosterone therapy, preferably a short-acting testosterone formulation (administered 1 h before sexual activity), is considered [43].

Novel Pharmacotherapy

The search for the ideal drugs for ejaculatory dysfunctions is still on. Emphasis has shifted from developing drugs targeting specific receptors such as α-1 adrenergic antagonists and oxytocin agonists to new targets such as the serotonin receptors. Efforts have also been made to develop new formulations and combinations of traditional therapeutic agents.

PSD502 is a novel compound of lidocaine-prilocaine delivered as an aerosolized metered spray. PSD502 has received marketing approval in Europe but is not yet available as a licensed prescription in the United States [13]. Its novel design allows only shallow penetration into the mucosa of the glans penis, and therefore the keratinized skin of the shaft is not affected. There are minimal reports of transfer to partners due to this non-penetrating unique formulation.

Dyclonine is a local anesthetic usually used in dentistry and alprostadil is a vasodilator/prostaglandin E1. A topical mixture of dyclonine and alprostadil in a cream formulation has been evaluated as a treatment for PE. The product is applied 5–20 min before intercourse to the tip of the penis in the region of the meatus and has been found to reduce the degree of stimulation to the penis. These topical formulations when used alone or when used as an adjunct to either SSRIs or PDE5 inhibitors have been reported to be more effective in PE than a placebo [32].

Because emission and ejaculation are under the control of the sympathetic component of the autonomic nervous system, α-adrenergic antagonists can delay ejaculation and increase IELT. Several α-adrenergic antagonists have been tried but only

Silodosin, a selective $\alpha 1$A-adrenoceptor antagonist is very effective in improving symptoms and increasing IELT in patients with PE following on-demand use of 4 mg silodosin orally 1 h before sexual intercourse [51].

Botulinum toxin is a biological exotoxin with high potency produced by gram-positive *Clostridium botulinum.* Out of the seven serotypes available, only type A and type B are useful clinically [9]. Botulinum toxin A can theoretically help patients with PE by inhibiting the rhythmic contractions of the bulbospongiosus muscle during ejaculation. More studies still need to be done to determine the efficacy and safety of Botulinum toxin A injection into the bulbospongiosus muscle for the management of PE as available studies show mixed results [3, 54].

For delayed ejaculation, efforts continue to be made by researchers to develop medications that increase neurotransmitters in the brain that promote ejaculation (dopamine or oxytocin) or decrease inhibitory neurotransmitters (serotonin) to treat this disorder. Drugs that have shown some positive results include amantadine, cyproheptadine, yohimbine, buspirone, and bethanechol [43].

Flibanserin is a drug that has been approved by the Food and Drug Administration (FDA) in the USA for the treatment of hypoactive sexual desire disorder in both pre and post-menopausal women. Flibanserin is both a serotonin agonist and antagonist. It is a serotonin 1A agonist and a serotonin 2A antagonist and can improve sexual desire by enhancing the downstream release of dopamine and norepinephrine that enhances sex desire while reducing the inhibitory effect of serotonin release in the brain circuits responsible for reduced sexual interest and desire [59]. Off-label use of flibanserin has been shown to be helpful for primary anorgasmia though with some side effects [48].

Surgical Interventions in Premature Ejaculation

Surgical or interventional methods may be indicated for patients with premature ejaculation who have no response or poor response to pharmacological, psychological, and behavioural therapies. These methods for the interventional treatment of premature ejaculation include selective penile dorsal nerve resection, cryoablation and pulsed radiofrequency, pudendal neuromodulation, injection of materials into the glans penis with hyaluronic acid, Botulinum toxin A injection into the bulbospongiosus muscles, implantation of graft material under Buck fascia, neuromuscular electrical stimulation of the pelvic floor muscles and transcutaneous posterior tibial nerve stimulation [21, 23, 58, 62].

Selective Penile Dorsal Neurectomy

Penile sensitivity plays one of the key roles among the pathologic mechanisms of premature ejaculation. The number of dorsal nerve branches positively correlated with penile sensitivity [23]. Therefore, selective dorsal neurectomy for decreasing penile sensitivity is a promising treatment for patients with lifelong PE who have no or poor response to medical therapy or refuse oral medication. It is an invasive and irreversible treatment procedure and has been applied as a separate procedure or combined with penile glans augmentation. After circumcision incision, the dorsal nerve of the penis can be identified, and 3–4 branches of the penile dorsal nerve are removed at high magnification such as loop or microscope. Although the current guidelines do not suggest penile dorsal neurectomy as a treatment option in patients with premature ejaculation, it provides an efficacy rate of 90% with a significant increase in IELT [33, 64]. In a study by Liu et al., they demonstrated the dorsal penile nerve branches of patients with lifelong PE were larger in numbers and thicker than those without lifelong PE, and selective dorsal neurectomy was effective in improving lifelong PE by IELT prolongation and ejaculation controllability, with few post-operative complications. However, it has no widespread application areas, because of its side effects including penile numbness, penile pain and penile paresthesia [29].

Cryoablation and Pulsed Radiofrequency

It has been tried to treat resistant patients with PE by cryoablation or pulsed radiofrequency neuromodulation of the dorsal penile dorsal nerve to reduce hypersensitive peripheral sexual input signals and inhibit penile hypersensitivity [23]. In a study of 15 men with PE, IELT increased from 18.5 to 139.9 s at 3 weeks after the pulsed radiofrequency procedure with no side effects [12].

Implantation of Graft Materials

Penile sensitivity is considered to be one of the key pathologic mechanisms of PE. An acellular dermal matrix graft as an inner condom was inserted into Buck's fascia as the subcutaneous pocket of the penis in 20 men with PE [62]. After the procedure, the IELT significantly increased from 0.67 to 2.37 min with no serious complications or adverse effects.

Injections Materials into the Glans Penis

Injection materials have been considered to make bulky barriers that reduce the access of tactile stimuli to sensation receptors of the glandular penis. Hyaluronic acid is the mainly used injection material [49, 55, 66]. Glans penis augmentation using hyaluronic acid is proposed to act as a bulking agent that blocks accessibility and inhibits tactile stimulation of the dorsal nerve receptors to improve ejaculatory control and ejaculation latency time. After local anaesthesia to the skin of the glans penis for 30 min, approximately 2 ml of hyaluronic acid is injected into the different parts of the glans penis via a 30-gauge needle. The efficacy and safety of glans penis augmentation with hyaluronic acid has been demonstrated in the studies. However, most studies are low quality with no control group and lack of long-term follow-up. In the prospective controlled studies, the mean IELT highly significantly increased to approximately 350 s with the hyaluronic acid injections, compared to controls [49, 55, 66]. In addition to an increase in the IELT, hyaluronic acid provided approximately 2 cm girth enhancement compared to controls in a multicenter randomized controlled trial [2]. IELT also significantly increased from 5.36 ± 3.51 to 7.86 ± 4.73 min in the hyaluronic acid injection group and from 5.23 ± 3.55 to 6.43 ± 4.22 min in the controls with no serious adverse events in both group. Although studies reported no severe complications, some case reports showing glans necrosis, fibrosis and granuloma formations have been reported. Therefore, the possibility of such complications should be explained with caution to patients who desire such injections.

Botulinum Toxin A Injection

Botulinum toxin A injections have been used in the treatment of different urogenital disorders especially to increase bladder capacity and to decrease involuntary bladder contractions. The idea of using Botulinum toxin A injections into the bulbospongiosus muscle in the treatment of premature ejaculation is to inhibit rhythmic contractions of the bulbospongiosus and ischiocavernosus muscles, leading to a decreased expulsion phase of the ejaculation. The efficacy of injection usually starts at one week and lasts approximately 6–9 months. In a recent randomized controlled trial, 98 men with lifelong PE were randomized as a 100-unit injection into two bulbospongiosus muscles and saline injection as a placebo group [54]. The treatment group showed notably extended intravaginal ejaculatory latency times, compared to their initial performance after treatment. In addition, there were enhancements in PEP scores, and notably, no significant complications were reported. In another recently published prospective randomized study, the treatment group with the same injection (100 units of Botulinum toxin) failed to prove clinical efficacy for the treatment of lifelong premature ejaculation when compared to a placebo [3]. Therefore, the guidelines suggest the use of Botulinum toxin A injections as an experimental therapy, and should not be offered to patients with premature ejaculation in clinical practice.

Neuromuscular Electrical Stimulation

Electrical stimulation of pelvic floor muscles before planned sexual activity can prevent the rhythmic contractions necessary for completing the ejaculatory process by maintaining sub-tetanic continuous contraction and prolonging the ejaculation time in patients with PE. In an experimental rat study, low-frequency (2 Hz) electrical stimulation applied to the male rats significantly prolonged the ejaculation time [15]. A prospective, single-blinded, self-controlled study, consisting of 23 patients with lifelong PE, found 85% experienced prolonged masturbation ejaculatory latency time (MELT) under transcutaneous electrical stimulation (TES) compared with the sham treatment, with the mean MELT values increased 3.5-fold under TES [57]. In another prospective, randomized double-blind clinical study, 51 patients with lifelong PE were randomized as the treatment and control group to assess the feasibility, safety and efficacy of the vPatch, a miniaturized on-demand perineal transcutaneous electrical stimulation device for treating PE [56]. The baseline geometric mean IELT significantly increased from 67 to 123 s in the TES group, compared with an insignificant increase from 63 to 81 s in the control group.

Transcutaneous Posterior Tibial Nerve Stimulation

Transcutaneous posterior tibial nerve stimulation (TPTNS) has been introduced as a new treatment option for PE [21, 60]. The rationale for using TPTNS for premature ejaculation was to inhibit the emission and expulsion phases of ejaculation. In a phase II single-arm study to evaluate the efficacy and safety of TPTNS for PE treatment, 54.5% showed tripled baseline IELT scores at 12 weeks. The IELT increased 4.8-fold, 6.8-fold and 5.4-fold at 12, 24, and 48 weeks, respectively. One episode of constipation was reported, and one patient reported a sensation of heat in the leg during one therapy session. The findings suggest that TPTNS therapy delays ejaculation in patients with lifelong premature ejaculation, with no serious secondary effects [60]. However, controlled trials with many patients with PE or sample sizes are needed to verify these results.

Surgical Interventions in Delayed Ejaculation

Several surgical interventions for the treatment of delayed ejaculation (DE) exist, but none has been formally approved by the US Food and Drug Administration. Given the paucity of effective treatments for DE, some clinicians have explored non-pharmacological strategies such as pudendal nerve release, intracavernosal injections, platelet-rich plasma and surgical interventions [58]. No published, peer-reviewed data exists supporting any of these approaches. Given the risks and potential expense, the guidelines do not recommend the use of any invasive procedure for DE outside the context of an ethical board-approved clinical trial in which participants give informed consent for participation in research. Therefore, clinicians should counsel patients with delayed ejaculation that no currently available data indicates that invasive non-pharmacological strategies are of benefit.

Surgical Interventions in Anejaculation/ Retrograde Ejaculation

Fertility potentials for men with anejaculation/retrograde ejaculation include medication with α-agonist agents, penile vibratory stimulation (PVS), prostatic massage, electro-ejaculation (EEJ) and testicular/epididymal sperm retrieval procedures such as testicular sperm extraction/aspiration (TESE/TESA) and/or microsurgical epididymal sperm aspiration/ percutaneous epididymal sperm aspiration (MESA/PESA).

PVS and EEJ via rectal prob. are commonly used methods in the treatment of men with spinal cord injury who seek children. PVS is the first-line therapy for the treatment of patients in which all spinal cord components (both the sympathetic and the parasympathetic mechanisms) of the ejaculation reflex and the dorsal nerve of the penis are intact. The treatment with PVS consists of vibration applied to the penis, usually on the dorsum or the frenulum, for up to 10 min [19]. The treatment can be intermittent or continued until antegrade ejaculation occurs. Autonomic dysreflexia sometimes may occur in patients with spinal cord injuries above the level of T6. Sperm obtained with PVS can be used for intrauterine insemination (IUI) and in vitro fertilization/ intracytoplasmic sperm injection (IVF/ICSI), and therefore cost-effective and easy pregnancies can be achieved instead of more invasive testicular or epididymal sperm extraction. PVS is successful in 86% of men with SCI whose level of injury is T10 or rostral [25].

If PVS fails or the level is caudal to T10, the patients are referred for EEJ. EEJ consists of the electrical stimulation of the nerves and smooth muscle of the pelvic muscles, the prostate and seminal vesicles, through the rectum in patients affected by a complete SCI. Usually, EEJ is considered second-line therapy for patients who fail with PVS [19]. The change in retrograde ejaculation is higher for EEJ than for PVS; therefore, if an antegrade ejaculation is not obtained following the electrostimulation, a retrograde ejaculation may be suspected and a catheter can be placed to collect semen from the bladder. Sperm is obtained via EEJ in 95% of men with SCI, and outcomes of IVF/ICSI resulted in a 37.5% pregnancy rate per cycle, 50% pregnancy rate per couple, 33.3% live birth rate per cycle and 43.8% live birth rate per couple [25]. In cases PVS and EEJ failed, sperm can be obtained with TESE/TESA and/or MESA/PESA procedures. Theoretically, sperm retrieval rates with these methods are 100% to use for ICSI.

Surgical Treatment of Ejaculatory Duct Obstruction

Ejaculatory duct obstruction may cause hematospermia, decreased ejaculated volume and abnormal sperm parameters leading to infertility in males. The standard treatment of ejaculatory duct obstructive pathologies is transurethral resection of the ejaculatory duct (TURED). TURED can be performed via monopolar or bipolar cautery or laser incisions such as neodymium, holmium or thulium energy sources [28, 42, 44]. Alternative treatment methods for TURED include transutricular seminal vesiculoscopy, TRUS-guided re-canalization and balloon dilation and laparoscopic excision of the external prostatic ejaculatory duct cyst [1, 14].

Cystourethroscopy should be performed at the beginning of the TURED procedure to evaluate the anterior, bulbous and posterior urethra to exclude unusual cystoscopic findings such as distorted anatomy of the verumontanum, inflammatory calcifications, ejaculatory duct cysts and midline cysts.

Laser techniques include Holmium laser incision with wavelength 2140 nm, solid-state laser, absorbed by water, normal saline as irrigating fluid, 532 nm (Greenlight) vaporization, Diode laser vaporization and Thulium: yttrium–aluminium–garnet Laser (Tm: YAG). The advantages of the laser technologies include increased visibility, avoiding complications of monopolar TURED with functioning in normal saline instead of conventional non-conductive irrigation fluid, better hemostasis, early catheter removal and shorter hospitalization, and it can be performed under anti-coagulants. Its disadvantages include needing experience and endoscopic skills, and the most common post-operative complication is dysuria.

Several studies revealed that treatment of ejaculatory duct obstructive pathologies by TURED may lead to a 60–70% improvement in semen parameters and achieve spontaneous pregnancy in 20–34% of the cases [1]. In a systematic review, consisting of 29 studies with 634 patients with ejaculatory duct obstruction who had surgery with different techniques, the improvement rates in semen parameters were 83.0% in semen volume, 63.0% in sperm motility and 62.5% in sperm concentration [42]. The natural pregnancy rate across the studies was a median of 25.0%. Improvements in both outcomes were greater in patients with congenital etiologies and partial EDO. In the same systematic review, differences in surgical technique did not appear to affect outcomes. Complications range from 0 to 24% and include hematuria, infection (epididymoorchitis), retrograde ejaculation, reflux, fistula, ED and stenosis. Positive effects of TURED on ART are to obviate the need for ART (20–40%), to downstage the level of ART from IUI to spontaneous pregnancy (13%) or from IVF/ICSI to IUI (50%) [28].

Transurethral seminal vesiculoscopy is an alternative method with low cost especially in patients with hematospermia to show real-time images [14]. It is performed through the distal ejaculatory duct, not inserting into the opening of the ejaculatory duct, passing the inner wall of the utricle entrance. This method provided the disappearance or reduction of hematospermia in 68.06% and 12.5% of the patients, respectively. However, it has no widespread application areas, because the current guidelines do not recommend it as a first-line treatment.

Future Directions

While the actual prevalence of EjD is often under-reported and under-recognized, the experience of many clinicians suggests that the problem is not rare and can be a source of considerable embarrassment and dissatisfaction for patients. The interplay between the 'objective' (ejaculation) and 'subjective' (orgasm) elements of male sexual climax are complex and remain incompletely understood. It is thought that PE often affects younger men while DE and AE are more common in older men.

Over the past 20–30 years, the treatment armamentarium for EjD has expanded from behavioural psychotherapy to drug treatments and/or surgical interventions. Multiple well-controlled, evidence-based studies have demonstrated the efficacy and safety of various drugs in PE and to some extent DE, RE and AE too. Nonetheless, published literature supports the concurrent role of psychotherapeutic treatments in a holistic multi-disciplinary care model. The role of surgery as an effective (and safe) treatment for PE remains controversial since its longer-term outcomes are unknown and the risk of ED and glans numbness or hyperesthesia has serious consequences. Neuromyogenic (functional) pathologies, which impair peristalsis, lead to hypotonia/atonia in the male reproductive tract, and cause partial ejaculatory duct obstruction, are pathologies still to be investigated. Dynamic diagnostic methods to evaluate these pathologies and treatment with neuromodulation are the current topics of experimental research. Surgery remains largely ineffective in cases of DE, RE and AE. Patients with fertility issues relating to DE, RE or AE may benefit from mechanical devices or consider various sperm retrieval methods in the setting of IVF.

There is a pressing need for additional epidemiological data relevant to specific geographical regions and the development of evidence-based definitions in the current sociocultural environment. Appropriately designed studies to establish the prevalence and characteristics of EjD will enable better-designed clinical trials which will provide a more robust evidence basis for management. Further research is necessary to elucidate the neurobiology of various forms of EjD. Innovative assessment tools such as vibrational thresholds, somatosensory latency testing and functional imaging modalities will play a role in providing clinically usable data and may in the future have clinical relevance. Scientific advances in novel molecules, including melatonin, carbon monoxide and nitric oxide may also have relevance to ejaculation and orgasm that is not completely understood.

References

1. Abdel-Al I, Elatreisy A, Hassan GM, Gharib TM. Long-term success durability of transurethral resection of ejaculatory duct in treating infertile men with ejaculatory duct obstruction. J Endourol. 2022;36(7):982–8.
2. Ahn ST, Shim JS, Bae WJ, Kim SW, Kim JJ, Moon DG. Efficacy and safety of penile girth enhancement using hyaluronic acid filler and the clinical impact on ejaculation: a multicenter, patient/evaluator-blinded, randomized active-controlled trial. World J Mens Health. 2022;40(2):299–307.
3. Almekaty K, Ghaith A, Ragab M, Rashed A, Hagras A, Ghoneem A, Raheem AA, Zahran MH. Effect of bulbospongiosus muscle injection with botulinum-a toxin for treatment of lifelong premature ejaculation; a randomized controlled trial. Int J Impot Res. 2024; https://doi.org/10.1038/s41443-024-00831-8.
4. Alwaal A, Breyer BN, Lue TF. Normal male sexual function: emphasis on orgasm and ejaculation. Fertil Steril. 2015;104:1051–60.
5. Althof SE. Psychological approaches to the treatment of rapid ejaculation. J Men's Heal Gend. 2006;3:180–6.
6. Althof SE, McMahon CG. Contemporary Management of Disorders of male orgasm and ejaculation. Urol. 2016;93:9–21.
7. Althof SE, McMahon CG, Waldinger MD, et al. An update of the International Society of Sexual Medicine's guidelines for the diagnosis and treatment of premature ejaculation (PE). Sex Med. 2014;2(2):60–90.
8. American Psychiatric Association: Diagnostic and Statistical Manual of Mental Disorders, Fifth Edition (2013) American Psychiatric Publishing, Inc. Arlington, VA. https://doi.org/10.1176/appi.books.9780890425596. Last accessed 1 Apr 2024
9. Aoki KR, Guyer B. Botulinum toxin type A and other botulinum toxin serotypes: a comparative review of biochemical and pharmacological actions. Eur J Neurol. 2001;8:21–9.
10. Aversa A, Francomano D, Bruzziches R, Natali M, Spera G, Lenzi A. Is there a role for phosphodiesterase type-5 inhibitors in the treatment of premature ejaculation? Int J Impot Res. 2011;23(1):17–23.
11. Bai Y, Pu C, Han P, Li J, Yuan H, Tang Y, Wang X, Wei Q. Selective serotonin reuptake inhibitors plus phosphodiesterase-5 inhibitors for premature ejaculation: a systematic review and meta-analysis. Urol. 2015;86(4):758–65.
12. Basal S, Goktas S, Ergin A, Yildirim I, Atim A, Tahmaz L, Dayanc M. A novel treatment modality in patients with premature ejaculation resistant to conventional methods: the neuromodulation of dorsal penile nerves by pulsed radiofrequency. J Androl. 2010;31(2):126–30.
13. Busato W, Galindo CC. Topical anaesthetic use for treating premature ejaculation: a double-blind, randomized, placebo-controlled study. BJU Int. 2004;93(7):1018–21.
14. Chen WK, Yu DD, Chen ZX, Li PF, Cai J, Liu YP, Wu ZG. Transurethral seminal vesiculoscopy for intractable hematospermia: experience from 144 patients. BMC Urol. 2021;21:48–55.
15. Cizmeci S, Ongun S, Sarac A, Sel E, Tozburun S, Durmus N. Low frequency neuromuscular electrical stimulation applied to the bulbospongiosus muscle prolongs the ejaculation latency in a rat model. Int J Impot Res. 2023; https://doi.org/10.1038/s41443-023-00678-5. PMID: 36782022
16. Clement P, Giuliano F. Physiology and pharmacology of ejaculation. Basic Clin Pharmacol Toxicol. 2016;119:18–25.

17. Corona G, Jannini EA, Mannucci E, Fisher AD, Lotti F, Petrone L, et al. Different testosterone levels are associated with ejaculatory dysfunction. J Sex Med. 2008;5:1991–8.
18. Cruz R. Clomipramine side effects. J Am Acad Child Adolesc Psychiatry. 1992;31:1168–9.
19. Di Bello F, Creta M, Napolitano L, Califano G, Passaro F, Morra S, et al. Male sexual dysfunction and infertility in spinal cord injury patients: state-of-the-art and future perspectives. J Pers Med. 2022;12:873–84.
20. Dording CM, Mischoulon D, Petersen TJ, Kornbluh R, Gordon J, Nierenberg AA, Rosenbaum JF, Fava M. The pharmacologic management of SSRI-induced side effects: a survey of psychiatrists. Ann Clin Psychiatry. 2002;14(3):143–7.
21. Gul M, Bocu K, Serefoglu EC. Current and emerging treatment options for premature ejaculation. Nat Rev Urol. 2022;19(11):659–80.
22. Holstege G, Georgiadis JR, Paans AMJ, et al. Brain activation during human male ejaculation. J Neurosci. 2003;23(27):9185–93.
23. Hu QB, Zhang D, Ma L, Ng DM, Haleem M, Ma Q. Progresses in pharmaceutical and surgical management of premature ejaculation. Chin Med J. 2019;132(19):2362–72.
24. Huyghe E, Cuzin B, Grellet L, et al. Recommendations for the treatment of premature ejaculation. Prog Urol. 2023;33(5):237–46.
25. Ibrahim E, Aballa TC, Brackett NL, Lynne CM. Electroejaculation in men with spinal cord injury: a step-by-step video demonstration. Fertil Steril. 2021;115(5):1344–6.
26. International Classification of Diseases, Eleventh Revision (ICD-11), World Health Organization (WHO) 2019/2021. https://icd.who.int/browse11. Last accessed 1 Apr 2024
27. Jannini EA, Lenzi A. Ejaculatory disorders: epidemiology and current approaches to definition, classification and subtyping. World J Urol. 2005;23(2):68–75.
28. Kadıoglu A, Cayan S, Tefekli A, Orhan I, Engin G, Turek PJ. Does response to treatment of ejaculatory duct obstruction in infertile men vary with pathology. Fertil Steril. 2001;76:138–47.
29. Karsiyakali N, Sarikaya S, Karatas OF. Anatomic basis and clinical effect of selective dorsal neurectomy for patients with lifelong premature ejaculation: a randomized controlled trial. J Sex Med. 2019;16(7):1122.
30. Khan AH, Rasaily D. Tramadol use in premature ejaculation: daily versus sporadic treatment. Indian J Psychol Med. 2013;35:256–9.
31. Kim SW, Choi J, Kim S, et al. Tolerability and adequate therapeutic dosage of oral clomipramine for the treatment of premature ejaculation: a randomized, double-blind, placebo-controlled, fixed-dose, parallel-grouped clinical study. Int J Impot Res. 2018;30:65–70.
32. Lee HY, Pyun JH, Shim SR, Kim JH. Efficacy of various treatment in premature ejaculation: systematic review and network meta-analysis. World J Mens Health. 2024;42(2):338–46.
33. Liu Q, Li S, Zhang Y, Cheng Y, Fan J, Jiang L, Li S, Tang Y, Zeng H, Wang J, Zhu Z. Anatomic basis and clinical effect of selective dorsal neurectomy for patients with lifelong premature ejaculation: a randomized controlled trial. J Sex Med. 2019;16(4):522–34.
34. Li Y, Zhang Z, Xie J, Lian X, Zhang G, Wang C. Bioequivalence assessment of two Dapoxetine hydrochloride formulations in healthy Chinese males under fasted and fed conditions. Clin Pharmacol Drug Dev. 2024; https://doi.org/10.1002/cpdd.1393.
35. Marangell LB, Dennehy EB, Wisniewski SR, et al. Case-control analyses of the impact of pharmacotherapy on prospectively observed suicide attempts and completed suicides in bipolar disorder: findings from STEP-BD. J Clin Psychiatry. 2008;69:916–22.
36. Martin-Tuite P, Shindel AW. Management options for premature ejaculation and delayed ejaculation in men. Sex Med Rev. 2020;8(3):473–85.
37. Martyn-St James M, Cooper K, Kaltenthaler E, Dickinson K, Cantrell A, Wylie K, Frodsham L, Hood C. Tramadol for premature ejaculation: a systematic review and meta-analysis. BMC Urol. 2015;15:1–11.
38. Masters WH, Johnson VE. Human sexual inadequacy. Boston: Little, Brown and Company; 1971. p. 3–4.

39. McCabe MP, Sharlip ID, Atalla E, et al. Definitions of sexual dysfunctions in women and men: a consensus statement from the fourth international consultation on sexual medicine 2015. J Sex Med. 2016;13:135–43.
40. McMahon CG. Management of ejaculatory dysfunction. Intern Med J. 2014;44:124–31.
41. McMahon CG. Treatment of premature ejaculation with sertraline hydrochloride: a single-blind placebo controlled crossover study. J Urol. 1998;159:1935–8.
42. Mekhaimar A, Goble M, Brunckhorst O, Alnajjar HM, Ralph D, Muneer A, Ahmed K. A systematic review of transurethral resection of ejaculatory ducts for the management of ejaculatory duct obstruction. Turk J Urol. 2020;46(5):335–47.
43. Nguyen V, Dolendo I, Uloko M, Hsieh TC, Patel D. Male delayed orgasm and anorgasmia: a practical guide for sexual medicine providers. Intl J Impot Res. 2023;15:1–8.
44. Orhan I, Onur R, Cayan S, Koksal I, Kadıoglu A. Seminal vesicle sperm aspiration in the diagnosis of ejaculatory duct obstruction. BJU. 1999;84:1050–3.
45. Otani T. Clinical review of ejaculatory dysfunction. Reprod Med Biol. 2019;18(4):331–43.
46. Perelman MA. Reexamining the definitions of PE and DE. J Sex Marital Ther. 2017;43(7):633–44.
47. Sadovsky R, Waldinger E, Becher E, et al. International Society for Sexual Medicine's Guidelines for the diagnosis and treatment of premature ejaculation. J Sex Med. 2010;7:2947–69.
48. Saffati G, Naeem T, Kaaki B, Khera M. First-time orgasm in a young man with lifelong anorgasmia after flibanserin use: a case report. Sex Med. 2023;11(6):qfad066.
49. Sakr A, Elgalaly H, Seleem MM, Kamel M, El-Sakka AI, Ibrahim IM. Outcome of hyaluronic acid gel injection in glans penis for treatment of lifelong premature ejaculation: a pilot study. Arab J Urol. 2023;21(1):31–5.
50. Salonia A, Bettochi C, Boeri L, et al. European Association of Urology guidelines on sexual and reproductive health-2021 update: male sexual dysfunction. Eur Urol. 2021;80(3):333–57.
51. Sato Y, Otani T, Amano T, Araki T, Kondou N, Matsukawa M, Tobe M, Haga K, Uchida K, Honma I. Silodosin versus naftopidil in the treatment of premature ejaculation: a prospective multicenter trial. Int J Urol. 2017;24(8):626–31.
52. Serefoglu EC, McMahon CG, Waldinger MD, Althof SE, Shindel A, Adaikan G, et al. An evidence-based unified definition of lifelong and acquired premature ejaculation: report of the second international society for sexual medicine ad hoc committee for the definition of premature ejaculation. Sex Med. 2014;2:41–59.
53. Shah MD, Shah S, Nusrat NB, Zafar N, Rehman AU, SHAH MD, Nusrat N, Rehman AU. Topical anesthetics and premature ejaculation: a systematic review and meta-analysis. Cureus. 2023;15(8):e42913.
54. Shaher H, Noah K, Abdelzaher M, Kandil W, Ahmed IS, Nouh I S. Is bulbospongiosus muscle botox injection safe and effective in treating lifelong premature ejaculation? Randomized controlled study. World J Urol. 2024;42(1):218.
55. Shebl SE, Ali S, Shokr M. Hyaluronic acid injection in the glans penis for the treatment of refractory premature ejaculation: a prospective, controlled study. Andrologia. 2021;53(7):e14084.
56. Shechter A, Mondaini N, Serefoglu EC, Gollan T, Deutsch F, Appel B, Gruenwald I. A novel on-demand therapy for lifelong premature ejaculation using a miniature transperineal electrical stimulator-the vPatch: an as-treated analysis. J Sex Med. 2023;20(1):22–9.
57. Shechter A, Serefoglu EC, Gollan T, Springer S, Meiry G, Appel B, Gruenwald I. Transcutaneous functional electrical stimulation—a novel therapy for premature ejaculation: results of a proof of concept study. Int J Impot Res. 2020;32(4):440–5.
58. Shindel AW, Althof SE, Carrier S, et al. Disorders of ejaculation: an AUA/SMSNA guideline. J Urol. 2022;207(3):504–12.
59. Stahl SM. Mechanism of action of flibanserin, a multifunctional serotonin agonist and antagonist (MSAA), in hypoactive sexual desire disorder. CNS Spectr. 2015;20(1):1–6.

60. Uribe OL, Sandoval-Salinas C, Corredor HA, Martínez JM, Saffon JP. Transcutaneous electric nerve stimulation to treat patients with premature ejaculation: phase II clinical trial. Int J Impot Res. 2020;32(4):434–9.
61. Waldinger MD. What do men with premature ejaculation prefer: daily dosing or on-demand drug treatment? Sexologies. 2008;17:S44.
62. Wang H, Bai M, Zhang HL, Zeng A. Surgical treatment for primary premature ejaculation with an inner condom technique. Medicine. 2019;98:3–5.
63. Wu T, Yue X, Duan X, Luo D, Cheng Y, Tian Y, Wang K. Efficacy and safety of tramadol for premature ejaculation: a systematic review and meta-analysis. Urol. 2012;80:618–24.
64. Zhan GX, Yu LP, Bai WJ, Wang XF. Selective resection of dorsal nerves of penis for premature ejaculation. Int J Androl. 2012;35(6):873–9.
65. Zhang D, Cheng Y, Wu K, Ma Q, Jiang J, Yan Z. Paroxetine in the treatment of premature ejaculation: a systematic review and meta-analysis. BMC Urol. 2019;19:1–2.
66. Zhang C, Quan Y, Song Y, Bai W, Li Q, Xu T, Zhang X. Efficacy and safety assessment of glandular augmentation with hyaluronic acid for premature ejaculation. Andrologia. 2022;54(7):e14435.

Chapter 25
Chronic Orchialgia: New Treatment Paradigms

Ranjit Vishwakarma, Ravi Banthia, and Kasonde Bowa

Abbreviations

BOTOX	OnabotulinumtoxinA
CO	Chronic orchialgia
CSP	Chronic Epididymitis Symptoms
MDSC	Microsurgical Denervation of Spermatic Cord
NSAIDs	Non-steroidal anti-inflammatory drugs
PRF	Pulsed radiofrequency
QOL	Quality of life
TRAAD	Targeted robotic-assisted intra-abdominal denervation
TENS	Transcutaneous Electrical Nerve Stimulation
VAS	Visual Analogue Scale
WD	Wallerian degeneration

Introduction

Chronic orchialgia (CO) is defined as pain or discomfort of the testis or its surrounding tissues, lasting for more than three months and hampering the daily activities. It is known by several terminologies like chronic scrotal content pain, chronic

R. Vishwakarma (✉)
Department of Urology, Lilavati Hospital and Research Centre, Mumbai, India

R. Banthia
Global Andrology Forum, Moreland Hills, OH, USA

Department of Urology, Western General Hospital, Edinburgh, UK

K. Bowa
University of Zambia, School of Medicine, Lusaka, Zambia

E. Chung et al. (eds.), *Advances in Andrology*,
https://doi.org/10.1007/978-3-032-29112-7_25

testicular pain, chronic scrotal pain, testalgia, testicular pain syndrome. It is an extremely vexing condition affecting physical, mental, and psychological wellbeing of the patient. Although there are various etiologies proposed, however, significant number of cases are idiopathic. The absence of clear guidelines for diagnosis, evaluation, and management not only poses challenges for patients but also for the treating physician.

Epidemiology and Impact

Chronic orchialgia, or chronic testicular pain, is a condition that affects men of all ages, but the causes and rates vary. Regardless of age or cause, CO significantly reduces quality of life across physical, psychological, and social domains due to persistent pain, anxiety, depression, and sexual dysfunction [1, 2].

It is common in children, with a prevalence of 0.8–30%. Early recognition and prompt treatment are crucial to prevent complications like testicular loss. Timely diagnosis can be challenging in children due to difficulties in localizing and communicating the source of pain. In young adults, it's often due to trauma, vasculitis, or unknown reasons, occurring in 0.5–3% of cases [3, 4].

It is relatively uncommon in the elderly but can be associated with various underlying conditions. Common causes include inguinal hernia, varicocele, or epididymal cysts with rates increasing to 2–8% in those over 50 years [5, 6]. Age-related changes and comorbidities can complicate the clinical presentation and delay diagnosis.

In immunocompromised individuals, such as those with HIV/AIDS or receiving immunosuppressive therapy, CO may be associated with opportunistic infections like orchitis or epididymo-orchitis. Immunocompromised status may also increase the risk of testicular abscess formation, which requires prompt surgical intervention.

Diabetic men are at an increased risk of developing CO due to autonomic neuropathy and vascular dysfunction. Diabetic orchitis, epididymitis, and testicular infarction are more common in this population.

Access to healthcare and diagnostic resources can be limited in low-income settings, making evaluation and management more challenging. Delayed presentation is common, leading to increased risk of complications.

Etiology and Pathogenesis

Chronic orchialgia refers to persistent testicular or scrotal pain lasting at least three months. It mainly involves pain in the testicle, but can also affect other areas like the epididymis, paratesticular structures, and spermatic cord [7]. Its causes can be broadly categorized as direct, which arises from testicular and paratesticular pathologies, and indirect, which arises from intra-abdominal pathologies.

The somatic supply to the testes and scrotum originates from the L1–L2 and S2–S4 nerve roots through the iliohypogastric, ilioinguinal, genitofemoral, and pudendal nerves [8]. The testes are embryologically derived from the same level as the kidneys. As a result, they have 90% sympathetic autonomic innervation, originating from the T10–L1 segments, and 90% parasympathetic innervation, originating from the S2–S4 segments. Superior spermatic nerves, composed of fibers from the renal and intermesenteric plexuses, follow the testicular artery to the testis. Middle spermatic nerves arise from the superior hypogastric plexus, pass to the mid-ureter, and travel alongside the vas deferens to the internal ring, where they join the spermatic cord. Inferior spermatic nerves originate from the pelvic plexus (inferior hypogastric plexus) and join the middle spermatic nerves at the prostate-vesical junction. Some afferent and efferent fibers decussate to the contralateral pelvic plexus, which may explain how lesions in one testis affect the function of the other testis [9].

Chronic testicular pain often originates from the same causes as acute testicular discomfort. This includes torsion of the testicles, epididymitis, tumors, obstructions, varicocele, spermatocele, epididymal cysts, hydrocele, damage after hydrocele or hernia surgery, and post-vasectomy issues [7]. Scrotal pain may arise from intra-abdominal processes like ureteral calculi, inguinal hernia, abdominal vascular aneurysms, and retroperitoneal tumors. Symptoms like a new onset varicocele, inguinal bulge, abdominal bruit, or hematuria may indicate retroperitoneal or pelvic pathology. Spinal pathology should be considered in patients with concurrent back pain or neurological symptoms. Even though there are several potential causes of CO, around 25–50% of cases are idiopathic [8]. Psychological factors contributing to genital pain should be considered in CO. In a study of 48 men with no etiology, many showed signs of conditions like somatization disorder, depression, and substance dependency, along with low social support [10].

Parekattil and his colleagues retrospectively reviewed a prospective study comparing the spermatic cord biopsies obtained in mapped fashion in 56 patients with CO at a total of 57 Microsurgical Denervation of the Spermatic Cord (MDSC) procedures. Similar sampling was done in 10 controls without CO undergoing elective inguinal/cord surgery for other reasons, such as varicocele or testicular tumors. They found three primary locations (trifecta nerve complex) for significant Wallerian degeneration (WD) in the CO group. In decreasing order of nerve density, they were (1) cremasteric muscle fibers (mean 19.1 nerves per patient with 33% to 67% WD), (2) peri-vasal tissues and vasal sheath (mean 9.4 nerves per patient with 63% WD), and (3) posterior peri-arterial/lipomatous tissue (mean 3.3 nerves per patient with 35% WD). Another area of interest was the pericord (extra-cord) sheath and veins, with a mean of 2.4 nerves per patient with 23% WD. They concluded that the spermatic cord has a distinct anatomical distribution of nerves, with a unique pattern of WD, and targeting of these abnormal nerves may improve microsurgical cord denervation efficacy in CO patients [11].

Chronic orchialgia often begins after scrotal or testicular injury. This acute pain can cause nerve sensitization, leading to modulation of nerve pathways and hypersensitivity. Wallerian degeneration, a heightened immune cell response, may cause inflammation surrounding nerves, leading to neural hypersensitivity [12]. Parekattil and his colleagues found increased nerve density in the spermatic cord of patients with CO, supporting this hypothesis [11]. This hypersensitivity can result in allodynia or hyperalgesia, which can persist even months after the injury has healed. However, where there is no obvious trauma, the precise mechanism of WD activation remains unclear. Pain from nearby organs sharing the same nerve pathway with the scrotum can also contribute to chronic testicular pain. Additionally, CO might be part of a larger behavioral syndrome, starting with pain and being reinforced by internal or external factors, providing secondary benefits to the patient [13].

Diagnosis and Evaluation

Diagnosing CO relies on a thorough patient history to uncover possible triggers and associated factors. Standardized tools like the Chronic Epididymal Pain Scale or Pain Disability Questionnaire can help measure symptom severity objectively [3, 14]. Additionally, imaging such as ultrasound, MRI, or CT scans helps in identifying potential structural issues like lesions, torsion, inflammation, or neoplasm [4, 15].

Treatment Options

A multi-disciplinary approach to patients with CO is recommended. This may involve pain management specialists, psychiatrists, pelvic floor physical therapists, primary care physicians, and urologists. Conservative treatments should be attempted before considering invasive surgeries [16–18]. While there's no set consensus on treatment protocols, initial interventions typically focus on non-invasive methods. If these fail, referral to an urologist for procedural or surgical options may be considered (Table 25.1).

Table 25.1 Treatment options

Treatment approach	Details
Neural blockade	Local anesthetics (e.g., lidocaine, bupivacaine) or corticosteroids injected to temporarily relieve pain and aid in identifying the pain source
Cryoablation	Ultrasound-guided targeted micro-cryoablation of spermatic cord nerves to induce localized freezing and disrupt nociceptive signaling
Botulinum toxin injections	Injection of 100–300 units of botulinum toxin to induce temporary paralysis of cremaster muscle and spermatic cord, relieving muscular spasm-associated pain
Amniotic tissue injections	Injection of cryopreserved amniotic membrane and fluid to promote nerve/tissue regeneration and reduce inflammation
Pulsed radiofrequency ablation	Short bursts of high-frequency alternating current to modulate nociceptive nerve conduction and alleviate pain
Transcutaneous electrical nerve stimulation	Low-voltage electrical current delivered through skin electrodes to inhibit transmission of pain signals
Varicocelectomy	Surgical ligation or removal of dilated spermatic venous plexus in cases of varicocele-associated CO
Vasectomy reversal	Reversal of vasectomy procedure may alleviate CO in some cases of post-vasectomy pain syndrome
Microsurgical denervation of spermatic cord	Open or robotic-assisted surgical denervation of spermatic cord, disrupting testicular innervation from genitofemoral and ilioinguinal nerves; provides durable pain relief in 70–90% of cases
Epididymectomy	Surgical removal of the epididymis for isolated epididymal pathology like cysts or obstructive lesions
Orchidectomy	Removal of the testis via inguinal or high scrotal approach, considered a last resort for severe, intractable CO refractory to other treatments
Robotic intra-abdominal denervation	Emerging surgical technique targeting proximal denervation of spermatic cord at its origin, potentially providing long-term analgesia while preserving the testis

Conservative Management

The initial course of treatment involves dietary and lifestyle recommendations, which typically include avoiding chocolate, citrus, strong spices, caffeine, and constipation as well as extended periods of sitting.

Antibiotics prescribed are usually trimethoprim/sulfamethoxazole or a quinolone because of their lipid solubility. They are typically prescribed for two to four weeks. Antibiotic therapy is not recommended for empiric use, unless there are objective signs or a reasonable suspicion of an infection [7].

Non-steroidal anti-inflammatory drugs (NSAIDs) are typically used as the first line of pharmacological therapy. The mechanism of action of NSAIDs is well established, as are their analgesic and anti-inflammatory properties. Recurrence rates after successful NSAID use are as high as 50%; however, easy availability and relatively lesser side effects make NSAIDs the first choice of medications. Narcotic analgesics should be avoided except in cases of occasional breakthrough pain [19].

Tricyclic antidepressants work by blocking the reuptake of norepinephrine and serotonin in the brain. Their analgesic effect is thought to be due to inhibition of sodium and L-type calcium channel blockers in the dorsal horn of the spinal cord. Tertiary amines in this class (amitriptyline and clomipramine) are more effective for neuropathic pain than secondary amines (desipramine and nortriptyline) but are also more sedating and more likely to be associated with postural hypotension. They are usually given as a single dose at bedtime and will typically require at least two to four weeks to show effectiveness, although it may take up to eight weeks [20].

If tricyclic therapy is not successful, the next conservative therapy approach would be to add an anticonvulsant such as gabapentin and pregabalin. These are recommended due to their proven efficacy in neuropathic pain and their relative lack of side effects. In a small study, over 60% of patients with idiopathic CO showed significant pain relief. However, comprehensive large-scale studies are still needed to confirm these findings [20].

Pelvic floor physical therapy is useful for those with pelvic muscle dysfunction or identifiable myofascial trigger points. In properly selected patients, about 50% have noted improvement in their pain after 12 sessions. It also appears that physical therapy can improve pain and quality of life (QOL) scores for CO patients even after other treatments [21]. Nielsen and his colleagues found 85% reduction in orchialgia using trigger point dry needling after an average of 4.6 sessions. They also noted improvements in pain and QOL scores suggesting that dry needling could be an alternative treatment option in combination with other therapies [22].

Minimal Invasive Treatment

Minimally invasive techniques like nerve blocks using local anesthetics (e.g., lidocaine, bupivacaine) or corticosteroids can help diagnose and treat symptoms for certain patients. These blocks can temporarily relieve pain from a suspected source and also offer therapeutic benefits [5, 14]. They can predict how patients might respond to surgical treatments for CO. Another option, ultrasound-guided cryoablation, freezes and destroys nerves in the spermatic cord to reduce pain signaling [6, 22].

Botulinum toxin injections induce temporary paralysis of the cremaster muscle and spermatic cord to relieve muscular spasm-mediated pain. Typical doses range from 100 to 300 units [23]. A study by Khambati et al. found that onabotulinumtoxinA (Botox) cord blocks provide pain relief for men with Chronic Epididymitis Symptoms (CSP) for a three-month period. Up to 56% had sustained pain reduction and reduced tenderness even after three months. However, by six months, most men had returned to their baseline levels of pain and tenderness [24]. Dockrey et al. found no superiority of onabotulinumtoxinA plus local anesthesia for pain control in men with CSP. Botulinum may be a viable, minimally invasive treatment option for CSP patients, but may require frequent retreatment due to the likelihood of recurrence of pain [25].

Pulsed radiofrequency (PRF) ablation or transcutaneous electrical nerve stimulation (TENS) is additional minimally invasive options for modulation of afferent neurotransmission. Pulsed radiofrequency uses short bursts of high-frequency alternating current to modulate nociceptive signaling [26], providing a non-neurogenic, non-surgical treatment for various painful conditions. It alters pain signals through biological changes, reducing sensation in the affected area. While studies on PRF are limited, most focus on nerves like the ilioinguinal nerve or genital branch of the genitofemoral nerve. In a double-blind, sham-controlled clinical trial, 80% of patients treated with PRF experienced a 50% reduction in Visual Analogue Scale (VAS), pain score compared to 23.3% in the sham group [21, 27–29].

Transcutaneous electrical nerve stimulation uses low-voltage electrical current delivered through skin electrodes to inhibit pain signal transmission [1, 3]. A study by Tantawy et al. found that TENS reduced VAS pain scores and improved patients' quality of life two months after the intervention, indicating its potential for pain relief [30].

Vibratory treatment, a non-invasive method used for non-urological painful conditions like fibromyalgia, muscle pain, and diabetic neuropathy, has shown promising results in reducing daily pain and frequency in 78% of patients using a battery-operated massage ball for four weeks. However, further studies are needed to demonstrate their clinical benefits [31, 32].

Amniotic tissue injections using cryopreserved amniotic membrane and fluid may promote regeneration of damaged nerves/tissues and blunt inflammation via the tissue's anti-inflammatory properties [1, 2].

Surgical Management

When it comes to managing patients who do not respond to medical treatments, surgical intervention becomes a crucial consideration. Patient selection is crucial to the success of surgical treatment. One important criterion for surgical consideration is the patient's response to cord block. Those with 50% pain reduction are more likely to benefit from surgical intervention [33].

Varicoceles are present in 2–10% men with CO. Varicocelectomy with ligation or removal of dilated spermatic venous plexus may be indicated for CO arising from varicocele [5, 8]. Studies show that 72.4–94.3% of men experience either partial or complete pain reduction following varicocele surgery [34–37].

Vasectomy pain syndrome is a rare but common side effect of vasectomies, characterized by acute post-procedural pain lasting over two to four weeks and CO [38,

39]. It can be triggered by sexual activity, ejaculation, or physical exercise. The exact cause is unknown, but it is believed to be caused by back pressure from congestion during ejaculation. Perineural fibrosis, caused by fluid discharge into the caudal epididymis, raises back pressure and causes pain. If conservative treatments fail, MDSC may be recommended. Reversing a vasectomy can help treat post-vasectomy pain syndrome, which has shown significant pain relief rates. Nerve entrapment, post-operative scarring, persistent vasoconstriction, and neuropathic causes are the reasons for inadequate pain reduction after the procedure [40].

Microsurgical Denervation of the Spermatic Cord is the most extensively studied treatment option in CO. Excellent surgical outcomes have made it the surgical procedure of choice for unresponsive conservative therapies. Several studies indicate a success rate of 70–100% for MDSC, especially if patients have had a positive response to a spermatic cord block [41–45].

The procedure is technically challenging, requiring an advanced microscope to identify the small veins, arteries, and lymphatic vessels. The basic principle involves separating the trifecta nerve complex within the spermatic cord, which denerves the testis from hypersensitive nerves. This principle accounts for its consistently high satisfaction rates. The procedure is usually done through an inguinal incision, and the spermatic cord is exposed and delivered out of the wound. The peri-vasal fascia is stripped, and a vasectomy is typically performed if not previously performed. The procedure involves denuding the spermatic cord including cremasteric muscles leaving behind a bridge of internal spermatic artery, vein, and few lymphatic vessels.

Microsurgical Denervation of the Spermatic Cord can lead to surgical complications, including testicular atrophy, hydrocele, wound infection, incisional hematoma, and in severe cases, testicular loss. Around 70–80% of men experience complete relief of symptoms, and another 10–20% have partial pain relief after MDSC. While complete pain relief may take up to three months, approximately 40% reported complete pain relief immediately after the procedure.

Epididymectomy is a potent surgical option for chronic pain localized to the epididymis, such as from spermatocele or granuloma. It is also effective in controlling post-vasectomy pain as an alternative to vasectomy reversals. West and his colleagues in their study showed that 90% patients had a sustained improvement of their scrotal pain after three to eight years [46]. A separate study found significant improvements in pain scores in the post-vasectomy group, with 93.3% experiencing reduced or no pain compared to the non-vasectomy group [47, 48].

In stubborn cases unresponsive to other interventions, orchidectomy involving removal of the testis via inguinal or high scrotal approach may be required as a last resort, though it is associated with psychological impacts [4, 15]. The inguinal approach has better results than the scrotal approach. Patients should be informed and counseled accordingly, as even this last-resort treatment may not be 100% effective in treating chronic pain and may cause hypogonadism [49].

Emerging techniques like robotic intra-abdominal denervation target proximal denervation at the origin of the spermatic cord for potential long-term analgesia while preserving the testis [1, 50]. A study by Calixte et al. found that targeted robotic-assisted intra-abdominal denervation (TRAAD) of the genitofemoral and inferior hypogastric nerves proximal to the internal inguinal ring is a viable treatment option for patients with chronic groin pain refractory to MDSC/targeted MDSC or orchiectomy for CO. The technique preserves the ilioinguinal nerve and only ligates the genitofemoral and inferior hypogastric nerve within the abdomen above the internal inguinal ring. Seventy-one percent of patients experienced significant pain reduction, and 33% experienced complete relief. The study concluded that TRAAD of the genitofemoral and inferior hypogastric nerves is a viable treatment option for patients with chronic groin pain when MDSC or orchiectomy fails [51].

Conclusion

Chronic orchialgia presents a formidable challenge for both patients and healthcare providers. As our understanding of the underlying pathophysiology deepens, conservative and minimally invasive treatment options continue to evolve. These advancements aim to alleviate pain and enhance patients' quality of life.

References

1. Katz EE, Patel ND. Chronic orchalgia: Diagnostic and treatment considerations. Transl Androl Urol. 2021;10(3):1303–14.
2. Berdache N, et al. Use of local orthotics for the treatment of chronic orchialgia. Andrologia. 2020;53(2):e13901.
3. Alhajeri F, Majeed A. Chronic orchalgia: An updated review. J Clin Urol. 2020;13(5):312–21.
4. Levine LA, Hoyt CS. Chronic orchalgia: Current perspectives and treatment options. Asian J Androl. 2019;21(5):450–6.
5. Wampler SM, Brannigan RE. Chronic orchalgia: An overview. Andrology. 2017;5(2):275–82.
6. Masarani M, Cox R. The aetiology, pathophysiology and management of chronic orchalgia. BJU Int. 2018;121(4):494–501.
7. Levine L. Chronic orchialgia: evaluation and discussion of treatment options. Ther Adv Urol. 2010;2:209–14.
8. Davis BE, Noble MJ, Weigel JW, et al. Analysis and management of chronic testicular pain. J Urol. 1990;143:936–9.
9. Reynolds LW, Sills SM. Orchialgia. In: Waldman SD, editor. Pain management. Philadelphia: Elsevier; 2011.
10. Schover LR. Psychological factors in men with genital pain. Cleve Clin J Med. 1990;57:697–700.
11. Parekattil SJ, Gudeloglu A, Brahmbhatt JV, Priola KB, Vieweg J, Allan RW. Trifecta nerve complex—potential anatomic basis for microsurgical denervation of the spermatic cord for chronic orchialgia. J Urol. 2013;190(1):265–70.
12. Baron R. Mechanisms of disease: neuropathic pain—a clinical perspective. Nat Clin Pract Neurol. 2006;2:95–106.
13. Arnold LM, Choy E, Clauw DJ, et al. Fibromyalgia and chronic pain syndromes: a white paper detailing current challenges in the field. Clin J Pain. 2016;32:737–46.
14. Patel AP, Jarvi K. Management of chronic orchalgia. Transl Androl Urol. 2021;10(3):1391–402.

15. Nickel JC. Chronic epididymitis: a practical approach. Rev Urol. 2003;5(4):216–21.
16. Belanger GV, VerLee GT. Diagnosis and surgical management of male pelvic, inguinal, and testicular pain. Surg Clin North Am. 2016;96(3):593–613.
17. Tojuola B, Layman J, Kartal I, Gudelogul A, Brahmbhatt J, Parekattil S. Chronic orchialgia: Review of treatments old and new. Indian J Urol. 2016;32(1):21–6.
18. Tan WP, Levine LA. An overview of the management of post-vasectomy pain syndrome. Asian J Androl. 2016;18(3):332–7.
19. Ho KY, Gwee KA, Cheng YK, et al. Nonsteroidal anti-inflammatory drugs in chronic pain: implications of new data for clinical practice. J Pain Res. 2018;11:1937–48.
20. Sinclair AM, Miller B, Lee LK. Chronic orchialgia: consider gabapentin or nortriptyline before considering surgery. Int J Urol. 2007;14:622–5.
21. Basal S, Ergin A, Yildirim I, Goktas S, Atim A, Sizlan A, Irkilata HC, Kurt E, Dayanc M. A novel treatment of chronic orchialgia. J Androl. 2012;33(1):22–6.
22. Jarvi K, et al. Novel therapies for the treatment of chronic orchialgia. Urol Pract. 2021;8(6):619–28.
23. Khera M, Frey C, Toombs BD. Orchialgia and the chronic pelvic pain syndrome. Indian J Urol. 2005;21(3):126–33.
24. Khambati A, Lau S, Gordon A, Jarvi KA. OnabotulinumtoxinA (Botox) nerve blocks provide durable pain relief for men with chronic scrotal pain: a pilot open-label trial. J Sex Med. 2014;11(12):3072–7.
25. Dockray J, Aljumaily A, Lau S, Jarvi KA. A randomized, double-blind, controlled trial shows that onabotulinum toxin a nerve blocks do not provide improved pain control in men with chronic scrotal pain. J Urol. 2020;203(4):767–72.
26. Hetta DF, Mahran AM, Kamal EE. Pulsed radiofrequency treatment for chronic post-surgical orchialgia: a double-blind, sham-controlled, randomized trial: three-month results. Pain Physician. 2018;21(2):199–205.
27. Cohen SP, Foster A. Pulsed radiofrequency as a treatment for groin pain and orchialgia. Urology. 2003;61(3):645.
28. Rozen D, Parvez U. Pulsed radiofrequency of lumbar nerve roots for treatment of chronic inguinal herniorraphy pain. Pain Physician. 2006;9(2):153–6.
29. Venkataparthasarathy R, Ather MH. 592 Ilioinguinal and genitofemoral neuralgia: pulsed radiofrequency—a novel technique. Eur J Pain. 2006;10(S1):S155c–S156.
30. Tantawy SA, Kamel DM, Abdelbasset WK. Does transcutaneous electrical nerve stimulation reduce pain and improve quality of life in patients with idiopathic chronic orchialgia? A randomized controlled trial. J Pain Res. 2017;11:77–82.
31. Pujol J, Ramos-López D, Blanco-Hinojo L, et al. Testing the effects of gentle vibrotactile stimulation on symptom relief in fibromyalgia. Arthritis Res Ther. 2019;21(1):148.
32. Stillman BC. Vibratory motor stimulation: a preliminary report. Aust J Physiother. 1970;16(3):118–23.
33. Larsen SM, Benson JS, Levine LA. Microdenervation of the spermatic cord for chronic scrotal content pain: single institution review analyzing success rate after prior attempts at surgical correction. J Urol. 2013;189:554–8.
34. Abrol N, Panda A, Kekre NS. Painful varicoceles: Role of varicocelectomy. Indian J Urol. 2014;30:369–73.
35. Maghraby HA. Laparoscopic varicocelectomy for painful varicoceles: Merits and outcomes. J Endourol. 2002;16:107–10.
36. Kim HT, Song PH, Moon KH. Microsurgical ligation for painful varicocele: Effectiveness and predictors of pain resolution. Yonsei Med J. 2012;53:145–50.
37. Park HJ, Lee SS, Park NC. Predictors of pain resolution after varicocelectomy for painful varicocele. Asian J Androl. 2011;13:754–8.
38. Christiansen CG, Sandlow JI. Testicular pain following vasectomy: a review of postvasectomy pain syndrome. J Androl. 2003;24:293–8.

39. Tan WP, Tsambarlis PN, Levine LA. Microdenervation of the spermatic cord for post-vasectomy pain syndrome. BJU Int. 2018;121:667–73.
40. Sinha V, Ramasamy R. Post-vasectomy pain syndrome: diagnosis, management and treatment options. Transl Androl Urol. 2017;6(Suppl 1):S44–7.
41. Devine CJ, Schellhammer PF. The use of microsurgical denervation of the spermatic cord for orchalgia. Trans Am Assoc Genitourin Surg. 1978;70:149–51.
42. Choa RG, Swami KS, Testicular denervation. A new surgical procedure for intractable testicular pain. Br J Urol. 1992;70:417–9.
43. Levine LA, Matkov TG, Lubenow TR. Microsurgical denervation of the spermatic cord: a surgical alternative in the treatment of chronic orchialgia. J Urol. 1996;155:1005–7.
44. Levine LA, Matkov TG. Microsurgical denervation of the spermatic cord as primary surgical treatment of chronic orchalgia. J Urol. 2001;165:1927–9.
45. Oliveira RG, Camara C, Alves Jde M, Coelho RF, Lucon AM, et al. Microsurgical testicular denervation for the treatment of chronic testicular paininitial results. Clinics (Sao Paulo). 2009;64:393–6.
46. West AF, Leung HY, Powell PH. Epididymectomy is an effective treatment for scrotal pain after vasectomy. BJU Int. 2000;85:1097–9.
47. Siu W, Ohl DA, Schuster TG. Long-term follow-up after epididymectomy for chronic epididymal pain. Urology. 2007;70:333–5.
48. Hori S, Sengupta A, Shukla CJ, et al. Long-term outcome of epididymectomy for the management of chronic epididymal pain. J Urol. 2009;182:1407–12.
49. Lowe G. Extirpative surgery for chronic orchialgia: is there a role? Transl Androl Urol. 2017;6(Suppl 1):S2–5.
50. Davis BE, Noble MJ, Weigel JW, Foret JD, Mebust WK. Analysis and management of chronic testicular pain. J Urol. 1990;143:936–9.
51. Calixte N, Tojuola B, Kartal I, et al. Targeted Robotic Assisted Microsurgical Denervation of the Spermatic Cord for the Treatment of Chronic Orchialgia or Groin Pain: A Single Center. Large Series Review J Urol. 2018;199(4):1015–22.

Chapter 26
Chronic Prostatitis: Beyond the Triple A's (Antibiotics, Anti-inflammatory, and Alpha-Blockers)

Widi Atmoko, Halil İbrahim İvelik, and Ahmet Baris Altay

Introduction

Prostatitis is a commonly encountered disease in urology clinics, characterized by lower urinary tract symptoms (LUTS) and pain in the pelvic region. It is often associated with symptoms suggestive of lower urinary tract and sexual dysfunction, as well as negative cognitive, behavioral, or emotional outcomes [1]. According to the National Institutes of Health (NIH) recommendations, prostatitis, which is classified into four separate groups, including Type I and Type II prostatitis, is considered a clinical condition caused by bacterial pathogens [2]. Approximately 10% of cases of prostatitis, a common diagnosis, are associated with proven bacterial infection.

W. Atmoko (✉)
Department of Urology, Dr. Cipto Mangunkusumo Hospital, Faculty of Medicine, Universitas Indonesia, Jakarta, Indonesia

H. İ. İvelik
Department of Urology, Faculty of Medicine, Kütahya Health Sciences University, Kütahya, Türkiye

A. B. Altay
Global Andrology Forum, Moreland Hills, OH, USA

Ege University School of Medicine, Urology Department, Izmir, Turkey

E. Chung et al. (eds.), *Advances in Andrology*,
https://doi.org/10.1007/978-3-032-29112-7_26

Epidemiological Prevalence

The prevalence of prostatitis in population-based studies of men aged 20 to 79 years ranges from 2.2% to 9.7%, with an estimated overall prevalence of approximately 8.2% [3]. Prostatitis accounts for approximately 5% of outpatient visits and 8% of urologist visits among men aged 18 and older and 1% of primary care physician visits. In men experiencing symptoms of prostatitis, bacteria have been found to be positive in only about 10% of prostate fluid cultures [4]. Chronic bacterial prostatitis (CBP) can develop in approximately 10% of men with acute bacterial prostatitis (ABP) [5, 6].

Etiology

Prostatitis has long been considered a pathology associated with bacterial pathogens, but over the years, it has been categorized into different subgroups, such as Type III CP/CPPS, which include similar symptoms but lack a bacterial pathogen. The etiology and pathogenesis of the disease, classified into four separate groups according to the NIH, have not yet been fully elucidated.

NIH Category I: Acute Bacterial Prostatitis (ABP)

Escherichia coli is identified as the primary causative agent of acute bacterial prostatitis. Other potential pathogens include Pseudomonas aeruginosa, Enterococcus, Proteus, Klebsiella, Enterobacter, and Serratia species. In sexually active individuals, Neisseria gonorrhoeae and Chlamydia trachomatis should also be considered as possible pathogens.

NIH Category II: Chronic Bacterial Prostatitis (CBP)

CBP prevalence is very low, accounting for only 5–10% of all prostatitis cases. Pathogens responsible for this syndrome include both gram-positive and gram-negative bacteria, as well as pathogens causing complex urogenital system infections.

NIH Category III: Chronic Prostatitis and Chronic Pelvic Pain Syndrome (CP-CPPS)

Due to the inability to demonstrate positive cultures and identify the causative agent, the etiology of most CP/CPPS cases remains uncertain. In recent years, there has been an acceleration in research efforts in the field of molecular biology aimed at elucidating the etiology of this syndrome.

NIH Category IV: Asymptomatic Inflammatory Prostatitis

Studies have shown that men with asymptomatic inflammatory prostatitis can have semen containing a large number of bacteria from up to eight different organisms. The number of bacteria may be directly proportional to the white blood cell count.

Risk Factors

Risk factors for the development of prostatitis generally include prostatic infections resulting from ascending urinary tract infections. Microorganisms typically reach the prostate through ascending routes from the urethra, reflux of infected urine into prostatic ducts, direct or lymphatic spread of bacteria from the rectum, and hematogenous dissemination. Chronic prostatitis, classified under NIH Category III, comprises the largest and most complex group of patients with prostatitis, also posing the greatest challenge for treatment. It is a syndrome where a uropathogenic agent cannot be demonstrated using standard microbiological methods, forming a complex patient group for which etiology remains incompletely understood as research continues.

Pathophysiology

Prostatitis has long been considered a pathology associated with bacterial pathogens, but over the years, it has been categorized into different subgroups, such as Type III CP/CPPS, which include similar symptoms but lack a bacterial pathogen. The etiology and pathogenesis of the disease, classified into four separate groups according to the NIH, have not yet been fully elucidated. In this context, the etiopathogenesis will be evaluated in subgroups according to the NIH classification.

NIH Category I: Acute Bacterial Prostatitis (ABP)

Acute bacterial prostatitis is primarily caused by Escherichia coli. Other potential pathogens include Pseudomonas aeruginosa, Enterococcus, Proteus, Klebsiella, Enterobacter, and Serratia species. In sexually active individuals, Neisseria gonorrhoeae and Chlamydia trachomatis should also be considered as possible pathogens. Cryptococcus, Salmonella, and Candida species are possible causes in individuals with human immunodeficiency. In particular, infections that develop after transurethral procedures are mostly due to Pseudomonas species [7]. These species have a high resistance rate to carbapenems and cephalosporins. Postoperative infections can occur after transrectal prostate biopsies. A decrease in the rate of postoperative prostatitis has been observed due to perioperative antibiotics. However, the rate of prostatitis induced by fluoroquinolone-resistant pathogens and broad-spectrum beta-lactamase-producing E. coli has significantly increased [8].

Due to its acute clinical presentation, ABP is an acute inflammatory condition of the prostate, which is easier to diagnose and treat compared to other categories. ABP presents with sudden onset of moderate to high fever, weakness, chills, lower urinary tract symptoms, and most importantly, perineal prostatic pain. Arthralgia and myalgia are often present. On digital rectal examination, the prostate is edematous, firm, warm, and tender to palpation. The prostate is indurated and enlarged. The most serious complication of ABP is bacteremia and sepsis. Acute urinary retention may develop. A rare complication of ABP is prostatic abscess. Prostatic abscess typically occurs in immunocompromised patients. It can be caused by various bacteria, primarily Escherichia coli (70%), as well as Pseudomonas and other coliform bacteria. While Staphylococcus aureus can cause abscess formation by hematogenous spread to the prostate, anaerobic bacteria can rarely lead to abscess formation. Transurethral resection or drainage under radiological guidance can be performed for the treatment of these abscesses [9].

NIH Category II: Chronic Bacterial Prostatitis (CBP)

Patients in this category have recurrent urinary tract infections caused by a localized bacterial agent demonstrated by prostatic inflammation and localization testing. Unlike ABP, systemic symptoms are not present in this group. Localized symptoms described under ABP are present. The prostate may be normal on digital rectal examination or irregular induration may be palpated. Sometimes crepitation can be obtained.

CBP prevalence is very low, accounting for only 5–10% of all prostatitis cases. Pathogens responsible for this syndrome include both gram-positive and gram-negative bacteria, as well as pathogens causing complex urogenital system infections. Many animal studies have shown the formation of a biofilm layer in the prostatic acini in cases of chronic infection. This biofilm helps create suitable growth conditions for pathogens, which prolongs and supports this pathogenic condition [10]. Neisseria gonorrheae and Chlamydia trachomatis, as sexually transmitted diseases, along with Staphylococcus aureus, Trichomonas vaginalis, Klebsiella pneumoniae, Ureaplasma urealyticum, Mycoplasma hominis, Proteus mirabilis, Serratia marcescens, and Enterobacter cloacae, are among the possible pathogens [10, 11].

NIH Category III: Chronic Prostatitis and Chronic Pelvic Pain Syndrome (CP-CPPS)

This group constitutes the largest and most complex group of patients with prostatitis, including most prostatitis patients, and is also the most challenging to treat. CP-CPPS is characterized by prostatic pain and accompanying lower urinary tract symptoms, and it is a syndrome where a uropathogenic agent cannot be demonstrated using standard microbiological methods [12]. Due to the inability to demonstrate positive cultures and identify the causative agent, the etiology of most CP/CPPS cases remains uncertain. In recent years, there has been an acceleration in research efforts in the field of molecular biology aimed at elucidating the etiology of this syndrome. Studies suggest that CP/CPPS may be associated with infections (bacterial and viral pathogens, including Chlamydia, cytomegalovirus, and herpes simplex virus), as well as with uric acid levels, inflammation, autoimmunity, or neuromuscular mechanisms [13]. Some research studies suggest that CP/CPPS may be due to hidden prostatic bacterial infections [14]. It is also crucial to consider psychological factors as a contributing factor to the etiology of Type III prostatitis. Therefore, psychotherapy and behavioral support are recommended to benefit patients [15]. Since there are no definitive and accurate diagnostic tests for evaluating CP/CPPS patients, it is often challenging to propose therapeutic regimens for the treatment of this syndrome. CP/CPPS can be triggered by multiple factors. Studies suggest that intraprostatic reflux leads to chemical damage triggering an immune response, which may be a potential starting mechanism for chronic inflammation, and hyperalgesia develops in periprostatic nerve cells [16]. Furthermore, studies suggest that individual genetic characteristics and pain thresholds may be associated, and damage to antinociceptive pathways due to deficiencies in the norepinephrine pathway (such as patients with chronic fibromyalgia) may also be a contributing factor [16].

Prostate massage secretion (EPS) and urine samples taken after prostate massage (VB3) are divided into two subgroups based on the presence or absence of white blood cells (WBCs), inflammatory and non-inflammatory. The predominant symptom in patients with chronic pelvic pain syndrome is usually localized pain in the perineum, suprapubic area, and penis. This pain can also be present in the testicles, inguinal area, and hips. A history of pain associated with ejaculation is often obtained [17]. Additionally, lower urinary tract symptoms may be present. Symptoms tend to fluctuate over time.

Due to the diverse and varied complaints of patients in this group, the Chronic Prostatitis Collaborative Research Network (CPCRN) has defined a symptom index to investigate the impact of these complaints on patients' quality of life. This index is called the NIH-Chronic Prostatitis Symptom Index (NIH-CPSI) [18]. This index consists of 13 items grouped into three main scoring categories: Pain, Urinary

Symptoms, and Quality of Life. In the clinical evaluation of a patient with CP-CPPS, along with NIH-CPSI, the Meares–Stamey test, uroflowmetry or post-void residual urine measurement, and cytological evaluation of urine are recommended.

Patients in Category III are divided into two separate subgroups: inflammatory (IIIa) and non-inflammatory (IIIb). This differentiation is based on the findings of white blood cells in EPS, VB3, and seminal fluid samples. While the NIH system makes this distinction based on white blood cells, it has not defined a specific number for diagnosis. In the traditional system, the presence of 10 white blood cells in each high-power field suggests prostatic inflammation [19].

NIH Category IV: Asymptomatic Inflammatory Prostatitis

This condition is characterized by a significant presence of leukocytes and/or bacteria in prostatic specimens (EPS, semen, tissue biopsy) without typical symptoms. Patients are usually investigated due to benign prostatic hyperplasia (BPH) and high PSA levels, and inflammation is diagnosed during the examination of EPS. There is no consensus on its clinical significance. In cases like these, antimicrobial therapy should be initiated before procedures such as cystoscopy, prostate biopsy, and transurethral resection [20].

Clinical Phenotyping

Chronic prostatitis/chronic pelvic pain syndrome (CP/CPPS) is characterized by a complex clinical presentation involving a range of symptoms, including urinary complaints, pelvic pain, sexual dysfunction, and psychiatric issues. Unlike acute bacterial prostatitis, where patients exhibit similar symptoms and respond uniformly to treatment, CP/CPPS presents a significant challenge due to its heterogeneity. Recent insights underscore that individuals with CP/CPPS constitute a diverse group with distinct etiological mechanisms, necessitating personalized therapeutic approaches.

UPOINT Clinical Phenotyping

In response to this complexity, a practical clinical phenotyping system known as UPOINT (Urinary, Psychosocial, Organ-specific, Infection, Neurologic/Systemic, and Tenderness) has been proposed [21]. Derived from the work of Shoskes, this six-point classification system aids in categorizing patients with urologic chronic pelvic pain syndrome (UCPPS) into domains based on specific clinical manifestations. The domains include urinary (U), psychosocial (P), organ-specific (O), infection (I), neurological (N), and muscle tension/tenderness (T). Recent modifications to the UPOINT system have suggested the addition of an "S" domain, addressing sexual dysfunction. This addition, termed UPOINTs, reflects the recognition of the significant impact of CP/CPPS on sexual function, providing a more comprehensive approach to patient assessment [22]. The strength of the UPOINT system lies in its ability to quickly categorize patients into one or more domains, facilitating the design of individually tailored therapeutic plans which will be discussed later in this chapter.

Patients with the "Urinary" phenotype complain of LUTS, including bothersome nocturia, daytime frequency, or urinary urgency. They may have an NIH-CPSI urinary score > 4 and may experience incomplete emptying of the bladder. The "Urinary" domain is often among the most commonly positive domains in men with CPPS, ranging from 60–72% of CPPS populations [21, 23]. A postvoid bladder scan should be obtained in these patients to evaluate elevated residual urine or urinary retention.

Patients in the "Psychosocial" domain often have depression or depressive symptoms, anxiety, stress, and poor coping/adjustment mechanisms [21, 24]. Patients may also catastrophize, characterized by a sense of helplessness and hopelessness about the condition and rumination about their symptoms. Patients with CP/CPPS have a high prevalence of psychological issues and may have a history of sexual or other physical abuse, which is associated with poorer quality of life.

The "Organ-specific" patients have complaints that implicate the prostate and/or bladder as symptom drivers [21]. Prostate-related symptoms can include prostate tenderness to palpation, white blood cells in EPS, hematospermia, and prostate calcifications. Bladder-related symptoms can include pain with bladder filling that improves with voiding and Hunners' lesions seen on cystoscopy. These symptoms suggest a diagnosis of interstitial cystitis/bladder pain syndrome.

Patients with CP/CPPS are often prescribed empiric antibiotics, which are rarely effective at improving symptoms. The "Infection" domain refers to instances where patients have uropathogenic bacteria in urine, EPS, or the urethra without meeting criteria for UTI or Category I or II prostatitis. Mycoplasma and Ureaplasma may be such pathogens present that are not commonly tested [21, 25].

The "Neurological/systemic" patients can be characterized by pain outside the lower abdomen, genitals, and pelvis, fibromyalgia, chronic fatigue syndrome, irritable bowel syndrome, and/or other systemic pain complaints [21, 26].

Lastly, patients in the "Tenderness" domain have spasm, tenderness, and/or trigger points of the pelvis or abdominal muscles diagnosed on DRE and genital and abdominal examinations. [21].

Diagnosis

Chronic prostatitis/chronic pelvic pain syndrome (CP/CPPS) lacks definitive gold standard tests for diagnosis. Evaluation begins with a meticulous physical examination and a thorough review of medical history to identify symptoms associated with prostatitis. To achieve a comprehensive assessment, obtaining a complete list of other concurrent health issues is also advised [27].

Diagnosis Criteria

For the evaluation of CP/CPPS, the use of standardized questionnaires and forms can be beneficial. Presently, the National Institutes of Health (NIH) Chronic Prostatitis Symptom Index (NIH-CPSI) is widely employed for assessing chronic prostatitis symptoms. This questionnaire, consisting of nine sections providing information on urinary symptoms, pain, and quality of life, allows for independent or summarized scoring to analyze three specific domains. The symptom index is utilized to monitor changes in the disease process [18]. Alongside NIH-CPSI, the Meares-Stamey test, uroflowmetry, postvoid residual urine measurement, and cytological evaluation of urine are recommended.

Diagnostic Approach and Modality

Numerous studies have indicated that CP/CPPS patients often exhibit psychosocial symptoms and depression. Consequently, it is crucial to identify these symptoms alongside physical symptoms, emphasizing the recommendation for psychological counseling for CP/CPPS patients [28].

The NIH consensus panel suggests additional tests for the assessment of CP/CPPS. Patients with incomplete bladder emptying should be evaluated for postvoid residual urine. Assessment of urine retention is beneficial in cases of recurrent urinary tract infections and storage symptoms. Evaluation of urinary flow rates can provide valuable information about overall voiding status. A decrease in maximum flow rate may indicate reduced detrusor contractility or obstruction at the bladder outlet. Urine cytology can identify possible urological epithelial malignancies that may cause obstructive or irritative voiding symptoms [29].

Many research studies propose the performance of a quantitative prostatic localization study known as the Meares-Stamey four-glass test. However, due to its time-consuming nature, a study by Nickel et al. introduced a simpler screening test named the two-glass test. In a comparative study evaluating the two-glass test against the four-glass test in the initial assessment of men diagnosed with CP/CPPS, both tests yielded similar results [30].

For patients experiencing localized urethral or penile pain, dysuria symptoms, or those with a history of sexually transmitted diseases or unprotected sexual intercourse, obtaining urethral swabs is recommended [31].

Urodynamic studies should be conducted in patients predominantly presenting with voiding symptoms. The results of this study offer valuable information to support the assessment of postvoid residual urine and urinary flow. Urodynamics or video urodynamics can assist in detecting any obstruction and sphincter dyssynergia. Unlike prostatitis, these disorders can be treated with various therapeutic options, addressing the lower urinary system and pelvic pain symptoms experienced by patients [29].

Cystoscopy can also be utilized as a helpful tool for evaluating patients with CP/CPPS or as an additional method to assess urodynamic studies. Cystoscopy is recommended in patients with a history of hematuria or abnormal cytology. Additionally, in patients with irritative or obstructive symptoms, cystoscopy can be a valuable diagnostic method for assessing potential malignancy [31].

Imaging studies using Doppler ultrasonography have observed increased blood flow to the prostate in patients suffering from CP/CPPS. Abnormalities in the ejaculatory duct and seminal vesicle can be determined using transrectal ultrasonography (TRUS). This imaging technique can be useful in evaluating patients with hematospermia or ejaculation pain [10].

Serum PSA and CP/CPPS: Monitoring serum prostate-specific antigen (PSA) levels should not be considered a useful or reliable diagnostic tool for evaluating CP/CPPS patients. If S-PSA levels increase in men with CP/CPPS symptoms, assessment for chronic bacterial prostatitis (CBP) and prostate malignancy is recommended [32].

Differential Diagnosis

NIH Category I: Acute Bacterial Prostatitis (ABP)

Physical Examination: Acute bacterial prostatitis can be diagnosed through a physical examination. A comprehensive examination of the genital area, abdomen, perineum, and prostate should be conducted during the initial visit. Due to the potential pain and risk of bacteremia, the massage or localization examination of an acutely infected prostate is contraindicated.

Urinalysis and Culture: In cases of acute bacterial prostatitis, performing urinalysis and culture is crucial. A midstream urine culture should be obtained and analyzed for the presence of white blood cells. If the leukocyte count is greater than 10 per field, the diagnosis will be positive. In patients with compatible symptoms of a palpable bladder or discharge, an evaluation for residual urine should be conducted.

Imaging: Imaging studies are not routinely preferred during the initial evaluation. However, before initiating initial treatment, computed tomography scanning or transrectal prostate ultrasonography (TRUS) may be beneficial in determining prostatic abscess/pathology. For ABP patients with obstructive symptoms or post-micturition residual urine, bladder scanning or pelvic ultrasound is recommended [10, 33].

Serum PSA: Elevated prostate-specific antigen (PSA) levels associated with acute bacterial prostatitis can lead to confusion and anxiety in patients. Therefore, routine screening with PSA is not recommended for ABP patients [32].

NIH Category II: Chronic Bacterial Prostatitis (CBP)

Physical Examination: A physical examination should be conducted during the evaluation of chronic bacterial prostatitis. The examination should encompass the external genital area, pelvic floor, prostate, abdomen, and perineum.

4-Glass or 2-Glass Test: This method is still considered the "gold standard" for localizing prostatic infection. It is an accurate and simple method for screening bacteria. Aseptic technique should be used for sampling. Prostate secretions can be obtained by systematically massaging each lobe of the prostate [30].

Semen Cultures: Studies in the literature indicate that semen has higher sensitivity than expressed prostatic secretion (EPS) for diagnosing CBP. Therefore, semen analysis is recommended [34].

Transrectal Ultrasonography of the Prostate: TRUS is considered optional but not mandatory, as it provides information only about the structure of the prostate and does not reveal information about specific categories of prostatitis [10].

Urodynamic Examination: Urodynamic examination cannot be reliably used as a diagnostic test for prostatitis. However, it can be helpful in demonstrating bladder problems or obstruction [29].

NIH Category IV: Asymptomatic Inflammatory Prostatitis

Asymptomatic inflammatory prostatitis is most commonly diagnosed incidentally after a prostate biopsy or spermogram test. Evaluation of patients with asymptomatic inflammatory prostatitis can be performed using the prostate-specific antigen (PSA) test, which is the most commonly used diagnostic tool. Additionally, diagnoses can be made through tests such as semen analysis, prostate tissue, or expressed prostatic secretion (EPS) tests that provide information about inflammation in the absence of symptoms 10, 32].

Treatment

The multifactorial nature of CP/CPPS results in the absence of the gold standard of treatment. Holistic and multimodal therapy that covers the biopsychosocial aspects is generally preferred over monotherapy to alleviate the symptoms and improve the quality of life in patients with CP/CPPS [35]. Moreover, several meta-analyses have shown that monotherapies rarely result in clinically significant NIH-CPSI score reduction (>6) and limited long-term outcomes. The current management options for CP/CPPS are variable, ranging from pharmacological to non-pharmacological modalities. Previously, a combination of medical treatments, particularly the Triple As (α blockers, antibiotics, and anti-inflammatory), was often prescribed for CP/CPPS [35–37]. However, with the advancements in medical science and technology, several novel therapies emerged and were investigated, expanding the range of treatment options available for tailored approaches to each CP/CPPS case.

Pharmacological Treatment

The most commonly used first-line treatment options for CP/CPPS are antibiotics, analgesics/anti-inflammatory, with additional α blockers if there are obstructive symptoms of LUTS. Alpha-blockers can relieve the symptoms of LUTS by inhibiting type 1 alpha-adrenergic receptors, thus preventing smooth muscle contractions in the ureter, prostate, and bladder. This agent, specifically alfuzosin, was also found to have an anti-inflammatory effect in neurogenic inflammation [38].

Compared to other medications, α blockers are the most extensively studied. Based on a pooled analysis of 18 articles, α blockers could reduce the total NIH-CPSI score up to 5.01 (95% CI: −7.41 to −2.61) at short-term follow-up with tamsulosin as the one showing the biggest improvement (−5.89 decrease of CPSI score) [1]. In long-term follow-up, the improvement of NIH-CPSI score with α blockers was 5.60 (95% CI -10.89 to −0.32) based on only four studies. Nevertheless, the adverse events, such as dizziness and postural hypotension, seemed to be higher compared to the placebo, with a risk ratio of 1.60 (95% CI: 1.09 to 2.34). Due to the low quality of studies, the overall effect of α blockers for CP/CPPS is uncertain. In spite of that, the Prostatitis Expert Reference Group in 2015 suggested that CP/CPPS patients who experience substantial voiding LUTS may consider using α blockers, especially the uroselective ones such as tamsulosin, to minimize the risk of adverse effects [39]. It may be used for 4–6 weeks before considering other treatments. Similarly, the European Association of Urology (EAU) guidelines for chronic pelvic pain in 2024 also strongly recommend α blockers for patients with a duration of primary prostate pain syndrome (PPPS) of less than 12 months [40].

For antibiotics, in the case of chronic bacterial prostatitis (CBP), fluoroquinolone can generally be given as the first-line treatment. If intracellular bacteria are known to cause CBP, then macrolide or tetracycline can be given. Metronidazole is considered in the case of CBP due to *Trichomonas vaginalis* [41]. Similar to α blockers, in vitro studies showed that certain antibiotics (levofloxacin and ciprofloxacin) also have anti-inflammatory effects. Based on a meta-analysis of only 5 studies, the use of antibiotics, specifically quinolone, improves CP/CPPS symptoms with the improvement of NIH-CPSI score of −2.43 (95% CI −4.72 to −0.15) without additional risk of adverse events [1]. Alpha-blockers as adjunctive treatment to antibiotics did not result in any differences compared to antibiotics alone, at least for the first 6 weeks [42]. The EAU guidelines in 2024 continue to recommend the use of fluoroquinolone or tetracycline for a minimum of 6 weeks for individuals who have not received prior treatment and have experienced PPPS for less than 12 months [40]. Nevertheless, the repeated use of antibiotics is discouraged if there is no proof of infectious cause based on cultures and no significant symptom improvement by controlling infection.

Anti-inflammatories are the last “A” in Triple As a medication for CP/CPPS, which includes but is not limited to non-steroidal anti-inflammatory drugs (NSAIDs), corticosteroids, ibuprofen, and a muscle relaxant. Based on the pooled analysis of 585 participants in seven studies, anti-inflammatories had a small impact on total NIH-CPSI scores with a mean difference (MD) of −2.50 (95% CI −3.74 to −1.26) and no increased risk of adverse effects [1]. Similar results with MD of −2.56 (95% CI −4.50 to −0.62) were found in a pooled analysis of five studies that analyzed the efficacy of NSAIDs compared to placebo. Due to the limited quality of research and a small patient sample size, the EAU recommendations only provide a weak recommendation for the use of NSAIDs in treating PPPS [40]. Clinicians should also take into account the potential long-term impact of NSAIDs. Generally, NSAIDs use should be halted if there is no improvement in symptoms after 4–6 weeks of treatment initiation [39].

The other way to improve LUTS in CP/CPPS patients is to use 5-alpha reductase inhibitors (5-ARIs). These can regress the prostatic epithelium and suppress the angiogenesis in prostatic glands to decrease inflammation. However, the clinical studies are limited and underpowered, resulting in conflicting results of their efficacy. In a randomized trial of 64 participants, finasteride resulted in a non-significant improvement in the NIH-CPSI compared to placebo at MD of 4.60 but without any association to increased adverse events [43]. In the other study by Kaplan et al., a significant reduction of NIH-CPSI scores was found in the finasteride group but not in the saw palmetto (Serenoa repens) group [44]. Due to the limited evidence, 5-ARIs cannot be routinely recommended in CP/CPPS cases but may be considered in a selected cases, if there is a concomitant benign prostatic enlargement.

Phytotherapy, such as quercetin, pollen extract, cranberry juice, calendula and curcuma, pumpkin seed oil, terpene mixture, cernilton, eviprostat, saw palmetto extract, and multi-ingredient herbal formulations, is one of the emerging alternative therapies for CP/CPPS, especially due to the lack of proven efficacy of conventional therapies [45]. A meta-analysis of five studies found its possible efficacy to reduce prostatitis symptoms compared to placebo (MD −5.02; 95% CI −6.81 to −3.23) but without any improvement in sexual dysfunction [1]. Furthermore, the network meta-analysis demonstrated a favorable efficacy (Risk ratio [RR]: 1.6, 95% CI 1.1 to 2.3) for phytotherapy [46]. The majority of phytotherapy has anti-inflammatory and analgesic effects as a mechanism to improve prostatitis symptoms. As it is generally well-tolerated, phytotherapy can serve as a promising treatment as monotherapy or adjunctive treatment. However, more well-conducted research should be done before any specific recommendations about phytotherapy for CP/CPPS can be made.

Another pharmacological agent that can be offered for PPPS based on a weak recommendation from the EAU guidelines is pentosan polysulfate (PPS), a semi-synthetic drug from beech-wood hemicellulose. One clinical study found that the use of 300 mg of PPS orally three times a day for 16 weeks could significantly improve overall symptoms and QoL, with greater improvement compared to placebo in terms of QoL (22% vs 12%, $p = 0.031$) [47]. However, a meta-analysis of two studies of moderate to low quality only found a probable little to no impact of pentosane on prostatitis symptoms and adverse events [1]. The other therapies that have been investigated for CP/CPPS are allopurinol, traditional Chinese medicine, anticholinergic, antidepressants, phosphodiesterase-5 inhibitor, pregabalin (anti-epileptic that is approved for neuropathic pain), mepartricin (a compound known to decrease estrogen levels in the prostate), tanezumab (monoclonal antibody), and zafirlukast (leukotriene antagonist) [1]. However, the evidence of these agents is limited and, therefore, should be used in case of any indication according to the phenotypic profile of CP.

In a recent network meta-analysis published in 2022, a combination of anti-inflammatories (ibuprofen and thiocolchicoside—a muscle relaxant) with doxazosin was more effective than placebo (MD −4.80, 95% CI −9.20 to −0.40) [48]. In further Bayesian rank analysis, the combination of ibuprofen, thiocolchicoside, and doxazosin ranked first to improve total NIH-CPSI analysis, while the combination of tamsulosin and levofloxacin was found to be the most effective in terms of ranking first for both NIH—CPSI pain and urinary scores. However, despite the effectiveness of combining oral therapy, there was no significant statistical distinction between using a single therapy and using a combination of therapies, in general. Furthermore, the majority of trials exhibited a high risk of incomplete outcome data bias. Therefore, the authors have concluded that there is insufficient evidence to substantiate the efficacy of oral pharmacological treatments for CP/CPPS.

A more invasive pharmacological agent, intraprostatic injection of botulinum toxin A (BTA) and pelvic floor muscle BTA injections have been investigated in two trials. Theoretically, BTA will inhibit the release of the neurotransmitter acetylcholine from nerve ends, which consequently leads to muscular relaxation and pain reduction. The intraprostatic BTA injection was found to be well-tolerated and can significantly improve prostatitis symptoms with MD of −25.80 (95% CI −30.15 to −21.45) compared to placebo [49]. Significant improvements were seen in pain, urinary, and QoL domains. While the potential advantages of intraprostatic BTA injections appear promising, the existing evidence is insufficient to make any definitive recommendations regarding the use of BTA for treating CP/CPPS [50]. On the other hand, pelvic floor muscle BTA injections failed to show any efficacy for CP/CPPS based on NIH-CPSI score when compared to injection of normal saline [51].

Non-pharmacological Treatment

Lifestyle Modification

Based on the risk factors of CP/CPPS available in the literature, 13 recommendations in diet, sexual, and lifestyle habits were developed [52]. The recommendations included the following:

1. Abstain from consuming any form of alcoholic beverages.
2. Refrain from consuming spicy foods, including pepper, chili, and coffee.
3. Adhere to a proper diet that consists of 50% carbohydrates, 30% fats, and 20% proteins on a daily basis.

4. Enhance your consumption of fruits, vegetables, and foods abundant in natural fibers.
5. Refrain from having two ejaculations within a single day.
6. Avoid engaging in a period of sexual abstinence that exceeds 4 days.
7. Avoid attempting to delay the ejaculation during both sexual intercourse and masturbation.
8. Avoid using interrupted coitus as a form of contraception.
9. Walk and engage in relaxing physical activities.
10. Avoid sedentary activities and sitting for extended periods of time. Utilize a donut-shaped cushion when sitting for an extended period of time.
11. Avoid engaging in sports that may cause harm to your prostate, such as bicycling, motorcycling, and horse riding.
12. Avoid wearing constricting underpants or trousers.
13. Engage in regular hot baths or bidets to relax and release the muscles in the pelvic area.

In a study that included 100 participants, the group of patients who had a lifestyle modification for 3 months had a significant reduction in total NIH-CPSI score from 22.1 to 8.1, while the reduction in the control group was only at 4.3 [52]. Despite this, the quality of the study was flawed, with a high risk of bias in selection, detection, and performance, missing outcome data, and suspected selective outcome reporting, resulting in the uncertainty of efficacy. Moreover, no data exist in terms of adverse effects, sexual concern, QoL, and depression/anxiety. As a result, there is currently no universally accepted recommendation for making lifestyle changes in males with CP/CPPS.

Physical Activity

Physical activity is used in many chronic disease entities to improve QoL, decrease anxiety and stress, and improve overall health function. For CP/CPPS, physical activity was thought to help by improvements in pain sensitivity and changes in immune, neuroendocrine, and autonomic function. In a study of 85 subjects, physical activity significantly improved the total NIH-CPSI score, especially the pain and QoL domain, but not for the urinary symptoms score [53]. The study was not blinded and had a high risk of performance and attrition bias. Based on current evidence, the impact of physical activity on managing CP/CPPS is limited.

Prostate Massage

The exact mechanism of prostate massage for treating CP/CPPS is not yet fully understood. Aside from relieving muscle spasms, improving blood flow, and disrupting biofilm, it was once considered to expel inflammatory cells and fluid from the obstructed acini in the gland and, therefore, reduce prostate inflammation and congestion. In a study of 81 patients with CP, it was found that additional prostatic massage did not significantly improve the response of participants to antibiotics based on NIH-CPSI scores at 4 weeks follow-up [54]. Another study by Shen et al. investigated traditional Chinese medicine with or without a prostate massage to 72 participants and found that the combination group had lower scores for pain, urinary, and QoL domains [55]. Nevertheless, these studies also had very low quality due to bias. No recommendations about prostate messages are currently available. Therefore, it should only be used confined to clinical trial settings.

Acupuncture

Acupuncture is the emerging and most promising non-pharmacological therapy for CP/CPPS. It is now widely used globally for many chronic diseases including CP/CPPS. In the TCM philosophy, acupuncture augments pain perception and improves neuromuscular dysfunction by regulating and redistributing neurovascular flow (Qi) and energy flow through the meridians [56]. Another possible explanation is that acupuncture can promote tissue repair, modulate pain reflex arcs, and release neuropeptides and local endorphins to reduce local pain. Several studies have also demonstrated that acupuncture exhibits anti-inflammatory and immune-modulating effects [56].

There are a number of methods in acupuncture that have been developed, including manual to electronic acupuncture. A meta-analysis of ten high-quality trials involving 798 participants examined the effects of various acupuncture techniques, including scalp acupuncture, acupoint injection, electric acupuncture, acupuncture, and Tiaoshen acupuncture, on patients with chronic prostatitis/chronic pelvic pain syndrome (CP/CPPS) [57]. The analysis revealed that acupuncture demonstrated superior outcomes in terms of pain score, NIH-CPSI score, quality of life score, urinary symptoms, and efficacy rate when compared to sham treatment or Western medicine. The adverse effect of acupuncture was limited to a minor hematoma and transient soreness. With the current evidence, the EAU guidelines strongly recommend the use of acupuncture for PPPS. A recent study found that acupuncture may be more effective in treating CP/CPPS in patients who lead an active lifestyle, do not smoke, have no other health conditions, and experience severe symptoms [58]. More research on the long-term efficacy of acupuncture is warranted.

Extracorporeal Shockwave Therapy (ESWT)

Extracorporeal shockwave therapy (ESWT) is a low-intensity energy that has been used widely in urology and other fields of medicine. In the case of CP/CPPS, it has the potential to alleviate pain and other symptoms by various means, including nociceptor hyperstimulation, passive muscle tone reduction, increased nitric oxide synthesis, local angiogenesis, and interruption of pain nerve impulses [59]. ESWT can also change the threshold of pain by disrupting pain memories and remodeling neuroplasticity.

A recent meta-analysis of 651 patients from 12 randomized trials found that the Li-ESWT group had significantly lower total NIH-CPSI scores, pain domain scores, and QoL scores compared to baseline and the control group at the end of treatment, as well as at 1, 4, 12, and 24 weeks after treatment [60]. The reductions in these scores were more long-lasting and significant when Li-ESWT was paired with pharmacological treatment, compared to when Li-ESWT was used as monotherapy. Aside from that, erectile function and LUTS symptoms were also improved for at least 12 weeks after treatment based on the VAS score, IIEF score, and IPSS score, respectively. The improvement in IIEF score was postulated due to secondary effect from reduced pain and during transperineal ESWT application, and some energy is transmitted to the crura of the corpora cavernosa leading to further improvement of erectile function [59]. In terms of safety, no serious AEs were reported in any trials [60].

Despite the several positive impacts of ESWT proven in trials, the ideal protocol, ideal population, and cost-benefit analysis are unknown. Therefore, the EAU guidelines do not give any explicit recommendations on the use of ESWT for CP/CPPS. Lack of familiarity with ESWT beyond its use in treating ED among urologists also results in their hesitancy to recommend ESWT as a viable therapy option for CP/CPPS [60]. Prior to its general use in clinical practice, it is necessary to conduct a comprehensive study with a longer duration of follow-up to validate the effectiveness of ESWT.

Rehabilitation and Other Physical Treatment

Several other physiotherapy modalities are believed to be beneficial for CP/CPPS. The treatments mentioned are transrectal thermotherapy, transurethral thermotherapy, tibial nerve stimulation biofeedback, electromagnetic chair, sono-electromagnetic therapy, external radiofrequency hyperthermia, laser therapy, myofascial trigger point release therapy, osteopathy, tibial nerve stimulation, and transcutaneous electrical nerve stimulation [61]. Although the trial may have reported a favorable outcome, the effectiveness of these methods remains unknown, mostly due to the low quality and limited number of participants involved in the clinical investigation. Therefore, these modalities cannot be recommended as routine treatment, but they hold potential for future research and larger-scale trials.

Surgical Treatment

As the last resort of treatment, surgical treatment is often considered. There is a general agreement that if surgery is chosen, it is preferable to completely remove prostate tissue that is inflamed or infected. A pooled analysis of case series including 110 patients who underwent transurethral prostate resection and 21 patients who underwent radical prostatectomy found an improvement of symptoms in 85% and 95% of cases, respectively [62]. However, several patients develop erectile dysfunction and incontinence after radical prostatectomy. With the high risk of treatment, a limited amount of data, and the absence of randomized controlled trials, no recommendation for clinical decisions can be made. Further research with a more minimally invasive approach, such as prostate enucleation, may be beneficial.

A study by Zhao et al. found that if the foreskin length covered up the glans penis in more than half or completely, the odds for CP/CPPS were higher, with the odds ratio of 1.66 and 1.86, respectively [63]. The same group of researchers then analyzed the efficacy of circumcision combined with antibiotic, anti-inflammatory, and α-blocker therapy for CP/CPPS. They found that up to 84.6% of 385 participants in the circumcision group had a decrease of at least four points on the total NIH-CPSI score from baseline ($P < 0.001$) [64]. Overall reduction was also significantly greater in the circumcision group compared to the control group. However, the small effect size of the research and moderate-quality evidence cannot serve as the clinical base for further recommendation.

Psychological Treatment

The psychological aspect is an important domain in CP/CPPS as it is frequently associated with pain [65]. Patients with CP/CPPS often have higher levels of stress, depression, and anxiety compared to healthy populations. A number of positive coping mechanisms, such as relaxation training to self-hypnosis, can improve the psychosocial well-being of CPPS patients. A trial of cognitive behavioral therapy (CBT) for CP/CPPS has been conducted by asking the participants to use reaction records to report their feelings for 8 weeks. Through weekly 1-h sessions of CBT, the patients were guided to recognize their feelings and to engage in new positive thinking/behavioral responses. At the end of the trial, the researchers found that CBT can be used as an adjunctive therapy with other treatments but not as a sole modality [66]. Similarly, a preliminary study of 11 men with CPPS found a potential benefit of psychosocial management techniques. Due to its comprehensive advantages and minimal adverse effects, psychological treatment can be a justifiable approach for assisting in pain alleviation or addressing other mental health conditions, but further investigation is encouraged in this field.

Multimodal and Personalized Approach

Chronic prostatitis has a variety of causes and symptoms that can be categorized based on the UPOINT system. The UPOINT system plays a pivotal role in transforming CP/CPPS into a manageable condition. The tailored approach afforded by UPOINT allows physicians to address specific phenotypes present in each patient systematically. Managing expectations and focusing on improving the quality of life become the main approaches in the management of CP/CPPS. Thus, UPOINT stands as a valuable tool in navigating the intricate landscape of CP/CPPS, offering a path toward more effective and personalized management strategies [67].

A study analyzed the clinical response of multimodal treatment guided by UPOINT in 100 males [68]. Using this approach, it was found that almost 84% of patients throughout a median follow-up period of 50 weeks had a minimum 6-point reduction in the total NIH-CPSI score. The improvements were also seen in all pain, urinary, and QoL domains. The effectiveness of this approach appears to be unrelated to age, ethnicity, initial degree and severity of the disease, or the number of therapies used in the multimodal therapy strategy [69]. Classification and treatment options based on the UPOINTS phenotype are outlined in Table 26.1. An additional "S" for the sexual dysfunction domain was given as around a significant percentage of men with CP/CPPS, up to 62%, have concomitant sexual dysfunction, particularly erectile dysfunction, and premature ejaculation [71]. Incorporating a sexual dysfunction component into the UPOINT system could potentially enhance the overall well-being of men undergoing treatment for urological CPPS [72].

In addition to sexual dysfunction, it has been found that CP/CPPS may also be associated with reduced quality of sperm and fertility potential. Ranging from male accessory gland inflammation, metabolic syndrome, inflammatory bowel disease, and HPV co-infection to autoimmunity has been proposed to be the mechanism linking CP/CPPS to male infertility [73]. Therefore, patients with known CP/CPPS are encouraged to adopt a multidisciplinary approach. A recognition of the biopsychosocial components of CP/CPPS will help in creating a holistic approach [74].

Table 26.1 UPOINT phenotype system treatment guide

	Domain						
Treatment	U	P	O	I	N	T	S
Alpha-blockers	✓						
5-alpha-reductase inhibitors	✓						
Antimuscarinics	✓						
Beta 3 agonist	✓						
Dietary/behavioral changes	✓		✓				
Counseling, cognitive behavior therapy		✓					
Antidepressants, anxiolytics		✓					
Stress reduction		✓			✓	✓	
Interstitial cystitis/bladder pain syndrome therapies			✓				
Chronic pelvic pain syndrome therapies			✓				
Antibiotics				✓			
Neuromodulating medications					✓	✓	
Pelvic floor physical therapy						✓	
Trigger point injection						✓	
Shockwave therapy						✓	
Acupuncture						✓	
Phosphodiesterase-5 inhibitors							✓

Adapted and modified from Dewitt-foy et al. [26] and Maeda et al. [70]
U Urinary; *P* Psychological; *O* Organ-specific; *I* Infection; *N* Neurologic/systemic; *T* Tenderness; *S* Sexual

Prognosis

The overall QoL of patients with CP/CPPS is similar to that of those with angina, myocardial infarction, or Crohn's disease and even worse than that of patients with congestive heart failure or diabetes mellitus [75, 76]. Therefore, the primary objective in controlling CP/CPPS is to effectively mitigate the symptoms to the extent that they have minimal or no influence on the physiological and psychosocial aspects of patients' daily lives. Many patients with CP/CPPS can achieve a subjective cure and be completely satisfied with the treatment outcome, even when the CPSI score has not reached zero [77]. Significant alleviation of subjective symptoms, negative result in culture, no prostate tenderness, normal urine evaluation, and being able to engage in sexual activities without pain are several specific measures on the optimal treatment goal of CP/CPPS [78].

Conclusion

Male CP/CPPS affects a large number of individuals and has a substantial negative effect on their quality of life. The diagnosis of CP/CPPS is sometimes challenging, and treatment can be difficult due to the varying underlying etiology and symptoms, causing frustration for both clinicians and patients. Currently, there is no universally applicable therapy that can be applied to all cases. The UPOINT system is frequently used to determine the phenotypic type of CP/CPPS and direct the multimodal management. Currently, there are several therapy options available for managing CP/CPPS; however, many of them lack sufficient evidence to support their effectiveness. Additional clinical research will contribute to improved management of patients with CP/CPPS in the future.

References

1. Franco JVA, Turk T, Jung JH, Xiao YT, Iakhno S, et al. Pharmacological interventions for treating chronic prostatitis/chronic pelvic pain syndrome: a Cochrane systematic review. BJU Int. 2020;125(4):490–6.
2. Alexander RB, Ponniah S, Hasday J, Hebel JR. Elevated levels of proinflammatory cytokines in the semen of patients with chronic prostatitis/chronic pelvic pain syndrome. Urology. 1998;52(5):744–9.
3. Mody L, Krein SL, Saint S, Min LC, Montoya A, et al. A targeted infection prevention intervention in nursing home residents with indwelling devices: a randomized clinical trial. JAMA Intern Med. 2015;175(5):714–23.
4. Krieger JN, Lee SW, Jeon J, Cheah PY, Liong ML, Riley DE. Epidemiology of prostatitis. Int J Antimicrob Agents. 2008;31 Suppl 1(Suppl 1):S85–90.
5. de la Rosette JJ, Hubregtse MR, Meuleman EJ, Stolk-Engelaar MV, Debruyne FM. Diagnosis and treatment of 409 patients with prostatitis syndromes. Urology. 1993;41(4):301–7.

6. Yoon BI, Kim S, Han DS, Ha US, Lee SJ, Kim HW, Han CH, Cho YH. Acute bacterial prostatitis: how to prevent and manage chronic infection? J Infect Chemother. 2012;18(4):444–50.
7. Kim SH, Ha US, Yoon BI, Kim SW, Sohn DW, Kim HW, Cho SY, Cho YH. Microbiological and clinical characteristics in acute bacterial prostatitis according to lower urinary tract manipulation procedure. J Infect Chemother. 2014;20(1):38–42.
8. Ozden E, Bostanci Y, Yakupoglu KY, Akdeniz E, Yilmaz AF, Tulek N, Sarikaya S. Incidence of acute prostatitis caused by extended-spectrum beta-lactamase-producing Escherichia coli after transrectal prostate biopsy. Urology. 2009;74(1):119–23.
9. Ackerman AL, Parameshwar PS, Anger JT. Diagnosis and treatment of patients with prostatic abscess in the post-antibiotic era. Int J Urol. 2018;25(2):103–10.
10. Khan FU, Ihsan AU, Khan HU, Jana R, Wazir J, Khongorzul P, Waqar M, Zhou X. Comprehensive overview of prostatitis. Biomed Pharmacother. 2017;94:1064–76.
11. Nagy V, Kubej D. Acute bacterial prostatitis in humans: current microbiological spectrum, sensitivity to antibiotics and clinical findings. Urol Int. 2012;89(4):445–50.
12. A Pontari M. Inflammation and anti-inflammatory therapy in chronic prostatitis. Urology. 2002;60(6 Suppl):29–33; discussion 33–4.
13. Benson PJ, Smith CS. Cytomegalovirus prostatitis. Urology. 1992;40(2):165–7.
14. de la Rosette JJ, Hubregtse MR, Karthaus HF, Debruyne FM. Results of a questionnaire among Dutch urologists and general practitioners concerning diagnostics and treatment of patients with prostatitis syndromes. Eur Urol. 1992;22(1):14–9.
15. Yilmaz U, Liu YW, Berger RE, Yang CC. Autonomic nervous system changes in men with chronic pelvic pain syndrome. J Urol. 2007;177(6):2170–4; discussion 2174.
16. Dadabhoy D, Clauw DJ. Fibromyalgia: progress in diagnosis and treatment. Curr Pain Headache Rep. 2005;9(6):399–404.
17. Shoskes DA, Landis JR, Wang Y, Nickel JC, Zeitlin SI, Nadler R. Chronic Prostatitis Collaborative Research Network Study Group. Impact of post-ejaculatory pain in men with category III chronic prostatitis/chronic pelvic pain syndrome. J Urol. 2004;172(2):542–7.
18. Wagenlehner FM, van Till JW, Magri V, Perletti G, Houbiers JG, Weidner W, Nickel JC. National Institutes of Health Chronic Prostatitis Symptom Index (NIH-CPSI) symptom evaluation in multinational cohorts of patients with chronic prostatitis/chronic pelvic pain syndrome. Eur Urol. 2013;63(5):953–9.
19. Nickel JC, Downey J, Clark J, Casey RW, Pommerville PJ, et al. Levofloxacin for chronic prostatitis/chronic pelvic pain syndrome in men: a randomized placebo-controlled multicenter trial. Urology. 2003b;62(4):614–7.
20. Ramos JA, Salinas DF, Osorio J, Ruano-Ravina A. Antibiotic prophylaxis and its appropriate timing for urological surgical procedures in patients with asymptomatic bacteriuria: a systematic review. Arab J Urol. 2016;14(3):234–9.
21. Shoskes DA, Nickel JC, Rackley RR, Pontari MA. Clinical phenotyping in chronic prostatitis/chronic pelvic pain syndrome and interstitial cystitis: a management strategy for urologic chronic pelvic pain syndromes. Prostate Cancer Prostatic Dis. 2009;12(2):177–83.
22. Magri V, Boltri M, Cai T, Colombo R, Cuzzocrea S, De Visschere P, Giuberti R, Granatieri CM, Latino MA, Larganà G, Leli C, Maierna G, Marchese V, Massa E, Matteelli A, Montanari E, Morgia G, Naber KG, Papadouli V, Perletti G, Rekleiti N, Russo GI, Sensini A, Stamatiou K, Trinchieri A, Wagenlehner FME. Multidisciplinary approach to prostatitis. Arch Ital Urol Androl. 2019;90(4):227–48.
23. Guan X, Zhao C, Ou ZY, Wang L, Zeng F, Qi L, Tang ZY, Dun JG, Liu LF. Use of the UPOINT phenotype system in treating Chinese patients with chronic prostatitis/chronic pelvic pain syndrome: a prospective study. Asian J Androl. 2015;17(1):120–3.
24. Anderson RU, Wise D, Nathanson BH. Chronic prostatitis and/or chronic pelvic pain as a psychoneuromuscular disorder—a meta-analysis. Urology. 2018;120:23–9.
25. Shoskes DA, Nickel JC, Dolinga R, Prots D. Clinical phenotyping of patients with chronic prostatitis/chronic pelvic pain syndrome and correlation with symptom severity. Urology. 2009b;73(3):538–42; discussion 542–3.

26. DeWitt-Foy ME, Nickel JC, Shoskes DA. Management of chronic prostatitis/chronic pelvic pain syndrome. Eur Urol Focus. 2019;5(1):2–4.
27. McNaughton Collins M, MacDonald R, Wilt TJ. Diagnosis and treatment of chronic abacterial prostatitis: a systematic review. Ann Intern Med. 2000;133(5):367–81.
28. Wang J, Liang K, Sun H, Li L, Wang H, Cao J. Psychotherapy combined with drug therapy in patients with category III chronic prostatitis/chronic pelvic pain syndrome: a randomized controlled trial. Int J Urol. 2018;25(8):710–5.
29. Matsukawa Y, Funahashi Y, Ishida S, Naito Y, Yuba T, Matsuo K, Gotoh M. Clinical features and urodynamic findings in elderly men with chronic prostatitis. Int J Urol. 2022;29(5):441–5.
30. Nickel JC, Shoskes D, Wang Y, Alexander RB, Fowler JE Jr, Zeitlin S, O'Leary MP, Pontari MA, Schaeffer AJ, Landis JR, Nyberg L, Kusek JW, Propert KJ. How does the pre-massage and post-massage 2-glass test compare to the Meares-Stamey 4-glass test in men with chronic prostatitis/chronic pelvic pain syndrome? J Urol. 2006;176(1):119–24.
31. Nickel JC, Alexander RB, Schaeffer AJ, Landis JR, Knauss JS, Propert KJ. Chronic Prostatitis Collaborative Research Network Study Group. Leukocytes and bacteria in men with chronic prostatitis/chronic pelvic pain syndrome compared to asymptomatic controls. J Urol. 2003a;170(3):818–22.
32. Terrone C, Poggio M, Bollito E, Cracco CM, Scarpa RM. Prostatite asintomatica: una frequente causa di elevazione del PSA [Asymptomatic prostatitis: a frequent cause of raising PSA]. Recenti Prog Med. 2005;96(7–8):365–9. Italian. PMID: 16209120.
33. La Vignera S, Crafa A, Condorelli RA, Barbagallo F, Mongioì LM, Cannarella R, Compagnone M, Aversa A, Calogero AE. Ultrasound evaluation of patients with male accessory gland inflammation: a pictorial review. Andrology. 2021;9(5):1298–305.
34. Budía A, Luis Palmero J, Broseta E, Tejadillos S, Benedicto A, Queipo JA, Gobernado M, Fernando Jiménez Cruz J. Value of semen culture in the diagnosis of chronic bacterial prostatitis: a simplified method. Scand J Urol Nephrol. 2006;40(4):326–31.
35. Thakkinstian A, Attia J, Anothaisintawee T, Nickel JC. α-blockers, antibiotics and anti-inflammatories have a role in the management of chronic prostatitis/chronic pelvic pain syndrome. BJU Int. 2012;110(7):1014–22.
36. Nickel JC. Classification and diagnosis of prostatitis: a gold standard? Andrologia. 2003;35(3):160–7.
37. Nickel JC. The three As of chronic prostatitis therapy: antibiotics, alpha-blockers and anti-inflammatories. What is the evidence? BJU Int. 2004;94(9):1230–3.
38. Khattak AS, Raison N, Hawazie A, Khan A, Brunckhorst O, Ahmed K. Contemporary management of chronic prostatitis. Cureus. 2021;13(12):e20243.
39. Rees J, Abrahams M, Doble A, Cooper A. Prostatitis Expert Reference Group (PERG). Diagnosis and treatment of chronic bacterial prostatitis and chronic prostatitis/chronic pelvic pain syndrome: a consensus guideline. BJU Int. 2015;116(4):509–25.
40. Engeler D, Baranowski AP, Parsons B, Berghmans B, Birch J, et al. EAU guidelines on chronic pelvic pain. Arnhem: EAU Guidelines; 2024.
41. Bonkat G, Bartoletti R, Bruyère F, Cai T, Geerlings SE, et al. EAU guidelines on urological infection. Arnhem: EAU Guidelines; 2024.
42. Widia F, Atmoko W, Agung NP, Rahardjo HE, Rasyid N, Birowo P, Taher A. The efficacy of antibiotic and alpha-blocker combination therapy versus antibiotic monotherapy in chronic prostatitis/chronic pelvic pain syndrome: a systematic review. Low Urin Tract Symptoms. 2023;15(4):107–15.
43. Leskinen M, Lukkarinen O, Marttila T. Effects of finasteride in patients with inflammatory chronic pelvic pain syndrome: a double-blind, placebo-controlled, pilot study. Urology. 1999;53(3):502–5.
44. Kaplan SA, Volpe MA, Te AE. A prospective, 1-year trial using saw palmetto versus finasteride in the treatment of category III prostatitis/chronic pelvic pain syndrome. J Urol. 2004;171(1):284–8.

45. Hu M, Wazir J, Ullah R, Wang W, Cui X, Tang M, Zhou X. Phytotherapy and physical therapy in the management of chronic prostatitis-chronic pelvic pain syndrome. Int Urol Nephrol. 2019;51(7):1081–8.
46. Anothaisintawee T, Attia J, Nickel JC, Thammakraisorn S, Numthavaj P, McEvoy M, Thakkinstian A. Management of chronic prostatitis/chronic pelvic pain syndrome: a systematic review and network meta-analysis. JAMA. 2011;305(1):78–86.
47. Nickel JC, Forrest JB, Tomera K, Hernandez-Graulau J, Moon TD, Schaeffer AJ, Krieger JN, Zeitlin SI, Evans RJ, Lama DJ, Neal DE Jr, Sant GR. Pentosan polysulfate sodium therapy for men with chronic pelvic pain syndrome: a multicenter, randomized, placebo controlled study. J Urol. 2005;173(4):1252–5.
48. Qin Z, Zhang C, Guo J, Kwong JSW, Li X, Pang R, Doiron RC, Nickel JC, Wu J. Oral pharmacological treatments for chronic prostatitis/chronic pelvic pain syndrome: a systematic review and network meta-analysis of randomised controlled trials. EClinicalMedicine. 2022;48:101457.
49. Falahatkar S, Shahab E, Gholamjani Moghaddam K, Kazemnezhad E. Transurethral intraprostatic injection of botulinum neurotoxin type A for the treatment of chronic prostatitis/chronic pelvic pain syndrome: results of a prospective pilot double-blind and randomized placebo-controlled study. BJU Int. 2015;116(4):641–9.
50. Parsons BA, Goonewardene S, Dabestani S, Pacheco-Figueiredo L, Yuan Y, et al. The benefits and harms of botulinum toxin-A in the treatment of chronic pelvic pain syndromes: a systematic review by the European Association of Urology Chronic Pelvic Pain Panel. Eur Urol Focus. 2022;8(1):320–38.
51. Gottsch HP, Yang CC, Berger RE. A pilot study of botulinum toxin A for male chronic pelvic pain syndrome. Scand J Urol Nephrol. 2011;45(1):72–6.
52. Gallo L. Effectiveness of diet, sexual habits and lifestyle modifications on treatment of chronic pelvic pain syndrome. Prostate Cancer Prostatic Dis. 2014;17(3):238–45.
53. Giubilei G, Mondaini N, Minervini A, Saieva C, Lapini A, Serni S, Bartoletti R, Carini M. Physical activity of men with chronic prostatitis/chronic pelvic pain syndrome not satisfied with conventional treatmentsDOUBLEHYPHENcould it represent a valid option? The physical activity and male pelvic pain trial: a double-blind, randomized study. J Urol. 2007;177(1):159–65.
54. Ateya A, Fayez A, Hani R, Zohdy W, Gabbar MA, Shamloul R. Evaluation of prostatic massage in treatment of chronic prostatitis. Urology. 2006;67(4):674–8.
55. Shen SL, He DL, Luo Y. Clinical trials of combined therapy of an oral Chinese medicine with massage for chronic nonbacterial prostatitis. Zhonghua Nan Ke Xue. 2006;12(9):851–3. Chinese
56. Chang S. The meridian system and mechanism of acupuncture—a comparative review. part 2: mechanism of acupuncture analgesia. Taiwanese J Obstetr Gynecol. 2013;52(1):14–24.
57. Pan J, Jin S, Xie Q, Wang Y, Wu Z, Sun J, Guo TP, Zhang D. Acupuncture for chronic prostatitis or chronic pelvic pain syndrome: an updated systematic review and meta-analysis. Pain Res Manag. 2023;2023:7754876.
58. Wang X, Zhu L, Yang M, Chen Y, Liu Z. Factors related to acupuncture response in patients with chronic prostatitis/chronic pelvic pain syndrome: secondary analysis of a randomized controlled trial. World J Urol. 2024;42(1):112.
59. Mykoniatis I, Pyrgidis N, Sokolakis I, Sountoulides P, Hatzichristodoulou G, Apostolidis A, Hatzichristou D. Low-intensity shockwave therapy for the management of chronic prostatitis/chronic pelvic pain syndrome: a systematic review and meta-analysis. BJU Int. 2021;128(2):144–52.
60. Kong X, Hu W, Dong Z, Tian J, Wang Y, Jin C, Liang C, Hao Z, Wang Z. The efficacy and safety of low-intensity extracorporeal shock wave treatment combined with or without medications in Chronic prostatitis/chronic pelvic pain syndrome: a systematic review and meta-analysis. Prostate Cancer Prostatic Dis. 2023;26(3):483–94.
61. Franco JV, Turk T, Jung JH, Xiao YT, Iakhno S, Garrote V, Vietto V. Non-pharmacological interventions for treating chronic prostatitis/chronic pelvic pain syndrome. Cochrane Database Syst Rev. 2018;5(5):CD012551.

62. Schoeb DS, Schlager D, Boeker M, Wetterauer U, Schoenthaler M, Herrmann TRW, Miernik A. Surgical therapy of prostatitis: a systematic review. World J Urol. 2017;35(11):1659–68.
63. Zhao YY, Xu DL, Zhao FJ, Han BM, Shao Y, Zhao W, Xia SJ. Redundant prepuce increases the odds of chronic prostatitis/chronic pelvic pain syndrome (CP/CPPS). Asian J Androl. 2014;16(5):774–7.
64. Zhao Y, Zhao W, Lang G, Chen Y, Liu J, Wang G, Ma X, Gong M, Xu D, Xia S. Circumcision plus antibiotic, anti-inflammatory, and α-blocker therapy for the treatment for chronic prostatitis/chronic pelvic pain syndrome: a prospective, randomized, multicenter trial. World J Urol. 2015;33(5):617–22.
65. Huang X, Qin Z, Cui H, Chen J, Liu T, Zhu Y, Yuan S. Psychological factors and pain catastrophizing in men with chronic prostatitis/chronic pelvic pain syndrome (CP/CPPS): a meta-analysis. Transl Androl Urol. 2020;9(2):485–93.
66. Nickel JC, Mullins C, Tripp DA. Development of an evidence-based cognitive behavioral treatment program for men with chronic prostatitis/chronic pelvic pain syndrome. World J Urol. 2008;26(2):167–72.
67. Bryk DJ, Shoskes DA. Using the UPOINT system to manage men with chronic pelvic pain syndrome. Arab J Urol. 2021;19(3):387–93.
68. Samplaski MK, Li J, Shoskes DA. Inclusion of erectile domain to UPOINT phenotype does not improve correlation with symptom severity in men with chronic prostatitis/chronic pelvic pain syndrome. Urology. 2011;78(3):653–8.
69. Majzoub A, Mahdi M, Khalil I, Saeedi AA, Rumaihi KA. Clinical phenotyping and multimodal treatment of men with chronic prostatitis/chronic pelvic pain syndrome from the Middle East and North Africa: determining treatment outcomes and predictors of clinical improvement. Urology. 2022;167:179–84.
70. Maeda K, Shigemura K, Fujisawa M. A review of current treatments for chronic prostatitis/chronic pelvic pain syndrome under the UPOINTS system. Int J Urol. 2023;30(5):431–6.
71. Li HJ, Kang DY. Prevalence of sexual dysfunction in men with chronic prostatitis/chronic pelvic pain syndrome: a meta-analysis. World J Urol. 2016;34(7):1009–17.
72. Davis SN, Binik YM, Amsel R, Carrier S. Is a sexual dysfunction domain important for quality of life in men with urological chronic pelvic pain syndrome? Signs "UPOINT" to yes. J Urol. 2013;189(1):146–51.
73. Graziani A, Grande G, Martin M, Ferraioli G, Colonnello E, Iafrate M, Dal Moro F, Ferlin A. Chronic prostatitis/chronic pain pelvic syndrome and male infertility. Life (Basel). 2023;13(8):1700.
74. Sandler MD, Ledesma B, Thomas J, Ben-Ezra L, Lokeshwar SD, Paz LA, White J, Ramasamy R, Masterson TA. Biopsychosocial approach to male chronic pelvic pain syndrome: recent treatments and trials. Sex Med Rev. 2023;12(1):59–66.
75. Wenninger K, Heiman JR, Rothman I, Berghuis JP, Berger RE. Sickness impact of chronic nonbacterial prostatitis and its correlates. J Urol. 1996;155(3):965–8.
76. McNaughton Collins M, Pontari MA, O'Leary MP, Calhoun EA, Santanna J, Landis JR, Kusek JW, Litwin MS. Chronic Prostatitis Collaborative Research Network. Quality of life is impaired in men with chronic prostatitis: the Chronic Prostatitis Collaborative Research Network. J Gen Intern Med. 2001;16(10):656–62.
77. Reichard CA, Makovey I, Shoskes DA. Phenotype, symptom severity and treatment in a 'cured' cohort of chronic pelvic pain syndrome patients. Can J Urol. 2015;22(1):7623–6.
78. Zhang J, Liang C, Shang X, Li H. Chronic prostatitis/chronic pelvic pain syndrome: a disease or symptom? Current perspectives on diagnosis, treatment, and prognosis. Am J Mens Health. 2020;14(1):1557988320903200.

Chapter 27
Wearable Devices in Male Sexual Dysfunction

Charles A. Loeb, Dongsuk Kim, and Faysal A. Yafi

Introduction

Male sexual dysfunction (MSD) is an increasingly common condition that can significantly impact patient quality of life. Its prevalence has surged in recent years, in both older demographics as well as younger men [1]. A combination of lifestyle adjustments, environmental influences, and social pressures have come together to worsen this trend, increasing the urgency to find effective interventions [2–4].

Pharmacologic and surgical interventions have long been the mainstay of the medical treatment of MSD, but wearable male devices (WMDs) have emerged as a promising non-invasive alternative designed to enhance sexual function and pleasure during intercourse. These devices are often overlooked by patients and clinicians, but offer many advantages over traditional methods, foster patient engagement, and allow for highly personalized treatments.

In this chapter, we explore the realm of WMDs tailored to address MSD. Drawing from thorough research on current literature and market insights, our goal is to investigate the landscape of these innovative products and provide readers with the knowledge they need to improve patient care in MSD.

C. A. Loeb (✉)
Hoag Specialty Clinic, Hoag Memorial Hospital Presbyterian, Newport Beach, CA, USA

D. Kim
Department of Urology, Ilsan Hospital, National Health Insurance Service, Goyang, South Korea
e-mail: dskim100@cha.ac.kr

F. A. Yafi
Department of Urology, University of California Irvine, Irvine, CA, USA

E. Chung et al. (eds.), *Advances in Andrology*,
https://doi.org/10.1007/978-3-032-29112-7_27

Wearable Devices in Male Sexual Medicine

Constriction Bands

Commonly known as penile rings, constriction bands are wearable devices designed to enhance erections by applying pressure to the base of the penis and restrict penile venous outflow. These bands are a non-invasive, user-friendly, and generally affordable solution for men seeking to address MSD [5, 6]. They present discreet options that work independently of the underlying cause of erectile dysfunction, potentially reducing anxiety levels during sexual encounters.

Studies investigating the efficacy of constriction bands have been limited, but they suggest a potential role in managing mild-moderate ED, particularly when used in conjunction with vacuum erection devices (VEDs) in post-prostatectomy patients [5]. Additionally, these devices may alleviate the severity of climacturia, a common issue following certain urologic surgeries [6].

While generally considered safe, improper use of constriction bands may pose risks such as injury to the penis or urethra and reduced sensation due to prolong constriction. Extended wear beyond recommended time limits can lead to venous occlusion, increasing the risk of complications such as venous thrombosis and paresthesia due to decreased arterial perfusion. Some rigid materials used in devices may also carry the risk of penile entrapment, necessitating emergency intervention [7–9].

Some popular constriction bands include the Maintain Ring Loop, Eddie by Giddy, Xialla, and the FirmTech Performance Ring, each offering unique designs aimed at improving functionality and comfort.

The Maintain Loop Ring is an excellent example of an adjustable constriction band. It is made from a medical-grade, latex-free loop that allows for customization of fit and comfort with a very low cost. Although clinical trials or investigatory evidence specifically for this device are lacking, its safety profile is expected to be similar to other penile constriction devices [8]. Made of a softer material and adjustable for easier removal, the risks of complications such as penile strangulation are theoretically much lower.

The Eddie by Giddy is a reusable constriction band that utilizes a patented omega shape that conforms to the male anatomy to work with the natural shape and physiology while avoiding urethral obstruction [10]. The product advertises clinical trial regulatory evidence in which 59 male patients were surveyed and noted significant improvements in erectile function, self-esteem, quality of life, and sexual satisfaction, with overall 95% positive results [10]. The trials referenced are not readily available for review, and while the structural design of an open-bottom makes the device easy to remove and penile strangulation likely mitigated, this was not specifically investigated.

The Xialla device consists of a soft silicone ring that fits around the base of the penis designed to improve function compared to conventional penile rings through a discrete band that anchors the ring to the base of the spine, offering enhanced stability and the benefit not requiring an erection to have occurred before placing the device [11]. Clinical trials have demonstrated its efficacy in improving erectile function across various ED etiologies. One study of 21 men with ED caused by corporal veno-occlusive dysfunction reported significant benefit to erectile function and sexual enhancement in 66% of patients [12]. Another study of 11 men with post radical prostatectomy ED reported a 54% improvement in penile rigidity sufficient for intercourse, and partners reported improved comfort, satisfactory penetrative rigidity, and acceptable aesthetics when compared to intracavernosal injections [13].

The FirmTech Performance ring employs an asymmetrical latch-and-loop design for easy placement and removal while applying pressure to the base of the penis to maintain erectile rigidity [14]. Physician testimonials are available through the product website, and the website states the device is backed by scientific research. However, no peer-reviewed articles with data to support this claim are currently published, and specific safety data are currently unavailable as clinical trials are underway.

Constriction bands offer a promising avenue for managing MSD, providing a convenient and effective solution with proper usage. However, caution must be exercised to mitigate potential risks associated with their use beyond recommended guidelines.

Vibratory Stimulation

Vibratory stimulation devices improve sexual performance by stimulating penile blood flow and enhancing sensation [15]. Vibratory stimulation can aid in sexual dysfunction and promote pelvic health by creating involuntary contractions of the pelvic floor muscles [16]. Clinical data specific to these devices are limited, but literature on the use of penile vibratory stimulation in spinal cord injury patients shows promising results [5]. Vibratory devices are non-invasive, easy to use, and can be worn discreetly under clothing. Potential risks include discomfort from intense vibration and local skin irritation [6, 15].

Prolong Climax Control is a vibratory stimulation device used in a 6-week training program. The program utilizes the "start-stop" technique during masturbation or sexual activity, with gradually increasing the intensity of the stimulation over time [17]. Clinical trials have shown promising results, with significant delays in time to ejaculation and improvements in sexual satisfaction reported. An initial study of the training program found a delay in time to ejaculation from 48 seconds to 8 minutes 48 seconds on average in 61% of men, compared to cognitive behavioral therapy which achieved a delay of 2 minutes 36 seconds on average in 40% of men [18]. In a study on lifelong sufferers of premature ejaculation who failed to respond to antidepressants submitted to the FDA, participants using Prolong achieved a median increase in time to ejaculation of 3 minutes and reported an improvement in all aspects of sexual satisfaction with no reported side effects [19]. Further research is needed to understand their long-term effectiveness (Fig. 27.1).

While vibratory stimulation may offer a useful tool for managing MSD, more robust clinical studies are required to ascertain their efficacy and safety profiles comprehensively.

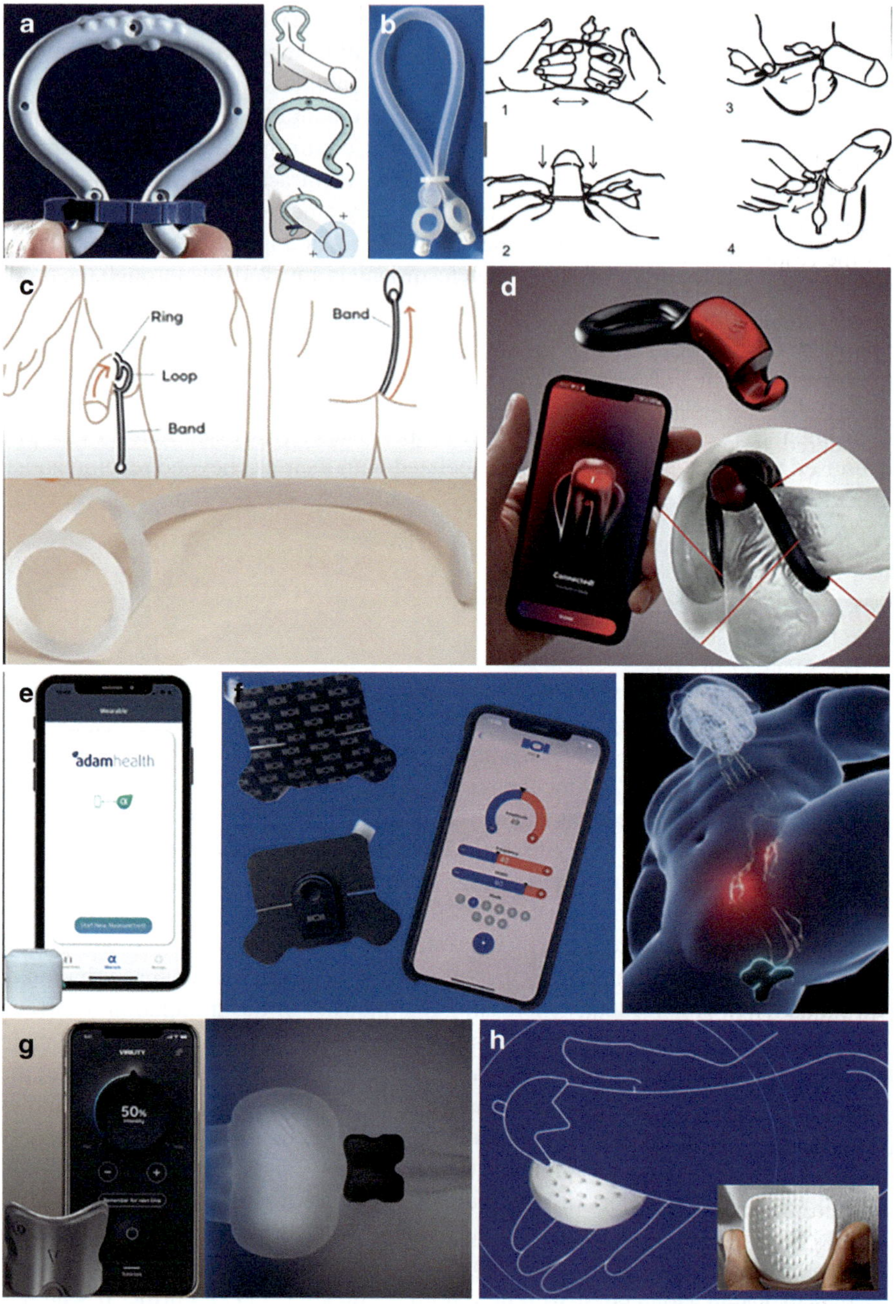

Fig. 27.1 Reviewed devices: (**a**) Eddie by Giddy, (**b**) Maintain Loop Ring, (**c**) Xialla, (**d**) FirmTech Performance Ring, (**e**) Adam sensor, (**f**) Morari Patch, (**g**) Virility Medical in2 Patch, and (**h**) Prolong Climax Control. (All images obtained directly from product websites)

Neuromodulatory Devices

Neuromodulation utilizes electrical stimulation to influence nerve activity and improve sexual response in men with MSD. These devices primarily target the pudendal nerve to delay ejaculation and enhance sexual performance [20]. Notable examples include the Morari Patch and the vPatch / in2 Patch by Virility Medical.

One advantage of neuromodulation devices is that they provide a noninvasive, discreet treatment option for MSD. Most are designed as adhesive patches worn on the perineum during sexual activity, allowing therapy to be delivered with minimal disruption to intimacy [20]. These devices often come with smartphone applications that allow users to adjust stimulation intensity, offering personalized treatment and data-driven insights into sexual function. However, potential risks such as skin irritation, decreased sensation, and rare instances of pudendal nerve injury should be considered, though these risks are generally minor and infrequent.

The Morari Patch is a disposable adhesive patch placed on the perineum, intended to treat premature ejaculation by blocking neurotransmitter signals from the brain, and retrain the brain of men who may have "learned" to ejaculate before they lose their erection [21]. While clinical data specific to this device are pending, it is currently being evaluated in clinical trials, and safety and adverse event profile are yet to be fully assessed.

The vPatch / in2 patch is a wearable skin patch designed to delay ejaculation in patients with premature ejaculation by enhancing the contraction of pelvic floor muscles through intermittent transcutaneous neuromuscular electrical stimulation (TES) to the superficial muscles of the perineum to trigger muscle contraction. The mechanism of action of this device, TES, has been studied in a randomized placebo-controlled trial as a proof of concept. In this study, 23 patients with lifelong premature ejaculation were randomized to TES or sham applied to the perineum at two visits separated by one week and found that masturbation ejaculatory latency time increased in 85% of patients using TES compared to sham. There was also a 73.5% self-reported sense of improvement compared to 41.2% in the sham group. It demonstrated a high safety profile, with a 1.08% minor adverse event rate [20]. A recent sham-controlled, randomized, double-blind study on the device itself from two international centers looked at 51 patients with lifelong premature ejaculation and found that intravaginal ejaculatory latency time increased significantly from 67 seconds to 123 seconds in the active group over a two week period, compared to an insignificant increase from 63 to 81 seconds in the sham group. Intravaginal ejaculatory latency time increased by 3.1 times in the active versus sham group, and no serious adverse events were reported [22].

Neuromodulation devices offer a promising approach to treating MSD, providing personalized treatment options with evolving safety and clinical data. Further research is warranted to fully understand their effectiveness and long-term safety profiles.

Penile Support / External Penile Prostheses

Penile support devices provide external assistance to men who seek to enhance their sexual experience or participate in penetrative intercourse. Devices such as the belted prosthetic phallus, penis sleeve, penis sheath, and penis extender are designed to complement the user's natural anatomy. They slide over the penis to provide support and potentially improve satisfaction. These devices are often constructed from silicone or elastomer materials and can be custom fitted to the user's anatomy. They come in various forms, including sleeves that cover the penile shaft, sheaths that enclose the entire penis, and extenders that elongate the penis. Some variants may incorporate vibratory elements for added stimulation [23].

Traditionally marketed as "strap-on dildos," these devices have gained attention in various communities, although efforts to medicalize their terminology, such as "belted prosthetic phallus," remain limited in adoption. Despite their historical association with the lesbian community, these devices are increasingly recognized for their potential benefits in diverse sexual contexts [23]. These devices are not well tested or promoted in the medical literature, and healthcare providers may be unaware of how using an external penile prosthesis can lead to rewarding sex [24].

While these devices do not address erectile dysfunction directly, they can facilitate penetrative intercourse and enhance tactile stimulation. Small clinical studies suggest that they may improve sexual performance and patient and partner satisfaction, but such studies are limited to case series and anecdotal reports with limited sample sizes and follow-up data [23, 25, 26].

Penile support devices are easy to use, non-invasive, and generally affordable. Users should be aware of potential discomfort, decreased sensation, and local skin irritation associated with prolonged use. Despite these considerations, penile support devices off a promising avenue for individuals seeking to enhance their sexual experience.

Wearable Smart Sexual Devices

The world of wearable smart devices is not just about tracking steps or monitoring heart rates anymore. Fitness trackers, smartwatches, and heart rate monitors have become a mainstay for monitoring various aspects of health, and now wearable smart sexual devices are emerging as the newest frontier in sexual health.

These devices can provide real-time information regarding sexual performance, offer feedback on sexual performance metrics, and even the ability to customize the sexual experience. Advances in sensor technology and data analytics offer detailed insights into sexual function [27–29]. They can be used like a personal sexual health coach to allow users to customize their experience in the bedroom. By integrating sensors and performance tracking, users can quantify sexual function in their natural environment, allowing for remote monitoring and tracking of changes over time

[28]. With a growing body of literature suggesting a link between cardiovascular fitness and ED, smart sexual devices may provide data relating to erectile health and cardiac functioning as an early indicator of cardiovascular event risk [30, 31]. Much like how fitness trackers monitor activity levels and sleep patterns to provide insights into overall health, wearable smart sexual devices provide valuable information for assessing sexual health and well-being.

The ADAM sensor by Adam Health is a ring-like device worn at the base of the penis overnight to provide continuous monitoring of changes in penile tumescence during sleep [32, 33]. These data are then transmitted to a mobile app, where algorithms analyze and provide a report on erectile quality. The sensor tracks the number of erection episodes, total erection time, and Tumescence Activity Units, giving users valuable insights into their nocturnal erections and overall sexual health. The ADAM sensor represents a novel approach to monitoring erectile function, offering an easy-to-use solution for patients with MSD [32]. While the device is not yet commercially available, research suggests its potential as a valuable clinical and research tool, although further evaluation on safety and adverse events is needed [32].

Many of the devices discussed above come with smart options that enhance their functionality. The FirmTech Tech Ring includes sensors to track vital signs of erectile fitness, such as the number of nocturnal erections, duration of erection, and firmness of the penis. The vSmart / in2 smart version offers customizable stimulation intensity via a mobile application, allowing users to personalize their experience [14].

The integration of technology with sexual health represents a significant advancement that can allow people to take control of their sexual health and improve their experience. Wearable smart sexual devices can offer more insight and control over sexual health than ever before. Wearable technology has revolutionized other areas of healthcare, and smart sexual devices are poised to play a crucial role in improving sexual health outcomes.

Future Developments

Looking ahead, wearable devices for managing MSD are on the brink of significant advancement. More precise, personalized interventions and improved outcomes can be achieved by integrating artificial intelligence into data from wearable sexual devices. Integrating telemedicine with wearable devices can help expand access to sexual health care, and remote monitoring can allow for real-time assessment of sexual function. Patients can be more proactive, and clinicians can remotely monitor patient progress and adjust treatment as needed, enhancing patient care and optimizing outcomes.

Further technological advancement in wearable sensors can contribute to the development of more sophisticated wearable devices that capture a broader range of physiological parameters related to sexual function. Enhanced penile tumescence monitoring and biometric sensors can provide a comprehensive picture of sexual health and its relationship to overall well-being [27, 28, 32].

The future of wearable devices holds the potential for revolutionizing the diagnosis, treatment, and monitoring of MSD. As technology continues to evolve, wearable devices will become key tools in the field of sexual wellness, offering personalized insights, improved outcomes, and accessibility to sexual health care.

Conclusion

Wearable devices for managing MSD offer several advantages, ranging from non-invasive treatment options to discreet solutions for enhancing sexual performance. Wearable sexual devices provide a variety of options for addressing different aspects of MSD and make sexual health more accessible to a wider range of individuals with MSD.

The future of wearable devices in managing MSD holds promise with ongoing advancements in smart devices. These developments are poised to enhance the accuracy and effectiveness of wearable devices, enabling better assessment and management of sexual health issues.

Encouraging clinician utilization of wearable devices in managing MSD is vital. Emphasizing the benefits of these devices in clinical practice, such as improved patient monitoring and tailored interventions, can foster their integration into routine assessments and treatment plans. Education and training can equip clinicians with the knowledge and skills needed to effectively incorporate wearable devices into patient care, ultimately leading to better sexual wellness.

References

1. Calzo JP, Austin SB, Charlton BM, et al. Erectile dysfunction in a sample of sexually active young adult men from a U.S. cohort: demographic, metabolic and mental health correlates. J Urol. 2021;205(2):539–44. https://doi.org/10.1097/JU.0000000000001367.
2. Yafi FA, Jenkins L, Albersen M, et al. Erectile dysfunction. Nat Rev Dis Primers. 2016;2(1):16003. https://doi.org/10.1038/nrdp.2016.3.
3. Feldman HA, Goldstein I, Hatzichristou DG, Krane RJ, McKinlay JB. Impotence and its medical and psychosocial correlates: results of the Massachusetts Male Aging Study. J Urol. 1994;151(1):54–61. https://doi.org/10.1016/S0022-5347(17)34871-1.
4. Tomlinson J, Wright D. Impact of erectile dysfunction and its subsequent treatment with sildenafil: qualitative study. BMJ. 2004;328(7447):1037. https://doi.org/10.1136/bmj.38044.662176.EE.
5. Levine LA. External devices for treatment of erectile dysfunction. Endocrine. 2004;23(2–3):157–60. https://doi.org/10.1385/ENDO.23.2-3.157.
6. Miranda EP, Taniguchi H, Cao DL, Hald GM, Jannini EA, Mulhall JP. Application of sex aids in men with sexual dysfunction: a review. J Sex Med. 2019;16(6):767–80. https://doi.org/10.1016/j.jsxm.2019.03.265.

7. Harris E, Llompart D, Izquierdo G, Aziz MA. Patient with penile and scrotal strangulation due to prolonged use of a metal ring device. Cureus. 2020;12(12):e11928. https://doi.org/10.7759/cureus.11928.
8. Silberstein J, Grabowski J, Lakin C, Goldstein I. Penile constriction devices: case report, review of the literature, and recommendations for extrication. J Sex Med. 2008;5(7):1747–57. https://doi.org/10.1111/j.1743-6109.2008.00848.x.
9. Dawood O, Tabibi S, Fiuk J, Patel N, El-Zawahry A. Penile ring entrapment - a true urologic emergency: grading, approach, and management. Urol Ann. 2020;12(1):15–8. https://doi.org/10.4103/UA.UA_16_19.
10. Eddie® Makes All the Difference. Erectile dysfunction management & ED treatment - Eddie by Giddy. https://eddiebygiddy.com
11. Xialla. Xialla. https://xialla.com
12. Littlemore AM, Laing L, Bella AJ. 109 evaluation of a FDA and Health Canada compliant novel medical device for improving erectile function across erectile dysfunction etiologies. J Sex Med. 2017;14(Supplement_1):S27–8. https://doi.org/10.1016/j.jsxm.2016.11.062.
13. Littlemore AM, Laing L, Bella AJ. 106 salvage of post-prostatectomy injection therapy (with and without Venoseal for Cvod) treatment failures by injection therapy coupled with novel silicone loop occlusion device. J Sex Med. 2017;14(Supplement_1):S26–7. https://doi.org/10.1016/j.jsxm.2016.11.059.
14. Male enhancement erection band: Penoscrotal & constriction rings. FirmTech Inc. https://myfirmtech.com/
15. Muncey W, Sellke N, Kim T, Mishra K, Thirumavalavan N, Loeb A. Alternative treatment for erectile dysfunction: a growing arsenal in men's health. Curr Urol Rep. 2021;22(2):11. https://doi.org/10.1007/s11934-020-01023-9.
16. Dubinskaya A, Horwitz R, Scott V, Anger J, Eilber K. Is it time for doctors to Rx vibrators? A systematic review of pelvic floor outcomes. Sex Med Rev. 2023;11(1):15–22. https://doi.org/10.1093/sxmrev/qeac008.
17. Last longer in bed and boost your sexual performance today. Prolong Device. https://prolongdevice.com/
18. Porst H, Burri A. Novel treatment for premature ejaculation in the light of currently used therapies: a review. Sex Med Rev. 2019;7(1):129–40. https://doi.org/10.1016/j.sxmr.2018.05.001.
19. Jern P. Evaluation of a behavioral treatment intervention for premature ejaculation using a handheld stimulating device. J Sex Marital Ther. 2014;40(5):358–66. https://doi.org/10.1080/0092623X.2013.857376.
20. Gruenwald I, Serefoglu EC, Gollan T, et al. Transcutaneous neuromuscular electrical stimulation may be beneficial in the treatment of premature ejaculation. Med Hypotheses. 2017;109:181–3. https://doi.org/10.1016/j.mehy.2017.10.008.
21. Morari Patch. Morari Medical. https://www.morarimedical.com.
22. Shechter A, Mondaini N, Serefoglu EC, et al. A novel on-demand therapy for lifelong premature ejaculation using a miniature transperineal electrical stimulator-the vPatch: an as-treated analysis. J Sex Med. 2023;20(1):22–9. https://doi.org/10.1093/jsxmed/qdac012.
23. Wassersug R, Wibowo E. Non-pharmacological and non-surgical strategies to promote sexual recovery for men with erectile dysfunction. Transl Androl Urol. 2017;6(Suppl 5):S776–94. https://doi.org/10.21037/tau.2017.04.09.
24. Tatem A, Kovac JR. External penile prosthesis as a novel approach to the treatment of erectile dysfunction. Transl Androl Urol. 2017;6(Suppl 5):S795–6. https://doi.org/10.21037/tau.2017.11.01.
25. Krzastek SC, Bopp J, Smith RP, Kovac JR. Recent advances in the understanding and management of erectile dysfunction. F1000Res. 2019;8:F1000 Faculty Rev-102. https://doi.org/10.12688/f1000research.16576.1.
26. Santos-Longhurst A. These are the 12 best penis sleeves, according to experts. Healthline. https://www.healthline.com/health/erectile-dysfunction/best-penis-sleeve. Accessed 3 Feb 2023.

27. Levine LA, Lenting EL. Use of nocturnal penile tumescence and rigidity in the evaluation of male erectile dysfunction. Urol Clin North Am. 1995;22(4):775–88.
28. Edgar R, Trip EJ, Wolterink GJW, Veltink PH, Beck JJH. New methods for the monitoring of nocturnal erections. Int J Impot Res. 2022;34(1):1–7. https://doi.org/10.1038/s41443-020-00365-9.
29. Li CY, Larsen S, Yap T. Nocturnal penile tumescence study. In: Minhas S, Mulhall J, editors. Male sexual dysfunction. John Wiley & Sons, Ltd; 2016. p. 129–32. https://doi.org/10.1002/9781118746509.ch15.
30. Raheem OA, Su JJ, Wilson JR, Hsieh TC. The association of erectile dysfunction and cardiovascular disease: a systematic critical review. Am J Mens Health. 2017;11(3):552–63. https://doi.org/10.1177/1557988316630305.
31. Miner M, Parish SJ, Billups KL, Paulos M, Sigman M, Blaha MJ. Erectile dysfunction and subclinical cardiovascular disease. Sex Med Rev. 2019;7(3):455–63. https://doi.org/10.1016/j.sxmr.2018.01.001.
32. Konstantinidis CV, Alexandrou S, Alexandrou M, Raheem AA. Adam sensor: a novel nocturnal penile tumescence wearable device - technology overview & applications. J Sex Med. 2022;19(11, Supplement 4):S133–4. https://doi.org/10.1016/j.jsxm.2022.10.073.
33. Adam Sensor. Adam Health. https://talktoadam.com/adam-sensor.

Chapter 28
Penile Enlargement: Current Treatments and Controversies

Christopher C. K. Ho and M. Falcone

Introduction

There are different groups of men who come for penile enlargement and this distinction is important since one form of treatment may be very appropriate and useful for one group of men, but not the other [1]. These include:

(a) *Acquired False Penile Shortness*—acquired adult buried penis (AABP) is widely recognized as the only acquired false penile shortness condition.
(b) *Congenital Intrinsic Penile Shortness*—this includes isolated microphallus and microphallus in association with corrected severe hypospadias, epispadias or ectopia vesicae. The latter present at adulthood with short broad corpora, and chordee with shortening due to inadequate length of the precarious, skin-tube-neo-urethra fashioned in childhood.
(c) *Acquired Intrinsic Penile Shortness*—it includes Peyronie's disease, surgical trauma/amputation, fracture pelvis and multiple urethroplasties.
(d) *Body Dysmorphic Disorder (BDD)*—clinical diagnosis defined by the American Psychiatric Association (APA) [40] as the strong distress generated by perceived defect (s) or flaw(s) in an individual's physical appearance. This flaw is not observable to others, or, if it exists, it appears only slightly [2].
(e) *Normal but Short Penis*—this is another group of men who have a penile length within 2SD and are therefore labelled normal and not needing treatment, but they are still at the lower end of the normal, and many of them face rejection or

C. C. K. Ho (✉)
Department of Surgery, Taylor's University, Subang Jaya, Selangor, Malaysia

M. Falcone
Urology Department, Città della Salute e della Scienza, University of Torino, Torino, Italy

Urology Department, Biruni University, Istanbul, Turkey
e-mail: marco.falcone@unito.it

E. Chung et al. (eds.), *Advances in Andrology*,
https://doi.org/10.1007/978-3-032-29112-7_28

a disparaging remark from a sexual partner that leaves them emotionally shattered.

Due to the controversies of the indications as well methods, penile enlargement has been a hot topic in andrology.

Indication

Stretched penile length (SPL) is the maximum length of the penis while stretched, measured from the base of the penis, under the pubic symphysis to the tip of the glans, and is thought to approximate erect penile length within 10% [3].

Congenital and acquired micropenis are the classic surgical indications for penile elongation surgery after excluding hormonal causes (and after giving testosterone therapies).

True micropenis is defined as a normally formed penis that has an SPL that falls below two standard deviations of normal for a patient's age and race. Normal values for preterm infants born between the 24th and 36th week of gestation can be calculated using the formula: $(0.16 \times \text{weeks of gestation}) - 2.27$ [4].

The goal of intervention in these patients is to restore a functional penis size in order to allow normal standing micturition, enable satisfying sexual intercourse and improve patient quality of life.

Non-invasive Therapies

(a) *Penile Traction Devices*

Also called penile stretchers, penile traction devices are designed to stretch the penis over time and provide increased length through tissue modification and healing. They require regular use and expected results are modest, usually accounting for 1–2 cm of increased length. These techniques have been studied primarily in men with penile shortening from radical prostatectomy for prostate cancer. Results are often temporary and patient satisfaction has been poor [5].

(b) *Vacuum Erection Pump*

These consist of a plastic cylinder placed over the penis and a suction pump to create a vacuum in the tube to stretch the penis. While the expected increase in length is similar to the traction devices, some increase in girth is also observed. To achieve the desired result, the vacuum erection device must be used daily for several months [5]. As with traction devices, the length increase is usually transient.

(c) *Penile Exercises*

Exercises such as jelqing are often reported as natural methods for penile enhancement [6]. Jelqing involves rhythmic stretching and massaging of the penis. While some men claim to have experienced improvements, evidence-based medical data for effectiveness are lacking.

(d) *Endocrinological Therapies*

(i) Testosterone Therapy

Testosterone enanthate 25 mg every 4 weeks has been used in prepubertal boys with isolated micropenis and has been shown to increase in penile length of over 100% [7]. Testosterone cream has also been tried and there was a significant increase in SPL in 50 prepubertal boys treated with testosterone cream 5% (10 mg/daily applied directly to the phallus) for a duration of 30 days [8]. It remains unclear whether such early use of androgens has any benefit on penile length in adulthood [9–11].

However, in male patients with late-onset hypogonadism, testosterone therapy has not been shown to cause any significant change in penile length [12].

(ii) Topical Dihydrotestosterone Gel Treatment

In Clinical Practice, an Increase in Penile Length Has Been Reported in Partial Androgen Insensitivity Syndrome (PAIS) [13] and 5α-Reductase deficiency [14] in Pre- and Peripubertal Patients but Not in Adults. There Are no Standardized Guidelines or Consensus on Therapeutic Regimen for DHT Transdermal Gel Application to Genital Skin

(e) *Psychotherapy*

There are patients who think they have small penis although clinically it is normal. This condition could be due to penile dysmorphophobia disorder (PDD) or small penis anxiety (SPA). This patient would benefit from referral to psychiatrist for psychotherapy.

Penile Enlargement Surgeries

Penile Lengthening

Ligamentolysis and Dorsal Skin Plasty

This technique involves an infrapubic surgical incision and the release of the ligament attaching the penis to the pubic bone. A combined elongating V-Y skin plasty may also be considered. Overall, a variable increase in SPL was observed (1.1–4.3 cm) in the current published series [15, 16]. Postoperative complications were deemed to be minimal (Table 28.1).

Table 28.1 Ligamentolysis and dorsal skin plasty

Author (year)	Year	n	Study design	Age, years	Follow-up, months	Stretched penile length gain, cm
Deskoulidi et al. [17]	2023	75	Retrospective	NA	NA	3
Littara et al. [16]	2019	21	Retrospective	38.08 ± 1.1	12	1.1
Zhang et al. [18]	2019	15	Retrospective	33.2 ± 4.6	3	4.3 ± 1.6
Li et al. [15]	2006	27	Retrospective	NR	16	1.1 ± 1.1
Spyropoulos et al. [19]	2005	11	Retrospective	25–25	Not reported	1.6 (1–2.3)

Ventral Phalloplasty/Scrotoplasty

This intervention involves a ventral shaft skin plasty to move the peno-scrotal angle proximally, thereby increasing the exposure of the penile shaft. Chen et al. performed ventral phalloplasty on 12 patients with satisfactory results and no complications [20]. Yu et al. reported outcomes for 62 patients with an increase in penile length of 2.6 cm. Most patients (93.5%) were satisfied with the surgical results [21]. No significant complications in postoperative settings were reported.

Suprapubic Lipoplasty/Lipectomy

This intervention aims to reduce the size of the suprapubic fat pad either via a minimally invasive approach (liposuction) or surgically (lipectomy). The removal of the suprapubic fat pad aims to increase penile shaft exposure. Ghanem et al. performed liposuction on 10 patients [22]. The reported complications included oedema in 50%, oedema and ecchymosis in 10% and oedema and hematoma in 10%. Overall, 80% of patients were satisfied following the procedure. The Shaeer's monsplasty technique was evaluated in 20 patients [23]. Pre-operatively, flaccid length was 3 ± 0.9 cm, and erect length was 8 ± 4.6 cm. At three months post-operatively, the flaccid length was 7.1 ± 2.1 cm, with a 57.9% improvement in length, and erect length was 11.8 ± 2.1 cm, a 32% improvement.

Penile Prosthesis Implantation

The literature fails to show a direct relationship between PPI and penile length in men with ED and no concomitant Peyronie's disease (PD). In a study by Deveci et al., SPL was evaluated in men undergoing primary implant surgery due to diabetes or RP [24]. Seventy two % of patients reported a subjective decrease in penile length although no statistically significant difference was demonstrated in measured SPL. In another study, 45 patients with PD and no deformity or penile curvature <30° or severe penile fibrosis/scarring were implanted with an AMS 700 LGX [25]. The mean SPL improved from 13.1 ± 1.2 cm to 13.7 ± 1.1 cm and 14.2 ± 1.2 cm at

6 and 12 months, respectively. Complications related to PPI were infection (0.8% in high volume centre) and mechanical failure.

Corporal Lengthening Manoeuvres

Penile length restoration using the sliding technique (ST) and concomitant PPI was first described in a small series of 3 patients with end-stage PD associated with severe shortening and further supported by a larger series of 28 patients in a multicentre study [26, 27]. Overall, 95% of men were satisfied with their increase in length with an average penile lengthening of 3.2 cm. The outcomes of these procedures are limited, and their utility in clinical practice is questioned due to severe complications such as penile prosthesis infection and glans necrosis [28].

Penile Disassembly

This technique involves the separation of the penis into its anatomical components and the insertion of autologous cartilage into the space created between the glans cap and the tip of the corpora cavernosa. Perovic et al., in a study with 19 patients, reported an increase of 3 cm in SPL and 3.1 cm in erect length [29]. The results of this surgery are poorly documented, and significant complications such as glans necrosis have led to controversy over its value as a surgical option.

Penile Enlargement

Filler Injections

Injectable filling materials can be classified according to their different properties. They can be autologous, biological or synthetic in nature. The fat injection material is obtained from the patient's own tissue (autologous), usually by liposuction. Biological fillers can be of human and animal (collagen) or bacterial (hyaluronic acid) origin. Poly-l-lactic acid (PLA), hydroxyethyl methacrylate, polyalkylimide hydrogel (PAAG), polymethylmethacrylate (PMMA), calcium hydroxyapatite (CHA), silicone and paraffin constitute filler materials of synthetic origin.

HA gel is one of the most commonly used injectable fillers in plastic surgery. Its application for penile girth enhancement has gained popularity due to its biocompatibility and infrequent mild temporary side effects. Cross-linked HA has a more lasting effect over time. Studies have reported an increase of 1.4 to 3.78 cm in penile girth with HA injection. Patient satisfaction is high (78–100%), with no severe side effects reported [30–36]. Minimal complications were detected in up to 9.1% of patients.

Other Fillers (Silicone, Paraffin)

Foreign body injections are still frequently practiced in many countries, either by patients themselves or by healthcare workers, using various substances such as paraffin, silicone or petroleum jelly (Vaseline) to increase penile circumference [37–40].

This results in a chronic granulomatous inflammatory foreign body reaction. The resultant pathological condition, known as sclerosing lipogranuloma of the penis (also referred to as paraffinoma or siliconoma), can range from oedema and infection to Fournier's gangrene. Penile reconstructive surgeries may be required to remove lipogranulomas [41–43].

Autologous Fat Injection

This surgical technique involves thinning the lower abdomen with liposuction and injecting the harvested fat tissue into the penile shaft. Retrospective studies have reported an average increase of 2 to 3.5 cm in penile circumference [44, 45].

No statistically significant decrease in IIEF scores was observed, and no serious adverse events were reported. More than 75% of patients were satisfied with the procedure. Minimal complications such as penile oedema and lipogranuloma formation were reported in up to 14.7% of patients.

Subcutaneous Penile Implant (Penuma—Himplant)

Recently, the silicone penile implant 'Penuma®' (International Medical Devices [Beverly Hills, CA, USA]) has received FDA approval and has shown promising results for penile girth enhancement. Penuma® is a soft silicone subcutaneous implant placed on 3/4 of the penile shaft and fixed to the glans with a polyester mesh. Studies have reported an average increase in penile circumference of 2 to 5 cm with Penuma® insertion [46, 47]. Recently, the device has been renewed and renamed as Himplant®.

Total Phallic Reconstruction

This represents the most complex form of genital reconstruction, aimed at creating a new phallus with a neo-urethra, and is reserved for severe penile insufficiency (e.g. congenital micropenis, bladder exstrophy-epispadias complex). Various flaps can be considered to address total phallic reconstruction. Any perceived benefits must be carefully weighed against potential complications [48–51].

Controversies/Ethics

When considering the ethics of penile augmentation, several principles in medical decision-making must be addressed, including personal, clinical and social factors. For men with micropenis and functional issues, surgical intervention may be beneficial. However, those with body dysmorphic disorder should first receive psychological or psychiatric treatment. Social considerations are multifaceted and must be weighed to prevent unnecessary suffering. The primary ethical question is whether prioritizing such surgeries is appropriate given limited health resources and societal pressures. Professionally, doctors have a duty to uphold public trust in the medical profession and promote patients' best interests. This involves careful evaluation of patients' overall health, especially psychological aspects, rather than simply fulfilling requests for surgery with limited evidence of benefit. A multidisciplinary approach that is sensitive to patient needs while maintaining ethical standards and safeguarding mental health is crucial. Transparent doctor–patient communication about expectations, risks, benefits and alternatives is essential for achieving better outcomes in this complex field.

Current Status

The Sexual Medicine Society of North America issued the following position statement and guidelines: 'The Society for the Study of Impotence has found no peer reviewed, objective or independently monitored studies, or other data, which prove the safety or efficacy of penile lengthening and girth enhancement surgery. The Society believes that, in men who do not have congenital anatomical anomalies of the penis, the safety and efficacy of penile lengthening and girth enhancement surgery have not been established. Therefore, penile lengthening and girth enhancement surgery can only be regarded as experimental surgery. The Society is aware of complications and adverse outcomes which should be clearly disclosed to patients considering such surgery. The Society believes that those government agencies charged with the regulation of medical practice and the enforcement of laws prohibiting false or unsubstantiated advertising claims should give careful attention to claims made with regard to these surgical procedures [52].

The European Association of Urology Guidelines on Penile Size Abnormalities and Dysmorphophobia statement is as follows: 'Patients with normal penile size who are seeking penile augmentation should be referred for psychological evaluation for potential dysmorphophobic disorders. Penile length and girth enhancements can be achieved via a multitude of treatments, but a personalized management plan is crucial for satisfactory results. Endocrinological therapies, when indicated, are effective in the prepubertal setting only. Vacuum therapy has a limited evidence base in treatment protocols, although acceptable outcomes have been reported for penile traction therapy. Surgical techniques to enhance penile length and girth have limited evidence and should only be proposed after extensive patient counselling' [1].

The Clinical recommendations on penile reconstructive and prosthetic surgery: a consensus statement from the Asia-Pacific Society of Sexual Medicine (APSSM): Patients should be provided with information regarding potential complications related to surgery, and strict adherence to safe surgical principles. Preoperative optimization of medical comorbidities and stringent postoperative care are important to improve patient satisfaction rates. For complex patients, surgical intervention should ideally be referred and performed by expert high-volume surgeons to maximize clinical outcomes. The APSSM advocates for surgeons in AP to individualize surgical options based on patient condition(s) and needs, surgeon expertise, and local resources [53].

Conclusion

Due to the controversies and lack of data regarding penile enlargement treatment, careful counselling of patient is mandatory before embarking on any treatment.

References

1. Falcone M, Bettocchi C, Carvalho J, Ricou M, Boeri L, Capogrosso P, Cocci A, Corona G, Gül M, Hatzichristodoulou G, Jones TH, Kadioğlu A, Kalkanli A, Martinez-Salamanca JI, Milenkovic U, Morgado LA, Russo GI, Serefoğlu EC, Tharakan T, Verze P, Minhas S, Salonia A. European Association of Urology guidelines on penile size abnormalities and dysmorphophobia: summary of the 2023 guidelines Eur Urol Focus. 2023:S2405-4569(23)00197-9. https://doi.org/10.1016/j.euf.2023.08.012. Epub ahead of print. PMID: 37709592.
2. American Psychiatric Association. Diagnostic and statistical manual of mental disorders. 5th ed. Arlington: APA Publishing; 2013.
3. Wessells H, Lue TF, McAninch JW. Penile length in the flaccid and erect states: guidelines for penile augmentation. J Urol. 1996;156:995–7.
4. Aaronson IA. Micropenis: medical and surgical implications. J Urol. 1994;152:4–14; Wiygul J, Palmer LS. Micropenis. ScientificWorldJournal 2011;11:1462–9; Ghanem H, Glina S, Assalian P, et al. Position paper: management of men complaining of a small penis despite an actually normal size. J Sex Med. 2013;10:294–303.
5. Hehemann MC, Towe M, Huynh LM, et al. Penile girth enlargement strategies: what's the evidence? Sex Med Rev. 2019;7:535–47.
6. www.mayoclinic.org/healthy-lifestyle/sexual-health/in-depth/penis/art-20045363. Accessed 10 Jul 2023.
7. Nerli RB, Guntaka AK, Patne PB, Hiremath MB. Penile growth in response to hormone treatment in children with micropenis. Indian J Urol. 2013;29(4):288–91.
8. Arisaka O, Hoshi M, Kanazawa S, et al. Systemic effects of transdermal testosterone for the treatment of microphallus in children. Pediatr Int. 2001;43(2):134–6.
9. van der Zwan YG, Nina C, van Jet K, et al. Long-term outcomes in males with disorders of sex development. J Urol. 190(3):1038–42.

10. Tietjen DN, Uramoto GY, Tindall DJ, Husmann DA. Characterization of penile androgen receptor expression in micropenis due to hypogonadotropic hypogonadism. J Urol. 1998;160(3 Pt2):1075–9.
11. Money J, Lehne GK, Pierre-Jerome F. Micropenis: adult follow-up and comparison of size against new norms. J Sex Marital Ther. 1984;10(2):105–16.
12. Park KK, Lee SH, Chung BH. The effects of long-term androgen deprivation therapy on penile length in patients with prostate cancer: a single centre, prospective, open-label, observational study. J Sex Med. 2011;8:3214–9.
13. Becker D, Wain LM, Chong YH, et al. Topical dihydrotestosterone to treat micropenis secondary to partial androgen insensitivity syndrome (PAIS) before, during, and after puberty-a case series. J Pediatr Endocrinol Metab. 2016;29(2):173–7.
14. Sasaki G, Ishii T, Hori N, et al. Effects of pre- and post-pubertal dihydrotestosterone treatment on penile length in 5α-reductase type 2 deficiency. Endocr J. 2019;66(9):837–42.
15. Li CY, et al. Penile suspensory ligament division for penile augmentation: indications and results. Eur Urol. 2006;49:729.
16. Littara A, et al. Cosmetic penile enhancement surgery: a 3-year single-centre retrospective clinical evaluation of 355 cases. Sci Rep. 2019;9:6323.
17. Deskoulidi PI, Caminer D. Lengthening phalloplasty with division of the suspensory ligament and distally based fat flaps in penis enlargement operations. Plast Reconstr Surg. 2023;152(3):434e–7e. https://doi.org/10.1097/PRS.0000000000010313. Epub 2023 Mar 22. PMID: 36943707.
18. Zhang X, et al. Suspensory ligament release combined with acellular dermal matrix filler in infrapubic space: a new method for penile length augmentation. Andrologia. 2019;51:e13351.
19. Spyropoulos E, et al. Augmentation Phalloplasty patient selection and satisfaction inventory: a novel questionnaire to evaluate patients considered for augmentation phalloplasty surgery because of penile dysmorphophobia. Urology. 2007;70:221.
20. Chen YB, et al. A new plastic surgical technique for adult congenital webbed penis. J Zhejiang Univ Sci B. 2012;13:757.
21. Yu W, et al. Minimally invasive technique for the concealed penis lead to longer penile length. Pediatr Surg Int. 2010;26:433.
22. Ghanem H, et al. Infrapubic liposuction for penile length augmentation in patients with infrapubic adiposities. Aesth Plast Surg. 2017;41:441.
23. Shaeer O, et al. Revealing the buried penis in adults. J Sex Med. 2009;6:876.
24. Deveci S, et al. Penile length alterations following penile prosthesis surgery. Eur Urol. 2007;51:1128.
25. Negro CL, et al. Implantation of AMS 700 LGX penile prosthesis preserves penile length without the need for penile lengthening procedures. Asian J Androl. 2016;18:114.
26. Rolle L, et al. A new, innovative, lengthening surgical procedure for Peyronie's disease by penile prosthesis implantation with double dorsal-ventral patch graft: the "sliding technique". J Sex Med. 2012;9:2389.
27. Rolle L, et al. A prospective multicentric international study on the surgical outcomes and patients' satisfaction rates of the 'sliding' technique for end-stage Peyronie's disease with severe shortening of the penis and erectile dysfunction. BJU Int. 2016;117:814.
28. Falcone M, Preto M, Morgado AR, Sokolakis I, Sarıkaya S, Capece M, Capogrosso P, Manfredi C, Tsampoukas G, Russo G. Risk and benefits of penile length preservation techniques during penile prosthesis implantation: a systematic review by the young academic urologists sexual and reproductive health working group. Ther Adv Urol. 2024 Jan;8(16):17562872231215177.
29. Perovic SV, et al. New perspectives of penile enhancement surgery: tissue engineering with biodegradable scaffolds. Eur Urol. 2006;49:139.

30. Ahn ST, et al. Efficacy and safety of penile girth enhancement using hyaluronic acid filler and the clinical impact on ejaculation: a multi-center, patient/evaluator-blinded, randomized active-controlled trial. World J Mens Health. 2022;40:299.
31. Yang DY, et al. A comparison of the efficacy and safety between hyaluronic acid and Polylactic acid filler injection in penile augmentation: a multicenter, patient/evaluator-blinded, randomized trial. J Sex Med. 2019;16:577.
32. Kwak TI, et al. The effects of penile girth enhancement using injectable hyaluronic acid gel, a filler. J Sex Med. 2011;8:3407.
33. Yang DY, et al. A comparison between hyaluronic acid and polylactic acid filler injections for temporary penile augmentation in patients with small penis syndrome: a multicenter, patient/evaluator-blind, comparative, randomized trial. J Sex Med. 2020;17:133.
34. Yang DY, et al. Comparison of clinical outcomes between hyaluronic and polylactic acid filler injections for penile augmentation in men reporting a small penis: a multicenter, patient-blinded/evaluator-blinded, non-inferiority, randomized comparative trial with 18 months of follow-up. J Clin Med. 2020;9:1024.
35. Zhang CL, et al. Penile augmentation with injectable hyaluronic acid gel: an alternative choice for small penis syndrome. Asian J Androl. 2022;24:601–6.
36. Quan Y, et al. Complications and management of penile augmentation with hyaluronic acid injection. Asian J Androl. 2021;23:392.
37. Dellis AE, et al. Paraffinoma, siliconoma and Co: disastrous consequences of failed penile augmentation-a single-centre successful surgical management of a challenging entity. Andrologia. 2018;50:e13109.
38. Karakan T, et al. Injection of vaseline under penis skin for the purpose of penis augmentation. Case Rep Urol. 2012;2012:510612.
39. Dellis AE, et al. Minimal surgical management of penile paraffinoma after subcutaneous penile paraffin injection. Arab J Urol. 2017;15:387.
40. Eandi JA, et al. Penile paraffinoma: the delayed presentation. Int Urol Nephrol. 2007;39:553.
41. Fakin R, et al. Reconstruction of penile shaft defects following silicone injection by bipedicled anterior scrotal flap. J Urol. 2017;197:1166.
42. Murányi M, et al. A new modified bipedicle scrotal skin flap technique for the reconstruction of penile skin in patients with paraffin-induced Sclerosing Lipogranuloma of the penis. J Urol. 2022;208:171.
43. Sedigh O, et al. Penile injection of aedile silicone: a dangerous shortcut. Urologia. 2022;89:456.
44. Kang DH, et al. Efficacy and safety of penile girth enhancement by autologous fat injection for patients with thin penises. Aesth Plast Surg. 2012;36:813.
45. Panfilov DE. Augmentative phalloplasty. Aesth Plast Surg. 2006;30:18.
46. Elist JJ, et al. A single-surgeon retrospective and preliminary evaluation of the safety and effectiveness of the Penuma silicone sleeve implant for elective cosmetic correction of the flaccid penis. J Sex Med. 2018;15:1216.
47. Siegal AR, et al. Outcomes of a single center's initial experience with the Penuma® penile implant. Urology. 2022;171:236–43.
48. Lumen N, et al. Phalloplasty: a valuable treatment for males with penile insufficiency. Urology. 2008;71:272.
49. Lumen N, et al. Reconstructive surgery for severe penile inadequacy: phalloplasty with a free radial forearm flap or a pedicled anterolateral thigh flap. Adv Urol. 2008;2008:704343.
50. Perovic SV, et al. Total phalloplasty using a musculocutaneous latissimus dorsi flap. BJU Int. 2007;100:899.
51. Garaffa G, et al. Total phallic reconstruction using radial artery based forearm free flap phalloplasty in patients with epispadias-exstrophy complex. J Urol. 2014;192:814.
52. Y. Krakowsky, Matta R, Grober E. 043 Complications and surgical management of vaseline injection into the penis for girth enhancement—a photo documentary: support for the SMSNA's position on penile lengthening and girth enhancement. J Sex Med. 2016;13(Suppl 1):S21.

53. Chung E, Moon D-G, Hui J, Chang H-C, Hakim L, Nagao K, Tan R, Mak SK, Tantiwongse K, Lin H, Mai DBT, Nguyen Q, Tan HM, Sato Y, Jiann B-P, Park K, Xin ZC, Park H-J. Clinical recommendations on penile reconstructive and prosthetic surgery: a consensus statement from the Asia-Pacific Society of Sexual Medicine. Sex Med. 2023;11(2):qfad003. https://doi.org/10.1093/sexmed/qfad003.

Index

E. Chung et al. (eds.), *Advances in Andrology*,
https://doi.org/10.1007/978-3-032-29112-7

B

C

T

GPSR Compliance

The European Union's (EU) General Product Safety Regulation (GPSR) is a set of rules that requires consumer products to be safe and our obligations to ensure this.

If you have any concerns about our products, you can contact us on ProductSafety@springernature.com

In case Publisher is established outside the EU, the EU authorized representative is:

Springer Nature Customer Service Center GmbH
Europaplatz 3
69115 Heidelberg, Germany

Batch number: 10664975

Printed by Printforce, the Netherlands